Revision MCQs and EMIs for the MRCPsych

Practice questions and mock exams for the written papers

An evidence-based approach

Basant K Puri MA, PhD, MB, BChir, BSc (Hons)
MathSci, FRCPsych, DipMath, PG Cert Maths, MMath
Professor and Honorary Consultant, Hammersmith Hospital, London, UK

Roger C M Ho MBBS (Hong Kong), DPM (Ireland), GDip Psychotherapy
(Singapore), MMed (Psych) (Singapore), MRCPsych (UK)
Assistant Professor and Associate Consultant, Psychoneuroimmunology (PNI)
Research Programme and Department of Psychological Medicine, University Medical
Cluster, Yong Loo Lin School of Medicine and National University Health System,
National University of Singapore, Singapore

Ian H Treasaden MB BS MRCS LRCP FRCPsych LLM
Consultant Forensic Psychiatrist, West London Mental Health NHS Trust; Honorary
Senior Lecturer, Imperial College London; Head of Forensic Neurosciences,
Hammersmith Hospital, London, UK

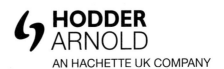

HODDER
ARNOLD
AN HACHETTE UK COMPANY

First published in Great Britain in 2011 by
Hodder Arnold, an imprint of Hodder Education, a division of Hachette UK
338 Euston Road, London NW1 3BH

http://www.hodderarnold.com

Hachette UK's policy is to use papers that are natural, renewable and recyclable products and made from
wood grown in sustainable forests. The logging and manufacturing processes are expected to conform to
the environmental regulations of the country of origin.

Whilst the advice and information in this book are believed to be true and accurate at the date of going to
press, neither the authors nor the publisher can accept any legal responsibility or liability for any errors or
omissions that may be made. In particular (but without limiting the generality of the preceding disclaimer)
every effort has been made to check drug dosages; however it is still possible that errors have been
missed. Furthermore, dosage schedules are constantly being revised and new side-effects recognized.
For these reasons the reader is strongly urged to consult the drug companies' printed instructions before
administering any of the drugs recommended in this book.

British Library Cataloguing in Publication Data
A catalogue record for this book is available from the British Library

Library of Congress Cataloging-in-Publication Data
A catalog record for this book is available from the Library of Congress

ISBN   978-1-444-11864-3

1 2 3 4 5 6 7 8 9 10

Commissioning Editor: Caroline Makepeace
Project Editor: Joanna Silman
Production Controller: Kate Harris
Cover Design: Lynda King
Index: Jan Ross

Cover images: Main image © Science Photo Library; inset images © Wellcome Images

Typeset in 9.5 pt Rotis Serif by Phoenix Photosetting, Chatham, Kent, ME4 4TZ
Printed and bound in the UK by MPG Books Ltd

What do you think about this book? Or any other Hodder Arnold title?
Please visit our website: **www.hodderarnold.com**

Contents

PREFACE   vii

PART 1: THE FOUNDATIONS OF MODERN PSYCHIATRIC PRACTICE

1   History of psychiatry   3
2   Introduction to evidence-based medicine   9
3   History and philosophy of science   11
4   Research methods and statistics   15
5   Epidemiology   31
6   How to practise evidence-based medicine   33
7   Psychological assessment and psychometrics   37

PART 2: DEVELOPMENTAL, BEHAVIOURAL, AND SOCIOCULTURAL PSYCHIATRY

8   Human development   43
9   Introduction to basic psychology   49
10   Awareness   51
11   Stress   55
12   Emotion   59
13   Information-processing and attention   63
14   Learning theory   67
15   Motivation   73
16   Perception   77
17   Memory   83
18   Language and thought   87
19   Personality   91
20   Social psychology   95
21   Social science and sociocultural psychiatry   99
22   Cultural psychiatry   103

PART 3: NEUROSCIENCE

23   Neuroanatomy   111
24   Basic concepts in neurophysiology   117
25   Neurophysiology of integrated behaviour   121
26   Neurogenesis and cerebral plasticity   127
27   The neuroendocrine system   129
28   The neurophysiology and neurochemistry of arousal and sleep   133
29   The electroencephalogram and evoked potential studies   137
30   Neurochemistry   141
31   Neuropathology   151
32   Neuroimaging   155
33   Genetics   159

PART 4: MENTAL HEALTH PROBLEMS AND MENTAL ILLNESS

34	Classification and diagnostic systems	165
35	Cognitive assessment	169
36	Neurology for psychiatrists	173
37	Organic disorders	179
38	Schizophrenia and paranoid psychoses	187
39	Mood disorders/affective psychoses	191
40	Neurotic and stress-related disorders	195
41	Dissociative (conversion), hypochondriasis and other somatoform disorders	199
42	Eating disorders	203
43	Personality disorders	205
44	Perinatal psychiatry	207
45	Psychosexual medicine	211
46	Gender identity disorders	215
47	Paraphilias and sexual offenders	217
48	Psychiatric assessment of physical illness	221
49	Overlapping multi-system, multi-organ illnesses/syndromes	225
50	Multiple chemical sensitivity	227
51	Mental health problems in patients with myalgic encephalomyelitis	231
52	Pain and psychiatry	233
53	Sleep disorders	237
54	Suicide and deliberate self-harm	243
55	Emergency psychiatry	249
56	Care of the dying and bereaved	251

PART 5: APPROACHES TO TREATMENT

57	Clinical psychopharmacology	257
58	Electroconvulsive therapy	265
59	Transcranial magnetic stimulation and vagus nerve stimulation	267
60	Psychotherapy: an introduction	269
61	Dynamic psychotherapy	273
62	Family therapy	275
63	Marital therapy	279
64	Group therapy	283
65	Cognitive-behavioural therapy	287
66	Other individual psychotherapies	291
67	Therapeutic communities	295
68	Effectiveness of psychotherapy	297

PART 6: CLINICAL SPECIALITIES

69	Addiction psychiatry	301
70	Child and adolescent psychiatry	307
71	Learning disability psychiatry	313
72	Old-age psychiatry	317
73	Rehabilitation psychiatry	321

PART 7: MENTAL HEALTH SERVICE PROVISION

74 Management of psychiatric services   327
75 Advice to special medical services   329

PART 8: LEGAL AND ETHICAL ASPECTS OF PSYCHIATRY

76 Forensic psychiatry   333
77 Legal aspects of psychiatric care, with particular reference to England and Wales   343
78 Ethics and law   347
79 Risk assessment   349

MOCK EXAMINATION PAPERS

MRCPsych Paper 1   353
MRCPsych Paper 2   383
MRCPsych Paper 3   409

INDEX   443

Preface

This book consists of over 1500 questions and answers.

The first part of the book acts as a study guide and is divided into different subject areas of psychiatric knowledge. It consists of 'best of five' multiple choice questions (MCQs) and extended matching item questions (EMIs) in a ratio of approximately two to one. When readers have studied a particular area of psychiatric knowledge, they can test themselves on their understanding by trying to answer the questions set on that topic. The standard of the questions has in general been set to at least that of the Royal College of Psychiatrists' MRCPsych examinations. Those preparing for other examinations might also find this book of value. However, this particular part of the book is designed to be more than mere preparation for the MRCPsych examination and is aimed at generally developing the knowledge that a practising psychiatrist requires. These questions are designed to test for an *understanding* of the material, rather than for pure rote learning of the answers and eidetic recall. We recommend that readers make the effort to answer the questions on a given topic before turning to the answers. This, together with developing understanding further by studying relevant content of a psychiatric textbook, will make for a far more valuable study experience. To aid this study process, the answers are sometimes fairly detailed in this section of the book and extensive cross reference is made to our textbook *Psychiatry: An Evidence-Based Text* upon which most of the questions and answers in this part of the book are based.

The second section of the book consists of 600 questions and answers set out as three revision mock examinations. They correspond to Papers 1, 2 and 3 of the MRCPsych, according to the Royal College of Psychiatrists' examinations regulations in force in 2011. The questions (a mixture of MCQs and EMIs) have been set to reflect the type and standard of questions of the MRCPsych examinations at the time of writing. As these are revision papers, the answers given are, in general, less detailed than those supplied in the first part of this book. Readers who are preparing for the MRCPsych examinations are urged always to keep themselves up to date with the latest regulations and guidance issued by the Royal College, which have significantly changed in recent years.

We would welcome feedback from those using this book as a study aid or revision guide. Please do let us know if there are any further types of questions you would like to see in the next edition of this book.

We wish to thank again all the authors who contributed to our textbook *Psychiatry: An Evidence-Based Text.*

Basant K Puri, Roger CM Ho and Ian H Treasaden
Cambridge, Singapore & London
2011

PART 1

The foundations of modern psychiatric practice

Chapter   **1**

History of psychiatry

QUESTIONS

Note that for answers to extended matching items (EMIs), each option (denoted a, b, c, etc.) might be used once, more than once or not at all. For multiple-choice questions (MCQs), please select the best answer.

1. **MCQ** – Which of the following works was written by Michel Foucault?
   (a) *A History of Clinical Psychiatry: the Origin and History of Psychiatric Disorders*
   (b) *A History of Psychiatry: from the Era of the Asylum to the Age of Prozac*
   (c) *Madness and Civilization: a History of Insanity in the Age of Reason*
   (d) *Moses and Monotheism*
   (e) *The Myth of Mental Illness.*

2. **MCQ** – Select one correct statement regarding Andrew Scull:
   (a) He wrote *George III and the Mad Business*.
   (b) He favoured a 'meliorist' history of psychiatry.
   (c) He introduced a radically new take on psychiatry as representing social power and social control.
   (d) He postulated that a 'great confinement' took place in the seventeenth and eighteenth centuries.
   (e) He was the famed eighteenth-century 'mad-doctor' and physician to Bethlem Hospital.

3. **MCQ** – Which of the following works was written by Carl Jung?
   (a) *Beyond the Pleasure Principle*
   (b) *Envy and Gratitude*
   (c) *Illustrations of Madness*
   (d) *Memories, Dreams, Reflections*
   (e) *Mind and Madness in Ancient Greece.*

4. **EMI** – Classic texts in psychiatry (1)
   (a) Andrews *et al.*
   (b) Berrios
   (c) Bleuler
   (d) Ellenberger
   (e) Freud
   (f) Fuller Torrey and Miller
   (g) Hunter and Macalpine
   (h) Kraeplin
   (i) Maudsley
   (j) Pinel
   (k) Sargant and Slater
   (l) Scull

   (m) Tuke
   (n) Von Krafft-Ebbing
   (o) Zilboorg and Henry

   Who of the above wrote, or co-wrote, the following works?
   (i) *Chapters in the History of the Insane*
   (ii) *The Most Solitary of Afflictions: Madness and Society in Britain 1700–1900*
   (iii) *The History of Bethlem*
   (iv) *The Discovery of the Unconscious.*

5. **EMI** – Classic texts in psychiatry (2)
   (a) Anthony
   (b) Berrios
   (c) Bleuler
   (d) Ellenberger
   (e) Freud
   (f) Fuller Torrey and Miller
   (g) Hunter and Macalpine
   (h) Kraeplin
   (i) Maudsley
   (j) Pinel
   (k) Sargant and Slater
   (l) Scull
   (m) Tuke
   (n) Von Krafft-Ebbing
   (o) Zilboorg and Henry

   Who of the above wrote, or co-wrote, the following works?
   (i) *Museums of Madness*
   (ii) *A Manual of Psychological Medicine*
   (iii) *The Interpretation of Dreams*
   (iv) *The Physiology and Pathology of the Mind.*

6. **EMI** – Classic texts in psychiatry (3)
   (a) Anthony
   (b) Berrios
   (c) Bleuler
   (d) Ellenberger
   (e) Freud
   (f) Fuller Torrey and Miller
   (g) Hunter and Macalpine

(h) Kraeplin
(i) Maudsley
(j) Pinel
(k) Sargant and Slater
(l) Scull
(m) Tuke
(n) Von Krafft-Ebbing
(o) Zilboorg and Henry

Who of the above wrote, or co-wrote, the following works?
(i) *Psychopathia Sexualis*
(ii) *Dementia Praecox or The Group of Schizophrenias*
(iii) *An Introduction to Physical Methods of Treatment in Psychiatry*
(iv) *A Treatise on Insanity.*

7. **EMI** – Major developments
(a) Eliot Slater
(b) Henry Maudsley
(c) John Conolly
(d) John Monro
(e) Julius Wagner-Jauregg
(f) Philippe Pinel
(g) Sigmund Freud
(h) William Harvey

Who of the above are best associated with the following developments in the history of psychiatry?
(i) Introducing non-restraint to the Hanwell asylum
(ii) Unchaining the insane in the 1790s
(iii) The use of pyrotherapy, with malaria inoculation, to treat dementia paralytica.

8. **EMI** – Historical events/themes (1)
(a) Criminal anthropology
(b) Described neurasthenia
(c) Moral insanity
(d) Murdered the prime minister's secretary
(e) Phrenology
(f) Shot at King George III
(g) Shot at Queen Victoria
(h) Wrote an early textbook of forensic psychiatry

Which of the above events or historical themes in the history of psychiatry are best associated with each of the following individuals?
(i) George Beard
(ii) Franz Gall
(iii) James Hadfield
(iv) Cesare Lombroso.

9. **EMI** – Key dates in psychiatry (1)
(a) 1860–1880
(b) 1880–1900
(c) 1900–1920
(d) 1920–1940
(e) 1940–1960
(f) 1960–1980

Which of the above time periods are best associated with inception date of each of the following?
(i) Lunacy Acts (England and Wales)
(ii) The first publication of the term 'schizophrenia' by Bleuler
(iii) Mental Health Act (England and Wales).

10. **EMI** – Historical events/themes (2)
(a) Criminal anthropology
(b) Described neurasthenia
(c) Moral insanity
(d) Murdered the prime minister's private secretary
(e) Phrenology
(f) Shot at King George III
(g) Shot at Queen Victoria
(h) Wrote an early textbook of forensic psychiatry

Which of the above events or historical themes in the history of psychiatry are best associated with each of the following individuals?
(i) Henry Maudsley
(ii) Daniel McNaughton
(iii) Johann Spurzheim
(iv) James Pritchard.

11. **MCQ** – Which of the following medications was not available for use during the nineteenth century?
(a) Apomorphine
(b) Chloral hydrate
(c) Chlorpromazine
(d) Hyoscine
(e) Opium.

12. **EMI** – Key dates in psychiatry (2)
(a) 1930–1940
(b) 1940–1950
(c) 1950–1960
(d) 1960–1970
(e) 1970–1980
(f) 1980–1990
(h) 1990–2000
(i) 2000–2010

Which of the above time periods are best associated with the date of introduction of each of the following antipsychotic drug treatments?
(i) Haloperidol
(ii) Clozapine
(iii) Second-generation antipsychotics, apart from clozapine.

13. **MCQ** – Which of the following psychopharmacological treatments was included by Sargant and Slater in their 1944 textbook?
(a) Amisulpride
(b) Amitriptyline
(c) Amphetamine
(d) Chlordiazepoxide
(e) Diazepam.

14. **MCQ** – Select the person most closely associated with the development of theories about archetypes:
    (a) Adler
    (b) Freud
    (c) Jung
    (d) Klein
    (e) Winnicott.

ANSWERS

1. c

It was published in an abridged version by the French historian, philosopher and sociologist in an English translation in 1965, following the original 1961 publication as *Folie et déraison: Histoire de la folie à l'âge classique*, and begins in the Middle Ages. *A History of Clinical Psychiatry: The Origin and History of Psychiatric Disorders* was edited by Professor German Berrios (University of Cambridge) and the late Professor Roy Porter (1995). *A History of Psychiatry: From the Era of the Asylum to the Age of Prozac* was written by Professor Edward Shorter (1997); *Moses and Monotheism* was written by Professor Sigmund Freud (1939); and *The Myth of Mental Illness* was written by Professor Thomas Szasz.

Reference: *Psychiatry: An evidence-based text*, pp. 3–4.

2. c

Professor Andrew Scull (Department of Sociology, University of California, San Diego) published the ground-breaking *Museums of Madness* in 1979, which introduced a radically new taken on psychiatry as representing social power and social control, thus reinforcing the status quo via an often doubtful construct of 'mental illness'. In 2009 he published *Hysteria: The Biography (Biographies of Disease)* (Oxford University Press).

George III and the Mad Business was written by Hunter and Macalpine (1969). The 'meliorist' history of psychiatry – things getting better, in terms of more accurate diagnoses, more thoughtful doctors (and attendants/nurses) and more humane treatments – was challenged by Prof. Scull. Michel Foucault postulated a 'great confinement' in the seventeenth and eighteenth centuries, whereby the world of free-thinking and imaginative 'unreason' had been corralled by the mechanistic warriors of reason and social control. The famed eighteenth-century 'mad-doctor' and physician to Bethlem Hospital was John Monro (1715–91).

Reference: *Psychiatry: An evidence-based text*, pp. 3–4.

3. d

Published in 1963, *Memories, Dreams, Reflections* represents a summation of the theories and work of Carl Jung (1875–1961). *Beyond the Pleasure Principle* was published by Sigmund Freud in 1920. In it Freud described his tripartite model of the human psyche into the id, the ego and the superego. A more detailed account followed in his 1923 work *The Ego and the Id*.

Envy and Gratitude represents the third (of four) volumes of the collected writings of Melanie Klein, published by Hogarth Press (London). *Illustrations of Madness: Exhibiting a Singular Case of Insanity and a No Less Remarkable Difference in Medical Opinion* was the 1810 work of John Haslam. It was a book-length account of a contended case, illustrating a 'first-rank' series of colourful symptoms typical of florid paranoid schizophrenia.

Mind and Madness in Ancient Greece: The Classical Roots of Modern Psychiatry is the 1978 classic exposition, by Bennett Simon, of Greek ideas, with chapters on 'tragedy and therapy' and 'Plato and Freud'.

Reference: *Psychiatry: An evidence-based text*, pp. 5–6.

4.

(i) m – Tuke's nineteenth-century history was written as a celebration of Victorian achievement in building asylums and rescuing 'lunatics' from the neglect and abuse of whips, chains and supernatural beliefs.

(ii) l – Scull's book was published in 1993.

(iii) a – Andrews, Briggs, Porter, Tucker and Waddington published this highly detailed and extensively researched 750-page modern social history in 1997, to celebrate the 750th anniversary of Bethlem Hospital, which was founded in 1247 as a priory for the sisters and brethren of the Order of the Star of Bethlehem (hence the name).

(iv) d – Ellenberger's *The Discovery of the Unconscious: The History and Evolution of Dynamic Psychiatry* was published in 1970 and contains over 900 pages on the development of psychological approaches to mental illness, and how Sigmund Freud rose successfully above numerous rivals.

Reference: *Psychiatry: An evidence-based text*, pp. 4–5.

5.

(i) l – Scull's 1979 ground-breaking work introduced a radically new taken on psychiatry as representing social power and social control. The 1993 work, *The Most Solitary of Afflictions: Madness and Society in Britain 1700–1900*, was an updated version of the 1979 work by the same author.

(ii) m – *A Manual of Psychological Medicine* was written by Bucknill and Tuke and published in 1858. It was the first proper English treatise of psychiatry, indicating the growing size of the speciality and the need for a student's textbook. Treatment is divided into 'hygienic', 'moral' and 'medical'.

(iii) e – *The Interpretation of Dreams* was published in 1900 and represents Sigmund Freud's classic text on his theory of the unconscious, dreams being considered essential to understand one's inner mental life. Freud referred to dreams as being the 'royal road to the unconscious'.

(iv) i – Henry Maudsley's *The Physiology and Pathology of the Mind* was published in 1867 in London. It was a much admired textbook which outlined the physical basis of mental disease as opposed to the 'metaphysical' theorizing that tended to dominate public discussion. Other works by Maudsley include *Body and Mind: An Inquiry into their Connection and Mutual Influence* (1870), *Responsibility in Mental Disease* (1874), *Body and Will: in its Metaphysical, Physiological and Pathological Aspects* (1883) and *Life in Mind and Conduct: Studies of Organic in Human Nature* (1902).

Reference: *Psychiatry: An evidence-based text*, **pp. 4–6.**

6.

(i)   n – *Psychopathia Sexualis: With Especial Reference to Contrary Sexual Instinct – A Medico-Legal Study* was published in 1886 (with an English translation first published in 1892). It contained the first detailed description of abnormal sexual behaviours, including sadism, masochism, 'congenital inversion' (that is, homosexuality) and fetishism.

(ii) c – Bleuler's *Dementia Praecox or The Group of Schizophrenias* was published in 1911 and in it Paul Eugen Bleuler first introduced the term 'schizophrenia', fusing psychoanalytical theory derived from Freud with the clinical descriptions of Kraeplin. The Bleulerian outline of schizophrenia dominated psychiatry until the 1960s.

(iii) k – William Sargant and Eliot Slater's 1944 book, *An Introduction to Physical Methods of Treatment in Psychiatry*, was the (wartime) classic of biological psychiatry. It trumpeted the use of insulin therapy, electroconvulsive therapy (ECT), chemical sedation, malaria treatment and prefrontal leucotomy, as opposed to psychotherapy, to which the authors barely paid lip service.

(iv) j – *A Treatise on Insanity*, published in 1801, contained an outline of 'maniacal disorders', including an attempt at classification and numerous case histories.

Reference: *Psychiatry: An evidence-based text*, **p. 6.**

7.

(i)   c – John Conolly introduced, against mocking scepticism, non-restraint to the enormous Hanwell asylum. His monograph on non-restraint was published in 1856.

(ii) f – Philippe Pinel, the father of French psychiatry, is said to have started to unchain the insane in the middle of the chaos of the French Revolution, with a battalion of soldiers hiding round the back of the hospital in case all hell broke loose. Paintings depicted this in France. However, there is some debate as to who was really the first person to start this trend of unchaining the insane. Some sources argue that Jean-Baptiste Pussin may first have started to remove iron shackles from insane inmates.

(iii) e – Julius Wagner-Jauregg won the Nobel Prize in Physiology or Medicine in 1927 for this therapy. His Nobel lecture was entitled 'The treatment of dementia paralytica by malaria inoculation', and began as follows: 'Two paths could lead to a cure for progressive paralysis: the rational and the empirical. The rational path appeared to be practical, as since Esmarch and Jessen, in 1858, attention had been drawn to a connection between progressive paralysis and syphilis. If incontestable proof that progressive paralysis was a syphilitic brain disease was first given much later (I mention in this connection the names Wassermann and Noguchi), therapeutic attempts to apply anti-syphilitic treatments were nevertheless instituted much earlier.'

Reference: *Psychiatry: An evidence-based text*, **p. 7.**

8.

(i)   b – George Beard described 'neurasthenia' in 1869.

(ii) e – Franz Gall was a leading exponent of phrenology, which considered the brain as the organ of the mind, different activities being located in different areas, therefore demanding careful examination of the shape of the head.

(iii) f – When James Hadfield shot at King George III in a theatre in 1800 and was charged with 'high treason', he stated that he had been acting on God's instructions. Deemed not responsible, he was sent to Bethlem, and deciding on whether someone is 'mad' or 'bad' has subsequently dominated public attitudes to mental illness. (Dyte, who had struck Hadfield's arm as he pulled the trigger, had saved the life of the King and as a reward was granted a monopoly on the sale of opera tickets.)

(iv) a – Cesare Lombroso founded the Italian School of Positivist Criminology. His theory of criminal anthropology suggested that criminals inherited their predisposition to crime and could be identified via various physical atavistic stigmata, such as a large jaw and chin, high cheekbones and a low sloping forehead.

Reference: *Psychiatry: An evidence-based text*, **Table 1.4.**

9.

(i)   b – The 1890 Lunacy Act incorporated changes introduced in the 1889 Lunatics Law Amendment Act. Both it and the 1891 Lunacy Act were repealed by the 1959 Mental Health Act.

(ii) c – *Dementia Praecox or The Group of Schizophrenias* was published in 1911 and in it Paul Eugen Bleuler first introduced the term 'schizophrenia', fusing psychoanalytical theory derived from Freud with the clinical descriptions of Kraeplin. Eugen Bleuler's 'four As' were autism, affective impairment, ambivalence and impaired associations; they made reliable diagnosis of schizophrenia rather difficult.

(iii) **e** – The first Mental Health Act in England and Wales that appears within the options given in this question is that of 1959. The more recent 1983 Act is outside the given options.

> Reference: *Psychiatry: An evidence-based text*, **Figure 1.2 and Table 1.11.**

10.

(i) **h** – Henry Maudsley's *Responsibility in Mental Disease*, published in 1874, was the first forensic psychiatry textbook.

(ii) **d** – The McNaughton Rules, determining criminal insanity (e.g. 'knowing the nature of the act'), derive from the 1843 trial of Daniel McNaughton who murdered the then prime minister's private secretary.

(iii) **e** – Like Franz Gall, Johann Spurzheim was a leading exponent of phrenology. Initially, the two doctors co-authored publications on this subject.

(iv) **c** – James Pritchard's descriptions of cases of 'moral insanity', in 1835, would be diagnosed today as either personality disorder or bipolar disorder.

> Reference: *Psychiatry: An evidence-based text*, **Table 1.4.**

11. c

Chlorpromazine was introduced in the 1950s. It was synthesized by Paul Charpentier and was tested in non-human mammals by Simone Courvoisier. Henri Laborit and Pierre Huguenard used it on surgical patients and noted how relaxed it made them. Jean Delay and Pierre Denikar then began to use it in psychiatric patients. They began treating psychotic patients with chlorpromazine in 1952, following reports of its successful use in the treatment of a manic patient by psychiatrist colleagues of Laborit. During the nineteenth century, apomorphine, chloral hydrate and opium were available for use as medications. Hyoscine (also known as scopolamine) has a similar molecular structure to that of atropine and was also in medicinal use during the nineteenth century.

> Reference: *Psychiatry: An evidence-based text*, **Figure 1.2 and Table 1.5.**

12.

(i) **c** – Haloperidol was introduced during the 1950s.

(ii) **e** – Clozapine was introduced in the 1970s but was withdrawn owing to agranulocytosis-related mortality. It was then reintroduced in the late 1980s, with mandatory regular blood monitoring.

(iii) **h** – These were introduced during the 1990s.

> Reference: *Psychiatry: An evidence-based text*, **Table 1.7.**

13. c

In their 1944 textbook, Sargant and Slater included discussion of stimulation via amphetamine (Benzedrine). The other options given in the question were not available as treatments in 1944.

> Reference: *Psychiatry: An evidence-based text*, **p. 12.**

14. c

Carl Jung (1875–1961) was the founder of analytical psychology and theories about archetypes.

> Reference: *Psychiatry: An evidence-based text*, **p. 13.**

Chapter 2

Introduction to evidence-based medicine

QUESTIONS

Note that for answers to extended matching items (EMIs), each option (denoted a, b, c, etc.) might be used once, more than once or not at all. For multiple-choice questions (MCQs), please select the best answer.

1. **MCQ** – Select the option that is likely to be the most effective way of developing competence in evidence-based medicine:
   (a) Attending courses
   (b) Listening to pharmaceutical company representatives
   (c) Reading case reports
   (d) Reflective practice
   (e) Studying textbooks.

2. **EMI** – Evidence-based medicine in practice (1)
   (a) Application of results in practice (empowering patients to make clinical decisions)
   (b) Critical appraisal of evidence for validity, clinical relevance and applicability
   (c) Evaluation of performance
   (d) Systematic retrieval of best available evidence
   (e) Translation of uncertainty to an answerable question
   (h) None of the above

To which of the above steps of evidence-based medicine does each of the following activities by clinicians belong?
   (i) Having knowledge and understanding of basic epidemiology

   (ii) Being aware of one's own limitations and uncertainties
   (iii) Being motivated to seek guidance from published literature and colleagues.

3. **EMI** – Evidence-based medicine in practice (2)
   (a) Application of results in practice (empowering patients to make clinical decisions)
   (b) Critical appraisal of evidence for validity, clinical relevance and applicability
   (c) Evaluation of performance
   (d) Systematic retrieval of best available evidence
   (e) Translation of uncertainty to an answerable question
   (h) None of the above

To which of the above steps of evidence-based medicine does each of the following activities by clinicians belong?
   (i) Having knowledge and understanding of the hierarchy of evidence
   (ii) Being able to assess patients and formulate a management plan
   (iii) Having knowledge and understanding of basic biostatistics.

ANSWERS

1. d

Books and courses can help us to develop our knowledge base, but the most effective way of developing competence in evidence-based medicine is through reflective practice – that is, learning embedded in clinical practice. Note that case reports lie relatively low down in the hierarchy of evidence.

Reference: *Psychiatry: An evidence-based text*, **pp. 16–17.**

2.

(i) **b** – This is a skill that is part of being able to appraise evidence critically.

(ii) **e** – This attitude forms part of being able to translate one's clinical uncertainty into answerable questions.

(iii) **e** – This attitude forms part of being able to translate one's clinical uncertainty into answerable questions.

Reference: *Psychiatry: An evidence-based text*, **p. 17.**

3.

(i) **d** – This is part of being able to retrieve the best available evidence systematically. Recognizing the inherent strengths and weaknesses of different study designs for different types of question is essential for the efficient identification of the best available evidence.

(ii) **e** – These skills form part of being able to translate one's clinical uncertainty into answerable questions.

(iii) **b** – This skill is part of being able critically to appraise evidence.

Reference: *Psychiatry: An evidence-based text*, **pp. 16–17.**

Chapter 3

History and philosophy of science

QUESTIONS

Note that for answers to extended matching items (EMIs), each option (denoted a, b, c, etc.) might be used once, more than once or not at all. For multiple-choice questions (MCQs), please select the best answer.

1. **EMI** – History of science
   (a) Alzheimer
   (b) Durkheim
   (c) Griesinger
   (d) Jaspers
   (e) Meynert
   (f) Nissl
   (g) Wernicke
   (h) Windelband

   Who of the above is best associated with each of the following?
   (i) Positivism
   (ii) Showed that the neurohistological changes in general paralysis were different from those in dementia
   (iii) A phenomenological approach to psychopathology
   (iv) 'Mental illnesses are brain illnesses'.

2. **MCQ** – In the history and philosophy of science, who of the following was a positivist?
   (a) Dilthey
   (b) Mill
   (c) Rickert
   (d) Weber
   (e) Windelband.

3. **MCQ** – According to Karl Jaspers, which of the following are subjective symptoms?
   (a) Delusional ideas
   (b) The brain mythologies
   (c) The Methodenstreit
   (d) Those understood by empathy
   (e) Verbal expression.

4. **MCQ** – According to Jaspers, genetic understanding is associated with an understanding of which of the following?
   (a) Logarithm of odds (LOD) scores
   (b) Phenomenology
   (c) The connection between one psychic imperative and another
   (d) The neutral theory

   (e) The role of single nucleotide polymorphisms (SNPs).
   Reference: Kimura, M. (1983) *The Neutral Theory of Molecular Evolution.* Cambridge: Cambridge University Press.

5. **MCQ** – Which of the following is not a form of primary delusion according to Jaspers?
   (a) An understandable delusion
   (b) A delusional atmosphere
   (c) A delusional awareness
   (d) A delusional idea
   (e) A delusional perception.

6. **EMI** – Philosophy
   (a) Davidson
   (b) Jaspers
   (c) Plato
   (d) Schopenhauer
   (e) Wernicke
   (f) Windelband

   Who of the above is best associated with each of the following concepts?
   (i) Nomothetic approaches
   (ii) Static understanding
   (iii) Anomalous monism
   (iv) Idiographic understanding.

7. **EMI** – Philosophy
   (a) Jaspers
   (b) Morris
   (c) Sabat
   (d) Stanghellini
   (e) Warnock
   (f) Widdershoven

   Who of the above is best associated with each of the following?
   (i) His/her work has found clinical application to improved decision-making in old-age psychiatry.
   (ii) His/her work has found clinical application to the interpretation of language difficulties in Alzheimer's disease.
   (iii) Wrote *Disembodied Spirits and Deanimated Bodies*.

8. **EMI** – History of science
   (a) Jaspers
   (b) Morris
   (c) Sabat
   (d) Stanghellini
   (e) Warnock
   (f) Widdershoven

Who of the above is best associated with each of the following?
   (i) His/her work has found clinical application to body dysmorphic disorders.
   (ii) Wrote *The Object of Morality*.
   (iii) The study of the way in which coenaesthia, sensus communis and attunement are related to each other.

9. **MCQ** – Select one correct statement regarding values-based practice:
   (a) It is derived purely from philosophical sources.
   (b) It is outcome-based rather than process-based.
   (c) Its theory predicts that the implicit values driving medical decision-making are often far more diverse than is generally recognized.
   (d) The theory underpinning values-based practice is based on work in linguistic analytical philosophy carried out by the 'Cambridge school'.
   (e) Values were strongly supported by Jaspers.

ANSWERS

1.

(i) b – Positivists, such as Emile Durkheim and Auguste Comte in France, argued that the human sciences were no different from the natural sciences.

(ii) f – Franz Nissl was a professor in the Heidelberg department of psychiatry. He was a neurohistologist who discovered the dye that allowed the structure of nerve cells to be clearly seen for the first time. Using this technique, he showed that the neurohistological changes in general paralysis were different from the changes described by Alois Alzheimer in dementia.

(iii) d – Karl Jaspers developed phenomenological psychopathology.

(iv) c – Psychiatry at the turn of the nineteenth century in Germany had moved out of the large institutions into university clinics. There was considerable resentment among the institutional psychiatrists that their discipline had been taken over by academic neuroscientists, whose knowledge of clinical psychiatry was scant, and whom they perceived as being under the spell of a crudely natural scientific model, epitomized by the German psychiatrist Wilhelm Griesinger's famous aphorism 'Mental illnesses are brain illnesses'.

Reference: *Psychiatry: An evidence-based text*, **pp. 19–21.**

2. b

John Stuart Mill (1806–1873) was a positivist. Positivists argued that the human sciences were no different from the natural sciences. Others argued that the human or cultural sciences were different from the natural sciences, in terms of either the nature of their subject matter or their methodology, or both. The latter, in Germany, included Heinrich Rickert, Wilhelm Dilthey, Wilhelm Windelband and Max Weber.

Reference: *Psychiatry: An evidence-based text*, **p. 20.**

3. d

According to Karl Jaspers, 'Objective symptoms can all be directly and convincingly demonstrated to anyone capable of sense-perception and logical thought; but subjective symptoms, if they are to be understood, must be referred to some process which, in contrast to sense perception and logical thought, is usually described by the same term "subjective". Subjective symptoms cannot be perceived by the sense-organs, but have to be grasped by transferring oneself, so to say, into the other individual's psyche; that is, by empathy. They can only become an inner reality for the observer by his participating in the other person's experiences, not by any intellectual effort.' Conversely, he described objective symptoms as follows:

'Objective symptoms include all concrete events that can be perceived by the sense, e.g. reflexes, registrable movements, an individual's physiognomy, his motor activity, verbal expression, written productions, actions and general conduct, etc.; all measurable performances... It is also usual to include under objective symptoms such features as delusional ideas, falsifications of memory, etc., in other words, the rational contents of what the patient tells us. These, it is true, are not perceived by the senses, but only understood; nevertheless, this "understanding" is achieved through rational thought, without the help of any empathy into the patient's psyche.'

Reference: *Psychiatry: An evidence-based text*, **pp. 20–21.**

4. c

Karl Jaspers distinguished between two forms of understanding of subjective phenomena: static understanding, which he also called phenomenology, and genetic understanding. He characterized the differences as follows: '"Genetic understanding" [is] the understanding of the meaningful connections between one psychic experience and another, the "emergence of the psychic from the psychic". Now phenomenology itself has nothing to do with this "genetic understanding" and must be treated as something entirely separate.' The LOD score is a statistical test used in linkage analysis. The neutral theory asserts that the great majority of evolutionary changes at the molecular level are caused by random drift of selectively neutral or nearly neutral mutant.

References: *Psychiatry: An evidence-based text*, **p. 22.**

5. a

Karl Jaspers argued that the key feature of primary delusions is that they are un-understandable. While secondary delusions or delusion-like ideas are, in principle, understandable in the context of a person's life history, personality, mood state or presence of other psychopathology, primary delusions have a kind of basic status. According to Jaspers, 'We can distinguish between two large groups of delusion according to their *origin*: one group *emerges understandably* from preceding affects, from shattering, mortifying, guilt-provoking or other such experiences, from false perception or from the experience of derealisation in states of altered consciousness etc. The other group is for us *psychologically irreducible*; phenomenologically it is something final. We give the term "*delusion-like ideas*" to the first group; the latter we term "*delusions proper*".' Jaspers divided primary delusions into four kinds: delusional atmosphere, delusional perceptions, delusional ideas and delusional awareness. Definitions of these terms are given on page 23 of the textbook.

Reference: *Psychiatry: An evidence-based text*, **pp. 23–24.**

6.

(i) **f** – Wilhelm Windelband was a Kantian philosopher of science. He first introduced the distinction between 'idiographic' and 'nomothetic' in his rectorial address of 1894. Key components of the distinction between them are that it is a distinction of method and not of subject matter, that it concerns treating events as unrepeated, and that it is a reaction against an over-reliance on an essentially general conception of knowledge.

(ii) **b** – Karl Jaspers distinguished between two forms of understanding of subjective phenomena: static understanding, which he also called phenomenology, and genetic understanding.

(iii) **a** – Jaspers suggested that understanding and explanation do not have two distinct subject matters. Rather, the difference between them is one of method or of the kind of intelligibility that they deploy. The idea that neural events might be susceptible to two distinct patterns of intelligibility was articulated by the American philosopher of mind Donald Davidson (1917–2003). On his model of the mind, 'anomalous monism', the very same events that comprise mental events and that – according to Davidson – stand in essentially rational relations also comprise physical events and can be subsumed under nomological causal explanations.

(iv) **f** – See the answer to (i).

Reference: *Psychiatry: An evidence-based text*, **Ch. 3**.

7.

(i) **f** – The work of the Dutch philosopher Guy Widdershoven has found clinical application to improved decision-making in old-age psychiatry.

(ii) **c** – The work of the American philosopher and psychologist Steven Sabat has found clinical application to the interpretation of language difficulties in Alzheimer's disease.

(iii) **d** – In his book of essays, *Disembodied Spirits and Deanimated Bodies*, the Italian psychiatrist and phenomenologist Giovanni Stanghellini has argued that some understanding of the experiences of sufferers of schizophrenia is possible on the hypothesis that they experience a threefold breakdown of common sense.

Reference: *Psychiatry: An evidence-based text*, **p. 26**.

8.

(i) **b** – The work of the Oxford philosopher of mind, Karen Morris, has found clinical application to body dysmorphic disorders.

(ii) **e** – This book, by the Oxford philosopher Sir Geoffrey Warnock (known as G. J. Warnock), was published in 1971 (his widow is Baroness Warnock).

(iii) **d** – In his book of essays, *Disembodied Spirits and Deanimated Bodies*, the Italian psychiatrist and phenomenologist Giovanni Stanghellini has argued that some understanding of the experiences of sufferers of schizophrenia is possible on the hypothesis that they experience a threefold breakdown of common sense. This involves a breakdown of three distinct areas: the ability to synthesize different senses into a coherent perspective on the world (coenaesthesia); the ability to share a common world view with other members of a community (sensus communis); and a basic pre-intellectual grasp of, or attunement to, social relations (attunement).

Reference: *Psychiatry: An evidence-based text*, **pp. 26–27**.

9. c

A key prediction of the theory of values-based practice is that the implicit values driving medical decision-making are often far more diverse than is generally recognized. This prediction has been tested by the British social scientist Anthony Colombo in a major study of the models of disorder (including values and beliefs) guiding decisions in the management of people with long-term schizophrenia in the community.

Values-based practice is distinctive theoretically in that it is derived from both philosophical and empirical sources. It is process- rather than outcome-based. Therefore values-based practice is most directly complementary to the sciences as a resource for clinical decision-making.

The theory underpinning values-based practice is based on work in linguistic analytical philosophy of the 'Oxford school' in the middle decades of the twentieth century, on the meanings of key value terms, such as 'good', 'ought' and 'right'.

Jaspers rather dismissed values.

Reference: *Psychiatry: An evidence-based text*, **Ch. 3**.

Chapter 4

Research methods and statistics

QUESTIONS

Note that for answers to extended matching items (EMIs), each option (denoted a, b, c, etc.) might be used once, more than once or not at all. For multiple-choice questions (MCQs), please select the best answer.

1. **EMI** – Types of data (1)
   (a) Binomial
   (b) Interval
   (c) Logarithmic
   (d) Nominal
   (e) Ordinal
   (f) Ratio

For each of the following examples select the most appropriate corresponding category of data type from the above list:
   (i) Likert scale
   (ii) Age
   (iii) Ethnic group (measured in several categories).

2. **EMI** – Types of data (2)
   (a) Binomial
   (b) Interval
   (c) Logarithmic
   (d) Nominal
   (e) Ordinal
   (f) Ratio

For each of the following examples select the most appropriate corresponding category of data type from the above list:
   (i) Visual analogue pain score
   (ii) Body temperature (in °C)
   (iii) The distribution of heads and tails after a given number of tosses of a coin.

3. **MCQ** – Which of the following does Cohen's kappa primarily index?
   (a) Construct validity
   (b) Inter-observer reliability
   (c) Intra-observer reliability
   (d) Item consistency
   (e) Sensitivity.

4. **MCQ** – The internal consistency of a measuring instrument, for continuous data, is best calculated using which of the following?
   (a) Cronbach's alpha
   (b) Kuder–Richardson Formula 20

   (c) Recombination fraction
   (d) Spearman–Brown formula
   (e) Weighted kappa.

5. **MCQ** – A psychiatric researcher wishes to assess whether a new measure is consistent with what we already know and expect. Which of the following types of validity would be the best one to use for this?
   (a) Content
   (b) Criterion
   (c) Discriminant
   (d) Face
   (e) Predictive.

6. **MCQ** – An evaluation of a new screening questionnaire for anorexia nervosa in primary care is conducted. The most important single feature of this questionnaire that would encourage you to use it is:
   (a) It has a positive predictive value of 24 per cent.
   (b) It has a sensitivity of 82 per cent.
   (c) It has a specificity of 58 per cent.
   (d) It has been tested in different countries.
   (e) It takes only 8–10 minutes, on average, to administer.

7. **EMI** – Statistics
   (a) 0
   (b) 5
   (c) 6
   (d) 20
   (e) 30
   (f) 43
   (g) 50
   (h) 56
   (i) 70
   (j) 80
   (k) 90
   (l) 100
   (m) Infinity
   (n) Insufficient information

For each of the following questions, select the most appropriate answer from the above list:
   (i) A commonly used lower limit of the risk of a

type I error (expressed as a percentage) in power calculations for randomized trials

(ii) The specificity of a test, expressed as a percentage, in which 70 people were classified 'true negative' and 30 were classified 'false positive'

(iii) The negative predictive power, expressed as a percentage, of a screening test in which 40 people were classified 'true positive', 10 as 'false positive', 26 as 'true negative' and 24 as 'false negative'

(iv) The odds of an event occurring if it happens five-sixths of the time

(v) The sensitivity of a test, expressed as a percentage, in which 80 people were classified 'true positive' and 20 were classified 'false positive'.

8. **EMI** – Diagnostic test measures
   (a) 0
   (b) 0.05
   (c) 0.09
   (d) 0.1
   (e) 0.25
   (f) 0.41
   (g) 0.7
   (h) 1
   (i) 7
   (j) 25
   (k) 70
   (l) 100
   (m) Infinity
   (n) Insufficient information

The prevalence of a psychiatric disorder in the population of interest is 1/11 (= 0.09 to two decimal places) and a patient tests positive using a test which has a sensitivity of 0.7 and a specificity of 0.9. For each of the measures below for a positive test, select the nearest appropriate correct answer, if any, from the above list (note that percentages are not being used):
   (i) The pre-test probability
   (ii) The pre-test odds
   (iii) The likelihood ratio (for a positive test)
   (iv) The post-test odds
   (v) The post-test probability.

9. **MCQ** – An evaluation is conducted of a new screening tool which produces a score on a continuous scale. Which of the following is the most important single feature that would encourage you to use it?
   (a) It is quick to carry out.
   (b) It has a receiver operator curve (ROC) that is close to the diagonal from the bottom left-hand side to the top right-hand side.
   (c) It has a ROC that strongly deviates towards the left-hand top corner.
   (d) It has a ROC that strongly deviates towards the right-hand bottom corner.
   (e) The area under the ROC is 0.6.

10. **MCQ** – Which of the following research methods is best suited to comparing cognitive-behaviour therapy with a selective serotonin reuptake inhibitor (SSRI) in anxiety disorders?
   (a) Double-blind and placebo-controlled
   (b) Open-label and randomized
   (c) Patient preference trial
   (d) Randomized and placebo-controlled (un-blinded)
   (e) Randomized and triple-blind.

11. **MCQ** – Which of the following is the least adequate method of randomization?
   (a) Minimization
   (b) Odd/even last digit of date of birth
   (c) Odd/even random number table
   (d) Odd/even roll of a fair unbiased die
   (e) Permuted block.

12. **EMI** – CONSORT diagram

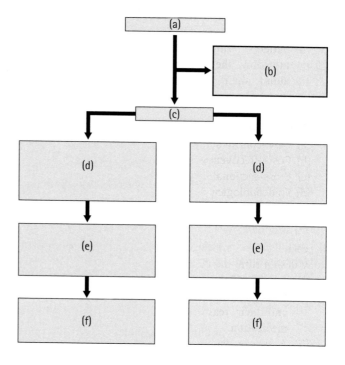

For each of the following labels, select the appropriate option from the above CONSORT diagram:
   (i) Analysed
   (ii) Randomized
   (iii) Assessed for eligibility
   (iv) Excluded
   (v) Lost to follow-up
   (vi) Allocated to an intervention.

13. **MCQ** – Which of the following is a clinical trial design that can be used when the randomization of individual patients is not possible?
   (a) Cluster randomized trial
   (b) Copy number variation
   (c) Crossover trial
   (d) Intention-to-treat
   (e) Randomized controlled trial.

14. **EMI** – Study design (1)
    (a) Case–control study
    (b) Cost-effectiveness analysis
    (c) Cross-sectional study
    (d) Epidemiological study
    (e) Qualitative study
    (f) Randomized controlled trial

For each study described below, select the most appropriate study design from the above list:
    (i) A study was conducted to assess the attitudes to their diagnosis of patients with depression.
    (ii) The efficacy of a new second-generation antipsychotic in the pharmacotherapy of schizophrenia is compared with that of haloperidol.
    (iii) To investigate the relationship between cannabis use and schizophrenia, a group of patients attending a psychiatric outpatient clinic with a diagnosis of schizophrenia were questioned about their use of cannabis. A group of age- and gender-matched patients, without a diagnosis of schizophrenia, attending the same clinic were also questioned about their cannabis use using an identical protocol.

15. **EMI** – Study design (2)
    (a) Case–control study
    (b) Cost-effectiveness analysis
    (c) Cross-sectional study
    (d) Epidemiological study
    (e) Qualitative study
    (f) Randomized controlled trial

For each study described below, select the most appropriate study design from the above list:
    (i) A group of patients with schizophrenia are invited to describe their views of oral antipsychotic medication and their reasons for not complying with their medication.
    (ii) A survey was conducted of a random sample of psychiatric trainee doctors attending a postgraduate psychiatry course. The questionnaire included questions about the number of years of postgraduate training the doctor had undergone and his/her satisfaction with the current psychiatry course.
    (iii) A study is conducted of a new second-generation antipsychotic for schizophrenia, to determine the average extra cost per unit reduction in symptom score.

16. **MCQ** – Which of the following is a feature of before–after (pre–post) patient intervention studies?
    (a) Loss to follow-up is appropriately dealt with using the last observation carried forward method.
    (b) Regression to the mean.
    (c) The effect of intervention is readily distinguished from natural improvement over time.

(d) The outcome is measured on different groups of patients before and after an intervention.
(e) There are no controls.

17. **EMI** – Study design (3)
    (a) Case–control study
    (b) Cross-sectional study
    (c) Ecological study
    (d) Prospective cohort study
    (e) Retrospective cohort study

For each study described below, select the most appropriate study design from the list above:
    (i) A study of retired people comparing time to death between those having a diagnosis of Alzheimer's disease and those without such a diagnosis.
    (ii) The aim of the study is to investigate whether birth trauma is a risk factor in the development of schizophrenia. Cases of schizophrenia are identified and an individually matched control subject is found for each patient, matched for age (within ± 2 years), ethnicity and birth postcode (zip code) area. The birth records are examined to determine whether birth trauma had occurred.
    (iii) A study is conducted of students in whom previous neurotic symptoms in adolescence have been self-reported. Current diagnosis of schizophrenia (if present) is made by a psychiatrist. The association between any earlier self-reported symptoms and a present diagnosis of schizophrenia is estimated.
    (iv) A survey is conducted to detect all people in contact with mental health services in a specific area over a 6-month period.
    (v) The unit of observation is a GP's (family doctor's) practice.

18. **MCQ** – Select one correct statement from the following regarding health economic studies:
    (a) A cost-effectiveness plane should not contain bootstrapped data.
    (b) A specific disease-related outcome cannot be used in a cost-effectiveness analysis.
    (c) If the incremental cost-effectiveness ratio is greater than a maximum willingness to pay, the corresponding therapy is considered cost-effective at that level.
    (d) One quality-adjusted life year (QALY) is equivalent to 2 years in a health state valued at 0.25.
    (e) The cost-effectiveness acceptability curve plots the probability of cost-effectiveness against various choices of minimum willingness to pay.

19. **MCQ** – Which of the following is the best quantitative estimate of the precision of a parameter estimate?
    (a) Bias
    (b) Confidence interval
    (c) Kurtosis

(d) Sample size
(e) Skewness.

20. **EMI** – Study bias
(a) Attrition
(b) Ascertainment
(c) Berkson's
(d) Interview
(e) Recall
(f) Selection

For each study described below, select the most appropriate type of bias that may occur from the list above:
(i) A study in which advertisements are placed in the press for subjects.
(ii) A prospective cohort study of Alzheimer's disease (defined properly only postmortem).
(iii) A study in which there is loss to follow-up resulting from patient death (which is not the primary outcome).
(iv) A study in which in-patients with schizophrenia are matched with controls, also in hospital, in order to investigate cannabis use as a risk factor for developing schizophrenia.

21. **MCQ** – Which of the following is not a Bradford-Hill criterion for causal inference?
(a) Analogy
(b) Biological gradient
(c) Plausibility
(d) Residual confounding
(e) Strength of association.

22. **MCQ** – Which of the following is not true of the normal distribution?
(a) It is the limit of the distribution of the mean when the distribution from which the means are derived do not follow a normal distribution.
(b) It is the limit of the distribution of the mean when the distribution from which the means are derived follow a normal distribution.
(c) Ninety-five per cent of the cases in a population that follows a normal distribution lie within $\pm$ 1.96 $\times$ (population standard deviation, SD) from the population mean.
(d) The formula for a normal distribution with mean 0 is a function of e^r.
(e) The variance of the standard normal distribution (z-scores) is 1.

23. **MCQ** – Select one correct statement regarding a Poisson distribution with a mean value of 4:
(a) It is also known as a Gaussian distribution.
(b) It is unimodal with a mode of 4.
(c) Sixty-eight per cent of cases lie within one standard deviation of 4.
(d) The distribution has a standard deviation of 2.

(e) The distribution is symmetrical about the mean value of 4.

24. **MCQ** – If E refers to the expected number of cases and O to the number actually observed, select one correct statement regarding the standardized mortality ratio (expressed as a percentage):
(a) It is E/O.
(b) It is $E/O \times 100$.
(c) It is O/E.
(d) It is $O/E \times 100$.
(e) There is insufficient information given in the question from which to calculate the standardized mortality ratio.

25. **EMI** – Binomial distribution model
(a) 0
(b) 0.5
(c) 1
(d) 2
(e) 4
(f) 8
(g) 16
(h) 20
(i) Infinity
(j) None of the above

A researcher decides to model the number of patient admissions to a specialist psychiatric ward by a binomial distribution. From past records, he decides to allocate a value of 0.2 to the probability of a patient being admitted to the ward in any one week. For each of the following, select the most appropriate answer from the list above:
(i) What is the mean number of patient admissions over 100 weeks?
(ii) What is the numerical value of the standard deviation of the number of patient admissions over 100 weeks?
(iii) After how many weeks would this distribution be well modelled by a normal distribution?
(iv) After how many weeks would this distribution be well modelled by a Poisson distribution?

26. **EMI** – Research methods
(a) 0
(b) 10 mg/day
(c) 20 mg/day
(d) 23.5 mg/day
(e) 26 mg/day
(f) 44 mg/day
(g) 47 mg/day
(h) 63 mg/day
(i) 70.5 mg/day
(j) 84 mg/day
(k) 94 mg/day
(l) None of the above

A study is conducted of seven patients taking the same antipsychotic medication. In order, from lowest to highest, the values of the doses are found to be: 10, 26, 26, 26, 63, 63 and 94 mg/day. They are plotted as the following type of box plot (which is not to scale):

Dose (mg/day)

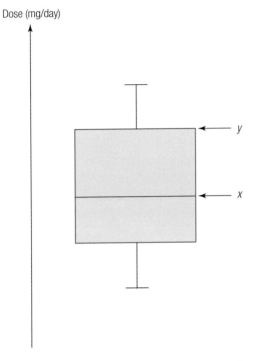

For each of the following questions relating to these data, select the most appropriate answer from the list above:
   (i)   What is the range?
   (ii) What is the value of x in the above box plot?
   (iii) What is the value of y in the above box plot?
   (iv) What is the mean?
   (v)   What is the mode?

27. **MCQ** – If the numerical value of the standard error of A is 6 and the numerical value of the standard error of B is 2, what is the numerical value of the standard error of $A - B$?
   (a) 4
   (b) $\sqrt{32}$
   (c) $\sqrt{40}$
   (d) 8
   (e) None of the above.

28. **EMI** – Statistics
   (a) 0
   (b) 0.01
   (c) 0.02
   (d) 0.03
   (e) 0.04
   (f) 0.05
   (g) 0.2
   (h) 0.5
   (i) 1.00
   (j) 1.64
   (k) 1.96
   (l) 2.00
   (m) Infinity

A manufacturer who supplies microarray chips to researchers in psychiatric genetics finds that, of a random sample of 1600 chips, 320 are faulty. For each of the following questions, select the nearest correct answer from the above list:
   (i)   What is the point estimate, $\hat{p}$, of the proportion of microarray chips that is faulty?
   (ii) What is the standard error of the point estimate found in (i)?
   (iii) What is the numerical value of the appropriate z-score to use in calculating the two-sided 95 per cent confidence interval for the proportion of microarray chips that is faulty?
   (iv) Using the notation of part (i), if the 95 per cent confidence interval for $\hat{p}$ is $(\hat{p} - x) - (\hat{p} + x)$, what is the value of x (to two decimal places)?

29. **EMI** – Statistics
   (a) 0
   (b) 0.05
   (c) 0.1
   (d) 0.2
   (e) 0.4
   (f) 0.8
   (g) 1
   (h) 2
   (i) 3
   (j) 4
   (k) 5
   (l) Infinity

For each of the following questions, select the nearest correct answer from the above list:
   (i)   In a small pilot study, a random sample of size four is found to have a standard deviation of 0.4 (arbitrary units). What is the numerical value of the standard error of the mean?
   (ii) Continuing on from part (i), a 95 per cent confidence interval for the mean can be constructed using the t-distribution with how many degrees of freedom?
   (iii) A study is proposed in which α will be set to 0.05 and the power will be 80 per cent. What is the probability of accepting the null hypothesis even though the alternative hypothesis is in reality true?
   (iv) Continuing on from part (iii), what is the probability of rejecting the null hypothesis even though the null hypothesis is true?
   (v)   What is the null hypothesis value for a comparison of proportions in two groups using odds ratios?

30. **MCQ** – Which of the following is the best test for homogeneity of variance?
   (a) ANOVA
   (b) Bartlett's test
   (c) Cohen's d
   (d) Levene's test
   (e) QQ plot.

31. **MCQ** – Which of the following is not an appropriate use of the square root function?
    (a) The calculation of the standard deviation from the variance.
    (b) The calculation of the standard error of a rate based on count data from a/N, where a events occur in N person-years.
    (c) The calculation of the standard error of the natural logarithm of an odds ratio from the sum of the reciprocals of the values of the four cells of the corresponding 2×2 table.
    (d) The transformation of count data prior to analysis using a parametric test.
    (e) The transformation of negatively skewed data prior to analysis using a parametric test.

32. **EMI** – Statistical tests
    (a) ANOVA
    (b) Chi-squared goodness-of-fit test
    (c) Chi-squared test
    (d) Chi-squared test for homogeneity
    (e) Kruskal–Wallis test
    (f) Log-rank test
    (g) Mann–Whitney U-test
    (h) McNemar test
    (i) One-sample t-test
    (j) Paired-sample t-test
    (k) Two-sample t-test
    (l) Wilcoxon signed rank test

For each of the following hypothesis tests, select the most appropriate test from the list above:
    (i) To check if three independent groups are age-matched.
    (ii) To assess whether two independent groups are gender-matched.
    (iii) A non-parametric comparison is to be conducted of Hamilton Depression Rating Scale (HAM-D) scores of a group of patients before and after cognitive-behaviour therapy.

33. **MCQ** – To which of the following distributions is $F_{1,y}$ equivalent?
    (a) χ^2_y
    (b) $F_{y,1}$
    (c) $N(\bar{x}, y)$
    (d) $N(\bar{x}, y/\sqrt{n})$
    (e) t_y.

34. **MCQ** – The appropriate number of degrees of freedom for a chi-squared test applied to a 2×2 contingency table is:
    (a) 0
    (b) 1
    (c) 2
    (d) 3
    (e) >3.

35. **MCQ** – The chi-squared test is to be applied to the following contingency table:

Test result	Gender	
	Male	Female
Positive	10	10
Negative	30	50

What is the expected value for the number of female subjects who have a positive test result?
    (a) 8
    (b) 9
    (c) 10
    (d) 11
    (e) 12.

36. **EMI** – t-test
    (a) 0
    (b) 0.5
    (c) 1
    (d) 1.5
    (e) 2
    (f) 2.5
    (g) 3
    (h) 3.5
    (i) 4
    (j) 6
    (k) 8
    (l) 14
    (m) 15
    (n) 16
    (o) 26
    (p) 29
    (q) No
    (r) Yes

A new putative rating scale for quality of life has been developed by a psychiatric trainee. She tests it on a randomly chosen sample of 16 healthy volunteers and finds that the mean score is 29 (SD = 8). Assuming that the scores follow a normal distribution, and using $\alpha = 0.05$, the trainee wishes to use a t-test to calculate whether or not her data suggest that the mean score on her scale is greater than 26. For each of the following questions, select the most appropriate answer from the list above:
    (i) Under the null hypothesis, what is the value of the mean score being tested?
    (ii) When a t-test is to be used to carry out the hypothesis testing, what is the corresponding standard error for the test statistic?
    (iii) What is the value of the test statistic?
    (iv) The critical value to use in the hypothesis testing is $t_{\alpha,v} = t_{0.05,v}$, where v is the number of degrees of freedom. What is x?
    (v) If the value of the test statistic is found to be less than $t_{0.05,v}$, can the trainee reject the null hypothesis?

37. **MCQ** – In the analysis of a single 2×2 contingency table, which of the following is least likely to be appropriate?
    (a) Bonferroni correction
    (b) Continuity correction
    (c) Fisher's exact probability test
    (d) Pearson residuals
    (e) Yates' correction.

38. **MCQ** – A psychiatric study is to be conducted of patients with stage 4 pancreatic cancer, one group of whom are to receive an active treatment and a second group a placebo. The patients are to be followed up to the time of death. Which of the following is correct?
    (a) A parametric survival analysis method that may be used is a Kaplan–Meier analysis.
    (b) Cox regression does not allow for the effects of covariates.
    (c) Survival distributions for the two groups can be compared using the log-rank test.
    (d) The corresponding Kaplan–Meier curves are smooth.
    (e) The data should not be censored.

39. **EMI** – Statistics
    (a) 0
    (b) 0.01
    (c) 0.05
    (d) 1
    (e) 1.5
    (f) 2
    (g) 4
    (h) 6
    (i) 8
    (j) 10
    (k) 20
    (l) 50
    (m) 100
    (n) Infinity

A psychiatric researcher wishes to determine if the levels of a particular neurotrophin are associated with those of a cytokine in healthy volunteers. The distributions of these levels do not differ significantly from normality, nor do their standard deviations differ significantly. He finds that the product–moment correlation coefficient is 0.1. For each of the following questions, select the most appropriate answer from the list above.
    (i) What value of the correlation coefficient is associated with a perfect positive relationship between the neurotrophin and cytokine levels?
    (ii) What is the percentage variance in the neurotrophin levels that is explained by the cytokine levels in this sample?
    (iii) What value would the correlation coefficient have under H_0?
    (iv) The researcher wishes to conduct a hypothesis test for the population correlation coefficient, using Fisher's transformation. The test statistic based on

this transformation follows $N(x,y)$. What is the value of x?
    (v) In part (iv), what is the value of y?

40. **MCQ** – Which of the following is the most likely reason for choosing to calculate Kendall's tau correlation coefficient rather than Spearman's correlation coefficient?
    (a) One of the variables is based on a linear Likert scale.
    (b) The assumption of equidistance cannot be made.
    (c) The data do not follow a normal distribution.
    (d) The square of Spearman's correlation coefficient cannot be interpreted in the same way as r^2.
    (e) They have different ranges of values.

41. **MCQ** – Which of the following is least likely to be used in a logistic regression analysis?
    (a) A linear predictor
    (b) ANCOVA
    (c) Chi-squared test
    (d) Maximum-likelihood estimation
    (e) The logit.

42. **EMI** – Regression analysis
    (a) Cox regression
    (b) Multinomial logistic regression
    (c) Ordered logistic regression
    (d) Poisson regression
    (e) None of the above

For each of the following studies, select the most appropriate type of regression, if any, from the above list:
    (i) The dependent variable is psychiatric diagnosis.
    (ii) The dependent variable is the grade of illness.
    (iii) The dependent variable is the number of admissions to a psychiatric hospital.
    (iv) A cohort study in which the rate ratio over a follow-up period is to be estimated after controlling for confounders.
    (v) Survival analysis.

43. **MCQ** – Which of the following is least likely to be used in model-building in regression?
    (a) Backward selection
    (b) Forward selection
    (c) Stepwise
    (d) The Akaike information criterion
    (e) The McNemar test.

44. **MCQ** – Which of the following is least likely to be used in a factor analysis?
    (a) Co-transcriptional processing
    (b) Oblimin rotation
    (c) Path diagram
    (d) Principal components analysis
    (e) Varimax rotation.

45. **EMI** – Types of analysis
    (a) Canonical correlation analysis
    (b) CART

(c) Cluster analysis

(d) Correspondence analysis

(e) None of the above

For each of the following, select the most appropriate method, if any, from the above list:

(i) Finding interactive effects and producing a tree-like diagram.

(ii) Graphically displaying cross-tabulated data.

(iii) Investigating linear functions that maximize the correlation between the variables in one set with the variables in another set.

(iv) To find subgroups within a dataset.

46. **EMI** – Statistical plots/diagrams

(a) Box

(b) Forest

(c) Funnel

(d) Path

(e) ROC

For each of the following, select the most appropriate plot/diagram from the above list:

(i) To display a structural equation model.

(ii) Informally to assess publication bias.

(iii) To check the sensitivity and specificity of a screening tool.

(iv) A scatterplot of sample sizes of studies versus their estimated effect sizes.

(v) In a meta-analysis, a graphical summary of effect sizes from individual trials and their confidence intervals, with an indication of the overall effect.

ANSWERS

1.

(i) e – In a Likert scale, a declarative sentence is given along with a number of response options. An example is given in the middle of Figure 4.1 in the accompanying textbook; it can be seen that the response values are ordered. The categories are therefore ranked. However, the differences between responses are not absolute (the value of the 'difference' between 'strongly agree' and 'agree' in the Likert scale in Figure 4.1 is not necessarily the same as the 'difference' between 'no opinion' and 'disagree', for example). Thus the corresponding type of scale is ordinal (see Table 4.1 in the accompanying textbook).

(ii) f – Age is a continuous variable for which zero has real meaning and in which absolute differences and proportions apply. The difference between the ages of 8 and 6 years is the same as the difference between the ages of 62.3 and 60.3 years, namely 2 years. The ratio of an age of 8 years to one of 4 years is the same as the ratio of an age of 20 years to one of 10 years, say.

(iii) d – Ethnic group measured in several categories is a variable consisting of discrete categorical data. Although historically there have been many times when, and many parts of the world in which, these categories were ranked (e.g. during the Nazi era in Nazi-occupied countries, 'Aryan' was ranked higher than Jewish), at the time of writing ethnic categories are not considered to have any particular order from a scientific viewpoint in civilized countries. Also, clearly there is no 'equal distance' between adjacent categories. Thus ethnic group is a nominal variable.

Reference: *Psychiatry: An evidence-based text,* **pp. 34–35.**

2.

(i) b – An example is given in Figure 4.1 in the main textbook, from which it can be seen that the response values are continuous.

(ii) b – At first sight it might appear that in this case there is a true zero. However, in this temperature scale the value of 0 is arbitrary and not a 'real' zero. It corresponds to the freezing point of water (which, in terms of thermodynamics, is an arbitrary choice). Thus, a temperature of 80°C cannot be said to be truly 'twice' a temperature of 40°C. (On the other hand, since 0 K represents absolute zero, then temperatures measured in kelvins are indeed measured on a scale in which 0 has real meaning.)

(iii) a – Let n denote the number of tosses of the coin, and let p be the probability of the coin landing heads face-up. Then the probability of the coin landing tails face-up is $1 - p = q$, say. (We are discounting the possibility that the coin might land on its edge.) The distribution of heads (and therefore of tails) after a given number of tosses of the coin is the binomial distribution $B(n, p)$, with mean np and variance npq. If the coin is fair, then $p = q = 0.5$; here the expected value of the number of heads would be the mean $np = n/2$. So if the coin were tossed 16 times, one would expect around eight of these to be heads. The corresponding variance of this distribution is $npq = n/4$, and so the corresponding standard deviation of the distribution would be $(\sqrt{n})/2$.

Reference: *Psychiatry: An evidence-based text,* **pp. 34–35, 45.**

3. c

The test–retest or intra-observer reliability of categorical variables is evaluated using Cohen's kappa. This is a measure of chance-adjusted agreement that takes a value of one when there is perfect agreement and of zero when observed agreement is equal to chance.

Reference: *Psychiatry: An evidence-based text,* **p. 36.**

4. a

For internal consistency, a common approach is to calculate Cronbach's alpha for continuous data, which is the average of all possible split-half reliabilities (where the items are divided in half and the reliabilities computed for the two halves).

If the data are binary, the formula is the same but the index is known as the Kuder–Richardson Formula 20 (KR20). Because reliability increases with the number of items, the index can be adjusted by the Spearman–Brown formula, so that the reliability of scales with different lengths can be compared directly. The recombination fraction is a measure of how often alleles at two genetic loci are separated during meiotic recombination.

The test–retest or intra-observer reliability of ordinal categorical variables, such as symptom scores with possible scores of low, medium or high, can be assessed using a weighted kappa, which penalizes according to the extent of disagreement.

Reference: *Psychiatry: An evidence-based text,* **p. 36.**

5. b

The validity of a test or measuring instrument is the term used to describe whether it measures what it purports to measure. Criterion validity assesses whether the measure is consistent with what we already know and what we expect.

Content validity is a subjective assessment that the instrument samples all the important contents or domains of the attribute. Discriminant validity is established when measures discriminate successfully between other measures of unrelated constructs.

Face validity is a subjective assessment that the instrument or item appears to measure the desired qualities.

Predictive validity assesses whether the measure predicts outcome accurately.

Reference: *Psychiatry: An evidence-based text*, pp. 36–37.

6. b

The sensitivity of a test or measuring instrument is the proportion of positive results out of the cases correctly identified. That is, sensitivity is equal to (true positives)/(true positives plus false negatives). Here, a sensitivity of 82 per cent is certainly more desirable than a specificity of only 58 per cent or a positive predictive value of just 24 per cent. The speed of administration, although a factor to consider, will not be the overriding one in this case; after all, a screening questionnaire could be devised that takes far less time to administer but that also has poorer sensitivity.

Reference: *Psychiatry: An evidence-based text*, Ch. 4.

7.

(i) **b** – This corresponds to $\alpha = 0.05$.

(ii) **i** – Using the notation of Table 4.4 (in the accompanying textbook), we are given that $b = 30$ and $d = 70$. Therefore the specificity = $d/(b + d)$ (from Table 4.5) = $70/(30 + 70) = 70/100 = 0.7 = 0.7 \times 100\% = 70\%$.

(iii) **j** – Using the notation of Table 4.4, we are given that $a = 40$, $c = 24$, and $d = 26$. Therefore the negative predictive power = $a/(c + d)$ (from Table 4.5) = $40/(24 + 26) = 40/50 = 0.8 = 0.8 \times 100\% = 80\%$.

(iv) **b** – If an event happens five-sixths of the time then we may take its probability of occurrence as being $p = 5/6$. The corresponding odds are given by $p/(1 - p) = (5/6)/(1 - 5/6) = (5/6)/(1/6) = (5/6) \times 6 = 5$.

(v) **n** – In the notation of Table 4.4, we are not given the value of c and we are given insufficient information from which to calculate this missing value. Hence we are unable to calculate the sensitivity of the test.

Reference: *Psychiatry: An evidence-based text*, Ch. 4.

8.

(i) **c** – The pre-test probability = the prevalence in the population of interest = $1/11 = 0.09$ to two decimal places (given).

(ii) **d** – The pre-test probability, $p = 1/11$. (It is better to work with exact values if possible, rather than using the 0.09 approximation.) Therefore the pre-test odds = $p/(1 - p) = (1/11)/(1 - 1/11) = (1/11)/(10/11) = (1/11) \times (11/10) = 1/10 = 0.1$.

(iii) **i** – The likelihood ratio (for a positive test) = sensitivity/(1 - specificity) (from Table 4.5 in the accompanying textbook) = $0.7/(1 - 0.9)$ (given) = $0.7/0.1 = 7$.

(iv) **g** – The post-test odds = pre-test odds × likelihood ratio for a positive test = 0.1×7 (from the results of (ii) and (iii) above) = 0.7.

(v) **f** – The post-test probability = (post-test odds)/(1 + post-test odds) = $(7/10)/(1 + 7/10)$ (from part iv) = $(7/10)/(17/10) = 7/17 = 0.41$ to two decimal places. If your long division is rusty (and this is an easy quotient to calculate) then it is reassuring to know that, in practice, you do not need to calculate 7/17 to two decimal places to determine that the correct answer is option f. Clearly $1/4 < 7/17 < 7/10$, and so the correct response must lie between 'e' and 'g', which means it must be 'f'.

Reference: *Psychiatry: An evidence-based text*, pp. 37–38.

9. c

The ROC is a plot of sensitivity vs (1 – specificity) for situations in which the screening tool produces a continuous score. The further the curve is towards the left-hand top corner, the better [high sensitivity and high specificity, i.e. a low value of (1 – specificity)]. An area under the curve of 0.6 is not particularly good; perfection would be 1, while 0.5, the diagonal line, is no better than chance. The reader is referred to Figure 4.2 in the accompanying textbook for an example for which the area under the curve is only 0.609.

Reference: *Psychiatry: An evidence-based text*, p. 38.

10. b

In open-label studies, both the patient and the therapist know the group to which the patient has been assigned. In this example of comparing cognitive-behaviour therapy with drug treatment for an anxiety disorder, clearly neither the patient nor the therapist will be blind to the treatment arm. Therefore in this case use of a placebo is not straightforward.

Reference: *Psychiatry: An evidence-based text*, p. 38.

11. b

This will tend to cluster together similar years of birth. Minimization tries to achieve appropriate balance between different treatment assignments. It is not a truly random method, but nevertheless it is generally acceptable. Random number tables are also not truly random, but, for many purposes, the pseudo-random numbers they contain give adequate randomization. Sequential numbers (or some other selection formula) chosen from a random number table will give rise to a set of numbers. When these are classed according to whether they are odd or even, these pseudo-random numbers will fall into the following two groups: {those numbers ending in the digits 1, 3, 5, 7 or 9} and {those numbers ending in the digits 0, 2, 4, 6 or 8}. Odd or even outcomes from the roll of a die will randomize into the following two groups: {1, 3, 5} and {2, 4, 6}. Permuted block randomization produces sequences of codes (e.g.

ABBA) that are generated at random and used to allocate subjects to treatment arms A and B in small blocks (in this case, four).

Reference: *Psychiatry: An evidence-based text*, **p. 38.**

12.

(i) **f** – Refer to Figure 4.3 in the accompanying textbook.
(ii) **c** – Refer to Figure 4.3 in the accompanying textbook.
(iii) **a** –Refer to Figure 4.3 in the accompanying textbook.
(iv) **b** –Refer to Figure 4.3 in the accompanying textbook.
(v) **e** – Refer to Figure 4.3 in the accompanying textbook.
(vi) **d** –Refer to Figure 4.3 in the accompanying textbook.

Reference: *Psychiatry: An evidence-based text*, **pp. 38–39.**

13. a

A cluster randomized trial may be used when the randomization of individual patients is not possible. If you were studying the effectiveness of a programme to encourage the wearing of helmets while cycling, you might find it difficult to arrange randomization of individual subjects. However, it might be relatively easy to arrange that certain school classes are presented with this material. In such a case, the schoolchildren in attendance would form a cluster that had been randomized together to this particular intervention. Outcomes may be measured at the subject level or the group level, or both. This type of design is relatively common in psychiatry, since therapies are often administered to whole groups at a time.

Copy number variation refers to variation in the number of copies of a genomic segment; maps of copy number variation are proving useful in studying complex disease genetics. Thus copy number variation is not a clinical trial design.

In crossover trials, subjects are individually randomized to a sequence of different treatments. For instance, a trial may begin by comparing A with B, for a time period *t*. Then the two groups might spend the next time period, *t*, being treated with B and A, respectively. This would be a two-way crossover trial. Sometimes, during the second period all the subjects receive one treatment (e.g. A vs placebo for a time period *t*, followed by A vs A for the next for a time period *t*); this constitutes a one-way crossover.

Intention-to-treat refers to the practice of analysing subjects as randomized, whether or not they are receiving the allocated treatment. It is not a clinical trial design. A randomized controlled trial cannot be used when the randomization of individual patients is not possible.

Reference: *Psychiatry: An evidence-based text*, **p. 38.**

14.

(i) **e** – It would be appropriate to consider the data collected from the patients to be qualitative rather than quantitative.

(ii) **f** – A randomized double-blind trial, with the established first-generation antipsychotic haloperidol acting as the control intervention, would be a gold-standard study design here.

(iii) **a** – In case–control studies, a group of cases is identified and then a comparison group of controls is assembled. A control would be a case if they had the outcome of interest, in this case a diagnosis of schizophrenia. By comparing the two groups with respect to the hypothesized risk factor of cannabis use, one may be able to infer something about the relationship between cannabis use and schizophrenia.

Reference: *Psychiatry: An evidence-based text*, **pp. 38–40.**

15.

(i) **e** – It would be appropriate to consider the data collected from the patients to be qualitative rather than quantitative.

(ii) **c** – Cross-sectional studies are observational studies that take a snapshot in time.

(iii) **b** – Cost-effectiveness analyses are health economic studies that are usually focused on comparing the costs and consequences of competing courses of action, such as, in this case, the use of a new second-generation antipsychotic in the treatment of schizophrenia.

Reference: *Psychiatry: An evidence-based text*, **pp. 40–41.**

16. b

Before-after, or pre-post, studies measure an outcome on the same group of patients before and after an intervention. Regression to the mean is a major disadvantage of such studies and occurs where improvement of some patients is inevitable because their initial symptoms were high by chance.

The last observation carried forward (LOCR) method has traditionally been used to deal with loss to follow-up in intervention studies (particularly randomized, double-blind, placebo-controlled trials), but this is now discredited, and principled methods of dealing with missing values are now recommended.

In before-after, or pre-post, studies, one cannot distinguish the effect of the intervention from natural improvement over time (this is another major disadvantage of such studies).

Reference: *Psychiatry: An evidence-based text*, **pp. 38–40.**

17.

(i) **d** – This type of study looks forwards in time and collects data on patients as they become exposed to the risk factor, comparing the outcomes after the passage of time.

(ii) **a** – Higher odds of birth trauma among those with schizophrenia compared with the controls might suggest that birth trauma was a risk factor.

(iii) e – This type of study compares outcomes in a group of people who have been exposed to a risk factor and another group who have not been so exposed.

(iv) b – This type of study takes a snapshot in time in order to investigate associations between risk factors and outcomes or, as in this case, to estimate the prevalence of a condition; given the total population figures for the area, in this case the survey could yield an estimate of the period prevalence of severe mental illness.

(v) c – Where the unit of observation is an area or group of people, as in this case, rather than an individual, the study is termed ecological. Such studies are most useful for health service provision, where conclusions are sought at an institutional level so that changes might be implemented at that level.

Reference: *Psychiatry: An evidence-based text*, pp. 40–41.

18. e

The use of the cost-effectiveness acceptability curve (CEAC) is an increasingly widespread technique. Bootstrapping is a technique whereby many subsamples are taken from the observed data in which some cases are dropped and some replicated; each subsample supplies point estimates, the variation in which indicates the uncertainty in the data. It is used in cases in which distributional assumptions of standard statistics cannot be met – as is often the case for cost data. Figure 4.5 in the main textbook shows results displayed in a cost-effectiveness plane; many samples consistent with the data have been bootstrapped to indicate the degree of uncertainty in the overall cost-effectiveness figure (shown by the bold dot in the figure).

Cost-effectiveness analysis tends to be performed where there is a specific disease-related outcome. For example, if a new drug to lessen symptoms in schizophrenia were tested, the effectiveness might be the reduction in a symptom score.

If the incremental cost-effectiveness ratio (ICER) is less than a maximum willingness to pay, the corresponding therapy is considered cost-effective at that level.

One QALY is equivalent to 2 years in a health state valued at 0.5.

Reference: *Psychiatry: An evidence-based text*, pp. 41–42.

19. b

Two measures are commonly reported to quantify the precision of parameter estimates: standard errors and 95 per cent confidence intervals. Bias is a systematic error in results or inference.

From a geometrical viewpoint, kurtosis is a measure of how peaked the shape of a distribution is. For a symmetrical continuous distribution that has a positive kurtosis, the shape of the distribution is more peaked than the corresponding normal distribution. Conversely, for a symmetrical continuous distribution that has a negative kurtosis, the shape of the distribution is more flat-topped than the corresponding normal distribution. (For the more mathematically inclined reader, the kurtosis of a data set can be considered to be a measure of the fourth moment of the sample about the sample mean.)

Confidence interval is a function of sample size. From a geometrical viewpoint, skewness is a measure of how symmetrical the shape of a distribution is. For a continuous distribution with positive skewness, the distribution has an extended upper tail (low values are relatively close to the mean but high values broaden out a longer distance from the mean). Conversely, for a continuous distribution with negative skewness, the distribution has an extended lower tail. (For the more mathematically inclined, the skewness is the third moment about the mean.)

Reference: *Psychiatry: An evidence-based text*, pp. 42–43.

20.

(i) f – The section of society who read these particular newspapers are most likely to be recruited.

(ii) b – This source of bias arises in this case because of the difficulty of diagnosing Alzheimer's disease other than at postmortem.

(iii) a – This type of bias refers to the loss to follow-up of subjects from a study (once the population to which the study applies has been defined).

(iv) c – In this type of bias, also known as admission rate bias, spurious association may be inferred because the case data arise from a special source. In this particular case, cannabis use itself may tend to lead to admissions and therefore may be seen more frequently among those in hospital.

Reference: *Psychiatry: An evidence-based text*, pp. 43 and 75.

21. d

The epidemiologist Bradford-Hill suggested several criteria for causal inference. These, together with interpretations, are listed in Table 4.7 of the main textbook. Residual confounding is not a Bradford-Hill criterion for causal inference, but can occur when a particular factor has not been controlled for (perhaps because it was never measured or recognized or because it was measured inaccurately).

Reference: *Psychiatry: An evidence-based text*, pp. 43–44.

22. d

Even if you are not familiar with the correct formula, you could have arrived at this correct answer in either of the following two ways. First, you would be expected to be able to work out that the other four options are correct, so it readily follows that 'd' is the correct answer to this question. Second, you should know that the normal distribution is symmetrical about its mean. With a mean of zero (given in this option), this means that a plot of the normal distribution would be symmetrical about the vertical (y-axis). But, a plot of e^r definitely does not have such symmetry. For example, e^{-2} does not equal e^2. In contrast, the graph of e to the power x^2, for example, is symmetrical about the vertical axis. For example, e to the power 2^2 is equal to e to the power $(-2)^2$, which is equal to e^4. (In fact, the formula in this case is indeed a function of e to the power x^2.)

Options 'a' and 'b' are correct by the central limit theorem. Option 'c' is given on page 44 of the main textbook. The standard normal distribution has a mean of 0 and a SD of 1 (see Fig. 4.7 in the main textbook). The variance is the square of the mean and so, in this case, is equal to $1^2 = 1$.

Reference: *Psychiatry: An evidence-based text*, **pp. 44–45.**

23. d

For a Poisson distribution, the variance is equal to the mean. Therefore the standard deviation of this Poisson distribution is the positive square root of 4, which is 2.

Options 'a' and 'c' apply to the normal distribution. This Poisson distribution has two modes, at 3 and 4. (For a positive integer λ, representing the mean or variance of such a distribution, the modes are at λ and $\lambda - 1$.)

As can be inferred from Figure 4.8 of the main textbook, a Poisson distribution with a mean value of 4 is not symmetrical about its mean value (although, as the mean value increases, so the distribution becomes more symmetrical).

Reference: *Psychiatry: An evidence-based text*, **pp. 44–46.**

24. d

Remember to multiply by 100 to obtain the standardized mortality ratio expressed as a percentage.

Reference: *Psychiatry: An evidence-based text*, **pp. 46.**

25.

(i)   h – The mean number of patient admissions over 100 weeks = 100 × (the mean number of patient admissions per week) = 100 × (the probability of a patient being admitted in any one week) = 100 × 0.2 = 20.

(ii) e – Omitting units, we have: variance = $np(1 - p)$ = 100 × 0.2 × (1 − 0.2) = 100 × 0.2 × 0.8 = 100 × 0.16 = 16. Therefore the numerical value of the required standard deviation = the positive square root of the corresponding variance = the positive square root of 16 = 4.

(iii) i – The higher the value of n, the better the modelling by a normal distribution. (The option of $n = 20$ is too small.)

(iv) j – Here, $p = 0.2 \gg 0.05$.

Reference: *Psychiatry: An evidence-based text*, **pp. 44–45.**

26.

(i)   j – The range = (highest value) – (lowest value) = (94 mg/day) – (10 mg/day) = 84 mg/day.

(ii) e – In the box plot, x corresponds to the median. There are seven data points. Seven is an odd number. So in this case the median value is the value of the middle (or fourth) ordered data point. This is 26 mg/day.

(iii) h – In the box plot, y corresponds to the upper quartile. There are seven data points, i.e. $n = 7$. Now, $(3/4) \times (n + 1) = (3/4) \times (7 + 1) = (3/4) \times (8) = 6$. So the upper quartile is the value of the sixth data point (in numerical order). This is 63 mg/day.

(iv) f – The value of the mean is the sum of the individual doses divided by the number of doses. So the numerical value of the mean is $[10 + 3(26) + 2(63) + 94]/n = 308/7 = 44$.

(v) e – The dose which occurs with greatest frequency in this sample is 26 mg/day.

Reference: *Psychiatry: An evidence-based text*, **pp. 46–47.**

27. c

The required standard error = $\sqrt{}$ (the square of the standard error of A plus the square of the standard error of B) = $\sqrt{(6^2 + 2^2)} = \sqrt{(36 + 4)} = \sqrt{40}$.

Reference: *Psychiatry: An evidence-based text*, **p. 49.**

28.

(i)   g – $\hat{p} = 320/1600 = 0.2$.

(ii) b – The standard error of $\hat{p} = \sqrt{(\hat{p}(1 - \hat{p})/n)} = \sqrt{(0.2 \times 0.8/1600)} = \sqrt{0.16/1600} = \sqrt{0.0001} = \sqrt{10^{-4}} = 10^{-2} = 0.01$.

(iii) k – Here we require $z_{0.05/2} = z_{0.025} = 1.96$.

(iv) c – Here, $x = 1.96 \times$ standard error of $\hat{p} = 1.96 \times 0.01 = 0.02$ (to two decimal places).

Reference: *Psychiatry: An evidence-based text*, **pp. 45–51.**

29.

(i)   d – We are given that, for a sample of size $n = 4$, the sample standard deviation, s, has numerical value 0.4. So the required standard error of the mean = $s/\sqrt{n} = 0.4/\sqrt{4} = 0.4/2 = 0.2$.

(ii) i – The corresponding number of degrees of freedom = $n - 1 = 4 - 1 = 3$.

(iii) d – The power = 80 per cent = 0.8. The required probability is the probability of a type II error = $\beta = 1 - $ power = $1 - 0.8 = 0.2$.

(iv) b – The required probability is the probability of a type I error = $\alpha = 0.05$.

(v) g – Remember that the null hypothesis value here is 1 and not 0.

Reference: *Psychiatry: An evidence-based text*, **pp. 49–52.**

30. d

ANOVA is analysis of variance. Options 'b' and 'e' test for normality. Option 'c' relates to the standardized difference.

Reference: Psychiatry: An evidence-based text, **p. 52.**

31. e

For negatively skewed data, an appropriate transformation to consider might be the squared function. The variance is the square of the standard deviation. The standard error of a rate based on count data, where a events occur in N person-years, is given by $\sqrt{\{a/N\}}$, as shown in Table 4.10 of the main textbook.

Option 'c' is an appropriate use of the square root function, as can be seen from the last formula in Table 4.9 of the main textbook. The square root function can be used for the transformation of count data before using a parametric test, although it is usually preferable to use methods based on the Poisson distribution rather than to transform and assume normality.

Reference: Psychiatry: An evidence-based text, **pp. 51–53.**

32.

(i) a – Number of independent groups being compared = 3 > 2. Scale of measurement is ratio (for age). So we use analysis of variance.

(ii) c – Number of independent groups being compared = 2. Scale of measurement is nominal (for gender). So we use the chi-squared test. (If the numbers are small enough, we could use Fisher's exact test instead, but this is not an available option in this question.)

(iii) l – This is a non-parametric available option for use instead of the parametric paired *t*-test.

Reference: Psychiatry: An evidence-based text, **pp. 54–57.**

33. e

Note that $F_{1,y} \uparrow F_{y,1}$.

Reference: Psychiatry: An evidence-based text, **p. 54.**

34. b

Here, the number of degrees of freedom = $(2 - 1) \times (2 - 1)$ = $1 \times 1 = 1$.

Reference: Psychiatry: An evidence-based text, **p. 58.**

35. e

The column total for the column that contains the corresponding cell is 10 + 50 = 60. The row total for the row that contains this cell is 10 + 10 = 20. The overall total (sum of all four cells) = 10 + 10 + 30 + 50 = 100. So the required expected value = (row total × column total)/(overall total) = (20 × 60)/100 = 1200/100 = 12.

Reference: Psychiatry: An evidence-based text, **pp. 58–59.**

36. o

(i) In this and the following explanations, conventional notation, as used in the main textbook, is employed. The trainee wishes to calculate whether or not her data suggest that the mean score on her scale is greater than 26. So the null hypothesis is that $\mu = 26$. This should not be confused with the mean score actually found in her sample, which is the sample mean, $\bar{x} = 29$.

(ii) e – The sample standard deviation, $s = 8$ and the sample size, $n = 16$. Therefore the required standard error = $s/\sqrt{n} = 8/\sqrt{(16)} = 8/4 = 2$. (Only the positive square root is taken.)

(iii) d – The test statistic = $(\bar{x} - \mu)/(s/\sqrt{n}) = (29 - 26)/2 = 3/2$ = 1.5.

(iv) m – Here, $v = n - 1 = 16 - 1 = 15$.

(v) q – [In fact, from the appropriate statistical table, $t_{0.05,15}$ = 1.753 (to three decimal places).] Since the test statistic $< t_{0.05,v}$ (which is given in the question), we cannot reject the null hypothesis.

Reference: Psychiatry: An evidence-based text, **pp. 54–55.**

37. a

This correction is used for multiple comparisons, which does not apply here, where a single 2 × 2 contingency table is being analysed. The remaining four options may indeed have a role in this analysis, as explained in the main textbook. Note that Fisher's exact probability test is another common name for Fisher's exact test; the latter rendering is used in the accompanying textbook.

Reference: Psychiatry: An evidence-based text, **pp. 58–59.**

38. c

This is a chi-squared test on one degree of freedom. It compares the observed numbers of events at each time point with the number expected if the survival curves were the same for the two groups. It does this by ordering the survival times of all participants and hence dividing the follow-up time into intervals in which events occur. In each time interval, the number of events is recorded and the number of participants who remain at risk is reduced accordingly. The numbers observed and expected under the null hypothesis of no difference between the groups are accumulated over the whole time period.

Kaplan–Meier analysis is a non-parametric survival method. Cox regression does allow the effects of covariates to be taken into account. The Kaplan–Meier curves are stepped rather than smooth, as can be seen in Figure 4.13 in the accompanying textbook.

If a participant withdraws or the study ends before the event occurs, the data are described as censored. For instance, suppose that this is an 8-week study; if a cancer patient has only been observed for 8 weeks and is alive at the end of this period, then this patient has a censored survival time (and clearly his survival time > 8 weeks). Survival analysis methods are used to analyse such censored data.

Reference: *Psychiatry: An evidence-based text*, **pp. 59–60.**

39.

(i) **d** – For a perfect negative relationship, the correlation coefficient would be –1.

(ii) **d** – The correlation coefficient, $r = 0.1$. The required value is $r^2 = (0.1)^2 = 0.01$. This is 0.01×100 per cent = 1 per cent.

(iii) **a** – Under the null hypothesis of there being no relationship between the two variables, the correlation coefficient would be zero.

(iv) **a** – The test statistic based on Fisher's transformation follows the standard normal distribution, $N(0,1)$. Therefore $x = 0$.

(v) **d** – This follows from the explanation just given for part (iv).

Reference: *Psychiatry: An evidence-based text*, **p. 61.**

40. b

Spearman's rank correlation coefficient, ρ, is the equivalent to r calculated on the ranked data and it detects any monotonic relationship. Spearman's ρ assumes that the difference between ranks is the same. If this assumption of equidistance cannot be made, then Kendall's tau correlation coefficient, τ, is an alternative for ordinal-level variables.

The assumption of equidistance is commonly made for linear Likert scales used in psychiatric measurement scales. Both ρ and τ are non-parametric alternatives to r, and so if the data do not follow a normal distribution the use of τ would also not be appropriate.

$(100 \times \rho^2)$ per cent cannot be interpreted as a percentage of variance in one variable explained by the other, in the same way as $(100 r^2 \%.)$ The range of values for both ρ and τ is the same, namely $-1 \le \rho, \tau \le 1$.

Reference: *Psychiatry: An evidence-based text*, **p. 62.**

41. b

A linear predictor can be used to form predictions of the odds and hence the probabilities for individuals, as shown in the example on page 64 of the accompanying textbook. If one wished to compare groups in terms of a binary variable then an approach would be a chi-squared test to compare proportions followed by logistic regression to control for other variables. Maximum-likelihood estimation and calculation of the logit are part of the logistic regression analysis.

Reference: *Psychiatry: An evidence-based text*, **p. 63–64.**

42.

(i) **b** – This is appropriate in cases in which the dependent variable is categorical and non-ordered, as is the case here.

(ii) **c** – This is appropriate in cases in which the dependent variable is categorical and ordered, as is the case here.

(iii) **d** – This is appropriate in cases in which the dependent variable takes the form of count data, as is the case here.

(iv) **d** – Poisson regression is commonly used in cohort studies to estimate rate ratios over a follow-up period after controlling for confounders and produces rate ratios.

(v) **a** – This is appropriate when the outcome is time to an event, as in survival analysis.

Reference: *Psychiatry: An evidence-based text*, **p. 64.**

43. e

This test appears in Table 4.12 and is described further on page 59 of the accompanying textbook. Backward selection, forward selection and stepwise (a mixture of the first two) are possible automatic methods used in model-building in regression.

An increasingly popular alternative to model selection based on significance testing is the use of information criteria, such as option 'd'.

Reference: *Psychiatry: An evidence-based text*, **pp. 64–65.**

44. a

This is a term from molecular genetics and refers to the transcription and concurrent processing of eukaryotic pre-mRNA. Varimax and oblimin rotations refer, respectively, to orthogonal and oblique rotations of extracted factors.

Figure 4.15 in the accompanying textbook shows an example of a path diagram. Principal components analysis transforms the data variables into components that explain decreasing proportions of the variance in the data and that are uncorrelated. It can be used as the first step in a factor analysis.

Reference: *Psychiatry: An evidence-based text*, **pp. 65–66.**

45.

(i) **b** – CART is classification and regression tree analysis and focuses on finding interactive effects (i.e. combinations of variables) rather than linear functions and produces a tree-like diagram.

(ii) **d** – Although this method is currently little used in psychiatry, it is potentially very useful for exploratory analysis of large cross-tabulations.

(iii) **a** – Again, this method is currently little used in psychiatry, perhaps because the results are difficult to interpret.

(iv) c – This is a vast set of methods that seek subgroups within a data set. It is a data-driven exploratory method, overlapping with data-mining, neural networks and pattern recognition.

Reference: *Psychiatry: An evidence-based text,* **pp. 66–67.**

46.

(i) d – Figure 4.15 in the accompanying textbook shows an example of this.

(ii) c – Figure 4.17 in the accompanying textbook shows an example of this.

(iii) e – Figure 4.2 in the accompanying textbook shows an example of such a receiver operator curve.

(iv) c – This is a simple scatterplot of the sample sizes (or precision) of studies against their estimated effect sizes. An example is shown in Figure 4.17.

(v) b – An example is shown in Figure 4.16 in the accompanying textbook; the lengths of the blue lines indicate the confidence intervals, the sizes of the boxes are proportional to the sample size and the vertical black dashed line together with the rhomboid shape indicate the overall effect.

Reference: *Psychiatry: An evidence-based text,* **Ch. 4.**

Chapter 5

Epidemiology

QUESTIONS

Note that for answers to extended matching items (EMIs), each option (denoted a, b, c, etc.) might be used once, more than once or not at all. For multiple-choice questions (MCQs), please select the best answer.

1. **MCQ** – Which of the following best gives the number of entirely new cases of an illness per unit of time?
   (a) Inception rate
   (b) Incidence rate
   (c) Period prevalence
   (d) Point prevalence
   (e) Population at risk.

2. **MCQ** – A birth cohort logistic regression analysis is conducted. Which of the following findings relating to female 45-year-olds versus male 45-year-olds is most likely to be consistent with the conclusion that females are more likely to have depression at 45 years of age than males?
   (a) Women vs men for depression at 45 years: odds ratio = 1.63 [95 per cent confidence interval (CI), 1.33–2.57]
   (b) Women vs men for depression at 45 years: odds ratio = 1.85 (95 per cent CI, 0.97–2.63)
   (c) Women vs men for depression at 45 years: odds ratio = 0.55 (95 per cent CI, 0.26–0.94)
   (d) The coefficient for being female is 0.05
   (e) The coefficient for being female and depressed is less than 0.05.

3. **MCQ** – A researcher carries out a factor analysis. Using the eigenvalues, which of the following factors should be identified as being worth examining?
   (a) Factors with eigenvalues < 0
   (b) Factors with eigenvalues = 0

   (c) Factors with eigenvalues lying between 0 and 1 (exclusive)
   (d) Factors with eigenvalues = 1
   (e) Factors with eigenvalues > 0.

4. **EMI** – Gender ratios for psychiatric disorders
   (a) Male to female ratio is significantly greater than 1
   (b) Male to female ratio is approximately equal to 1
   (c) Male to female ratio is significantly less than 1

   For each of the following psychiatric disorders, select the corresponding male to female ratio from the above list:
   (i) Bipolar I disorder
   (ii) Suicide
   (iii) Generalized anxiety disorder
   (iv) Panic disorder.

5. **MCQ** – Select one incorrect statement:
   (a) Agoraphobia is associated with comorbid major depression.
   (b) Bipolar disorder appears to be unrelated to ethnicity in terms of its prevalence.
   (c) Patients with drug dependence are at higher risk for bipolar disorder.
   (d) Schizophrenia is not associated with a significantly higher SMR.
   (e) The onset of specific phobias is usually between the ages of 5 and 8 years.

ANSWERS

1. a

Strictly, for entirely new cases of an illness, the term 'inception rate' rather than 'incidence rate' is correct, because incidence may include recurrent episodes.

Reference: *Psychiatry: An evidence-based text*, **pages 72–73.**

2. a

The odds ratio here > 1 and the 95 per cent CI does not cross 1. Option 'b' has a 95 per cent CI that crosses 1, and so there is no significant effect of being female on reports of depression at the age of 45 years.

Option 'c' has an odds ratio < 1 and the corresponding 95 per cent CI covers a range below 1. This would indicate support for the hypothesis that males were more likely than females to suffer from depression at the age of 45 years.

Options 'd' and 'e' relate to the value of coefficients in the logistic regression equation; the values of the coefficients, on their own, do not answer the question.

Reference: *Psychiatry: An evidence-based text*, **p. 77.**

3. e

Factors with eigenvalues greater than 1 are typically thought to be worth examining.

Reference: *Psychiatry: An evidence-based text*, **p. 79.**

4.

(i) b – According to the DSM-IV-TR, 'Recent epidemiological studies in the United States indicate that Bipolar I Disorder is approximately equally common in men and women (unlike Major Depressive Disorder, which is more common in women).'

(ii) a

(iii) c

(iv) c

References: American Psychiatric Association (2000) *Diagnostic and Statistical Manual of Mental Disorders, Fourth Edition, Text Revision (DSM-IV-TR).* **American** Psychiatric Association, Washington, DC, **p. 385;** *Psychiatry: An evidence-based text*, **pp. 80–81.**

5. d

The median standardized mortality ratio is around 2.6 for all-cause mortality.

Reference: *Psychiatry: An evidence-based text*, **pp. 80–81.**

Chapter 6

How to practise evidence-based medicine

QUESTIONS

Note that for answers to extended matching items (EMIs), each option (denoted a, b, c, etc.) might be used once, more than once or not at all. For multiple-choice questions (MCQs), please select the best answer.

1. **MCQ** – In the PICO model for translating uncertainty into an answerable question, the C stands for:
   (a) Comparison
   (b) Competence
   (c) Conclusion
   (d) Cost-effectiveness
   (e) Cue.

2. **MCQ** – A psychiatrist wishes to conduct a search using an electronic database of all studies that contain the term 'depression' or the term 'suicide', or both 'depression' and 'suicide'. Which of the following Boolean logic symbols would be the best one to insert between 'depression' and 'suicide' in the search?
   (a) *
   (b) ?
   (c) …
   (d) AND
   (e) OR.

3. **MCQ** – In the GATE frame for critical appraisal, the G stands for:
   (a) Gaussian
   (b) Gender
   (c) Generalized
   (d) Graphic
   (e) Gold-standard.

4. **EMI** – Effect measures
   (a) Absolute risk reduction
   (b) Control event risk
   (c) Experimental event risk
   (d) Number needed to treat
   (e) Risk ratio
   (f) Relative risk reduction

For each of the following definitions, select the corresponding effect measure from the above list:
(i) Proportion with the event of interest in the intervention group
(ii) Risk of experiencing the event in the experimental group relative to the control group
(iii) Difference in risk between the control and experimental groups
(iv) Proportion of events that would have been avoided in the control group had they been allocated the intervention.

5. **MCQ** – The second A in RAAMbo, within the GATE frame in critical appraisal, stands for:
   (a) Accounted
   (b) Allocation
   (c) Appraisal
   (d) Application
   (e) Assessment.

6. **EMI** – EBM
   (a) 0
   (b) 1
   (c) 2
   (d) 4
   (e) 8
   (f) 9
   (g) 10
   (h) 11
   (i) 12
   (j) 13–20
   (k) 21–30
   (l) 31–40
   (m) 41–50
   (n) 51–60
   (o) 61–70
   (p) 71–80
   (q) 81–90
   (r) 91–100

In a multicentre, double-masked, randomized, placebo-controlled trial, outpatients in the secondary progressive phase of multiple sclerosis, having scores of 3.0–6.5 on the Expanded Disability Status Scale (EDSS), received either 8 million IU interferon β-1b every other day subcutaneously, or placebo, for up to 3 years. The primary outcome was the time to confirmed progression in disability as measured by a 1.0 point increase on the EDSS, sustained for at least 3 months, or a 0.5 point increase if the baseline EDSS was 6.0 or 6.5. By 33 months, confirmed progression in disability has occurred in 39 per cent of the patients allocated to the active group and in 50 per cent of the patients allocated to the placebo group. Based on these results, for each of the following questions, which refer to this 33-month time-point, select the nearest answer from the above list:

(i) What is the corresponding risk ratio (as a percentage)?

(ii) What is the relative risk reduction (as a percentage)?

(iii) What is the absolute risk reduction (as a percentage)?

(iv) What is the number of patients we need to treat for 33 months with interferon β-1b to prevent one additional bad outcome?

ANSWERS

1. a

PICO stands for patient, intervention, comparison, outcome. An example of its application is given on page 83 of the accompanying textbook.

Reference: Psychiatry: An evidence-based text, **p. 83.**

2. e

A OR B includes all studies that contain term A or term B, or both A and B.

Reference: Psychiatry: An evidence-based text, **p. 85.**

3. d

GATE stands for Graphic Appraisal Tool for Epidemiological studies. The GATE frame is shown in Figure 6.1 of the accompanying textbook.

Reference: Psychiatry: An evidence-based text, **p. 86.**

4.

(i) c
(ii) e – This is also known as the relative risk.
(iii) a
(iv) f

Reference: Psychiatry: An Evidence-Based Text, **p. 87.**

5. a

Ideally, by the end of the study, all participants should be accounted for, but this is rarely the case and typically some participants will drop out, switch treatment or be lost to follow-up.

Option 'b' refers to the first A in RAAMbo. Option 'c' refers to the A in GATE.

Reference: Psychiatry: An Evidence-Based Text, **p. 86.**

6.

(i) **p** – The risk ratio (or relative risk) = (EER)/(CER), where EER is the experimental event risk (= 39 per cent), and CER is the control event risk (= 50 per cent). Therefore the risk ratio = 39 per cent/50 per cent = 78/100 = 78 per cent.

(ii) **k** – The relative risk reduction = (CER – EER)/(CER) = (0.50 – 0.39)/0.50 = 0.11/0.50 = 11/50 = 22/100 = 22 per cent.

(iii) **h** – The absolute risk reduction, ARR = CER – EER = (50 – 39) per cent = 11 per cent.

(iv) **f** – Here, we require the number needed to treat, which is given by 1/(ARR) = 1/0.11 = 100/11 which is approximately 9.

References: Kappos L and European Study Group on Interferon β-1b in Secondary Progressive MS (1998) Placebo-controlled multicentre randomised trial of interferon β-1b in treatment of secondary progressive multiple sclerosis. *Lancet* **352**: 1491–7; *Psychiatry: An evidence-based text*, **p. 87.**

Chapter 7

Psychological assessment and psychometrics

QUESTIONS

Note that for answers to extended matching items (EMIs), each option (denoted a, b, c, etc.) might be used once, more than once or not at all. For multiple-choice questions (MCQs), please select the best answer.

1. **MCQ** – A male 39-year-old patient with chronic schizophrenia gives his age as 26 years during a mental-state examination. There is no history of alcohol abuse. What is the most likely cause of this error?
   (a) A delusion
   (b) Cognitive impairment
   (c) Confabulation
   (d) Paranoia
   (e) Somatic passivity.

2. **MCQ** – A 52-year-old man with a frontal lobe disorder is seen to be wearing three pairs of spectacles, one on top of the other, at interview. This is most likely to be associated with which of the following?
   (a) A catastrophic reaction
   (b) Absent-mindedness
   (c) Auditory hallucinations
   (d) Utilization behaviour
   (e) Visual hallucinations.

3. **EMI** – Specific cognitive assessment
   (a) Being asked to generate the names of as many animals as can be thought of in one minute
   (b) Being asked to 'guesstimate' how fast racehorses gallop
   (c) Digit span
   (d) General knowledge questions
   (e) Mental arithmetic
   (f) Proverb interpretation

Regarding specific cognitive assessment in the mental-state examination, select which of the above bedside tests best assesses each of the following:
   (i) Attention and concentration
   (ii) Working memory
   (iii) Semantic memory
   (iv) Initiation
   (v) Reasoning and judgement.

4. **MCQ** – Which of the following is not part of the MMSE?
   (a) Being asked to demonstrate how to comb one's hair
   (b) Being asked to name a watch
   (c) Following a written instruction
   (d) Serial subtraction
   (e) Writing a sentence (spontaneously).

5. **EMI** – Tests
   (a) MMSE
   (b) NART
   (c) Quick test
   (d) VNR
   (e) WAIS
   (f) WISC-R

For an adult patient, select the test from the above list that would enable you best to carry out each of the following:
   (i) Estimate the pre-morbid IQ
   (ii) Estimate the current IQ relatively rapidly
   (iii) Formally assess the current IQ
   (iv) Screen for clinically significant cognitive impairment.

6. **EMI** – Types of memory
   (a) Episodic memory
   (b) Procedural memory
   (c) Semantic memory
   (d) Working memory
   (e) None of the above

Select the type of memory, if any, from the above list which is best associated with each of the following:
   (i) Driving a car
   (ii) Keeping a few items of verbal material in conscious awareness for about half a minute
   (iii) Recalling what you did yesterday
   (iv) Remembering that the capital of the United States is Washington DC
   (v) Conditioned reflexes.

7. **MCQ** – Which of the following parts of the brain is most likely, on the basis of lesion studies, to be associated with semantic memory?
   (a) Basal ganglia
   (b) Cerebellum
   (c) Dominant temporal neocortex
   (d) Non-dominant occipital lobe
   (e) Phonological loop.

8. **MCQ** – Which of the following tests is the best for assessing anterograde episodic memory function?
   (a) Famous Faces Test
   (b) Graded Naming Test
   (c) Hodges Semantic Memory Battery
   (d) Rivermead Behavioural Memory Test
   (e) Silly Sentences Test.

9. **EMI** – Frontal lobe function
   (a) Cognitive Estimates Test
   (b) Continuous Performance Test
   (c) Stroop Test
   (d) Wisconsin Card Sorting Test
   (e) Tower of London

Select the test from the above list that best assesses each of the following:
   (i) Set maintenance and shifting
   (ii) Planning and sequencing
   (iii) Reasoning and judgement
   (iv) Attentional capacity and focus.

10. **EMI** – Psychological assessment
   (a) Dysgraphia
   (b) Expressive dysphasia
   (c) Gerstmann's syndrome
   (d) Receptive dysphasia

Select the impairment from the above list that best corresponds to each of the following:
   (i) Dominant posterior superior temporal lobe lesion
   (ii) Speech is fluent but unintelligible with neologisms and grammatical errors
   (iii) Dominant inferior frontal lobe lesion
   (iv) Dominant parietal lobe lesion
   (v) Angular gyrus lesion.

11. **MCQ** – Which of the following is not classically part of Gerstmann's syndrome?
   (a) Acalculia
   (b) Agraphia
   (c) Apraxia
   (d) Finger agnosia
   (e) Right–left disorientation.

12. **MCQ** – Which of the following is least likely to be a cause of dysarthria in psychiatric practice?
   (a) Antipsychotic medication
   (b) Basal ganglia pathology
   (c) Cerebellar pathology
   (d) Cranial nerve palsies
   (e) Non-dominant parietal lobe lesions.

13. **MCQ** – Select one correct statement regarding the measurement of IQ:
   (a) Learning disability is defined by an IQ one standard deviation (SD) below the mean.
   (b) The mean is 120.
   (c) The measurement error is 5.
   (d) The range is between 0 and 150.
   (e) The standard deviation is 20.

ANSWERS

1. b

In age disorientation in schizophrenia, patients may say that they are many years younger than their chronological age. This is considered cognitive rather than delusional.

Reference: *Psychiatry: An evidence-based text,* **pp. 90–91.**

2. d

Perseverative utilization behaviour is seen in patients with frontal lobe disorders, in which objects are used repeatedly.

Reference: *Psychiatry: An evidence-based text,* **p. 90.**

3.

(i)   e – Mental arithmetic is a way of testing attention and concentration (plus the specific ability to calculate). Many patients find 'serial sevens' rather challenging.

(ii) c – Working memory can be tested by digit span, i.e. repeating a series of digits after the doctor says them.

(iii) d – Semantic memory may be assessed by asking the patient some general knowledge questions, such as the name of the current monarch or president, and the years during which World War II took place. Some questions may be so easy as to exclude the effects of incomplete education and disinterest in current affairs.

(iv) a – To test initiation, patients can be asked to generate as many animals as they can think of in 1 min. Ten or fewer indicates impairment, as does perseveration (repeating an answer).

(v)   b

Reference: *Psychiatry: An evidence-based text,* **pp. 91–92.**

4. a

This is a test of basic praxis, and is a useful addition to a screening assessment based on the Mini-Mental State Examination. The MMSE includes the following assessments: orientation; attention; serial subtraction or spelling a word backwards; immediate recall; short-term memory; naming common objects; following simple verbal commands; following simple written commands; writing a sentence spontaneously; and copying a figure.

Reference: *Psychiatry: An evidence-based text,* **p. 92.**

5.

(i)   b – This provides the best established pre-morbid IQ evaluation.

(ii) c – This is shown in Table 7.1 and Figure 7.2 in the accompanying textbook.

(iii) e – Note that option 'f' is for the assessment of children.

(iv) a

Reference: *Psychiatry: An evidence-based text,* **Ch. 7.**

6.

(i)   b – Implicit memory includes the learning and retention of motor skills, which is known as procedural memory.

(ii) d – The working memory system serves to keep small amounts (five to nine items) of verbal, auditory or visual material present in conscious awareness for recall or manipulation, or both, for a brief period of up to about 30 s.

(iii) a – This type of memory is associated with the recollection of personal experience.

(iv) c

(v)   e – This is associated with implicit memory (but not procedural memory).

Reference: *Psychiatry: An evidence-based text,* **p. 94.**

7. c

Semantic memory is lost with lesions of this part of the brain.

Reference: *Psychiatry: An evidence-based text,* **p. 94.**

8. d

The Rivermead Behavioural Memory Test is the standard measure of episodic memory function in anterograde terms. It includes both non-verbal and verbal elements and tests of both recall and recognition.

Reference: *Psychiatry: An evidence-based text,* **p. 94.**

9.

(i)   d – Here, cards are sorted according to different rules (e.g. by number or shape of symbols). (Originally it involved the use of physical cards. These days, electronic versions are also available, with computerized recording of the results.)

(ii) e – Alternatives include the Tower of Hanoi and the Socks of Cambridge.

(iii) a – This test comprises ten 'guesstimate' questions.

(iv) c

Reference: *Psychiatry: An evidence-based text,* **pp. 95–96.**

10.

(i)   d – In receptive dysphasia there is a lesion affecting Wernicke's area in the dominant posterior superior temporal lobe.

(ii) d

(iii) b – In expressive dysphasia there is a lesion affecting Broca's area in the dominant inferior frontal lobe, usually extending into the frontoparietal regions served by the superior middle cerebral artery.

(iv) a – Dominant parietal lobe damage may be associated with dyspraxic dysgraphia, in which the motor control of writing is impaired.

(v) c – Rostral to Wernicke's area is the angular gyrus, which connects the temporal, parietal and occipital lobes. Lesions here produce Gerstmann's syndrome.

Reference: *Psychiatry: An evidence-based text*, **p. 96.**

11. c

Note that acalculia is referred to as dyscalculia, and agraphia as dysgraphia, in the accompanying textbook.

Reference: *Psychiatry: An evidence-based text*, **p. 96.**

12. e

The most common cause of dysarthria in psychiatric practice is probably extrapyramidal side-effects of antipsychotic medication.

Reference: *Psychiatry: An evidence-based text*, **p. 96.**

13. c

Learning disability is defined by an IQ that is two SDs below the population mean, which is theoretically 100. The range is 0–200 and the SD is 15.

Reference: *Psychiatry: An evidence-based text*, **p. 97.**

PART 2

Developmental, behavioural, and sociocultural psychiatry

Chapter 8

Human development

QUESTIONS

Note that for answers to extended matching items (EMIs), each option (denoted a, b, c, etc.) might be used once, more than once or not at all. For multiple-choice questions (MCQs), please select the best answer.

1. **EMI** – History of concepts in human development
   (a) Bandura
   (b) Bowlby
   (c) Piaget
   (d) Scarr and McCartney
   (e) Freud
   (f) Tanner

Select the person(s) from the above list most closely associated with the following concepts:
   (i)   Growth charts
   (ii) The model of gene–environment interaction in behavioural development
   (iii) Social learning
   (iv) Attachment theory
   (v)   Theory of cognitive development.

2. **MCQ** – In the development of attachment behaviours, which of the following is most likely to develop at or by the 12th month, but not before the 11th month?
   (a) A single (usually) attachment figure is established.
   (b) Early attachment behaviour is related to later emotional development.
   (c) Fear of strangers.
   (d) Substitute attachment figures are accepted in the absence of the primary attachment figure.
   (e) The attachment figure is of primary importance.

3. **MCQ** – Which of the following statements regarding attachment behaviour (in humans unless otherwise stated) is most likely to be correct?
   (a) Attachment depends primarily on obtaining food from the attachment figure.
   (b) Attachment depends primarily on proximity to and affection from the attachment figure.
   (c) During the first six months, the infant displays selectivity in the direction of relevant behaviours.
   (d) Rhesus monkeys separated from their mother will spend the majority of time clinging to a wire doll rather than to a wool one, if the former is the one that provides food.

   (e) The primary attachment figure is always the mother.

4. **EMI** – Attachment behaviours
   (a) Insecure-ambivalent attachment behaviour
   (b) Insecure-avoidant attachment behaviour
   (c) Secure attachment behaviour
   (d) None of the above

Select the type of attachment behaviour, if any, from the above list which is most closely associated with the following descriptions of behaviour that may be seen during early human development:
   (i)   Separation from the attachment figure results in distress, which rapidly subsides on reunion.
   (ii) Separation from the attachment figure results in a relative lack of distress and there is a general tendency for affection to be muted.
   (iii) The least common attachment style.
   (iv) Distress continues for some time after the return of the attachment figure.

5. **MCQ** – Which of the following is likely to be persistent in the longer term, rather than just an immediate effect of physical or sexual abuse during childhood?
   (a) Anxiety
   (b) Development of a phobia
   (c) Eating disturbance
   (d) Low self-esteem
   (e) Sleep disturbance.

6. **EMI** – Childhood temperamental typology
   (a) Difficult
   (b) Easy
   (c) Slow-to-warm-up
   (d) None of the above

Select the childhood temperamental typology, if any, from the above list that is most closely associated with the following descriptions.
   (i)   Applies to about 15 per cent of young children
   (ii) Irregular sleeping and feeding patterns
   (iii) Slowness to adapt to new situations.

7. **MCQ** – With which of the following types of attachment is the difficult children category of temperament in young children most likely to be associated?
   (a) Anxious-ambivalent
   (b) Anxious-avoidant
   (c) Secure
   (d) All of the above
   (e) None of the above.

8. **EMI** – Childhood temperamental typology
   (a) Difficult
   (b) Easy
   (c) Slow-to-warm-up
   (d) None of the above

Select the childhood temperamental typology, if any, from the above list that is most closely associated with each of the following descriptions:
   (i) Enjoyment of physical contact
   (ii) Emotional lability
   (iii) Found to apply to about half of young children in the original study.

9. **EMI** – Piaget's model of cognitive epistemology
   (a) Concrete operations
   (b) Formal operational
   (c) Preoperational
   (d) Sensorimotor

Select the stage in Piaget's model of cognitive epistemology from the above list that is most closely associated with each of the following descriptions:
   (i) Knowledge of the world is primarily acquired through sensory experience and basic motor actions.
   (ii) The child begins to engage in symbolic thought.
   (iii) Usually occurs between the ages of 18 months and 7 years.
   (iv) Complex self-identity develops.

10. **EMI** – Piaget's model of cognitive epistemology
    (a) Concrete operations
    (b) Formal operational
    (c) Preoperational
    (d) Sensorimotor

Select the stage in Piaget's model of cognitive epistemology from the above list that is most closely associated with each of the following descriptions:
   (i) The child acquires the ability to see situations from the viewpoint of others.
   (ii) The child acquires reversible thinking.
   (iii) Focus is on static states rather than transformations.
   (iv) Only towards the end of this stage does the child begin to form internal mental representations of the world and begin to engage in intentional behaviour.

11. **MCQ** – The structure and rules of language are best associated with which of the following?
    (a) Linguistics
    (b) Phonology
    (c) Pragmatics
    (d) Semantics
    (e) Syntax.

12. **MCQ** – According to Kohlberg's stage theory of moral development, which of the following stages is best associated with the level of conventional moral reasoning?
    (a) Acquisition of rewards (for self or others)
    (b) Acquisition of social reward (approval)/avoidance of disapproval
    (c) Conscience, individual moral code, abstract personal ethics
    (d) Defined by the 'public good', a social contract
    (e) Obedience and avoidance of punishment.

13. **EMI** – Erikson's model of psychosocial development
    (a) First year
    (b) Second to third years
    (c) Fourth to fifth years
    (d) Sixth to 13th years
    (e) Adolescence
    (f) Adulthood
    (g) Middle age
    (h) Later life

Select the stage in Erikson's model of psychosocial development from the above list that is most closely associated with each of the following crises:
   (i) Identity/confusion
   (ii) Trust/mistrust
   (iii) Initiative/guilt
   (iv) Generativity/stagnation.

14. **EMI** – Erikson's model of psychosocial development
    (a) First year
    (b) Second to third years
    (c) Fourth to fifth years
    (d) Sixth to 13th years
    (e) Adolescence
    (f) Adulthood
    (g) Middle age
    (h) Later life

Select the stage in Erikson's model of psychosocial development from the above list that is most closely associated with each of the following favourable outcomes:
   (i) Development of self-identity
   (ii) Commitment to others, career, etc.
   (iii) Self-control and self-efficacy
   (iv) Sense of satisfaction, completion.

15. **EMI** – Erikson's model of psychosocial development
    (a) First year
    (b) Second to third years
    (c) Fourth to fifth years
    (d) Sixth to 13th years
    (e) Adolescence
    (f) Adulthood

(g) Middle age
(h) Later life

Select the stage from the above list that is most closely associated with each of the following crises:
(i) Integrity/despair
(ii) Intimacy/isolation
(iii) Autonomy/self-doubt
(iv) Competence/inferiority.

16. **EMI** – Erikson's model of psychosocial development
(a) First year
(b) Second to third years

(c) Fourth to fifth years
(d) Sixth to 13th years
(e) Adolescence
(f) Adulthood
(g) Middle age
(h) Later life

Select the stage from the above list that is most closely associated with each of the following favourable outcomes:
(i) Concern beyond self to family, society, future
(ii) Confidence in own ability to act/initiate
(iii) Trust and sense of security (attachment)
(iv) Competence in social and intellectual skills.

ANSWERS

1.

(i) f – An example of such a growth chart is given in Figure 8.1 in the accompanying textbook.

(ii) d – This is shown in Figure 8.2 in the accompanying textbook.

(iii) a – Studies by Albert Bandura in the 1960s and 1970s showed that children would mimic the behaviour of an observed model in the appropriate absence of any positive or negative reinforcer.

(iv) b

(v) c – Jean Piaget developed an epistemological account of intellectual development that transformed our understanding of the way in which children think.

Reference: *Psychiatry: An evidence-based text*, Ch. 8.

2. c

Reference: *Psychiatry: An evidence-based text*, p. 108.

3. b

Reference: *Psychiatry: An evidence-based text*, pp. 107–108.

4.

(i) c – Infants who display secure attachment behaviour use the attachment figure as a base from which to explore, occasionally returning to seek affection. Separation from the attachment figure induces anxiety and distress and interaction is sought when reunited, after which anxiety reduces and exploration resumes.

(ii) b – Insecure-avoidant behaviours are characterized by muted distress in the absence of the attachment figure and a minimal response when reunited.

(iii) a – Insecure-ambivalent behaviours represent the least common attachment style.

(iv) a

Reference: *Psychiatry: An evidence-based text*, pp. 108–109.

5. d

Reference: *Psychiatry: An evidence-based text*, p. 111.

6.

(i) c

(ii) a

(iii) c

Reference: *Psychiatry: An evidence-based text*, p. 112.

7. b

Reference: *Psychiatry: An evidence-based text*, p. 112.

8.

(i) b

(ii) a

(iii) d – Easy: about 40 per cent; difficult: about 10 per cent; slow-to-warm-up: about 15 per cent.

Reference: *Psychiatry: An evidence-based text*, p. 112.

9.

(i) d

(ii) c

(iii) c

(iv) b

Reference: *Psychiatry: An evidence-based text*, p. 113.

10.

(i) a

(ii) a

(iii) c

(iv) d

Reference: *Psychiatry: An evidence-based text*, p. 113.

11. e

This concerns the structure and rules of language and how to combine words to form sentences, understanding grammatical structure of language, including word order, use of pronouns, passive sentences, etc.

Reference: *Psychiatry: An evidence-based text*, p. 115.

12. b

This belongs to level 2. Options 'a' and 'e' are stages 1 and 2, respectively, of level 1. Options 'c' and 'd' are stages 6 and 5, respectively, of level 3.

Reference: *Psychiatry: An evidence-based text*, p. 118.

13.

(i) e

(ii) a

(iii) c

(iv) g

Reference: *Psychiatry: An evidence-based text*, p. 124.

14.

(i) e

(ii) f

(iii) b

(iv) h

Reference: *Psychiatry: An evidence-based text*, p. 124.

15.

(i)   h
(ii) f
(iii) b
(iv) d

Reference: *Psychiatry: An evidence-based text*, **p. 124.**

16.

(i)   g
(ii) c
(iii) a
(iv) d

Reference: *Psychiatry: An evidence-based text*, **p. 124.**

Chapter 9

Introduction to basic psychology

QUESTIONS

Note that for answers to extended matching items (EMIs), each option (denoted a, b, c, etc.) might be used once, more than once or not at all. For multiple-choice questions (MCQs), please select the best answer.

1. **MCQ** – In the history of psychology, Wilhelm Wundt is particularly associated with which of the following?
   (a) Behaviourism
   (b) Cognitive psychology
   (c) Gestalt psychology
   (d) Introspectionism
   (e) Psychoanalysis.

2. **MCQ** – In the history of psychology, John B. Watson is particularly associated with which of the following?
   (a) Behaviourism
   (b) Cognitive psychology
   (c) Gestalt psychology
   (d) Introspectionism
   (e) Psychoanalysis.

3. **MCQ** – Which of the following is least likely to be part of the process approach in psychology?
   (a) Biopsychology
   (b) Clinical psychology
   (c) Cognitive psychology
   (d) Comparative psychology
   (e) Physiological psychology.

4. **EMI** – Psychology
   (a) Developmental psychology
   (b) Individual differences
   (c) Process approach
   (d) Social psychology

Select the category from the above list that is most closely associated with the study of each of the following:
   (i)   Interpersonal perception
   (ii) Higher-order mental activities
   (iii) Prejudice and discrimination
   (iv) The ways in which people can differ from one another
   (v)   The lifespan approach.

ANSWERS

1. d

The aim of introspection was to analyse conscious thought into its constituent sensations, much as chemists analyse compounds into elements. The emergence of psychology as a separate discipline is generally dated to 1879, when Wilhelm Wundt, a German physiologist, opened the first psychology laboratory at the University of Leipzig. He and his co-workers attempted to investigate 'the mind' through introspection.

Reference: *Psychiatry: An evidence-based text*, **p. 127.**

2. a

Watson proposed that psychologists should confine themselves to studying behaviour, since only this is measurable and observable by more than one person. Watson's form of psychology was known as behaviourism. It largely replaced introspectionism and advocated that people should be regarded as complex animals to be studied using the same scientific methods as those used in physics and chemistry.

Reference: *Psychiatry: An evidence-based text*, **pp. 127–128.**

3. b

The process approach is typically confined to the laboratory (where experiments are the 'method of choice'). It makes far greater experimental use of non-human animals and assumes that psychological processes (particularly learning) are essentially the same in all species; any differences between species are only quantitative (differences of degree).

Reference: *Psychiatry: An evidence-based text*, **pp. 129–131 and 132.**

4.

(i)   d
(ii) c – This is particularly associated with cognitive psychology, which is part of the process approach.
(iii) d
(iv) b
(v)   a

Reference: *Psychiatry: An evidence-based text*, **pp. 129–132.**

Chapter 10

Awareness

QUESTIONS

Note that for answers to extended matching items (EMIs), each option (denoted a, b, c, etc.) might be used once, more than once or not at all. For multiple-choice questions (MCQs), please select the best answer.

1. **MCQ** – Which of the following is part of secondary consciousness rather than primary consciousness?
   (a) Attention
   (b) Memory
   (c) Perception
   (d) Self-consciousness
   (e) Sensory awareness.

2. **EMI** – Consciousness research
   (a) Allport
   (b) Greenfield
   (c) Hilgard
   (d) Libet
   (e) Passingham

Select the scientist from the above list who is most closely associated with each of the following aspects of consciousness research:
   (i) The concept of the epicentre.
   (ii) The ground-breaking finger-tapping functional magnetic resonance imaging (fMRI) experiment which concluded: 'It seems, having used the whole brain consciously to establish the individual finger movements, just the bare bones of the routine are left. The brain now has a template or habit that can produce the same behaviour "as if" it were still going through all the hoops of being consciously aware.'
   (iii) An EEG experiment in which participants' skin was pricked. There was a huge amount of activity in the somatosensory cortex, but participants reported no conscious experience of tingling or any other sensations. After about 500 ms, the activity evoked by the skin-prick spread away from the somatosensory cortex to a much larger brain area. Only at this stage did participants report feeling a tingle.
   (iv) The following definition of consciousness: 'Attention is the experimental psychologist's code name for consciousness.'
   (v) The neo-dissociation theory of hypnosis.

3. **MCQ** – Select one correct statement regarding EEG alpha rhythms:
   (a) They are most reliably recorded from the front of the scalp.
   (b) They correspond to a frequency range of 3–7 Hz.
   (c) They increase in the right brain hemisphere relative to the left on verbal tasks.
   (d) They increase in the waking adult brain when the eyes are opened rather than closed.
   (e) They indicate a 'turning on' of information processing.

4. **MCQ** – Select one incorrect statement regarding sleep in adult humans:
   (a) Chronic sleep loss is associated with increased calorie expenditure and therefore a reduced risk of obesity.
   (b) In the sleep laboratory, people who average 8 h of sleep a night and maintain that they are fully alert during the day, and who then get an extra hour's sleep at night, find that their productivity levels increase by around 25 per cent.
   (c) The endogenous circadian rhythm is normally not 24 h (plus or minus a few minutes).
   (d) The internal clock is likely to be the suprachiasmatic nucleus.
   (e) The metabolic and endocrine changes resulting from a significant sleep debt mimic many of the hallmarks of ageing.

5. **MCQ** – Select the best option. Slow-wave sleep consists of:
   (a) Stage 2 sleep
   (b) Stage 3 sleep
   (c) Stage 4 sleep
   (d) All of the above
   (e) None of the above.

6. **EMI** – Sleep stages
   (a) Stage 1
   (b) Stage 2
   (c) Stage 3
   (d) Stage 4

Select the sleep stage from the above list that is most closely associated with each of the following features of adult human sleep:

(i) Fifty per cent or more of a typical record consists of delta waves, and the person will spend up to 30 min in this stage.

(ii) It is fairly easy to wake the person. The EEG shows sleep spindles and occasional K complexes.

(iii) Theta waves accompanied by slow rolling eye movements occur, and the person can be woken up easily.

(iv) Spindles disappear and are replaced by delta waves for up to 50 per cent of the EEG.

7. **MCQ** – As an adult human passes through stages 1 to 4 of sleep (in that order), which of the following is most likely to occur?
(a) Muscle tone tends to increase.
(b) Sleep becomes less deep.
(c) The EEG wave amplitude tends to increase.
(d) The EEG wave frequency tends to increase.
(e) The EEG wave voltage tends to decrease.

8. **MCQ** – In which of the following stages of normal adult human sleep are PGO spikes/waves most characteristically seen?
(a) REM
(b) Stage 1
(c) Stage 2
(d) Stage 3
(e) Stage 4.

9. **MCQ** – Which of the following is least likely to be associated with NREM sleep?
(a) D-state
(b) Nightmares
(c) Sleeptalking
(d) Somnambulism
(e) Tossing and turning.

10. **EMI** – Sleep stages
(a) NREM sleep
(b) REM sleep
(c) Neither of the above

Select the sleep stage, if any, from the above list that is most closely associated with each of the following features of adult human sleep:
(i) Reduced blood pressure
(ii) Reduced respiratory rate
(iii) Clitoral engorgement.

11. **MCQ** – According to Hobson, which of the following modalities of hallucination is rarest during dreams?
(a) Auditory
(b) Movement sensations
(c) Tactile
(d) Taste
(e) Visual.

12. **MCQ** – Which of the following does not typically occur during dreams, according to Hobson?
(a) Amnesia
(b) Cognitive abnormalities
(c) Delusions
(d) Emotional intensification
(e) Pain.

13. **EMI** – Theories of sleep and dreaming
(a) Crick and Mitchison
(b) Hobson
(c) Horne
(d) Meddis
(e) Ornstein
(f) Oswald

Select the scientist(s) from the above list most closely associated with each of the following theories about sleep and dreaming:
(i) Reorganization of schemas occurs during sleep and dreaming.
(ii) Sleep can be analysed at the levels of behaviour, development and metabolism.
(iii) Mammalian sleep is an advantage because it keeps the animal immobilized for long periods, making it less conspicuous to would-be predators and, therefore, safer.

14. **EMI** – Theories of sleep and dreaming
(a) Crick and Mitchison
(b) Hobson
(c) Horne
(d) Meddis
(e) Ornstein
(f) Oswald

Select the scientist(s) from the above list most closely associated with each of the following theories about sleep and dreaming:
(i) The restoration theory
(ii) The core-optional theory
(iii) Reverse learning
(iv) The long periods of sleep of babies have evolved to prevent exhaustion in their mothers.

ANSWERS

1. d

In Edelman's terms, non-humans possess primary consciousness; this comprises sensory awareness, attention, perception, memory (or learning), emotion and action. What makes human beings distinct is their additional possession of secondary consciousness, i.e. self-consciousness or awareness. This, according to Singer, is the experience of one's own individuality, the ability to experience oneself as an autonomous individual with subjective feelings.

Reference: *Psychiatry: An evidence-based text*, **p. 137.**

2.

(i) b – According to Greenfield, the epicentre is like a stone thrown into a pond, causing ripples to spread out. The extent of neuronal 'ripples' would affect the degree of consciousness at any given time.

(ii) e – This fMRI study, supervised by Passingham (University of Oxford), was conducted at the Institute of Neurology (University College London) by McCrone and colleagues. It may have revolutionary implications for our understanding of what it means to experience something consciously. Details are given in Box 10.2 in the accompanying textbook.

(iii) d – Baroness Greenfield has cited these experimental results of Libet in support of her model of consciousness.

(iv) a

(v) c – According to this theory, the consciousness that solves a problem may be different from the consciousness that reports the solution: neither is 'higher' or 'lower' than the other; they are simply different.

Reference: *Psychiatry: An evidence-based text*, **pp. 138–141.**

3. c

The converse is true for spatial tasks.

Reference: *Psychiatry: An evidence-based text*, **pp. 141–142.**

4. a

Chronic sleep loss could not only speed up the onset but also increase the severity of age-related diseases such as obesity, type 2 diabetes mellitus, hypertension and memory loss.

Reference: *Psychiatry: An evidence-based text*, **pp. 142–143.**

5. d

Reference: *Psychiatry: An evidence-based text*, **p. 145.**

6.

(i) d
(ii) b
(iii) a
(iv) c

Reference: *Psychiatry: An evidence-based text*, **p. 145.**

7. c

Reference: *Psychiatry: An evidence-based text*, **p. 145.**

8. a

A feature of REM sleep is the appearance of pontine-geniculo-occipital (PGO) spikes/waves, which are generated in the pons and travel through the lateral geniculate nucleus. PGO spikes typically occur in bursts, often preceding individual eye movements.

Reference: *Psychiatry: An evidence-based text*, **p. 145.**

9. a

This refers specifically to REM sleep.

Reference: *Psychiatry: An evidence-based text*, **pp. 145–146.**

10.

(i) a
(ii) a
(iii) b

Reference: *Psychiatry: An evidence-based text*, **p. 149.**

11. d

The hallucinations are predominantly visual.

Reference: *Psychiatry: An evidence-based text*, **p. 149.**

12. e

The hallucination of pain is extremely rare during dreams, according to Hobson.

Reference: *Psychiatry: An evidence-based text*, **p. 149.**

13.

(i) e – According to Ornstein, REM sleep and dreaming may be involved in the reorganization of our schemas (mental structures), so as to accommodate new information.

(ii) b – Hobson proposes that sleep can be analysed at these levels.

(iii) d

Reference: *Psychiatry: An evidence-based text*, **pp. 148–150.**

14.

(i) **f** – Oswald maintains that both REM and NREM sleep serve a restorative, replenishing function. According to this theory, NREM restores bodily processes that have deteriorated during the day, while REM sleep is a time for replenishing and renewing brain processes, through the stimulation of protein synthesis.

(ii) **c** – In Horne's core-optional theory of sleep, a distinction is made between core sleep, which is said to be necessary, and optional sleep, which is not necessary. Based on experimental evidence, only the first 3 h or so of adult human sleep are said to be truly necessary (core sleep), while the rest is optional.

(iii) **a** – Their basic idea is that we dream in order to forget.

(iv) **d**

Reference: *Psychiatry: An evidence-based text*, **pp. 147–150.**

Chapter 11

Stress

QUESTIONS

Note that for answers to extended matching items (EMIs), each option (denoted a, b, c, etc.) might be used once, more than once or not at all. For multiple-choice questions (MCQs), please select the best answer.

1. **EMI** – Models related to stress
   - (a) Engineering model
   - (b) General adaptation syndrome
   - (c) Transactional model
   - (d) Vitamin model

   Select the model from the above list that is most closely associated with each of the following:
   - (i) Due to Warr, this model identifies several environmental factors that affect mental health.
   - (ii) Due to Selye, formulated after examination of the major physiological changes associated with illness and stress.
   - (iii) This model views external stress as giving rise to a stress reaction. Up to a point, stress is inevitable and can be tolerated; moderate levels may even be beneficial (eustress).
   - (iv) This model views stress as arising from an interaction between people and their environment, in particular when there is an imbalance between the person's perception of the demands being made of them by the situation and their ability to meet those demands.

2. **MCQ** – In the study by Coffey *et al.* on the influence of shifts on job performance and job-related stress in female nurses in the USA, which of the following shifts were associated with the best job performance?
   - (a) Afternoon shifts
   - (b) Day shifts
   - (c) Night shifts
   - (d) Rotating shifts
   - (e) More than one of the above were joint equal.

3. **MCQ** – In the study by Coffey *et al.* on the influence of shifts on job performance and job-related stress in female nurses in the USA, which of the following shifts were associated with the highest job-related stress?
   - (a) Afternoon shifts
   - (b) Day shifts
   - (c) Night shifts
   - (d) Rotating shifts
   - (e) More than one of the above were joint equal.

4. **EMI** – Social Readjustment Rating Scale (SRRS)
   - (a) 0
   - (b) 10–12
   - (c) 45–55
   - (d) 63
   - (e) 73
   - (f) 100

   Select the SRRS score or range from the above list which is most closely associated with each of the following life events:
   - (i) Death of spouse
   - (ii) Christmas
   - (iii) Divorce
   - (iv) Marriage
   - (v) Retirement.

5. **MCQ** – Select one incorrect statement regarding stress:
   - (a) Community mental health nurses have been found to have a relatively high rate of burnout.
   - (b) Hassles are related positively to undesirable psychological symptoms.
   - (c) Life-event stress is related more closely to psychiatric symptoms among people rated as high on internal locus of control than among those rated as high on external locus of control.
   - (d) Life events may be considered to be distal causes of stress.
   - (e) Psychiatrists have a very high rate of suicide among doctors.

6. **EMI** – Types of coping
   - (a) Avoidance
   - (b) Detached
   - (c) Emotional
   - (d) Rational
   - (e) None of the above

Select the option from the above list that is most closely associated with each of the following long-term consequences of maladaptive and adaptive coping:

(i) Prevents overidentification with the problem.

(ii) Increasingly overwhelmed by the problem.

(iii) Blocking out cannot be sustained.

(iv) Problems are put into perspective.

7. **EMI** – General adaptation syndrome

(a) Alarm reaction

(b) Exhaustion

(c) Resistance

(d) Retirement

(e) Stressor

Select the option from the above list that is most closely associated with each of the following concepts from the general adaptation syndrome:

(i) Shock phase

(ii) Countershock phase

(iii) ACTH stimulation of the adrenal gland

(iv) Hypoglycaemia.

8. **MCQ** – Which of the following is not a category of coping strategy in the classification by Cohen and Lazarus?

(a) Direct action response

(b) Emotion-focused coping

(c) Information-seeking

(d) Inhibition of action

(e) Intrapsychic coping.

9. **EMI** – Types of coping

(a) Avoidance

(b) Detached

(c) Emotional

(d) Rational

(e) None of the above

Select the option from the above list that is most closely associated with each of the following short-term consequences of maladaptive and adaptive coping:

(i) Logic determines resolution of the problem.

(ii) Expression of emotion.

(iii) Temporary relief occurs as the problem is blocked out.

(iv) Able to stand back and take stock of the problem.

10. **MCQ** – Select one incorrect statement regarding stress:

(a) IgA levels have been found to increase immediately after an oral examination (if it appeared to go well).

(b) In a study of women with breast cancer, those using guided imagery with progressive muscle relaxation suffered fewer side-effects from medical treatment than women in a control group.

(c) In mental health nurses, an inverse relationship has been found between self-esteem and symptoms of depression.

(d) In the study by Greer and colleagues of women who had had a mastectomy after being diagnosed with breast cancer, at 15-year follow-up it was found that survival was much lower in the stoical or 'giving up' women.

(e) Wound healing takes approximately the same time in highly stressed and relatively 'stress-free' groups of individuals.

ANSWERS

1.

(i)   d

(ii) b

(iii) a

(iv) c – Because it is the person's perception of this mismatch between demand and ability that causes stress, the model allows for important individual differences in what produces stress and how much stress is experienced.

Reference: *Psychiatry: An evidence-based text*, **p. 153**.

2. b

Reference: *Psychiatry: An evidence-based text*, **p. 154**.

3. d

Reference: *Psychiatry: An evidence-based text*, **p. 154**.

4.

(i)   f

(ii) b – The mean SSRS value is 12 for this life event.

(iii) e

(iv) c – The mean SSRS value is 50 for this life event.

(v) c – The mean SSRS value is 45 for this life event.

Reference: *Psychiatry: An evidence-based text*, **p. 155**.

5. c

Using Rotter's Locus of Control Scale, and devising a new scale – the Life Events Scale – Johnson and Sarason found that life-events stress was related more closely to psychiatric symptoms (in particular, depression and anxiety) among people rated as high on external locus of control than among those rated as high on internal locus of control. That is, people who believe that they do not have control over what happens to them are more vulnerable to the harmful effects of change than those who believe they do. This is related to Seligman's concept of learned helplessness.

Reference: *Psychiatry: An evidence-based text*, **pp. 155–157**.

6.

(i)   b – This is a type of adaptive coping in which the problem or situation is not seen as a threat.

(ii) c – This is a type of maladaptive coping in which the individual feels overpowered and helpless.

(iii) a – This is a type of maladaptive coping in which the individual sits tight and hopes it all goes away.

(iv) d – This is a type of adaptive coping in which past experience is used to work out how to deal with the situation.

Reference: *Psychiatry: An evidence-based text*, **p. 162**.

7.

(i)   a – In the alarm reaction stage, when a stimulus is perceived as a stressor, there is a brief, initial shock phase.

(ii) a – Also in the alarm reaction stage, the shock phase is followed by a countershock phase.

(iii) c – During the resistance stage, adrenocorticotrophic hormone (ACTH) stimulation of the adrenal (or suprarenal) cortex occurs.

(iv) b

Reference: *Psychiatry: An evidence-based text*, **pp. 157–158**.

8. b

This involves trying to reduce the negative emotions that are part of the experience of stress. Intrapsychic coping is also known as palliative coping.

Reference: *Psychiatry: An evidence-based text*, **pp. 162–163**.

9.

(i)   d – This is a type of adaptive coping in which past experience is used to work out how to deal with the situation. The situation is given full attention and treated as a challenge to be met.

(ii) c – This is a type of maladaptive coping in which the individual feels overpowered and helpless. The individual may become miserable, depressed or angry, and may take out his frustrations on other people.

(iii) a – This is a type of maladaptive coping in which the individual sits tight and hopes it all goes away. The individual may pretend that there is nothing the matter if people ask.

(iv) b – This is a type of adaptive coping in which the problem or situation is not seen as a threat. The individual takes nothing personally and sees the problem as being separate from herself.

Reference: *Psychiatry: An evidence-based text*, **p. 162**.

10. e

Kiecolt-Glaser *et al.* compared the rate of wound healing in two groups: (i) a group of 13 'high-stress' women caring for relatives with Alzheimer's disease; and (ii) a 'stress-free' matched control group. All the women underwent a 3.5-mm full-thickness punch biopsy on their non-dominant forearm. Healing took significantly longer in the first group.

Reference: *Psychiatry: An evidence-based text*, **pp. 159–161**.

Part 2 : Developmental, behavioural, and sociocultural psychiatry

Chapter 12

Emotion

QUESTIONS

Note that for answers to extended matching items (EMIs), each option (denoted a, b, c, etc.) might be used once, more than once or not at all. For multiple-choice questions (MCQs), please select the best answer.

1. **MCQ** – Several primary emotions have been identified according to the classic study by Ekman and Friesen. Select one option which is not included in their classification:
   (a) Anger
   (b) Anticipation
   (c) Disgust
   (d) Happiness
   (e) Surprise.

2. **EMI** – Primary and complex emotions
   (a) Aggressiveness
   (b) Awe
   (c) Contempt
   (d) Disappointment
   (e) Love
   (f) Optimism
   (g) Remorse
   (h) Submission

Select the complex emotion option from the above list that is most closely associated with each of the following combinations of primary emotions (as proposed by Plutchik):
   (i)   Anticipation and joy
   (ii) Anger and disgust
   (iii) Fear and surprise
   (iv) Fear and acceptance.

3. **EMI** – Primary and complex emotions
   (a) Aggressiveness
   (b) Awe
   (c) Contempt
   (d) Disappointment
   (e) Love
   (f) Optimism
   (g) Remorse
   (h) Submission

Select the complex emotion option from the above list that is most closely associated with each of the following combinations of primary emotions (as proposed by Plutchik):
   (i) Disgust and sadness
   (ii) Anger and anticipation

(iii) Sadness and surprise
(iv) Joy and acceptance.

4. **MCQ** – Select one incorrect statement regarding emotions:
   (a) Ego-focused emotions, according to Markus and Kitayama, are experienced more by people in individualist cultures with more independent selves.
   (b) Emotions appear to be innate.
   (c) In the James–Lange theory of emotions, emotional experience is the cause of perceived bodily changes.
   (d) In the Middle Ages, in the West, hope was classified as a basic emotion.
   (e) The emotion accida involved a mixture of boredom with one's religious duties, attempting to put off carrying them out, sadness about one's religious failings and a sense of loss of one's former religious enthusiasm.

5. **MCQ** – In the famous experiment by Ax, which of the following changes was more likely to be associated with anger than with fear?
   (a) Increased breathing rate
   (b) Increased cardiac rate
   (c) Increased muscle action potential frequency
   (d) Increased muscle action potential size
   (e) Increased skin conductance level.

6. **EMI** – Schachter and Singer adrenaline experiment
   (a) Participants were much less likely to join in with the stooge or to report feeling euphoric or angry.
   (b) Participants were much more likely to join in with the stooge or to report feeling euphoric or angry.
   (c) No significant change in behaviour or reported feeling.

In the Schachter and Singer adrenaline experiment, participants were given an injection of either adrenaline or saline but told that they were given a vitamin injection in order to see its effect on vision. Select the outcome from the above list that is most closely associated with each of the following experimental groups of participants:
   (i) Participants received an adrenaline injection and

were given false information about the side-effects of the injection (itching, headache).

(ii) Participants received an adrenaline injection and were given accurate information about the side-effects of the injection (palpitations, tightness in the throat, tremor, sweating).

(iii) Participants received an adrenaline injection and were given no information about the side-effects of the injection.

(iv) Participants received a saline injection and were given no information about the side-effects of the injection.

7. **MCQ** – Schachter and Wheeler carried out an experiment in which participants were injected with either adrenaline or chlorpromazine, while control subjects were injected with a placebo. Given that chlorpromazine inhibits arousal, how much would you expect the adrenaline- and chlorpromazine-injected participants to laugh compared with the placebo-injected individuals while watching a slapstick comedy?

(a) The adrenaline-injected participants would laugh less and the chlorpromazine-injected participants would laugh less than the placebo-injected individuals.

(b) The adrenaline-injected participants would laugh less and the chlorpromazine-injected participants would laugh more than the placebo-injected individuals.

(c) The adrenaline-injected participants would laugh more and the chlorpromazine-injected participants would laugh less than the placebo-injected individuals.

(d) The adrenaline-injected participants would laugh more and the chlorpromazine-injected participants would laugh more than the placebo-injected individuals.

(e) There would be no significant difference between the three groups.

8. **EMI** – Types of attrribution

(a) Negative outcome, external locus and controllable

(b) Negative outcome, external locus and uncontrollable

(c) Negative outcome, internal locus and controllable

(d) Negative outcome, internal locus and uncontrollable

(e) Positive outcome, external locus and controllable

(f) Positive outcome, external locus and uncontrollable

(g) Positive outcome, internal locus and controllable

(h) Positive outcome, internal locus and uncontrollable

Select the attribution set from the above list that is most closely associated with each of the following situations:

(i) Someone studies hard and passes an examination.

(ii) Someone fails to give you promised help with your examination preparation and you fail your examination.

(iii) You do not revise and go on to fail an examination.

(iv) Someone helps you revise and you pass your examination.

(v) Someone has a run of bad luck and fails an examination.

9. **EMI** – Types of attribution

(a) Negative outcome, external locus and controllable

(b) Negative outcome, external locus and uncontrollable

(c) Negative outcome, internal locus and controllable

(d) Negative outcome, internal locus and uncontrollable

(e) Positive outcome, external locus and controllable

(f) Positive outcome, external locus and uncontrollable

(g) Positive outcome, internal locus and controllable

(h) Positive outcome, internal locus and uncontrollable

Select the set of attributions from the above list that is most closely associated with producing each of the following emotions:

(i) Gratitude

(ii) Guilt

(iii) Pity

(iv) Anger

(v) Pride.

10. **MCQ** – Which, if any, of the following classical experiments on emotion most strongly supports the concept of the misattribution effect?

(a) Dutton and Aron's suspension-bridge experiment

(b) Hohmann's study of adult males with spinal cord injuries

(c) Laird's facial feedback experiment

(d) Valins' false feedback experiment

(e) None of the above.

ANSWERS

1. b

The others not included as options are fear and sadness.

Reference: *Psychiatry: An evidence-based text*, p. 166.

2.

(i)   f
(ii) c
(iii) b
(iv) h

Reference: *Psychiatry: An evidence-based text*, pp. 166–167.

3.

(i)   g
(ii) a
(iii) d
(iv) e

Reference: *Psychiatry: An evidence-based text*, pp. 166–167.

4. c

James and Lange argued that our emotional experience is the result, not the cause, of perceived bodily changes.

Reference: *Psychiatry: An evidence-based text*, pp. 166–168.

5. d

In this famous experiment, Ax measured electrodermal, electromyographic, cardiovascular and respiratory activity in participants who were deliberately frightened and made angry.

Reference: *Psychiatry: An evidence-based text*, p. 170.

6.

(i)   b
(ii) a
(iii) b
(iv) a – This was the control group.

Reference: *Psychiatry: An evidence-based text*, p. 172.

7. c

This was the result of their experiment.

Reference: *Psychiatry: An evidence-based text*, pp. 172–173.

8.

(i)   g
(ii) a
(iii) c
(iv) e
(v)   b

Reference: *Psychiatry: An evidence-based text*, p. 174.

9.

(i)   e
(ii) c
(iii) b
(iv) a
(v)   g

Reference: *Psychiatry: An evidence-based text*, p. 174.

10. a

Reference: *Psychiatry: An evidence-based text*, pp. 174–175.

Chapter 13

Information-processing and attention

QUESTIONS

Note that for answers to extended matching items (EMIs), each option (denoted a, b, c, etc.) might be used once, more than once or not at all. For multiple-choice questions (MCQs), please select the best answer.

1. **MCQ** – Which of the following models of attention is not based solely on serial processing but allows parallel processing?
   (a) Attenuation model
   (b) Central capacity theory
   (c) Filter model
   (d) Multi-channel theory
   (e) Pertinence model.

2. **MCQ** – Select one of the following options which is least likely to be used to study selective attention?
   (a) Cocktail party phenomenon study
   (b) Dichotic listening
   (c) Dual-task technique
   (d) Shadowing technique
   (e) Split-span procedure.

3. **EMI** – Types of recall
   (a) 123478
   (b) 123487
   (c) 123748
   (d) 123784
   (e) 783214
   (f) 783241
   (g) 821734
   (h) 872134

Select the sequence from the above list that is most closely associated with each of the following types of recall in a split-span study in which the digits 8, 2, 1 are presented, in that order, to one ear while the digits 7, 3, 4 are presented simultaneously, in that order, to the other ear:
   (i) Ear-by-ear recall.
   (ii) Pair-by-pair recall.

4. **EMI** – Types of recall
   (a) Ear-by-ear recall
   (b) Pair-by-pair recall
   (c) Serial recall

Select the correct type of recall from the above options:
   (i) Which of the above three types of recall tends to be the most accurate?
   (ii) In a split-span study, which type of recall is the more accurate?

5. **EMI** – Broadbent's theory of the flow of information between stimulus and response
   (a) Effectors
   (b) Limited-capacity channel
   (c) Selective filter
   (d) Senses
   (e) Short-term store
   (f) Store of conditional probabilities of past events
   (g) System for varying output until some input is secured

Select the option from the above list that is most closely associated with each of components of Broadbent's theory of the flow of information between stimulus and response in the diagram below:

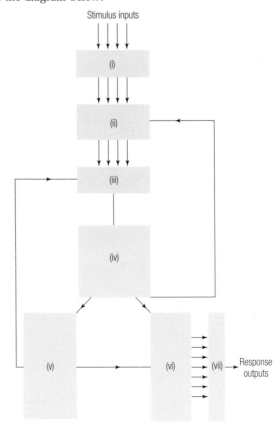

6. **EMI** – Treisman's attenuation model
   (a) Attenuated channels
   (b) Response processes
   (c) Selected channel
   (d) Selective filter (attenuator)
   (e) Semantic analysis (recognition processes)

Select the option from the above list that is most closely associated with each of components of Treisman's attenuation model in the diagram below:

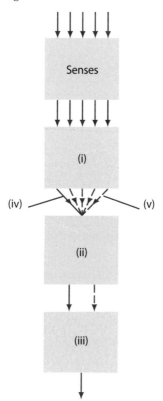

7. **EMI** – Deutsch–Norman theory of focused attention
   (a) Attention
   (b) Memory
   (c) Pertinence
   (d) Processing
   (e) Selection

Select the option from the above list that is most closely associated with each of components of the Deutsch–Norman theory of focused attention illustrated in the diagram below:

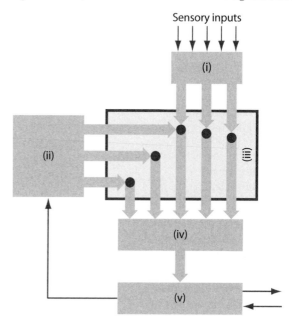

8. **MCQ** – Which of the following statements concerning focused visual attention is incorrect?
   (a) LaBerge asked participants to judge whether the middle letter of five letters came from the beginning or end of the alphabet. But on some occasions, a stimulus such as - 7 - - - was presented, and the task was to determine whether the 7 was one of two letters (T or Z). LaBerge found that the speed of judgement was a function of the distance from the centre of attention.
   (b) LaBerge found that when participants were required to attend to whole five-letter word strings rather than just one letter within such strings, the width of the internal spotlight's 'beam' increased, based on similarity of reaction times for items at the centre and periphery.
   (c) Participants were asked to search for the presence or absence of a single moving X among static Xs and moving Os. Decision times increased with an increasing number of distractors.

(d) When a picture is shown as the unattended stimulus on one trial, it slows the processing of an attended word with an identical or similar meaning on the next trial.

(e) When individuals are told to fixate on the outcome part of the visual field, it is still possible to attend to stimuli about seven degrees either side of the fixation point.

9. **MCQ** – Select one correct statement regarding dual-task performance:

(a) It is generally improved by practice.

(b) It is generally improved when the tasks make use of the same stages of processing (e.g. the input stage).

(c) It is generally improved when the tasks rely on related memory codes such as visual memory.

(d) It is generally improved when the tasks require similar responses to be made.

(e) It is generally more successful the more difficult the task.

10. **MCQ** – In the Kahneman limited-capacity theory of attention, which of the following is not an input into the central processor responsible for allocation policy?

(a) Arousal

(b) Enduring dispositions

(c) Evaluation of demands on capacity

(d) Momentary intentions

(e) Responses.

11. **MCQ** – Select one statement which is not true regarding Baddeley's working memory model:

(a) It contains a supervisory attentional system.

(b) It contains a visuospatial scratchpad.

(c) It contains an articulatory/phonological loop.

(d) It contains an episodic buffer.

(e) It is a synthesis model.

12. **EMI** – Types of action slip

(a) Discrimination failure

(b) Program assembly failure

(c) Storage failure

(d) Subroutine failure

(e) Test failure

(f) None of the above

Select the type of action slip, if any, from the above options that most closely corresponds to each of the following errors:

(i) A person intends to turn on the radio but walks past it and picks up the telephone instead.

(ii) In making a pot of 'tea' a person fails to put any tea into the pot.

(iii) A person pours a second kettle of boiling water into a teapot of freshly made tea without any recognition of having made the tea already.

(iv) Toothpaste is mistaken for shaving cream.

(v) A boiled sweet (candy) is unwrapped, the wrapping paper is placed in the mouth, and the sweet itself is thrown into a bin.

ANSWERS

1. d

Allport's theory of divided attention allowed for parallel processing.

Reference: *Psychiatry: An evidence-based text*, **p. 179.**

2. c

This method deliberately divides the participant's attention, and so is more suitable for studying divided attention.

Reference: *Psychiatry: An evidence-based text*, **p. 180.**

3.

(i) g – An alternative correct option would be 734821.
(ii) f – An alternative correct option would be 872314.

Reference: *Psychiatry: An evidence-based text*, **p. 180.**

4.

(i) c – When control subjects are given a list of six digits at a rate of one every 0.5 s, serial recall is typically 95 per cent accurate.
(ii) a – Broadbent found that pair-by-pair recall was considerably poorer than ear-by-ear recall in split-span studies.

Reference: *Psychiatry: An evidence-based text*, **p. 180.**

5.

(i)   d
(ii) e
(iii) c
(iv) b
(v)   f
(vi) g
(vii) a

Reference: *Psychiatry: An evidence-based text*, **p. 181.**

6.

(i)   d
(ii) e
(iii) b
(iv) c
(v)   a

Reference: *Psychiatry: An evidence-based text*, **p. 182.**

7.

(i)   d
(ii) c
(iii) b
(iv) e
(v)   a

Reference: *Psychiatry: An evidence-based text*, **p. 183.**

8. c

The finding given in the option is that which would be predicted by Treisman's theory, i.e. that serial attention is necessary for each item when searching for the target. In fact, the target was found easily, regardless of the display's size. This implies a parallel process.

Option 'b' is based on the global attention condition, and led to Eriksen's zoom-lens model of visual attention. Option 'd' refers to negative priming. Option 'e' was carried out by Posner and colleagues.

Reference: *Psychiatry: An evidence-based text*, **pp. 184–186.**

9. a

This could be because people develop new strategies for performing each task, minimizing interference between them. Another possibility is that practice reduces a task's attentional demands. Or practice may produce a more economical way of functioning that uses fewer resources.

Reference: *Psychiatry: An evidence-based text*, **p. 187.**

10. e

Further details are given in Figure 13.8, including its caption, in the accompanying textbook.

Reference: *Psychiatry: An evidence-based text*, **pp. 187–188.**

11. a

Baddeley does not consider the central executive to be purely an attentional system. He proposed the episodic buffer, sitting between the central executive and long-term memory, accepting information from any part of the system and holding it in a multidimensional code.

Reference: *Psychiatry: An evidence-based text*, **pp. 188–190.**

12.

(i)   e – Such slips presumably occur because a planned sequence of actions is not monitored sufficiently at some crucial point in the sequence.
(ii) d – In this type of action slip, one or more stages in a sequence of behaviours are either omitted or reordered.
(iii) c – An action that has already been completed is repeated.
(iv) a – There is failure to discriminate between two objects involved in different actions.
(v)   b – Actions are incorrectly combined.

Reference: *Psychiatry: An evidence-based text*, **p. 190.**

Chapter 14

Learning theory

QUESTIONS

Note that for answers to extended matching items (EMIs), each option (denoted a, b, c, etc.) might be used once, more than once or not at all. For multiple-choice questions (MCQs), please select the best answer.

1. **MCQ** – Select one incorrect statement regarding the behaviourist approach:
   (a) Behaviourists emphasize the role of environmental factors in influencing behaviour.
   (b) Behaviourists stress the use of operational definitions.
   (c) Behaviourism is sometimes referred to as S–R psychology.
   (d) Classical and operant conditioning are collectively theories of learning.
   (e) The aims of a science of behaviour include predicting and controlling behaviour.

2. **EMI** – Classical conditioning
   (a) CR
   (b) CS
   (c) UCR
   (d) UCS
   (e) None of the above

Select the most appropriate option that matches each of the numbered items (i) to (vi) in the diagram below, which represents the basic procedure involved in classical conditioning:

Stage 1 (before learning): (i) → (ii)
Stage 2 (during learning): (iii) + UCS → (iv)
Stage 3 (after learning): (v) → (vi)

3. **EMI** – Classical conditioning
   (a) Backward
   (b) Delayed or forward
   (c) Simultaneous
   (d) Trace
   (e) None of the above

Select the most appropriate type of classical conditioning, if any, from the above options, which matches each of the following:
   (i) The conditioned stimulus is presented and removed before the unconditioned stimulus is presented.
   (ii) The conditioned stimulus is presented before the unconditioned stimulus, and remains 'on' while the unconditioned stimulus is presented and until the unconditioned response appears.
   (iii) Conditioning has occurred when the conditioned stimulus on its own produces the conditioned response. This type of conditioning often occurs in real-life situations.
   (iv) The conditioned stimulus is presented after the unconditioned stimulus. This type of conditioning is often used in advertising.

4. **MCQ** – In an experiment with a dog, a buzzer, previously paired with food using Pavlovian conditioning, is paired with a black square. After ten pairings, the dog salivates a small but significant amount at the sight of the black square before the buzzer is sounded. The black square–buzzer pairing is referred to as which of the following types of conditioning?
   (a) Zero-order
   (b) First-order
   (c) Second-order
   (d) Third-order
   (e) Tenth-order.

5. **EMI** – Pavlovian conditioning
   (a) Discrimination
   (b) Discrimination training
   (c) Extinction
   (d) Generalization
   (e) Spontaneous recovery

This question relates to the Pavlovian conditioning of a dog, such that the dog salivates at the sound of a bell (which has been paired with food). Select the most appropriate option that matches each of the following findings:
   (i) If the dog is presented with bells that are increasingly different from the original, the conditioned response gradually weakens and eventually stops.
   (ii) The dog, having been trained using a bell of a particular pitch, is noted still to salivate when presented with a bell a little higher or lower in pitch.
   (iii) The bell is repeatedly presented without food.

The salivation response to the sound of the bell gradually becomes weaker and eventually stops.

(iv) The bell is repeatedly presented without food. The salivation response to the sound of the bell gradually becomes weaker and eventually stops. The dog is removed from the experimental situation and then put back a couple of hours later. It starts to salivate again in response to the presentation of the bell.

6. **MCQ** – Pavlov trained dogs to salivate to a circle but not to an ellipse, and then gradually changed the shape of the ellipse until it became almost circular. As this happened, which of the following phenomena was most likely to be observed?
   (a) Backward conditioning
   (b) Experimental neurosis
   (c) Law of effect
   (d) Systematic desensitization
   (e) Third-order conditioning.

7. **MCQ** – Select one incorrect statement regarding classical and operant conditioning:
   (a) Both are types of associative learning.
   (b) Extinction occurs in both types of conditioning.
   (c) Generalization occurs in both types of conditioning.
   (d) Spontaneous recovery occurs in both types of conditioning.
   (e) The strength of conditioning is measured mainly as a response rate in both types of conditioning.

8. **MCQ** – To which of the following does the law of effect refer best?
   (a) Behaviour is shaped and maintained by its consequences.
   (b) Completely new stimulus–response connections are formed.
   (c) The decreased speed with which an animal learns to escape from a puzzle-box in future trials after learning how to do so in the first trial.
   (d) The effect of random errors.
   (e) The reinforcer is presented regardless of what the animal does, and is presented before the response.

9. **EMI** – Reinforcement schedules
   (a) Continuous reinforcement
   (b) Fixed interval
   (c) Fixed ratio
   (d) Variable interval
   (e) Variable ratio

Select the most appropriate option from the above reinforcement schedules to which each of the following responses corresponds:
   (i)   There is a pronounced pause after each reinforcement, and then a very high rate of responding leading up to the next reinforcement.
   (ii) The response rate is slow but steady.

(iii) There is a very high response rate, which is very steady.
(iv) The response rate is very stable over long periods of time and there is some tendency to increase the response rate as time elapses since the last reinforcement.
(v) The response rate speeds up as the next reinforcement becomes available; there is a pause after each reinforcement; overall the response rate is fairly low.

10. **EMI** – Resistance to extinction
    (a) Very low
    (b) Fairly low
    (c) High
    (d) Very high

Select the most appropriate option from the above levels of resistance to extinction to which each of the following reinforcement schedules corresponds:
   (i)   Continuous reinforcement
   (ii) Fixed interval
   (iii) Fixed ratio
   (iv) Variable interval
   (v)   Variable ratio.

11. **EMI** – Reinforcement schedules
    (a) Continuous reinforcement
    (b) Fixed interval
    (c) Fixed ratio
    (d) Variable interval
    (e) Variable ratio

Select the most appropriate option from the above reinforcement schedules to which each of the following examples of human behaviour corresponds:
   (i)   Taking a short break of 10 min for every hour's concentrated studying achieved
   (ii) Being paid every month
   (iii) Gambling
   (iv) Receiving a high grade for every assignment.

12. **EMI** – Reinforcement schedules
    (a) Continuous reinforcement
    (b) Fixed interval
    (c) Fixed ratio
    (d) Variable interval
    (e) Variable ratio

Select the most appropriate option from the above reinforcement schedules to which each of the following examples of human behaviour corresponds:
   (i)   Being self-employed and receiving payment on an irregular basis, depending on when the customer pays for the product or service
   (ii) Piece work – the more work that is carried out, the more money is earned

(iii) Receiving a tip for every customer served

(iv) Being paid on a sales commission basis.

13. **MCQ** – In the Thorndike puzzle-box, which of the following is most likely to strengthen behaviours that result in their removal or avoidance?

(a) Blockers

(b) Negative reinforcers

(c) Positive primary reinforcers

(d) Positive secondary reinforcers

(e) Punishers.

14. **EMI** – Reinforcement schedules

(a) Continuous reinforcement

(b) Fixed interval

(c) Fixed ratio

(d) Variable interval

(e) Variable ratio

The figure below shows typical cumulative records for a response reinforced using five different schedules of reinforcement, labelled (i)–(v). Select the most appropriate option from the above reinforcement schedules to which each of these labels corresponds:

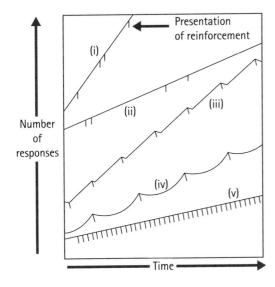

15. **MCQ** – In the two-factor theory of avoidance learning, on which of the following is the first factor based?

(a) Classical conditioning

(b) Negative reinforcement

(c) Positive reinforcement

(d) Punishment

(e) Shaping.

16. **MCQ** – In the two-factor theory of avoidance learning, on which of the following is the second factor based?

(a) Classical conditioning

(b) Negative reinforcement

(c) Positive reinforcement

(d) Punishment

(e) Shaping.

17. **MCQ** – In studies of the law of contiguity in laboratory rats, which of the following types of stimuli is most strongly associated with internal illness?

(a) Auditory

(b) Gustatory

(c) Tactile

(d) Visual

(e) More than one of the above.

18. **MCQ** – Which of the following is most likely to explain the persistence of human phobias?

(a) Avoidance learning

(b) Blocking

(c) Fixed ratio reinforcement schedules

(d) Forced reality testing

(e) Shaping.

19. **MCQ** – Of the following concepts from learning theory, which might best offer a partial explanation of depression?

(a) Aversive learning

(b) Contra-preparedness

(c) Learned helplessness

(d) Preparedness

(e) Shaping.

20. **MCQ** – Which of the following concepts is more closely associated with Skinner than with Tolman?

(a) Analysis of behaviour

(b) Cognitive map

(c) Latent learning

(d) Place learning

(e) Sign learning.

21. **MCQ** – Which of the following phenomena is most likely to explain why an addictive behaviour in a human occurs in the first place?

(a) Extinction

(b) Social learning theory

(c) Spontaneous recovery

(d) Stimulus generalization

(e) Variable ratio reinforcement.

ANSWERS

1. d

They may collectively be referred to as learning theory. Theories of learning usually imply theories other than conditioning theories, i.e. non-behaviourist theories (as discussed in the accompanying textbook).

Reference: *Psychiatry: An evidence-based text*, pp. 196–197.

2.

(i) d – In the classical Pavlovian example, this might be food acting as an unconditioned stimulus.

(ii) c – In the classical Pavlovian example, this might be salivation acting as an unconditioned response. (In this Pavlovian example, at this stage a bell does not produce salivation.)

(iii) b – Classically this is the sound of a bell, acting as a conditioned stimulus.

(iv) c

(v) b – In the classic Pavlovian example, the bell is now a conditioned stimulus.

(vi) a – The conditioned stimulus now produces the conditioned response (e.g. salivation, in the classical Pavlovian example).

Reference: *Psychiatry: An evidence-based text*, pp. 197–198.

3.

(i) d – Only a 'memory trace' of the conditioned stimulus remains to be conditioned.

(ii) b – Conditioning has occurred when the conditioned response appears before the unconditioned stimulus is presented.

(iii) c – The conditioned stimulus and unconditioned stimulus are presented together.

(iv) a – The accompanying textbook, in Table 14.1, gives a famous example of such an advertisement which has been shown in many countries and which the reader will probably recognize; such recognition is evidence of the power of this type of conditioning.

Reference: *Psychiatry: An evidence-based text*, p. 198.

4. c

Pavlov found with dogs that learning could not go beyond third- or fourth-order conditioning.

Reference: *Psychiatry: An evidence-based text*, pp. 198–199.

5.

(i) a

(ii) d – The conditioned response transfers spontaneously to stimuli similar to, but different from, the original conditioned stimulus.

(iii) c

(iv) e – This shows that extinction does not involve an 'erasing' of the original learning but rather a learning to inhibit or suppress the conditioned response when the conditioned stimulus is continually presented without an unconditioned stimulus.

Reference: *Psychiatry: An evidence-based text*, p. 199.

6. b

The dogs started to behave in 'neurotic' ways – whining, trembling, urinating and defecating, refusing to eat and so on. It was as if the dogs did not know how to respond: was the stimulus a circle (in which case, through generalization, they 'ought' to salivate), or was it an ellipse (in which case, through discrimination, they 'should not' salivate)?

Reference: *Psychiatry: An evidence-based text*, p. 199.

7. e

In operant conditioning, the strength of conditioning is indeed measured mainly as a response rate. However, in classical conditioning, the strength of conditioning is typically measured in terms of response magnitude (e.g. the number of drops of saliva) and/or latency (how quickly a response is produced by a stimulus).

Reference: *Psychiatry: An evidence-based text*, p. 201.

8. a

This was Skinner's version of this law. Options 'b' and 'e' refer to classical conditioning.

Reference: *Psychiatry: An evidence-based text*, pp. 201–202.

9.

(i) c

(ii) a

(iii) e

(iv) d

(v) b

Reference: *Psychiatry: An evidence-based text*, p. 202.

10.

(i) a

(ii) b

(iii) b

(iv) d

(v) d

Reference: *Psychiatry: An evidence-based text*, p. 202.

11.

(i) b
(ii) b
(iii) e
(iv) a

Reference: *Psychiatry: An evidence-based text*, **p. 202.**

12.

(i) d
(ii) c
(iii) a
(iv) c

Reference: *Psychiatry: An evidence-based text*, **p. 202.**

13. b

This is illustrated in Figure 14.7 in the accompanying textbook.

Reference: *Psychiatry: An evidence-based text*, **pp. 202–203.**

14.

(i) e
(ii) d
(iii) c
(iv) b
(v) a

Reference: *Psychiatry: An evidence-based text*, **p. 204.**

15. a

The animal first learns to be afraid (the warning signal elicits an anticipatory emotional response of fear/anxiety through classical conditioning).

Reference: *Psychiatry: An evidence-based text*, **p. 204.**

16. b

After learning to be afraid, the animal learns a response to reduce the fear; for example, in a shuttle box, jumping the barrier is negatively reinforced by avoiding the shock before it is switched on.

Reference: *Psychiatry: An evidence-based text*, **p. 204.**

17. b

Reference: *Psychiatry: An evidence-based text*, **pp. 204–205.**

18. a

Note that forced reality testing is a basis for the treatment of phobias in humans.

Reference: *Psychiatry: An evidence-based text*, **pp. 203–205.**

19. c

In Seligman's study of this, dogs learned that no behaviour on their part had any effect on the occurrence of a particular event (a painful shock). This has been demonstrated by Miller and Norman using human participants; Maier and Seligman have tried to explain human depression in terms of this phenomenon.

Reference: *Psychiatry: An evidence-based text*, **pp. 206–207.**

20. a

Skinner's analysis required an accurate but neutral representation of the relationship or contingencies between antecedents, behaviours and consequences.

Reference: *Psychiatry: An evidence-based text*, **pp. 201–208.**

21. b

This, through its emphasis on observational learning/modelling, together with its claim that mere exposure to the model is sufficient for learning to take place, can quite easily explain why someone would begin to engage in behaviour that leads to addiction.

Variable ratio reinforcement explains maintenance well, but it does not explain initiation well.

Reference: *Psychiatry: An evidence-based text*, **pp. 208–209.**

Chapter 15

Motivation

QUESTIONS

Note that for answers to extended matching items (EMIs), each option (denoted a, b, c, etc.) might be used once, more than once or not at all. For multiple-choice questions (MCQs), please select the best answer.

1. **EMI** – Maslow's hierarchy of needs
   (a) Aesthetic needs
   (b) Cognitive needs
   (c) Esteem needs
   (d) Love and belongingness
   (e) Physiological needs
   (f) Safety needs
   (g) Self-actualization

   Select the most appropriate option from the list of Maslow's hierarchy of needs (not listed in hierarchical order) to which each of the following examples corresponds:
   (i) The importance of routine and familiarity
   (ii) Realizing one's full potential
   (iii) Being part of a group
   (iv) Elimination
   (v) The need for meaning and predictability.

2. **EMI** – Hierarchy of needs
   (a) Behaviours related to self-actualization
   (b) Behaviours related to survival or deficiency needs
   (c) Neither of the above

   Select the most appropriate option, relating to the hierarchy of needs, with which each of the following corresponds:
   (i) A means to an end
   (ii) D-motives
   (iii) Intrinsically satisfying
   (iv) The ambition to be a good human being.

3. **MCQ** – Select one incorrect statement regarding Maslow's theory of the hierarchy of needs:
   (a) Higher-level needs are considered to be a later evolutionary development; self-actualization is a fairly recent need.
   (b) Needs lower down in the hierarchy must be satisfied before one can attend to needs higher up.
   (c) The higher up the hierarchy one goes, the easier it becomes to achieve the need.
   (d) The higher up the hierarchy one goes, the more the need becomes linked to life experience and the less 'biological' it becomes.

   (e) To reduce the full range of human motives to drives that must be satisfied or removed is mistaken.

4. **EMI** – Concept of motivation
   (a) Drive
   (b) Kibra
   (c) Negative reinforcement
   (d) Pleasure principle
   (e) Theory of hedonism

   Regarding the history of the concept of motivation, select the most appropriate option to which each of the following corresponds:
   (i) Proposed by the philosopher Hobbes
   (ii) Central to Freud's psychoanalytic theory
   (iii) Central to Skinner's operant conditioning
   (iv) Proposed by Woodworth.

5. **MCQ** – Select one incorrect statement regarding the hunger drive:
   (a) According to the glucostatic theory, the primary stimulus for hunger is a decrease in the level of blood glucose below a set-point.
   (b) According to Green, the lipostatic theory focuses on the end product of glucose metabolism.
   (c) According to Nisbett's version of the lipostatic theory, people have a body mass set-point about which their body mass fluctuates within relatively narrow limits; this is determined by the level of fat in adipocytes.
   (d) After depriving rats of food so that their body mass is substantially lowered, if lesions are made in the lateral hypothalamus they start eating more rather than less food, whereas this lesion lowers the body mass set-point in normal rats, which then eat less.
   (e) The hunger pangs theory of Cannon is a drive-reduction theory.

6. **MCQ** – Which of the following theories and models is/are least likely to be associated with encouraging the consumption of a varied diet?
   (a) Cephalic phase responses
   (b) Cultural evolution

(c) Food's incentive properties

(d) Leaky barrel model

(e) Sensory-specific satiety.

7. **MCQ** – In general, which of the following is most likely to be associated with being overweight in humans?

(a) Eating too quickly

(b) Hypothalamic dysfunction

(c) Lack of impulse control

(d) Low basal metabolic rate

(e) Poor ability to delay gratification.

8. **EMI** – Drive-reduction theory

(a) Drive reduction

(b) Drive reduction reinforces the drive-reducing behaviour

(c) Goal-directed behaviour

(d) Need reduction

(e) Tissue need

The figure below is a summary of drive-reduction theory. Select the most appropriate option from the above reinforcement schedules to which each of the labels corresponds:

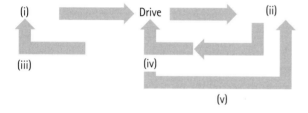

9. **MCQ** – Which of the following core social motives (after Fiske) underlies the others?

(a) Belonging

(b) Controlling

(c) Self-enhancing

(d) Trusting

(e) Understanding.

10. **MCQ** – Which of the following is least likely to be related to competence motives?

(a) Achievement motivation

(b) Curiosity drive

(c) Exploration

(d) Optimum-level theory

(e) Psychological reactance.

ANSWERS

1.

(i)   f
(ii) g
(iii) d
(iv) e
(v)   b

Reference: Psychiatry: An evidence-based text, **p. 214.**

2.

(i)   b
(ii) b
(iii) a
(iv) a

Reference: Psychiatry: An evidence-based text, **p. 214.**

3. c

The opposite is said to be the case. Many human goals are remote and long-term and can be achieved only in a series of steps. This pursuit of aims and goals that lie very much in the future is unique to human beings, although individuals differ in their ability to set and realize such goals.

Reference: Psychiatry: An evidence-based text, **pp. 214–215.**

4.

(i)   e – The seventeenth-century English philosopher Thomas Hobbes proposed this theory, according to which all behaviour is determined by the seeking of pleasure and the avoidance of pain.
(ii) d
(iii) c
(iv) a – This term was first used, in this context, by Robert Woodworth.

Reference: Psychiatry: An evidence-based text, **p. 215.**

5. e

The theory is a homeostatic drive theory.

Reference: Psychiatry: An evidence-based text, **pp. 216–218.**

6. d

Reference: Psychiatry: An evidence-based text, **pp. 216–220.**

7. d

Differences in basal metabolic rate largely determine our body mass.

Reference: Psychiatry: An evidence-based text, **p. 220.**

8.

(i)   e
(ii) c
(iii) d
(iv) a
(v)   b

Reference: Psychiatry: An evidence-based text, **p. 221.**

9. a

Reference: Psychiatry: An evidence-based text, **p. 226.**

10. a

The master reinforcer that keeps most of us motivated over long periods of time is, according to White, the need to confirm our sense of personal competence.

Reference: Psychiatry: An evidence-based text, **pp. 223–225.**

Chapter 16

Perception

QUESTIONS

Note that for answers to extended matching items (EMIs), each option (denoted a, b, c, etc.) might be used once, more than once or not at all. For multiple-choice questions (MCQs), please select the best answer.

1. **EMI** – Gestalt laws of perception
   (a) Closure
   (b) Common fate
   (c) Continuity
   (d) Part–whole relationship
   (e) Proximity
   (f) Similarity

From the above list of Gestalt laws of perception, select the most appropriate option to which each of the following examples corresponds:
   (i) The perception of a series of musical notes, occurring one after the other with little delay, as a single melody.
   (ii) A group of people running in the same direction appear to be unified in their purpose.
   (iii) The same music melody can be recognized when hummed, whistled or played with different instruments and in different ways.
   (iv) All the separate voices in a choir are heard as an entity.

2. **MCQ** – An experiment is conducted in which participants are shown the following diagram and have to match either the large or the small letter as quickly as possible. Which of the following results is most likely to occur?

```
H          H          H H H
H          H        H H    H H
H          H        H        H
H          H        H
H HHHHHHH H         H
H          H         H H H
H          H            H H H
H          H                   H
H          H        H          H
H          H         H        H
H          H           H H H H
```

   (a) The time to identify the large letter is significantly longer if the small component letters are matched to the large letter.
   (b) The time to identify the large letter is significantly longer if the small component letters are not matched to the large letter.
   (c) The time to identify the large letter is significantly shorter if the small component letters are matched to the large letter.
   (d) The time to identify the large letter is significantly shorter if the small component letters are not matched to the large letter.
   (e) None of the above.

3. **MCQ** – Regarding the importance of non-pictorial cues for depth perception, which of the following is not binocular?
   (a) Accommodation
   (b) Convergence
   (c) Retinal disparity
   (d) Stereopsis
   (e) None of the above.

4. **EMI** – Pictorial depth cues
   (a) Aerial perspective
   (b) Height in the horizontal plane
   (c) Linear perspective
   (d) Light and shadow
   (e) Motion parallax
   (f) Relative brightness
   (g) Relative size
   (h) Superimposition
   (i) Texture gradient

From the above list of pictorial depth cues, select the most appropriate option to which each of the following descriptions corresponds:
   (i) Railway tracks appear to converge as they recede into the distance.
   (ii) An object that blocks the view of another is seen as being nearer.
   (iii) Objects at a great distance appear to have a different colour.
   (iv) While sand looks rough close up, a stretch of beach looks more smooth and uniform.
   (v) Objects nearer to us seem to move faster than more distant objects.

5. **MCQ** – Suppose you stare at a bright light for a few seconds and then look away. You will experience an after-image. Now if you were quickly to look at a nearby object and then at an object further away, the after-image would seem to shrink and swell, appearing to be larger when you looked at the more distant object. Which of the following best accounts for this phenomenon?
   (a) Brightness constancy
   (b) Colour constancy
   (c) Location constancy
   (d) Shape constancy
   (e) Size constancy.

6. **EMI** – Perceptual illusions
   (a) Ambiguous figure
   (b) Distortion
   (c) Fiction
   (d) Light and shadow
   (e) Paradoxical figure
   (f) None of the above

From the above list, select the most appropriate perceptual illusion, if any, to which each of the following illusions corresponds:
   (i)   Ponzo illusion
   (ii) Twisted card illusion
   (iii) Necker cube
   (iv) Penrose impossible triangle
   (v)   Rubin's vase.

7. **EMI** – Apparent movement
   (a) Autokinetic effect
   (b) Induced movement
   (c) Motion after-effects
   (d) Phi phenomenon
   (e) Stroboscopic motion

From the above list of types of apparent movement, select the most appropriate option to which each of the following corresponds:
   (i)   When a number of separate lights are each turned on and off in quick succession, this can give the impression of a single light moving from one position to another.
   (ii) While sitting in a train at a railway station you might notice that you are 'moving backwards', when in fact it is the train on the next set of tracks that has started moving forwards.
   (iii) The mechanism by which motion pictures at the cinema operate.
   (iv) If you stare at a waterfall and then switch your gaze to the ground surrounding the water, the ground appears to be moving in the opposite direction.

8. **MCQ** – With respect to the visual perception of movement, select one incorrect statement:

   (a) According to Braddick, the human visual system seems to have two separate systems for measuring the speed and direction of individual features moving in the retinal image: a long-range feature-tracking system which seems to infer motion from one instant to the next; and a short-range motion-sensing system which seems to measure motion more directly by signalling changes in the image content over time.
   (b) If a lighted cigarette is moved about in a dark room, the cigarette will be perceived as moving, even though there are no background cues or frames of reference, because of the autokinetic effect.
   (c) M-type ganglion cells may respond to abrupt temporal changes.
   (d) The Rogers–Ramachandran illusion of shading reveals the assumption made by the visual system that light is expected to shine from above.
   (e) With respect to the apparent ability of the brain to distinguish between eye movements that signal movement of objects and eye (and head) movements that do not signal movement, Gregory has described two systems: the image–retina system, which responds to changes in the visual field that produce changes in the retinal image; and the eye–head system, which responds to movements of the head and eyes.

9. **MCQ** – Select one correct statement. A constructivist theory is:
   (a) Bottom-up
   (b) Direct
   (c) Essentially innate
   (d) Nativist
   (e) Traditional.

10. **MCQ** – Which of the following is least likely to influence perception through a direct influence on set?
   (a) Cultural factor
   (b) Expectation
   (c) Instruction
   (d) Interpreter
   (e) Reward and punishment.

11. **EMI** – Perceptual set
   (a) Beliefs
   (b) Cognitive style
   (c) Context and expectations
   (d) Emotion
   (e) Motivation
   (f) Values

From the above list relating to perceptual set, select the most appropriate option to which each of the following corresponds:
   (i)   A ufologist may perceive an ambiguous object in the sky differently from a person who is sure that there are no intelligent life forms in existence that visit the earth in UFOs.

(ii) Perceptual defence.

(iii) Hungry people are more likely to perceive vague or ambiguous pictures as relating to their hunger.

(iv) Perceptual accentuation.

(v) Subjects asked to copy the following briefly presented stimulus

PARIS
IN THE
THE SPRING

typically, incorrectly, write 'PARIS IN THE SPRING'.

12. **MCQ** – Select the option which is least likely to be correct. In the theory of direct visual perception (Gibson) the information provided by the optic array:
   (a) entails affordances
   (b) entails texture gradient
   (c) entails optic flow patterns
   (d) is essentially ambiguous
   (e) provides information for perception in a direct way involving little or no (unconscious) information-processing, computations or internal representations.

13. **MCQ** – Which of the following statements regarding visual perception is not true about both Gibson's and Gregory's theories?
   (a) Meaningless sensory cues must be supplemented by memory, habit, experience and so on in order to construct a meaningful world.
   (b) Perceptual experience can be influenced by learning.
   (c) Perception is an active process.

(d) Some kind of physiological system is needed in order to perceive.

(e) Visual perception is mediated by light reflected from surfaces and objects.

14. **EMI** – Neisser's analysis-by-synthesis model of perception
   (a) Affordances
   (b) Bottom-up
   (c) Feature analysis
   (d) Perceptual exploration search for expected features
   (e) Schema
   (f) Sensory cues/features from the stimulus environment
   (g) Top-down
   (h) Transactionalism

The figure below is a summary of Neisser's analysis-by-synthesis model of perception. Select the most appropriate option from the above reinforcement schedules to which each of the labels corresponds:

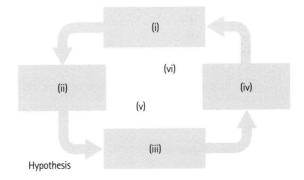

ANSWERS

1.

(i) e – Elements appearing close together in space or time tend to be perceived together.

(ii) b – Elements seen moving together are perceived as belonging together.

(iii) d

(iv) f

Reference: *Psychiatry: An evidence-based text*, **p. 231.**

2. e

The time to identify the large letter has been found to be unaffected by whether or not the small letters matched the large letter. On the other hand, the time taken to identify the small letters has been found to be affected by whether the large letter matched or not: when the large and small letters were different, response times were longer, as shown in Table 16.1 on page 231 of the accompanying textbook. This suggests that it is difficult to avoid processing the whole, and that global processing necessarily occurs before any more detailed perceptual analysis.

Reference: *Psychiatry: An evidence-based text*, **pp. 230–231.**

3. a

Reference: *Psychiatry: An evidence-based text*, **p. 232.**

4.

(i) c

(ii) h

(iii) a – An example is the hazy bluish tint of distant mountains.

(iv) i – Textured surfaces look rougher close up than from a distance.

(v) e – An example is how telegraph poles near the track may appear to flash by when the train is moving, compared with poles in the distance.

Reference: *Psychiatry: An evidence-based text*, **pp. 232–233.**

5. e

The after-image has a fixed size on the retina.

Reference: *Psychiatry: An evidence-based text*, **p. 233.**

6.

(i) b – This is illustrated in Figure 16.11(a) in the accompanying textbook.

(ii) b – This is illustrated in Figure 16.11(f) in the accompanying textbook.

(iii) a – This is illustrated in Figure 16.12(a) in the accompanying textbook.

(iv) e – This is illustrated in Figure 16.13(a) in the accompanying textbook.

(v) a

Reference: *Psychiatry: An evidence-based text*, **pp. 234–235.**

7.

(i) d – This can be explained by the law of continuity (see Box 16.1 on page 231 of the accompanying textbook).

(ii) b – Induced movement occurs when we perceive an object to be moving, although in reality the object is stationary and the surroundings are moving.

(iii) e – This can be explained by the law of continuity (see Box 16.1 on page 231 of the accompanying textbook).

(iv) c

Reference: *Psychiatry: An evidence-based text*, **pp. 231–236.**

8. b

The phenomenon described is correct, but the reason given for it is not. If you look at a stationary spot of light in an otherwise completely dark room, the light will appear to move; this apparent movement is the autokinetic effect.

The Rogers–Ramachandran illusion of shading is shown in Figure 16.15 on page 237 of the accompanying textbook.

Reference: *Psychiatry: An evidence-based text*, **pp. 236–238.**

9. e

It is top-down (not bottom-up), indirect (not direct), primarily the result of learning and experience (not essentially innate), empiricist (not nativist) and traditional (rather than ecological).

Reference: *Psychiatry: An evidence-based text*, **p. 238.**

10. d

Set acts as an interpreter and a selector. Several factors can influence or induce set, most being perceiver (or organismic) variables. But some relate to the nature of the stimulus or the conditions under which it is perceived. Both types of variable influence perception indirectly, through directly influencing set, which, as such, is a perceiver variable or characteristic (see also Fig. 16.18 in the accompanying textbook).

Reference: *Psychiatry: An evidence-based text*, **pp. 239–240.**

11.

(i) a – The beliefs we hold about the world can affect our interpretation of ambiguous sensory signals.

(ii) d – This refers to laboratory findings that subliminally perceived words that evoke unpleasant emotions take longer to be perceived at a conscious level than neutral words.

(iii) e

(iv) f – This refers to the phenomenon whereby, for example, children who were taught to value something more highly than they had done previously perceived the valued object as being larger.

(v) c

Reference: *Psychiatry: An evidence-based text,* **p. 240.**

12. d

The optic array provides unambiguous information about the layout and relevant properties of objects in space.

Reference: *Psychiatry: An evidence-based text,* **p. 241.**

13. a

This view is consistent with Gregory's theory but not with Gibson's theory of perception.

Reference: *Psychiatry: An evidence-based text,* **pp. 242–243.**

14.

(i) f
(ii) c
(iii) e
(iv) d
(v) b
(vi) g

Reference: *Psychiatry: An evidence-based text,* **p. 243.**

Chapter 17

Memory

QUESTIONS

Note that for answers to extended matching items (EMIs), each option (denoted a, b, c, etc.) might be used once, more than once or not at all. For multiple-choice questions (MCQs), please select the best answer.

1. **EMI** – Memory storage
   (a) Long-term
   (b) Sensory
   (c) Short-term
   (d) None of the above

   From the above list relating to forms of memory storage, select the most appropriate option to which each of the following corresponds:
   (i) It has an iconic memory.
   (ii) The acoustic similarity of words does not appear significantly to affect recall from this type of memory storage.
   (iii) It has an echoic memory.
   (iv) Its capacity is usually around 7±2 bits of information.
   (v) It has a primacy effect.

2. **MCQ** – Which of the following can be reduced to the least number of chunks?
   (a) DKSJLRXPQQDWNJB
   (b) RICHARDOFYORKGAVEBATTLEINVAIN
   (c) 19421967200120121948
   (d) 24681012141618202224...
   (e) 5, 7, 7, 2, 7, 0

3. **EMI** – Multi-store model of memory
   (a) Attention
   (b) Environmental input
   (c) Iconic memory and echoic memory
   (d) Long-term memory
   (e) Rehearsal
   (f) Response output
   (g) Retrieval
   (h) Short-term memory
   (i) Storage

   The figure below depicts the multi-store model of memory. Select the most appropriate option to which each of the labels corresponds:

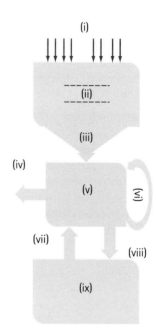

4. **MCQ** – Select one incorrect statement regarding memory:
   (a) The Brown–Peterson technique is one of rehearsal prevention.
   (b) The levels-of-processing approach includes a central processor that can carry out analysis at a phonemic level.
   (c) The levels-of-processing approach includes a central processor that can carry out analysis at a semantic level.
   (d) The multi-store model is also known as the dual-memory model.
   (e) The recency effect tends to be robust to the prevention of rehearsal.

5. **MCQ** – Which of the following would you least expect in a subject with anterograde amnesia?
    (a) An ability to learn motor skills
    (b) An ability to learn perceptual skills
    (c) An ability to remember perceptual skills
    (d) Poor recency effect
    (e) Relatively good procedural memory.

6. **EMI** – Forms of memory
    (a) Episodic
    (b) Semantic
    (c) Procedural
    (d) None of the above

From the above list relating to forms of memory, select the most appropriate option to which each of the following corresponds:
    (i) Autobiographical memory
    (ii) Correctly stating 'I know that bicycles have two wheels'.
    (iii) Knowing how to use a particular computer program.
    (iv) Flashback memory.

7. **MCQ** – Select one correct option to which declarative memory best refers:
    (a) Autobiographical memory and flashback memory
    (b) Episodic memory and semantic memory
    (c) Procedural memory and episodic memory
    (d) Procedural memory and semantic memory
    (e) Procedural memory and working memory.

8. **MCQ** – Which of the following is not part of working memory (Baddeley and Hitch)?
    (a) Articulatory loop
    (b) Central executive
    (c) Phonological driver
    (d) Slave system
    (e) Visuospatial scratchpad.

9. **MCQ** – Select one correct statement. Semantic memory is part of:
    (a) Episodic memory
    (b) Long-term memory
    (c) Sensory memory
    (d) Working memory
    (e) None of the above.

10. **MCQ** – Select one incorrect option regarding schemata:
    (a) They allow us to 'fill in the gaps' when our memories are incomplete.
    (b) They do not produce significant distortions in memory processes.
    (c) They have a powerful effect on the way in which memories for events are encoded.
    (d) They help us to make the world more predictable.
    (e) They provide us with ready-made expectations that help us to interpret the flow of information reaching the senses.

11. **EMI** – Theories of forgetting
    (a) Decay theory
    (b) Displacement theory
    (c) Interference theory
    (d) Motivated-forgetting theory
    (e) Retrieval-failure theory and cue-dependent forgetting

From the above list relating to theories of forgetting, select the most appropriate option to which each of the following corresponds:
    (i) Tip-of-the-tongue phenomenon
    (ii) Ego defence
    (iii) Changes in engrams through disuse
    (iv) Recall 8 h later of a list of ten nonsense syllables is on average higher in those who sleep immediately after learning them than in those who stay awake and continue with their normal activities.

ANSWERS

1.

(i)   b
(ii) a
(iii) b
(iv) c
(v)   a

Reference: *Psychiatry: An evidence-based text*, **pp. 246–251.**

2. d

This series results from the mapping $x \mapsto 2x$. This rule represents a single chunk. All the other options involve > one chunk.

Option 'a' clearly corresponds to many chunks. Option 'b' corresponds to seven chunks (for the words RICHARD OF YORK...). Option 'c' corresponds to five chunks (for the years 1942, 1967...). Option 'e' corresponds to at least three (5772 HC, 7, 0) and usually six (5, 7, 7, 2, 7, 0) chunks; in either case more than one.

Reference: *Psychiatry: An evidence-based text*, **p. 248.**

3.

(i)   b
(ii)   c
(iii) a
(iv)   f
(v)   h
(vi)   e
(vii) g
(viii) i
(ix)   d

Reference: *Psychiatry: An evidence-based text*, **p. 250.**

4. e

While the primacy effect is largely unaffected, the recency effect tends to disappear.

Reference: *Psychiatry: An evidence-based text*, **pp. 248–251.**

5. d

Reference: *Psychiatry: An evidence-based text*, **pp. 252–255.**

6.

(i)   a
(ii) b
(iii) c
(iv) a

Reference: *Psychiatry: An evidence-based text*, **pp. 254–255.**

7. b

Declarative memory is the type that corresponds to 'knowing that'. Table 17.2 on page 254 of the accompanying textbook makes the relationships between many of these different types of memory clear.

Reference: *Psychiatry: An evidence-based text*, **p. 254.**

8. c

There is a phonological (or articulatory) loop, which is not a driver but a slave system.

Reference: *Psychiatry: An evidence-based text*, **p. 255.**

9. b

As with Question 7, Table 17.2 on page 254 of the accompanying textbook makes the relationships between many different types of long-term memory clear.

Reference: *Psychiatry: An evidence-based text*, **pp. 254 and 256.**

10. b

They can produce significant distortions in memory processes, because they have a powerful effect on the way in which memories for events are encoded. This happens when new information conflicts with existing schemata.

Reference: *Psychiatry: An evidence-based text*, **p. 256.**

11.

(i)   e – This phenomenon illustrates the role of retrieval cues.
(ii) d – According to psychoanalytical theory, memories that are likely to induce guilt, embarrassment, shame or anxiety are actively, but unconsciously, pushed out of consciousness as a form of ego defence. (Motivated-forgetting theory corresponds to repression.)
(iii) a
(iv) c – These results are illustrated in Figure 17.8 on page 257 of the accompanying textbook.

Reference: *Psychiatry: An evidence-based text*, **pp. 256–261.**

Chapter 18

Language and thought

QUESTIONS

Note that for answers to extended matching items (EMIs), each option (denoted a, b, c, etc.) might be used once, more than once or not at all. For multiple-choice questions (MCQs), please select the best answer.

1. **EMI** – Relationship between language and thought
   (a) Language and thought are one and the same
   (b) Language is dependent on, and reflects, thought
   (c) Thought and language are initially quite separate activities
   (d) Thought is dependent on, or caused by, language

From the above list relating to theories of the relationship between language and thought, select the option with which each of the following is best associated:
   (i) Piaget
   (ii) Social constructionism
   (iii) Vygotsky
   (iv) Peripheralism.

2. **MCQ** – Select the most correct statement. The weakest version of the linguistic relativity hypothesis posits that:
   (a) Language affects perception
   (b) Language determines thought
   (c) Language influences memory
   (d) Language is not related at all to cognition and thought
   (e) Thought determines language.

3. **MCQ** – Of the following focal colours, which is the last to emerge in the history of languages?
   (a) Black
   (b) Green
   (c) Grey
   (d) Red
   (e) White.

4. **MCQ** – Select one correct statement. For cultures whose languages use only three basic colour terms, the three focal colours are most likely to be:
   (a) Black, white and red
   (b) Green, red and blue
   (c) Green, red and grey
   (d) Orange, red and blue
   (e) Orange, red and grey.

5. **EMI** – Linguistic codes
   (a) **Elaborated code**
   (b) **Restricted code**

From the above list, select the option with which each of the following characteristics is best associated:
   (i) Context-independent
   (ii) 'I' is used often
   (iii) Tends to stress the present
   (iv) Greater use of pronouns than nouns.

6. **EMI** – Pioneers in the study of language and thought
   (a) Berlin
   (b) Piaget
   (c) Vygotsky
   (d) Watson
   (e) Whorf
   (f) None of the above

From the above list of pioneers, select the option with which each of the following concepts relating to language and thought is best associated:
   (i) A child should begin talking about objects that are not present in his or her immediate surroundings only after object permanence has developed.
   (ii) Acquiring a language involves acquiring a *Weltanschauung.*
   (iii) Before the age of 2 years, pre-linguistic thought and pre-intellectual language exist as separate and independent activities.

7. **EMI** – Egocentric speech
   (a) Autistic speech
   (b) Concrete operational stage
   (c) Conservation of volume
   (d) Egocentric speech
   (e) Object permanence
   (f) Social origin of speech
   (g) Socialized speech
   (h) Speech for self
   (i) Speech for others

The figure below depicts the differences between Piaget and Vygotsky with respect to egocentric speech. Select the most appropriate option to which each of the labels above corresponds:

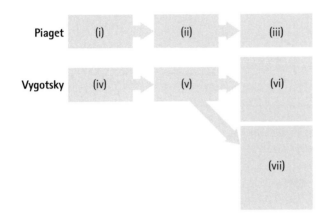

8. **MCQ** – Which of the following is least likely to be correct?
   (a) Babbling is an example of pre-intellectual language in Vygotsky's model.
   (b) Ebonics is a form of 'black English'.
   (c) Synpraxic is a primitive linguistic form in which words cannot be detached from the actions or objects they denote.
   (d) The strong version of the linguistic relativity hypothesis correctly predicts that form recognition should develop earlier in Navaho Indian children who speak both English and Navaho than in American children of European descent who speak only English (Navaho stresses the importance of form such that handling verbs involves different words depending on what is being handled).
   (e) The strong version of the linguistic relativity hypothesis correctly predicts that the form or shape recognition abilities of Navaho Indian children who speak either only Navaho, which stresses the importance of form (such that handling verbs involves different words depending on what is being handled), or Navaho and English should be greater than those of American children of European descent who speak only English.

ANSWERS

1.

(i) **b** – According to Piaget, language reflects the individual's level of cognitive development.

(ii) **d** – Social constructionists regard language as providing a basis for all our thought, a system of categories for dividing up experience and giving it meaning.

(iii) **c** – The view that thought and language are initially quite separate activities and then come together and interact at a later point in development (around the age of 2 years) is associated with this Russian psychologist.

(iv) **a** – This view is associated with Watson, the founder of behaviourism. His theory is called peripheralism, because Watson regarded 'thinking' as occurring peripherally in the larynx rather than centrally in the brain.

> **Reference:** *Psychiatry: An evidence-based text*, **p. 266.**

2. c

Information that is described more easily in a particular language will be better remembered than information that is more difficult to describe.

> **Reference:** *Psychiatry: An evidence-based text*, **p. 267–268.**

3. c

The colour terms appear to emerge in a particular sequence in the history of languages. This is illustrated in Figure 18.2 on page 270 of the accompanying textbook.

> **Reference:** *Psychiatry: An evidence-based text*, **pp. 268–270.**

4. a

For cultures with only three basic colour terms, these will be black, white and red. This finding suggests that there are certain focal colours which will always be labelled if colour terms are used at all. It is of interest that the Nazis chose these three visceral colours for their flags, with a black swastika (*Hakenkreuz*) on a white circular area surrounded by a red background (red presumably representing blood).

> **Reference:** *Psychiatry: An evidence-based text*, **pp. 268–269.**

5.

(i) **a** – Meaning is made explicit, e.g. 'James gave this book to me.'

(ii) **a** – This makes clear the speaker's intentions and emphasizes precise descriptions of experiences and feelings.

(iii) **b** – The here-and-now tends to be stressed.

(iv) **b** – Restricted code is characteristically grammatically crude, repetitive and rigid.

> **Reference:** *Psychiatry: An evidence-based text*, **pp. 271–272.**

6.

(i) **b** – According to Piaget, a child should begin talking about objects that are not present in his or her immediate surroundings only after understanding that things continue to exist even when they are not being perceived.

(ii) **e** – According to Whorf's linguistic determinism, language determines our concepts, and we can think only through the use of concepts. So, acquiring a language involves acquiring a 'world view'.

(iii) **c**

> **Reference:** *Psychiatry: An evidence-based text*, **pp. 267–274.**

7.

(i) a

(ii) d

(iii) g

(iv) f

(v) d

(vi) h or i.

(vii) i or h.

> **Reference:** *Psychiatry: An evidence-based text*, **p. 274.**

8. d

Further details are given in Box 18.1 on page 268 of the accompanying textbook.

> **Reference:** *Psychiatry: An evidence-based text*, **Ch. 18.**

Part 2 : Developmental, behavioural, and sociocultural psychiatry

Chapter 19

Personality

QUESTIONS

Note that for answers to extended matching items (EMIs), each option (denoted a, b, c, etc.) might be used once, more than once or not at all. For multiple-choice questions (MCQs), please select the best answer.

1. **MCQ** – Select one correct statement. The definition of personality in terms of 'enduring patterns of perceiving, relating to, and thinking about the environment and oneself that are exhibited in a wide range of social and personal contexts' is primarily from:
   (a) Cattell
   (b) DSM-IV
   (c) Eysenck Personality Questionnaire (manual)
   (d) ICD-9
   (e) ICD-10.

2. **MCQ** – It is said that we tend to explain our own behaviour as being reasoned, but ascribe that of others to enduring personality characteristics. Select one incorrect statement regarding this effect:
   (a) An illustrative example is that if we see you at a party telling jokes and ask you why, then you are likely to respond with a reason (e.g. 'To make people laugh' or 'To break the ice'); but if we point to someone else at the party who is telling jokes and ask you why he is doing that, you are much more likely to respond with a description relating to his personality (e.g. 'He's a funny man' or 'He's a real extravert').
   (b) It arises partly because we have ready access to our thoughts and motives.
   (c) It arises partly because we have ready access to the thoughts and motives of others.
   (d) It is also known as the correspondence bias.
   (e) It is also known as the fundamental attribution error.

3. **EMI** – Study of personality
   (a) Idiographic approach
   (b) Nomothetic approach

   Select the option from the above approaches with which each of the following is better associated:
   (i) Under this approach, it is possible, at least in theory, to identify the key personality dimensions common to every person.
   (ii) One can measure where an individual lies on each dimension using a standardized questionnaire or observation system.

(iii) A person can have unique characteristics.
(iv) Some people have characteristics that many others do not have.
(v) The belief that every human being has a sense of humour but that some people have a strong sense of humour while others have a weak sense of humour.
(vi) The belief that some people are greedy and some are not at all greedy.

4. **EMI** – Models of personality
   (a) Cognitive approach
   (b) Humanist approach
   (c) Trait model
   (d) Psychoanalytical theory

   From the above list relating to models of personality, select the option with which each of the following is best associated:
   (i) 16PF
   (ii) Kelly's construct theory
   (iii) EPQ
   (iv) Maslow's theory of self-actualization.

5. **MCQ** – Select one incorrect statement regarding trait models of personality:
   (a) They assume that traits are relatively stable over time.
   (b) They assume that traits influence behaviour.
   (c) They assume that trait levels differ among individuals.
   (d) They are fundamentally based on cluster analysis.
   (e) They are nomothetic theories.

6. **MCQ** – Who, of the following, is least associated with trait models of personality?
   (a) Carl Rogers
   (b) Cattell
   (c) Hippocrates
   (d) McCrae and John
   (e) Saucier and Goldberg.

7. **EMI** – Study of personality
   (a) Cattell's second-order factors
   (b) EPQ
   (c) Both of the above
   (d) None of the above

From the above list relating to the study of personality, select the option with which each of the following is best associated:
   (i) Lie scale
   (ii) Anxiety
   (iii) Exvia-invia
   (iv) Humanistic theory
   (v) Neuroticism
   (vi) Trait models
   (vi) Psychoticism.

8. **MCQ** – Which of the following is not a factor in the five-factor model of personality?
   (a) Aggressiveness
   (b) Conscientiousness
   (c) Extraversion
   (d) Neuroticism
   (e) Openness to experience.

9. **MCQ** – With which of the following are cognitive models of personality least associated?
   (a) The repertory grid
   (b) The theory that people's behaviour is determined by how they construe particular situations
   (c) The theory that people's behaviour is determined by how they interpret particular situations
   (d) The theory that people's behaviour is determined by their characteristic ways of thinking about the world
   (e) The theory that people's behaviour is determined by underlying traits.

10. **EMI** – Study of personality
    (a) Carl Roger's theory

(b) Eysenck's model of personality
(c) Kelly's construct theory
(d) None of the above

From the above list relating to the study of personality, select the option with which each of the following is best associated:
   (i) Aspects of personality are assessed along binary measures.
   (ii) Aspects of personality are assessed along dimensional measures.
   (iii) The model is that of 'humans as scientists'.
   (iv) Personality is about how people see themselves, their self-image and their interactions with others and the world.
   (v) It formed the basis of client-centred counselling.

11. **MCQ** – With which of the following is client-centred counselling least associated?
    (a) Clients can heal themselves.
    (b) The therapist offers advice to the client.
    (c) The therapist should react to the client with empathy.
    (d) The therapist should react to the client with warmth and genuineness.
    (e) Unconditional positive regard.

12. **MCQ** – Select one incorrect statement regarding the genetics of personality:
    (a) Heritability estimates of the factors of the five-factor model of personality are around 40–50 per cent.
    (b) Molecular genetic studies tend consistently to show significant linkage of *DRD4* and novelty-seeking behaviour.
    (c) Twin models in this field tend to assume no dominance effects.
    (d) Twin models in this field tend to assume no epistasis.
    (e) Twin models in this field tend to assume the existence ideally of many genes of small effect.

ANSWERS

1. b

Reference: *Psychiatry: An evidence-based text*, **p. 278.**

2. c

It is known that our subjective belief in personality is, at least in part, misleading.
Reference: *Psychiatry: An evidence-based text*, **p. 278.**

3.

(i) b
(ii) b
(iii) a
(iv) a
(v) b
(vi) a
Reference: *Psychiatry: An evidence-based text*, **p. 278.**

4.

(i) c – PF stands for personality factor.
(ii) a
(iii) c – EPQ stands for the Eysenck Personality Questionnaire.
(iv) b
Reference: *Psychiatry: An evidence-based text*, **pp. 279–282.**

5. d

They are based on the statistical technique of factor analysis.
Reference: *Psychiatry: An evidence-based text*, **p. 279.**

6. a

It is known that our subjective belief in personality is, at least in part, misleading.
Reference: *Psychiatry: An evidence-based text*, **pp. 279–281.**

7.

(i) b
(ii) a
(iii) a
(iv) d
(v) b
(vi) c
(vii) b
Reference: *Psychiatry: An evidence-based text*, **p. 279.**

8. a

The fifth, missing, factor is agreeableness.
Reference: *Psychiatry: An evidence-based text*, **pp. 279–280.**

9. e

Reference: *Psychiatry: An evidence-based text*, **pp. 280–281.**

10.

(i) c
(ii) b
(iii) c
(iv) a
(v) a
Reference: *Psychiatry: An evidence-based text*, **pp. 279–281.**

11. b

Rogers' theory is based around therapy and its importance and, essentially, around the idea that clients can heal themselves; it is the main job of the therapist to facilitate this rather than to offer advice.
Reference: *Psychiatry: An evidence-based text*, **p. 281.**

12. b

Distel *et al.* (2009) reported the following estimates for heritability for neuroticism, agreeableness, conscientiousness, extraversion and openness to experience: 43, 36, 43, 47 and 54 per cent, respectively.
References: Distel MA Trull TJ, Willemsen G, Vink JM, Derom CA, Lynskey M, Martin NG, Boomsma DI (2009). The five-factor model of personality and borderline personality disorder: a genetic analysis of comorbidity. *Biological Psychiatry* **66:** 1131–38; *Psychiatry: An evidence-based text*, **pp. 281–282.**

Chapter 20

Social psychology

QUESTIONS

Note that for answers to extended matching items (EMIs), each option (denoted a, b, c, etc.) might be used once, more than once or not at all. For multiple-choice questions (MCQs), please select the best answer.

1. **EMI** – Theories of aggression
   (a) Aggression arises out of inner drives
   (b) Frustration–aggression hypothesis
   (c) Social learning
   (d) None of the above

Select the option from the above list with which each of the following is best associated:
   (i) Albert Bandura
   (ii) Reciprocal determinism
   (iii) Oedipal complex
   (iv) John Dollard.

2. **MCQ** – Select one incorrect statement regarding social psychology:
   (a) A difficulty with the frustration–aggression theory is that not all people who are frustrated turn to aggression.
   (b) A positive association between aggression and watching violence on television is consistent with social learning theory.
   (c) Social exchange theory readily explains altruism.
   (d) The bystander effect might result from group influence.
   (e) The bystander effect might result from the diffusion of responsibility effect.

3. **EMI** – Theories of persuasion and influence
   (a) Door-in-the-face technique
   (b) Foot-in-the-door technique
   (c) Both of the above
   (d) None of the above

From the above list relating to social psychological theories of persuasion and influence, select the option with which each of the following is best associated:
   (i) Perceptual contrast
   (ii) The internal wish to be consistent
   (iii) One's newly established identity
   (iv) Reciprocating a concession.

4. **MCQ** – Select one incorrect statement regarding attitudes:
   (a) A popular method of measuring attitudes uses Likert scales.
   (b) Cognitive dissonance theory was mainly put forward by Osgood.
   (c) Semantic differential scales measure attitude factors.
   (d) The Implicit Association Test has revealed a pro-white bias in many Americans.
   (e) Thurstone scales represent an early attempt to measure attitudes.

5. **EMI** – Attitudes
   (a) Activity
   (b) Evaluation
   (c) Potency
   (d) None of the above

From the above list relating to general factors regarding attitudes, select the option with which each of the following adjective pairs is best associated:
   (i) Good–bad
   (ii) Strong–weak
   (iii) Active–passive.

6. **MCQ** – Select the strongest quality in the other that humans have been found to assess on meeting a stranger:
   (a) Competence
   (b) Industriousness
   (c) Intelligence
   (d) Skilfulness
   (e) Warmth.

7. **MCQ** – Select one incorrect statement regarding social skills:
   (a) A social skill component that is particularly strongly adversely affected in those who expect rejection is self-disclosure.
   (b) A vital social skill component is being able to assert displeasure with others.
   (c) Genetic factors account for around 50 per cent of how sensitive a person is to rejection.

(d) Interpersonal rejection sensitivity is associated with a state of social hypervigilance.

(e) Interpersonal rejection sensitivity is considered to lie at the heart of poor social skills.

8. **MCQ** – Select one incorrect statement regarding the ultimatum game:

(a) Less physically symmetrical men, in terms of their face and body, are more likely to make small initial offers.

(b) Male responders who reject a low offer tend to have a higher salivary testosterone level than the average of those who accept.

(c) Offers below 20 per cent are usually rejected by responders.

(d) Offers by proposers tend to be near the 50 per cent mark, which are much more generous than they need be.

(e) One reason those offered low sums might decline these is that they are thinking of what happens in the future of the relationship, in that acceptance may be associated with continued low offers in the future.

ANSWERS

1.

(i)   c – A social psychologist and Professor Emeritus of Stanford University.
(ii) c
(iii) a
(iv) b – He was an anthropologist/sociologist based at Yale.

Reference: *Psychiatry: An evidence-based text*, **pp. 285–286.**

2. c

Reference: *Psychiatry: An evidence-based text*, **pp. 285–286.**

3.

(i)   a
(ii) b
(iii) b
(iv) a

Reference: *Psychiatry: An evidence-based text*, **pp. 286–287.**

4. b

It was mainly put forward by Festinger.

Reference: *Psychiatry: An evidence-based text*, **pp. 287–289.**

5.

(i)   b
(ii) c
(iii) a

Reference: *Psychiatry: An evidence-based text*, **p. 288.**

6. e

Competence ranks second. Warmth and competence appear to account for over 80 per cent of our perceptions of everyday social life. When we try to interpret the behaviour or form impressions of others, warmth and competence account almost entirely for how we characterize them.

Reference: *Psychiatry: An evidence-based text*, **pp. 289–290.**

7. c

A collaboration led by Nathan Gillespie at the Queensland Institute of Medical Research found that just under a third of how sensitive you were to rejection was the proportion accounted for by genes.

Reference: *Psychiatry: An evidence-based text*, **p. 291.**

8. a

Indeed, it has been found that the degree of symmetry of face and body indexes physical attractiveness and the ability to cope with a wide range of environmental stressors during development.

Reference: *Psychiatry: An evidence-based text*, **pp. 292–293.**

Chapter 21

Social science and sociocultural psychiatry

QUESTIONS

Note that for answers to extended matching items (EMIs), each option (denoted a, b, c, etc.) might be used once, more than once or not at all. For multiple-choice questions (MCQs), please select the best answer.

1. **EMI** – NS-SEC
   (a) Class 1
   (b) Class 2
   (c) Class 3
   (d) Class 4
   (e) Class 5

From the above list relating to the five-class version of the NS-SEC, select the option with which each of the following occupations is best associated:
   (i)   The self-employed
   (ii) Lower supervisory and technical occupations
   (iii) Routine occupations
   (iv) Managerial occupations.

2. **EMI** – Social class and psychiatric illness
   (a) People from higher social classes
   (b) People from lower social classes
   (c) No significant social class difference

From the above list, select the option with which each of the following is best associated:
   (i)   More likely to receive electroconvulsive therapy
   (ii) More likely to be diagnosed as suffering from schizophrenia
   (iii) More likely to receive psychotherapy
   (iv) More likely to be treated on an outpatient basis.

3. **MCQ** – In industrialized societies, which of the following is the least likely to be a cause of increased rates of morbidity from psychiatric illness in women compared with men?
   (a) Double burden
   (b) Learned helplessness
   (c) Role accumulation
   (d) Role conflict
   (e) Sick role.

4. **EMI** – Rates of schizophrenia among UK immigrants
   (a) Higher than in the indigenous population
   (b) Lower than in the indigenous population
   (c) Not significantly different from that in the indigenous population

From the above list of comparison rates of schizophrenia in immigrant groups in the UK, select the option with which each of the following groups is best associated:
   (i)   Irish immigrants
   (ii) Afro-Caribbean immigrants
   (iii) South Asian immigrants
   (iv) Second-generation British-born Afro-Caribbean people.

5. **MCQ** – In a study of illness in society, if psychiatric symptoms in a person are normalized (in a social sciences context) which of the following is not considered to be a trigger to action?
   (a) Illness behaviour
   (b) Interference with work
   (c) Interpersonal crisis
   (d) Sanctioning
   (e) Temporalizing of symptomatology.

6. **MCQ** – Which of the following is least likely to be associated with total institutions and institutionalization?
   (a) Batch living
   (b) Binary management
   (c) Degradation rituals
   (d) Depersonalization
   (e) Gatekeeping.

7. **EMI** – Concepts in social science and sociocultural psychiatry
   (a) Illness behaviour
   (b) Myth of mental illness
   (c) Negotiated order
   (d) Sick role
   (e) Total institution
   (f) Triggers to action

From the above list of concepts in social science and sociocultural psychiatry, select the option with which each of the following is best associated:

(i) Parsons
(ii) Zola
(iii) Szasz
(iv) Strauss.

8. **MCQ** – Which of the following is not one of the vulnerability factors, identified by Brown and Harris, which were thought to increase the susceptibility to depression?
   (a) Absence of a confiding relationship with a partner
   (b) Increased expressed emotion in the family
   (c) Lack of employment outside the home
   (d) Loss of mother before 11 years of age
   (e) Three or more children under 15 years of age living at home.

9. **EMI** – Concepts in social science and sociocultural psychiatry
   (a) Illness behaviour
   (b) Myth of mental illness
   (c) Negotiated order
   (d) Sick role
   (e) Strain theory
   (f) Total institution
   (g) Triggers to action

Select the option from the above list with which each of the following is best associated:
   (i) Mechanic
   (ii) Goffman
   (iii) Merton.

10. **EMI** – Concepts in social science and sociocultural psychiatry
   (a) Discreditable
   (b) Discredited
   (c) Enacted stigma
   (d) Felt stigma
   (e) None of the above

Select the option from the above list with which each of the following is best associated:
   (i) A stigma bearer's experience of discrimination
   (ii) Deviance that is not immediately visible
   (iii) Deviance that is immediately visible to others
   (iv) A construct encompassing critical, hostile or emotionally over-involved attitudes towards a relative with a disorder or impairment
   (v) Fear of discrimination.

11. **MCQ** – Which of the following has been most strongly implicated as a cause of increased rates of schizophrenia in black members of predominantly non-black societies?
   (a) Increased anomie
   (b) Increased social capital
   (c) Long-term exposure to social defeat
   (d) Status frustration
   (e) Strain theory.

12. **MCQ** – In left realism, the square of crime does not include which of the following?
   (a) Offenders
   (b) Penal institutions
   (c) Society
   (d) The state
   (e) Victims.

13. **MCQ** – Which of the following is not considered a justification for judicial punishment?
   (a) Deterrence
   (b) Incapacitation
   (c) Rehabilitation
   (d) Restorative justice
   (e) Retribution.

ANSWERS

1.

(i) c – This includes small employers and own-account workers.
(ii) d
(iii) e
(iv) a – This includes managerial and professional occupations.
Reference: Psychiatry: An evidence-based text, **p. 297.**

2.

(i) b
(ii) b
(iii) a
(iv) a
Reference: Psychiatry: An evidence-based text, **p. 297.**

3. e

One set of explanations for these differences relates to women's disadvantaged position within society generally and the particular nature of their domestic roles. An increasing proportion of women work outside the home and may suffer from the double burden of employment and domestic roles, which generates stress as a result of both role accumulation and role conflict. It has also been argued that gender role socialization produces learned helplessness.

Illness may be regarded as a form of deviance in as much as it inhibits an individual's ability to perform his or her usual social roles and hence disrupts the smooth functioning of society. The sick role is an approved social role for the 'deviant'.
Reference: Psychiatry: An evidence-based text, **pp. 298–299.**

4.

(i) a
(ii) a
(iii) b
(iv) a
Reference: Psychiatry: An evidence-based text, **pp. 298–299.**

5. a

A fifth trigger is interference with personal relationships. Illness behaviour describes the way individuals perceive, evaluate and act upon pain, discomfort or other signals or organic malfunction.
Reference: Psychiatry: An evidence-based text, **pp. 299–300.**

6. e

The doctor has been viewed as society's gatekeeper, determining the official labelling of conditions as 'health' or 'sickness' and thus controlling access to the sick role. Note that the term depersonalization is not being used in the psychopathological sense here.
Reference: Psychiatry: An evidence-based text, **pp. 299–300.**

7.

(i) d
(ii) f
(iii) b
(iv) c
Reference: Psychiatry: An evidence-based text, **Ch. 21.**

8. b

This has been related to high levels of relapse in patients with schizophrenia.
Reference: Psychiatry: An evidence-based text, **pp. 301–302.**

9.

(i) a
(ii) f
(iii) e
Reference: Psychiatry: An evidence-based text, **Ch. 21.**

10.

(i) c
(ii) a – An example is a diagnosis of schizophrenia.
(iii) b
(iv) e – This is expressed emotion.
(v) d – This is more prevalent, and hence more disabling, than enacted stigma.
Reference: Psychiatry: An evidence-based text, **pp. 301 and 303.**

11. c

It has been observed that the relative risk of schizophrenia is especially high in groups with black skin colour and originating in a developing country or of second-generation immigrant status (for whom being treated as an 'outsider' in their country of birth may be particularly distressing). Incidence rates in this population are lower in neighbourhoods with higher proportions of ethnic minority residents, most likely because of the protection they offer against discrimination and isolation. The social defeat hypothesis also proposes that stress related to social rank may be particularly harmful.
Reference: Psychiatry: An evidence-based text, **p. 302.**

12. b

Left realism takes seriously the impact of crime on victims and seeks to produce realistic ways of dealing with crime. It sees deep structural inequalities as the root cause of crime and focuses on the square of crime, each element of which, and their inter-relationships, must be explored and addressed.

Reference: *Psychiatry: An evidence-based text*, p. 304.

13. d

This movement aims to abolish not only imprisonment but punishment generally, seeking to shift the focus from the offender to the victim, with the intention of securing recompense and reconciliation between offender and victim.

Reference: *Psychiatry: An evidence-based text*, p. 304.

Chapter 22

Cultural psychiatry

QUESTIONS

Note that for answers to extended matching items (EMIs), each option (denoted a, b, c, etc.) might be used once, more than once or not at all. For multiple-choice questions (MCQs), please select the best answer.

1. **EMI** – Acculturation strategies of ethnocultural groups
   (a) Assimilation
   (b) Integration
   (c) Marginalization
   (d) Separation

From the above list of acculturation strategies of ethnocultural groups, select the option with which (i), (ii), (iii) and (iv) in the following figure are best associated:

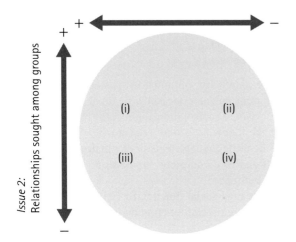

Issue 1:
Maintenance of heritage culture and identity

Issue 2:
Relationships sought among groups

2. **EMI** – Acculturation strategies of ethnocultural groups
   (a) Exclusion
   (b) Melting pot
   (c) Multiculturalism
   (d) Segregation

Select the option from the above list with which (i), (ii), (iii) and (iv) in the following figure are best associated:

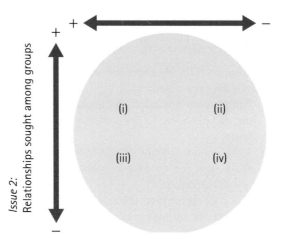

Issue 1:
Maintenance of heritage culture and identity

Issue 2:
Relationships sought among groups

3. **MCQ** – Which of the following is a description accounting for culturally neutral observations, in which the same entities can be identified across different cultures?
   (a) Edenics
   (b) Edic
   (c) Emic
   (d) Epic
   (e) Etic.

4. **EMI** – Effects on psychopathology
   (a) Pathoelaborating
   (b) Pathofacilitative
   (c) Pathogenic
   (d) Pathoplastic
   (e) Pathoreactive
   (f) Pathoselective

From the above list of the effects on psychopathology, select the option with which each of the following is best associated:
   (i) Culturally sanctioned suicide
   (ii) Heightened stress of cultural expectation leading to psychopathology
   (iii) Culture influences or models the manifestation.

5. **MCQ** – High rates of schizophrenia have been found in all but which one of the following?
   (a) Certain population isolates in northern Sweden
   (b) Daghestan
   (c) Hutterites in South Dakota
   (d) Palau islands
   (e) Several areas of Finland.

6. **EMI** – Effects on psychopathology
   (a) Pathoelaborating
   (b) Pathofacilitative
   (c) Pathogenic
   (d) Pathoplastic
   (e) Pathoreactive
   (f) Pathoselective

Select the option from the above list with which each of the following is best associated:
   (i) Culture does not affect the actual universalism of the disorder, but it does affect the frequency of onset.
   (ii) Although not directly affecting the disorder, it does affect how the disorder is viewed and dealt with within the culture.
   (iii) Universal behaviour reactions that may become exaggerated through reinforcement.

7. **MCQ** – High rates of psychiatric symptoms are found in all but which one of the following groups?
   (a) Chinese immigrants in the UK
   (b) Dutch Antillean immigrants in the Netherlands
   (c) Moroccan immigrants in the Netherlands
   (d) Surinamese immigrants in the Netherlands
   (e) Norwegian immigrants in the USA.

8. **EMI** – Forms of schizophrenia
   (a) 1–2 per cent
   (b) 10–11 per cent
   (c) 20–21 per cent
   (d) 30–31 per cent
   (e) 40–41 per cent

From the above list of potential percentages of patients with different forms of schizophrenia reported in the WHO ten-country study, select the option with which each of the following is best associated:
   (i) Acute-onset schizophrenia in developed countries
   (ii) Acute-onset schizophrenia in developing countries
   (iii) Catatonic schizophrenia in developed countries
   (iv) Catatonic schizophrenia in developing countries.

9. **MCQ** – Select one incorrect statement regarding hallucinations in patients with schizophrenia:
   (a) Auditory hallucinations have been found to be more common in non-European than in European patients in London.
   (b) Auditory hallucinations have been found to have similar rates in Pakistani patients in Pakistan and British Pakistanis.
   (c) Tactile hallucinations have been found to be more common in patients from the Middle East than in those from Europe.
   (d) Visual hallucinations have been found to be more common in patients from the Middle East than in those from Europe.
   (e) Visual hallucinations have been found to be more common in non-European than in European patients in London.

10. **EMI** – Schizophrenia outcomes
    (a) 0 per cent
    (b) 16 per cent
    (c) 37 per cent
    (d) 42 per cent
    (e) 63 per cent
    (f) 100 per cent

From the above list of potential percentages of patients with different outcome measures reported in the WHO ten-country study of schizophrenia, select the option with which each of the following is best associated:
   (i) Remitting/complete remission in developed countries
   (ii) Remitting/complete remission in developing countries
   (iii) Impaired social functioning in developed countries
   (iv) Impaired social functioning in developing countries.

11. **MCQ** – Select one incorrect statement:
    (a) In China it is more socially acceptable to receive the diagnosis of neurasthenia than depression.
    (b) In the WHO Collaborative Study on Standardized Assessment of Depressive Disorder, feelings of guilt were least common in Tehran compared with Basle, Montreal, Nagasaki and Tokyo.
    (c) The lifetime prevalence of depression has been found to be particularly low in Chinese American women.
    (d) The lifetime prevalence of depression has been found to be particularly low in Taiwan.
    (e) The lifetime prevalence of obsessive-compulsive disorder has been found to be particularly low in Taiwan.

12. **EMI** – Culture-bound disorders
    (a) Greenland
    (b) Japan
    (c) Korea
    (d) Nigeria
    (e) South-east Asia
    (f) South Africa

From the above list, select the option with which each of the following culture-bound disorders is best associated:
    (i)   Ode-ori.
    (ii) Taijinkyofusho
    (iii) Amok
    (iv) Hwa byung.

13. **EMI** – Culture-bound disorders
    (a) Amok
    (b) Ataque depression nervios
    (c) Hwa Byung
    (d) Koro
    (e) Latah
    (f) Ode-ori
    (g) Susto
    (h) Taijinkyofusho
    (i) Windigo.

From the above list of culture-bound disorders, select the option with which each of the following descriptions is best associated.
    (i)   A dissociative state in which patients exhibit echolalia, echopraxia and automatic obedience.
    (ii) Seen in South-east Asia, in these states there are severe episodes of violence and amnesia.
    (iii) A cultural variation of panic in which there are symptoms such as heat in the head or parasites crawling in the head at times of heightened fear.
    (iv) Seen in South-east Asia, men have an overwhelming fear that the penis is retracting into the abdomen and that death will occur immediately thereafter.
    (v)   Occurring in the Andes, patients suffer from a prolonged depressive episode which is believed by them to result from supernatural agencies.

14. **MCQ** – Select one incorrect statement regarding culture and psychiatric disorders:
    (a) Eating disorders have been considered as a culture-bound phenomenon, owing to a low prevalence rate within many non-Western cultures.
    (b) It has been argued that poverty gives rise to a culture that promotes and maintains substance abuse in Sri Lanka.
    (c) The prevalence of antisocial personality disorder has been reported to be much lower in Taiwan than in Canada.
    (d) There are multiple examples of studies from across the world in which high rates of post-traumatic stress disorder have been recorded in many different cultures with culturally validated tools.

    (e) Use of the International Personality Disorder Examination in a multinational study has reported an approximately equal rate of diagnosis of personality disorder using DSM-III-R and ICD-10.

15. **MCQ** – Select one incorrect statement regarding dementia and culture:
    (a) In the UK, the prevalence of dementia is higher in those of African-Caribbean origin than in those who are UK-born.
    (b) In the USA, the prevalence of dementia is higher in those who are African-American than in white Americans.
    (c) In the USA, the prevalence of dementia is higher in those who are Hispanic than in white Americans.
    (d) The prevalence of Alzheimer's disease is higher in China than in Western countries.
    (e) The prevalence of vascular dementia is higher in China than in Western countries.

16. **MCQ** – Select one correct statement regarding suicide and culture:
    (a) A study of suicide in New Delhi reported that poisoning was a more common method in young women and hanging was more common in young males.
    (b) Central American countries have higher rates of suicide than European countries.
    (c) In a study of Japanese suicides in the early part of the twenty-first century, suicide was found to account for a high proportion of all deaths of older men.
    (d) In China, overall more males than females die by suicide.
    (e) South American countries have higher rates of suicide than European countries.

17. **MCQ** – Age-specific rates of suicide for 20- to 44-year-olds in London were published in a 1997 study by Neeleman *et al*. Which of the following groups had the highest suicide rate?
    (a) African origin men
    (b) African-Caribbean women
    (c) Indian origin men
    (d) Indian women
    (e) White women.

18. **MCQ** – Which of the following groups had the highest suicide rate in the United States in 2002?
    (a) African-American males
    (b) American Indian/Alaskan native males
    (c) American Indian/Alaskan native females
    (d) Hispanic males
    (e) White males.

19. **MCQ** – There is a considerable variability in the CYP2D6 allele distribution among different ethnic groups. Depending on a large number of allelic variants, enzyme activity has been measured and grouped according to all but which one of the following types?
    (a) CM
    (b) EM

(c) IM

(d) PM

(e) UM.

20. **MCQ** – Select one incorrect statement regarding cultural aspects of pharmacokinetics and pharmacodynamics:

(a) Chinese patients have a higher CYP2D6 poor metabolizer frequency than white Caucasians.

(b) CYP3A4 is inhibited by black pepper from South Asia and *Piper cubeba* from Indonesia.

(c) CYP3A4 is inhibited by grapefruit juice.

(d) In clomipramine and antipyrine trials, significantly faster rates of metabolism have been found in South Asian subjects who switched to a 'British' diet, comparable with white British, than South Asians who followed 'Indian' vegetarian diets.

(e) There is an ethnocultural variation in the L allele frequency of *COMT*.

ANSWERS

1.

(i) b
(ii) a
(iii) d
(iv) c

Reference: *Psychiatry: An evidence-based text*, **p. 308.**

2.

(i) c
(ii) b
(iii) d
(iv) a

Reference: *Psychiatry: An evidence-based text*, **p. 308.**

3. e

Edenics refers to a theory regarding an original language. Emic accounts for culturally meaningful observations, which grow out of the culture and vary between cultures.

Reference: *Psychiatry: An evidence-based text*, **p. 309.**

4.

(i) f – This is the tendency to select certain culturally influenced reactions.
(ii) c – Culture is directly causative of psychopathology.
(iii) d – e.g. types of delusional beliefs such as 'I am the Christos.'

Reference: *Psychiatry: An evidence-based text*, **p. 309.**

5. c

They are a close-knit Protestant community with low rates of schizophrenia.

Reference: *Psychiatry: An evidence-based text*, **p. 310.**

6.

(i) b – e.g. excessive concern with body mass and association with onset of eating disorders.
(ii) e
(iii) a – e.g. types of suicidal act.

Reference: *Psychiatry: An evidence-based text*, **p. 309.**

7. a

Reference: *Psychiatry: An evidence-based text*, **Ch. 22.**

8.

(i) b – 10.9 per cent
(ii) e – 40.3 per cent
(iii) a – 1.2 per cent
(iv) b – 10.3 per cent.

Reference: *Psychiatry: An evidence-based text*, **p. 311.**

9. b

Reference: *Psychiatry: An evidence-based text*, **p. 311.**

10.

(i) c – 36.8 per cent
(ii) e – 62.7 per cent
(iii) d – 41.6 per cent
(iv) b – 15.7 per cent

Reference: *Psychiatry: An evidence-based text*, **p. 311.**

11. c

This group has a particularly high lifetime prevalence, reported in one study as being 21 per cent. With regard to (a), neurasthenia is a relatively common diagnosis in China. Concerning (b), it has been suggested that feelings of guilt are often associated with a Christian tradition.

In Taiwan, the lifetime prevalence of depression was only 1.5 per cent in one study (d), while the lifetime prevalence of obsessive-compulsive disorder was only 0.7 per cent in one study (e).

Reference: *Psychiatry: An evidence-based text*, **pp. 312–313.**

12.

(i) d
(ii) b
(iii) e
(iv) c

Reference: *Psychiatry: An evidence-based text*, **pp. 313–314.**

13.

(i) e
(ii) a
(iii) f
(iv) d
(v) g

References: *Psychiatry: An evidence-based text*, **Ch. 22;** Puri BK, Treasaden IH **(2011)** *Textbook of Psychiatry*, 3rd edn. Edinburgh: Churchill Livingstone, **Ch. 19.**

14. e

A twofold higher rate of diagnosis of personality disorder was found using DSM-III-R compared with ICD-10 in a 14-centre, 11-country, study using the International Personality Disorder Examination (IPDE), which is a semi-structured clinical interview.

In 'c', it should be noted that while the cause of such a difference may be a true difference in prevalence, it may instead reflect differences in how antisocial behaviour is defined in these two countries.

Reference: *Psychiatry: An evidence-based text*, **pp. 314–316.**

15. d

Reference: *Psychiatry: An evidence-based text*, **p. 316.**

16. c

Note that the question asks you to select one *correct* statement. (Always check the wording of the question carefully.) Traditionally Japan has a high rate of suicide, with complex cultural sanctioning of the behaviour in certain circumstances. This study was published in 2005 (Shiho *et al.*, 2005) and reported that the suicide rate had increased gradually since the early 1990s, reaching a post-war peak in 1998; the number of suicides had remained at about 30,000 every year since 1998, and middle-aged (55–59 years) and elderly men have especially high suicide rates.

References: *Psychiatry: An evidence-based text*, pp. 316–317; Shiho Y, Tohru T, Shinji S et al. (2005) Suicide in Japan: present conditions and prevention measures. *Crisis* **26:** 12–19.

17. d

The rate was 23.2 per 100 000 for Indian women. It was 15.0 per 100 000 for African origin men, 0.5 per 100 000 for African-Caribbean women, 18.1 per 100 000 for Indian origin men and 9.5 per 100 000 for white women.

References: Neeleman J, Mak V, Wessely S (1997) Suicide by age, ethnic group, coroners' verdicts and country of birth: a three-year survey in inner London. *British Journal of Psychiatry* **171:** 463–7; *Psychiatry: An evidence-based text*, p. 317.

18. e

The rate was 20.0 per 100 000 for white males. The rate was 9.8 per 100 000 for African-American males; 16.4 per 100 000 for American Indian/Alaskan native males; 4.1 per 100 000 for American Indian/Alaskan native females; and 8.3 per 100 000 for Hispanic males.

References: US Department of Health and Human Services, Centers for Disease Control and Prevention, National Center for Health Statistics (2004) *Health, United States, 2004*. Washington, DC: US Department of Health and Human Services, Centers for Disease Control and Prevention, National Center for Health Statistics; *Psychiatry: An evidence-based text*, p. 317.

19. a

EM, extensive metabolizer; IM, intermediate metabolizer; PM, poor metabolizer; UM, ultra-rapid metabolizer.

References: *Psychiatry: An evidence-based text*, p. 318; Zhou SF (2009) Polymorphism of human cytochrome P450 2D6 and its clinical significance: Part I. *Clinical Pharmacokinetics* **48:** 689–723.

21. a

The PM frequency in Chinese patients has been reported to be 1 per cent, compared with between 5 and 10 per cent in white Caucasians. CYP3A4 is involved in the metabolism of many antipsychotics, including clozapine, and benzodiazepines.

Reference: *Psychiatry: An evidence-based text*, pp. 319–320.

PART 3

Neuroscience

Chapter 23

Neuroanatomy

QUESTIONS

Note that for answers to extended matching items (EMIs), each option (denoted a, b, c, etc.) might be used once, more than once or not at all. For multiple-choice questions (MCQs), please select the best answer.

1. **EMI** – Frontal lobe areas
   (a) Broca's area
   (b) DLPFC
   (c) FEF
   (d) M1
   (e) Orbitofrontal cortex
   (f) PMd
   (g) PMv
   (h) Supplementary motor cortex
   (i) VLPFC

From the above list of frontal lobe areas, select the option with which each of the following is best associated:
   (i) Important in controlling ocular movements.
   (ii) Occupies the precentral gyrus and contains a somatotopic representation of the motor homunculus.
   (iii) PMv receives input from this area, which is involved in mnemonic processing and rule representation.
   (iv) Brodmann area 4.

2. **EMI** – Cranial fossae
   (a) Anterior
   (b) Middle
   (c) Posterior

From the above list of cranial fossae, select the option with which each of the following structures is best associated:
   (i) Sella turcica
   (ii) Cribriform plate
   (iii) Foramen caecum
   (iv) Optic canal.

3. **EMI** – Frontal lobe areas
   (a) Broca's area
   (b) DLPFC
   (c) FEF
   (d) M1
   (e) Orbitofrontal cortex
   (f) PMd
   (g) PMv
   (h) Supplementary motor cortex
   (i) VLPFC
   (j) None of the above

Select the option from the above list with which each of the following is best associated:
   (i) Involved with processes involving the motivational or emotional value of incoming information, including the representation of primary reinforcers, the representation of learned relationships between arbitrary neutral stimuli and rewards or punishments, and the integration of this information to guide response selection, suppression and decision-making
   (ii) Somatosensory association cortex
   (iii) Occupies Brodmann areas 44 and 45 in the dominant hemisphere
   (iv) A functional part of M1 which receives input from the DLPFC.

4. **MCQ** – Select one incorrect statement regarding the frontal lobe of the brain:
   (a) Electrical stimulation of M1 leads to contralateral muscular contraction.
   (b) It extends rostrally from the Sylvian fissure and superiorly from the fissure of Rolando.
   (c) PMd appears to be involved in decision circuits activated by free choice.
   (d) The dorsolateral prefrontal cortex is involved in self-ordered working memory, monitoring and the action of the central executive.
   (e) The frontal eye field receives afferent connections via the thalamus from the cerebellum.

5. **EMI** – Cranial fossae
   (a) Anterior
   (b) Middle
   (c) Posterior

Select the option from the above list with which each of the following structures is best associated:
   (i) Foramen magnum
   (ii) Foramen ovale
   (iii) Internal acoustic meatus
   (iv) Foramen spinosum
   (v) Ethmoid bone.

6. **MCQ** – Select one incorrect statement regarding neuroanatomy:
   (a) Brodmann area 17 is the primary visual cortex and is also known as the striate cortex.
   (b) The dominant temporal lobe contains Wernicke's area, which is a sensory speech area and may include part of the parietal cortex.
   (c) The middle temporal cortex, Brodmann area 21, has connections with different sensory modality pathways, including those related to vision, somatosensory input and auditory input.
   (d) The primary auditory cortex has a tonotopic cochlear representation, with low auditory frequencies being anterior and high frequencies posterior.
   (e) The primary visual cortex receives visual sensory input primarily from the medial geniculate nucleus via the optic radiation.

7. **EMI** – Cranial nerves
   (a) I
   (b) II
   (c) III
   (d) IV
   (e) V
   (f) VI
   (g) VII
   (h) VIII
   (i) IX
   (j) X
   (k) XI
   (l) XII

From the above list of cranial nerves, select the option with which the motor innervation of each of the following structures is best associated:
   (i) Superior oblique
   (ii) Stylopharyngeus
   (iii) Inferior oblique
   (iv) Muscles of facial expression.

8. **MCQ** – Which of the following cranial nerves carries a parasympathetic innervation to the ciliary ganglion?
   (a) Facial nerve
   (b) Oculomotor nerve
   (c) Optic nerve
   (d) Trigeminal nerve
   (e) Vagus nerve.

9. **EMI** – Cranial nerves
   (a) I
   (b) II
   (c) III
   (d) IV
   (e) V
   (f) VI
   (g) VII
   (h) VIII
   (i) IX
   (j) X
   (k) XI
   (l) XII

Select the option from the above list with which the sensory innervation of each of the following is best associated:
   (i) Retinal ganglion layer
   (ii) Gingivae
   (iii) Taste from the anterior two-thirds of the tongue
   (iv) Pharynx.

10. **MCQ** – Sensory innervation of the cornea is best associated with branches of which of the following nerves?
   (a) Facial nerve
   (b) Maxillary nerve
   (c) Oculomotor nerve
   (d) Ophthalmic nerve
   (e) Optic nerve.

11. **EMI** – Spinal cord ascending sensory pathways
   (a) Anterior spinothalamic tract
   (b) Lateral spinothalamic tract
   (c) Posterior column
   (d) Spinoreticular pathway.

From the above list of spinal cord ascending sensory pathways, select the option with which each of the following types of sensation is best associated:
   (i) Temperature
   (ii) Proprioceptive information
   (iii) Vibration.

12. **EMI** – Cranial nerves
   (a) I
   (b) II
   (c) III
   (d) IV
   (e) V
   (f) VI
   (g) VII
   (h) VIII
   (i) IX
   (j) X
   (k) XI
   (l) XII

Select the option from the above list with which the motor innervation of each of the following structures is best associated:
   (i) Almost all the muscles of the tongue
   (ii) Mylohyoid
   (iii) Lateral rectus
   (iv) Platysma
   (v) Levator palpebrae superioris.

13. **MCQ** – Which of the following is a descending spinal cord pathway that is particularly likely to have fibres originating in the superior colliculus?
   (a) Lateral spinothalamic tract
   (b) Rubrospinal tract

(c) Spinotectal tract

(d) Tectobulbar tract

(e) Tectospinal tract.

14. **MCQ** – Which of the following is a descending spinal cord pathway that is particularly likely to have fibres originating in the nucleus of Cajal?

(a) Interstitiospinal tract

(b) Lateral reticulospinal tract

(c) Lateral vestibulospinal tract

(d) Spinoreticular tract

(e) Solitariospinal tract.

15. **EMI** – Basal ganglia

(a) Corpus striatum

(b) Lentiform nucleus

(c) Paleostriatum

(d) Striatum

(e) None of the above.

From the above list of terms, select the option with which each of the following sets of basal ganglia components is best associated:

(i) Caudate nucleus and putamen

(ii) Globus pallidus and putamen

(iii) Globus pallidus

(iv) Globus pallidus and neostriatum.

16. **MCQ** – Which one of the following is not traditionally considered to be an Alexander basal ganglia–thalamocortical circuit?

(a) Anterior cingulate circuit

(b) Dorsolateral prefrontal circuit

(c) Medial orbitofrontal circuit

(d) Motor circuit

(e) Oculomotor circuit.

17. **MCQ** – Which of the following is not part of the (Alexander) basal ganglia–thalamocortical circuits?

(a) Cerebral cortex

(b) Globus pallidus

(c) Red nucleus

(d) Striatum

(e) Thalamus.

18. **MCQ** – Which of the following structures is not part of the hippocampal formation?

(a) CA3 pyramid

(b) Cingulate gyrus

(c) Parasubiculum

(d) Presubiculum

(e) Subiculum.

19. **MCQ** – Which of the following is not a sulcus seen on the surface of the medial temporal lobe?

(a) Collateral sulcus

(b) Hippocampal sulcus

(c) Rhinal sulcus

(d) Superior temporal sulcus

(e) Uncal sulcus.

20. **MCQ** – Select one incorrect statement regarding the fornix:

(a) Fibres of the fornix directly connect the hippocampal formation with the anterior thalamic nuclei.

(b) Fibres of the fornix directly connect the hippocampal formation with the hypothalamus.

(c) Fibres of the fornix directly connect the hippocampal formation with the perirhinal cortex.

(d) Fibres of the fornix directly connect the hippocampal formation with the septal nuclei.

(e) The fornix divides into a pre-commissural part and a post-commissural part.

21. **MCQ** – In which of the following central nervous system locations is neuromelanin not normally found in neuronal cytoplasm?

(a) Dorsal motor nucleus of the vagus

(b) Locus coeruleus

(c) Pars compacta

(d) Substantia nigra

(e) Superior colliculus.

22. **EMI** – Central nervous system (CNS) cells

(a) Astrocytes

(b) Choroid plexus cells

(c) Ependymal cells

(d) Neurones

(e) Oligodendrocytes

From the above list of cells found in the human CNS, select the option with which each of the following morphological descriptions is best associated:

(i) May be up to 1 m long in adult males

(ii) Possess few cell processes and lack cytoplasmic filaments

(iii) Cuboidal non-ciliated cells

(iv) Cuboidal ciliated cells.

23. **EMI** – Neuronal organelles

(a) Golgi apparatus

(b) Lipofuscin granule

(c) Nissl body

(d) Nucleolus

(e) None of the above

From the above list of neuronal organelles, select the option with which each of the following is best associated:

(i) Site of oxidative phosphorylation

(ii) Site of protein biosynthesis

(iii) Site of glycosylation and phosphorylation, and the biosynthesis of proteoglycans and carbohydrates

(iv) Site of transcription of rRNA by RNA pol I

(v) Contains non-metabolizable remnants of lysosomal digestion.

24. **EMI** – Neurochemical pathways in the CNS

(a) Cholinergic

(b) Dopaminergic

(c) Noradrenergic

(d) Glutamergic

(e) Serotonergic

(f) None of the above

Each of the following is a structure of the CNS and may be the origin of a major neurochemical pathway. From the above list of major neurochemical pathways in the CNS, select the option with which each of the following is best associated as an origin:

(i) Pars compacta of the substantia nigra

(ii) Locus coeruleus

(iii) Basal forebrain

(iv) Medullary raphe group

(v) Pontine raphe group.

25. **EMI** – Neurochemical pathways in the CNS
    (a) Cholinergic
    (b) Dopaminergic
    (c) Noradrenergic
    (d) Glutamergic
    (e) Serotonergic
    (f) None of the above

Each of the following is a CNS pathway and may be associated with a major neurochemical pathway. From the above list of major neurochemical pathways in the CNS, select the option with which each of the following is best associated as a pathway:

(i) Propiobulbar tract

(ii) Mesostriatal pathway

(iii) Corticofugal fibres

(iv) Coeruleospinal pathway.

26. **EMI** – Anatomical loops in the brain
    (a) Anterior cingulate cortex–nucleus accumbens–thalamic–anterior cingulate cortex
    (b) Anterior cingulate cortex–striatal–thalamic–anterior cingulate cortex
    (c) DLPFC–striatal–thalamic–DLPFC
    (d) Orbitofrontal cortex–caudate–thalamic–orbitofrontal cortex
    (e) None of the above

From the above list of anatomical loops in the brain, select the option with which each of the following functions is most likely to be associated:

(i) Executive function

(ii) Attention

(iii) Impulsivity.

27. **EMI** – Neurochemical pathways in the CNS
    (a) Cholinergic
    (b) Dopaminergic
    (c) Noradrenergic
    (d) Glutamergic
    (e) Serotonergic
    (f) None of the above

Each of the following is a pathway of the CNS and may be associated with a major neurochemical pathway. From the above list of major neurochemical pathways in the CNS, select the option with which each of the following is best associated as a pathway:

(i) Mesolimbic pathway

(ii) Corona radiata

(iii) Pontocerebellar tract

(iv) Nigrostriatal pathway.

ANSWERS

1.

(i)   c – FEF stands for frontal eye field, and occupies mainly Brodmann area 8.

(ii) d

(iii) i

(iv) d

Reference: *Psychiatry: An evidence-based text*, **pp. 332–333.**

2.

(i)   b

(ii) a

(iii) a

(iv) b

Reference: *Psychiatry: An evidence-based text*, **pp. 331–332.**

3.

(i)   e

(ii) j – This lies in the parietal lobe.

(iii) a – This is the motor speech area.

(iv) f

Reference: *Psychiatry: An evidence-based text*, **pp. 332–333.**

4. b

The fissure of Rolando is the central sulcus, while the Sylvian fissure is the lateral fissure. These fissures are shown well in Figure 23.5 on page 335 of the accompanying textbook.

Reference: *Psychiatry: An evidence-based text*, **pp. 332–333 and 335.**

5.

(i)   c

(ii) b – This transmits the mandibular division of the trigeminal nerve.

(iii) c

(iv) b – This transmits the middle meningeal artery.

(v)   a – This contains the cribriform plate.

Reference: *Psychiatry: An evidence-based text*, **pp. 331–332.**

6. e

It is primarily from the lateral geniculate nucleus. The optic radiation is shown in Figure 23.2 on page 333 of the accompanying textbook.

Reference: *Psychiatry: An evidence-based text*, **p. 333.**

7.

(i)   d

(ii) i

(iii) c

(iv) g

Reference: *Psychiatry: An evidence-based text*, **p. 336.**

8. b

Reference: *Psychiatry: An evidence-based text*, **p. 336.**

9.

(i)   b – The fibres of the optic nerve originate from the retinal ganglion layer.

(ii) e

(iii) g

(iv) j

Reference: *Psychiatry: An evidence-based text*, **pp. 336–337.**

10. d

Reference: *Psychiatry: An evidence-based text*, **pp. 336–337.**

11.

(i)   b

(ii) c

(iii) c

Reference: *Psychiatry: An evidence-based text*, **p. 338.**

12.

(i)   l – This cranial nerve supplies all the muscles of the tongue with the exception of palatoglossus.

(ii) e – Via the inferior alveolar branch of the mandibular nerve.

(iii) f

(iv) g

(v)   c

Reference: *Psychiatry: An evidence-based text*, **pp. 336–338.**

13. e

The lateral spinothalamic and spinotectal tracts are not descending spinal cord pathways, as indicated by their names. (The superior colliculus does receive afferent fibres from the contralateral spinal cord via the spinotectal and spinothalamic pathways.) The tectobulbar tract does originate in the superior colliculus but terminates in the pontine nuclei and in cranial nerve motor nuclei.

Reference: *Psychiatry: An evidence-based text*, **p. 338.**

14. a

Its fibres originate in the interstitial nucleus of Cajal (and also in the surrounding area in close proximity to this nucleus). Fibres descend to the lumbosacral level.

Reference: *Psychiatry: An evidence-based text*, **p. 338.**

15.

(i)   d – Also known as the neostriatum.
(ii) b
(iii) c
(iv) a

Reference: *Psychiatry: An evidence-based text*, **pp. 339–340.**

16. c

The lateral orbitofrontal circuit, on the other hand, is traditionally considered to be an Alexander basal ganglia–thalamocortical circuit.

Reference: *Psychiatry: An evidence-based text*, **pp. 340–341.**

17. c

A component missing from the given options is the substantia nigra, as shown in Figure 23.14 on page 342 of the accompanying textbook.

Reference: *Psychiatry: An evidence-based text*, **pp. 340–343.**

18. b

Its position is shown as label 14 in the coronal section of the brain in Figure 23.17(a) on page 344 of the accompanying textbook.

Reference: *Psychiatry: An evidence-based text*, **pp. 341–345.**

19. d

This sulcus is seen on the surface of the lateral temporal lobe. It is shown as label 12 in the superficial dissection of the brain viewed from the left side in Figure 23.5 on page 335 of the accompanying textbook.

Reference: *Psychiatry: An evidence-based text*, **pp. 335 and 343.**

20. c

See Figure 23.19 on page 345 of the accompanying textbook.

Reference: *Psychiatry: An evidence-based text*, **pp. 345, 347.**

21. e

Neuromelanin is a dark pigment derived from tyrosine.

Reference: *Psychiatry: An evidence-based text*, **p. 348.**

22.

(i)   d
(ii) e – Their name is derived from the fact that they possess few cell processes.
(iii) b
(iv) c

Reference: *Psychiatry: An evidence-based text*, **pp. 347–348.**

23.

(i)   e – This occurs in the mitochondria.
(ii) c
(iii) a
(iv) d
(v)   b

Reference: *Psychiatry: An evidence-based text*, **pp. 347–348.**

24.

(i)   b – In the mesencephalon.
(ii) c – In the pons.
(iii) a
(iv) e
(v)   e

Reference: *Psychiatry: An evidence-based text*, **pp. 348–351.**

25.

(i)   e
(ii) b
(iii) d
(iv) c

Reference: *Psychiatry: An evidence-based text*, **pp. 348–351.**

26.

(i)   c
(ii) b
(iii) d

Reference: *Psychiatry: An evidence-based text*, **p. 351.**

27.

(i)   b
(ii) d
(iii) e
(iv) b

Reference: *Psychiatry: An evidence-based text*, **pp. 348–351.**

Chapter 24

Basic concepts in neurophysiology

QUESTIONS

Note that for answers to extended matching items (EMIs), each option (denoted a, b, c, etc.) might be used once, more than once or not at all. For multiple-choice questions (MCQs), please select the best answer.

1. **MCQ** – Select one incorrect statement regarding basic concepts in the morphology and physiology of neurones in humans:
   (a) A neurone may make connections with as many as 1000–2000 other neurones by way of synapses.
   (b) A unipolar neurone has just one process extending from the cell body.
   (c) The adult brain contains in the order of 10 billion (10^{10}) neurones.
   (d) The contribution of sodium–potassium pumps to the resting membrane potential of a neurone is typically in the region of –3 mV.
   (e) The movement of substance across a surface in unit time is called flux.

2. **EMI** – Ion channels
   (a) Leakage
   (b) Ligand-gated
   (c) Mechanically gated
   (d) Voltage-gated
   (e) None of the above

   From the above list of ion channels found in cells in the human brain, select the option with which each of the following is best associated:
   (i) Movement of sodium and potassium ions through these channels is critical for the generation and propagation of action potentials.
   (ii) These open and close randomly and allow ions to pass through.
   (iii) Movement of calcium ions through these channels plays a role in the release of neurotransmitters at the presynaptic terminal.
   (iv) These open and close in response to a stimulus such as vibration.
   (v) These open or close in response to a chemical stimulus such as a neurotransmitter.

3. **MCQ** – Select one incorrect statement regarding ion concentrations across the plasma membrane of typical resting neurones in humans:
   (a) The extracellular chloride ion concentration is less than the intracellular chloride ion concentration.

   (b) The extracellular sodium ion concentration is greater than the intracellular sodium ion concentration.
   (c) The extracellular potassium ion concentration is less than the intracellular potassium ion concentration.
   (d) The membrane is more permeable to potassium ions than to sodium ions.
   (e) The sodium–potassium pump moves sodium ions out of and potassium ions into the cell in unequal proportions.

4. **MCQ** – Select one incorrect statement regarding human neuronal action potentials:
   (a) An action potential is initiated by a depolarizing stimulus which causes voltage-gated sodium ion channels to open.
   (b) During the early part of the absolute refractory period, voltage-gated sodium ion channel activation gates are open.
   (c) During the latter part of the absolute refractory period, voltage-gated potassium ion channels open while sodium ion channels are inactivating.
   (d) Potassium ion channels are slower to close than sodium ion channels, as a result of which there is a brief period following repolarization in which the membrane is transiently more permeable to potassium ions than it is during the resting state.
   (e) The depolarization and repolarization phases together constitute the relative refractory period.

5. **MCQ** – Select one incorrect statement regarding synapses in humans:
   (a) An IPSP is generated by the opening of chloride or potassium channels.
   (b) Electrical synapses are found in cardiac muscle.
   (c) If a presynaptic cell is stimulated in quick succession, it may induce EPSPs in a postsynaptic cell before the previous EPSPs have died away; this is known as spatial summation.
   (d) One EPSP causes facilitation for a brief period in the postsynaptic membrane.

(e) The release by the presynaptic cell of glutamate can induce an EPSP.

6. **MCQ** – Select one incorrect statement regarding neurotransmission in humans:

(a) Even under conditions of no stimulation, vesicles can release their contents into the synaptic cleft spontaneously.

(b) Fast axonal transport may allow transportation of transmitters at a speed of up to 400 mm/day.

(c) Neuropeptide transmitters are synthesized in the neuronal cell body and transported down the length of the axon via a cytoplasmic scaffold of microtubules using fast axonal transport.

(d) Small-molecule transmitters are transported down the neuronal axon using slow axonal transport of 0.5–5 mm/day to the nerve terminal.

(e) The size of mEPPs is altered by altering degrees of depolarization.

ANSWERS

1. c

There are probably around 10 times more neurones in the adult human brain. A diagram of a unipolar neurone is shown in Figure 24.2(c), on page 354 of the accompanying textbook.

Reference: *Psychiatry: An evidence-based text,* **pp. 354–356.**

2.

(i)   d
(ii)   a
(iii) d
(iv)   c –The mechanical stimulus distorts the membrane and thereby alters the physical properties of the channel and activates its gate.
(v)   b

Reference: *Psychiatry: An evidence-based text,* **p. 355.**

3. a

Typically, the extracellular chloride ion concentration is around 100 mM compared with an intracellular chloride ion concentration of around 7 mM. Typical values for sodium and potassium ions are shown in Table 24.1, on page 356 of the accompanying textbook.

Reference: *Psychiatry: An evidence-based text,* **pp. 355–356.**

4. e

As can be seen in Figure 24.4 on page 357 of the accompanying textbook, these two phases together are known as the absolute refractory period; this is followed by the relative refractory period.

Reference: *Psychiatry: An evidence-based text,* **pp. 356–357.**

5.c

This is temporal summation.

Reference: *Psychiatry: An evidence-based text,* **pp. 358–359.**

6. e

The size of mEPPs (miniature end-plate potentials) is not altered by altering degrees of depolarization, which implies that the release of neurotransmitter from the vesicle is an all-or-none phenomenon with a fixed amount (quantum) of neurotransmitter being released.

Reference: *Psychiatry: An evidence-based text,* **pp. 359–360.**

Chapter 25

Neurophysiology of integrated behaviour

QUESTIONS

Note that for answers to extended matching items (EMIs), each option (denoted a, b, c, etc.) might be used once, more than once or not at all. For multiple-choice questions (MCQs), please select the best answer.

1. **MCQ** – Select one incorrect statement regarding the human visual pathway:
   (a) Ganglion cells from the temporal retina project to the ipsilateral lateral geniculate nucleus and those from the nasal retina project to the contralateral lateral geniculate nucleus.
   (b) Light entering the eye passes through the ganglion cells and is imaged on the photoreceptor layer.
   (c) Signals from photoreceptors pass through bipolar cells to ganglion cells, the axons of which form the optic nerve, which projects principally to the lateral geniculate nucleus.
   (d) The horizontal and amacrine cell pathways within the retina allow spatial comparisons of cone signals.
   (e) Within the lateral geniculate nucleus, the projections from the two eyes are not aligned, so different topographical maps are found in different layers.

2. **EMI** – Human auditory pathway
   (a) Cochlear hair cells
   (b) Cochlear nuclear complex
   (c) Corpus callosum
   (d) Fornix
   (e) Lateral geniculate body
   (f) Medial geniculate body
   (g) Inferior colliculus
   (h) Nuclei of the lateral lemniscus
   (j) Primary auditory cortex
   (j) Spiral ganglion
   (k) Superior colliculus
   (l) Superior olivary complex

From the above list of cerebral structures, select the option with which each label (i–ix) in the following diagrammatic representation of the main stations of the human auditory pathway is best associated.

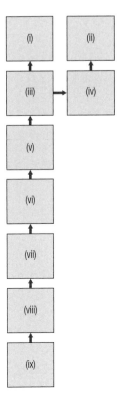

3. **EMI** – Auditory operational processing
   (a) Ascending auditory pathways to the primary auditory cortex
   (b) Auditory cortex
   (c) Cochlea
   (d) Higher cortices
   (e) Multimodal cortex

From the above list of anatomical structures, select the option with which each of the following types of auditory operational processing is best associated:
   (i) Profile analysis
   (ii) Invariance computation
   (iii) Spectrotemporal feature detection
   (iv) Object categorization
   (v) Multimodal association
   (vi) Modulation detection.

4. **EMI** – Auditory operational processing
   (a) Abstraction
   (b) Cross-modal analysis
   (c) Encoding
   (d) Feature analysis
   (e) Schema analysis

From the above list of types of processing, select the option with which each of the following examples of auditory operational processing is best associated:
   (i) Profile analysis
   (ii) Invariance computation
   (iii) Spectrotemporal feature detection
   (iv) Object categorization
   (v) Modulation detection.

5. **EMI** – Auditory operational processing
   (a) Abstraction
   (b) Cross-modal analysis
   (c) Encoding
   (d) Feature analysis
   (e) Schema analysis
   (f) None of the above

From the above list of types of processing, select the option with which each of the following examples of auditory operational processing is best associated:
   (i) Computational hub
   (ii) Auditory-image model
   (iii) Coincidence detection
   (iv) Sensory memory
   (v) Multimodal association
   (vi) Hierarchical analysis.

6. **MCQ** – Select one incorrect statement regarding pain:
   (a) AMN receptors respond primarily to mechanical and thermal stimuli.
   (b) Neurotransmitter release from the central terminal of peripheral afferents leads to activation of postsynaptic membrane receptor sites; activation of phospholipase C and adenylate cyclase leads to the biosynthesis of cAMP and DAG, mobilization of which may result in decreased potassium ion efflux and elevated intracellular calcium ions.
   (c) Peripheral inflammation leads to the production of opioid receptors by the dorsal root ganglion and their transport towards the peripheral terminal; these peripheral opioid receptors may be activated by endogenous opioid peptides released by monocytes, T-cells, B-cells and macrophages.
   (d) Regarding postsynaptic events following release of glutamate from central terminals of primary afferents in the spinal cord, in the presence of the co-factor NADPH, NOS uses citrulline as a substrate to produce nitric oxide and arginine.
   (e) Tissue damage leads to direct stimulation of nociceptors and the release of inflammatory mediators, including eicosanoids, cytokines, neurotransmitters and neuropeptides, which in turn reduce the nociceptor stimulation threshold and sensitize and stimulate the nociceptors further.

7. **EMI** – Neuroanatomy
   (a) CA1
   (b) CA2
   (c) CA3
   (d) CA4
   (e) CA5
   (f) Cerebellum
   (g) Corpus callosum
   (h) Inferior colliculus
   (i) Lateral entorhinal area
   (j) Medial entorhinal area
   (k) Parahippocampal cortex
   (l) Perirhinal cortex
   (m) Polymodal areas
   (n) Superior colliculus
   (o) Unimodal areas

From the above list of brain structures, select the option with which each label (i–viii) in the following diagrammatic representation of anatomical connections between the neocortex, parahippocampal region and hippocampus in the medial temporal lobe memory system is best associated:

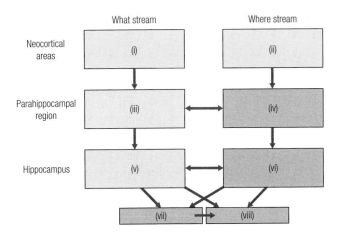

(f) Blood pressure
(g) DLPFC
(h) Hypothalamus
(i) Kidney
(j) Low-pressure receptors
(k) Orbitofrontal cortex
(l) Renin–angiotensin
(m) ↑ Sympathetic stimulation
(n) ↓ Sympathetic stimulation
(o) ↑ Vasoconstriction
(p) ↓ Vasoconstriction
(q) Water and Na⁺ reabsorption

From the above list, select the option with which each label (i–xii) in the following diagrammatic representation of the endocrine responses to hypovolaemia in humans is best associated:

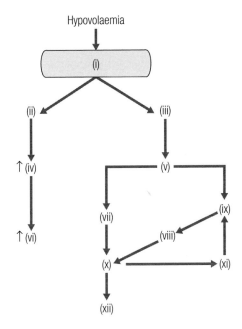

8. **MCQ** – Select the least correct statement regarding human sexual behaviour:

   (a) Higher levels of circulating testosterone are associated with increased sexual activity in both men and women.

   (b) In women, testosterone activity increases at around the time of ovulation and is associated with increased sexual desire.

   (c) Sexual behaviour is a regulatory form of behaviour.

   (d) Testosterone exposure during critical periods of early development produces permanent behavioural changes.

   (e) Testosterone masculinizes the brain in the male fetus, with particular effects in the preoptic area of the hypothalamus, which is much larger in males than females following testosterone exposure

9. **EMI** – Hormonal signals

   (a) Acts on the human brain to help decrease food intake

   (b) Acts on the human brain to help increase food intake

   (c) Acts on the human brain but does not affect food intake

   (d) Does not act directly on the human brain.

From the above list, select the option with which each of the following hormonal signals is best associated:

   (i) Thyroxine

   (ii) Insulin

   (iii) Glucocorticoid.

10. **EMI** – Endocrine responses to hypovolaemia

   (a) ↑ ADH

   (b) ↓ ADH

   (c) Adrenal cortex

   (d) Aldosterone

   (e) Baroreceptors

11. **EMI** – Hormonal signals

   (a) Acts on the human brain to help decrease food intake

   (b) Acts on the human brain to help increase food intake

   (c) Does not act on the human brain.

From the above list, select the option with which each of the following hormonal signals derived from the gastrointestinal tract is best associated:

   (i) GLP1

   (ii) PYY$_{3-36}$

   (iii) Ghrelin.

ANSWERS

1. e

Within the lateral geniculate nucleus, the projections from the two eyes are aligned, so the same topographic map of the contralateral half of the visual field is found in all layers. The axons of lateral geniculate nucleus neurones project almost exclusively to area V1, where they terminate primarily in layer 4 and form ocular dominance columns. The human visual pathway is shown in Figures 25.1 and 25.2 on pages 361 and 362, respectively, of the accompanying textbook.

Reference: *Psychiatry: An evidence-based text*, **pp. 361–362.**

2.

(i) k – This allows auditory stimuli to have an input into ocular movements, including reflex movements.
(ii) i
(iii) g
(iv) f – Note that the lateral geniculate nucleus is particularly associated with the visual pathway.
(v) h
(vi) l
(vii) b
(viii) j
(ix) a

Reference: *Psychiatry: An evidence-based text*, **pp. 362–363.**

3.

(i) c
(ii) b
(iii) a
(iv) d
(v) e
(vi) a

Reference: *Psychiatry: An evidence-based text*, **p. 363.**

4.

(i) c
(ii) a
(iii) d
(iv) e
(v) d

Reference: *Psychiatry: An evidence-based text*, **p. 363.**

5.

(i) a
(ii) c
(iii) c
(iv) a
(v) b
(vi) a

Reference: *Psychiatry: An evidence-based text*, **p. 363.**

6. d

As shown in Figure 25.10 on page 366 of the accompanying textbook, in the presence of NADPH, NOS nitric oxide synthase uses arginine as a substrate to produce nitric oxide (NO) and citrulline; NO has a role in normal cellular function, although increased production may be involved in hyperalgesia and may lead to neurotoxicity.

Reference: *Psychiatry: An evidence-based text*, **pp. 363–366.**

7.

(i) o
(ii) m
(iii) l
(iv) k
(v) i
(vi) j
(vii) c
(viii) a

Reference: *Psychiatry: An Evidence-Based Text*, **p. 366.**

8. c

Human sexual behaviour is a non-regulatory form of behaviour, i.e. it is not under the control of a homeostatic mechanism.

Reference: *Psychiatry: An evidence-based text*, **p. 367.**

9.

(i) b – This and the following answers are illustrated in Figure 25.16 on page 369 of the accompanying textbook.
(ii) a
(iii) b

Reference: *Psychiatry: An Evidence-Based Text*, **p. 369.**

10.

(i) f
(ii) e
(iii) j
(iv) m
(v) h
(vi) o
(vii) a
(viii) d
(ix) c
(x) i
(xi) l
(xii) q

Reference: *Psychiatry: An Evidence-Based Text*, **p. 373.**

11.

(i) **a** – This is glucagon-like peptide 1. This and the following answers are illustrated in Figure 25.16 on page 369 of the accompanying textbook.

(ii) **a** – This is peptide YY (3-36).

(iii) **b**

Reference: *Psychiatry: An Evidence-Based Text,* **p. 369.**

Chapter 26

Neurogenesis and cerebral plasticity

QUESTIONS

Note that for answers to extended matching items (EMIs), each option (denoted a, b, c, etc.) might be used once, more than once or not at all. For multiple-choice questions (MCQs), please select the best answer.

1. **MCQ** – Who among the following is least associated with making an important contribution to our understanding of corticoneurogenesis?
   (a) Cajal, Ramón y
   (b) Corti, Alfonso Giacomo Gaspare
   (c) His, Wilhelm
   (d) Rakic, Pasko
   (e) Retzius, Magnus Gustaf.

2. **MCQ** – In the human embryo, which layer of the developing cerebral cortex do migrating postmitotic neuroblasts form?
   (a) iz
   (b) Lateral zone
   (c) mz
   (d) pp
   (e) vz.

3. **MCQ** – From which layer of the human fetal cerebral cortex do most layers of the adult cerebral cortex derive?
   (a) cp
   (b) iz
   (c) mz
   (d) sp
   (e) vz.

4. **MCQ** – In humans, neurones in which developing cortical layer are the first to mature and are selectively vulnerable to early hypoxic-ischaemic brain injury in animal models?
   (a) cp
   (b) iz
   (c) mz
   (d) sp
   (e) vz.

5. **MCQ** – Select one incorrect statement regarding Huttenlocher and de Courten's 1987 postmortem study of synaptic density in the human striate cortex:
   (a) Analysis by individual cortical layers showed similar age-related changes in all strata, except for somewhat later synaptogenesis in cortical layers V and VI.
   (b) Synapse elimination occurred after 4 months, with loss of about 40 per cent of synapses between the ages of 8 months and 11 years.
   (c) Synapse numbers were relatively stable in adults.
   (d) Synaptogenesis was found to be most rapid between the ages of 2 and 4 months, a time that is also critical for the development of function in the visual cortex of the infant.
   (e) The total volume of the striate cortex reached adult size remarkably early, at about 4 years.

ANSWERS

1. b

In terms of mammalian neuroanatomy, he is particularly associated with the study of the cochlea. The organ of Corti is named after him.

Reference: *Psychiatry: An Evidence-Based Text,* **Ch. 26.**

2. d

This is the preplate.

Reference: *Psychiatry: An Evidence-Based Text,* **p. 374.**

3. a

This is the cortical plate. Layers II–VI of the cerebral cortex take their origin from the cortical plate.

Reference: *Psychiatry: An Evidence-Based Text,* **p. 374.**

4. d

Subplate neurones are the first cortical neurones to mature.

Reference: *Psychiatry: An Evidence-Based Text,* **p. 377.**

5. e

The total volume of the human striate cortex was indeed noted to reach adult size remarkably early – even earlier than 4 years, it actually reaches this size by about 4 months.

Reference: *Psychiatry: An Evidence-Based Text,* **p. 379.**

Chapter 27

The neuroendocrine system

QUESTIONS

Note that for answers to extended matching items (EMIs), each option (denoted a, b, c, etc.) might be used once, more than once or not at all. For multiple-choice questions (MCQs), please select the best answer.

1. **EMI** – Hypothalamus anatomy
   (a) Anterior
   (b) Central
   (c) Posterior
   (d) Not a nucleus of the hypothalamus

   From the above list of anatomical locations in the hypothalamus, select the option with which each of the following is best associated:
   (i)   Paraventricular nucleus
   (ii) Preoptic nucleus
   (iii) Red nucleus
   (iv) Mamillary.

2. **EMI** – Hypothalamic hormones
   (a) A hypothalamic hormone that is inhibitory
   (b) A hypothalamic hormone that is neither inhibitory nor stimulatory
   (c) A hypothalamic hormone that is stimulatory
   (d) Not a hypothalamic hormone

   From the above list, select the option with which each of the following is best associated:
   (i)   LH
   (ii) GHRH
   (iii) Somatostatin
   (iv) GnRH.

3. **EMI** – Hypothalamus anatomy
   (a) Anterior
   (b) Central
   (c) Posterior
   (d) Not a nucleus of the hypothalamus

   From the above list of anatomical locations in the hypothalamus, select the option with which each of the following is best associated:
   (i)   Supraoptic nucleus
   (ii) Posterior nucleus
   (iii) Dorsomedial nucleus

   (iv) Ventral anterior nucleus
   (v) Arcuate nucleus.

4. **EMI** – Hypothalamic hormones
   (a) A hypothalamic hormone that is inhibitory
   (b) A hypothalamic hormone that is neither inhibitory nor stimulatory
   (c) A hypothalamic hormone that is stimulatory
   (d) Not a hypothalamic hormone.

   From the above list, select the option with which each of the following is best associated:
   (i)   CRH
   (ii) CCK
   (iii) Dopamine
   (iv) AVP.

5. **MCQ** – Which of the following is not an anterior pituitary hormone?
   (a) ACTH
   (b) FSH
   (c) Oxytocin
   (d) Prolactin
   (e) TSH.

6. **MCQ** – Select one incorrect statement regarding cortisol receptors:
   (a) Centrally, the MR is mainly expressed either alone or together with the GR in hippocampal neurones, while the GR has a more ubiquitous distribution within brain neurones.
   (b) The GR becomes progressively occupied only at peaks of cortisol secretion and after a stressful stimulus.
   (c) The GR has a tenfold higher affinity for cortisol than does the MR.
   (d) The GR is believed to be more important than the MR in the regulation of the stress response when endogenous cortisol levels are high.
   (e) The MR monitors basal diurnal fluctuations in cortisol.

7. **EMI** – Hypothalamic–pituitary–adrenal axis (HPA) axis functioning in depression
   (a) Decreased
   (b) Increased
   (c) Neither decreased nor increased.

From the above list, select the option with which each of the following potential disturbances in HPA axis functioning, indicating an overactive axis, has been reported in major depression:
   (i) ACTH release in response to CRH when pre-treated with dexamethasone
   (ii) Cortisol levels
   (iii) Adrenal gland volume.

8. **MCQ** – Select one incorrect statement regarding the HPT axis:
   (a) T4 is more biologically active than T3.
   (b) T4 is the predominant form released from the thyroid, and subsequent de-iodination to T3 is performed by target organs including the brain.
   (c) The HPT axis is driven centrally by the secretion of TRH from the PVN.
   (d) TRH release is inhibited by serotonergic input to the hypothalamic nucleus, while dopamine has a net stimulatory effect.
   (e) TSH stimulates the synthesis and secretion of two thyroid hormones from the thyroid gland, namely T3 and T4.

9. **EMI** – HPA axis functioning in depression
   (a) Decreased
   (b) Increased
   (c) Neither decreased nor increased

From the above list, select the option with which each of the following potential disturbances in HPA axis functioning, indicating an overactive axis, has been reported in major depression:
   (i) CSF CRH
   (ii) Cortisol response to synacthen
   (iii) ACTH release in response to CRH.

10. **MCQ** – Select one incorrect statement regarding the DST:
   (a) Dexamethasone is a potent synthetic glucocorticoid that binds primarily to GRs in the anterior pituitary and thus suppresses ACTH and cortisol secretion via a negative feedback mechanism.
   (b) It allows the investigation of the functional integrity of negative feedback control of the HPA axis.
   (c) It is relatively specific to the diagnosis of major depression.
   (d) Its use in psychiatry was popularized by Carroll.
   (e) There are hundreds of published studies reporting on DST in depression, and they report that around a half of people with major depression fail adequately to suppress cortisol levels after administration of 1 mg dexamethasone.

11. **MCQ** – Select one incorrect statement regarding prolactin:
   (a) Abnormality high levels may be clinically silent for many years.
   (b) Antipsychotics can affect its levels by binding to dopamine receptors on the lactotroph cell membrane, with those having potent D2R antagonism and poorest blood–brain barrier permeability having the greatest and most sustained effect on blood levels.
   (c) Dopamine exerts a direct effect on pituitary lactotrophs by binding to D2Rs expressed on their cell membranes.
   (d) Dopamine exerts a tonic inhibitory influence on its synthesis and release.
   (e) It has a classical negative feedback loop.

ANSWERS

1.

(i)   b
(ii) a
(iii) d – This is found in the mesencephalon.
(iv) c

Reference: *Psychiatry: An Evidence-Based Text*, **p. 385.**

2.

(i)   d – Luteinizing hormone, or LH, is not a hypothalamic hormone.
(ii) c – This is a growth hormone-releasing hormone.
(iii) a
(iv) c – This is gonadotrophin-releasing hormone.

Reference: *Psychiatry: An Evidence-Based Text*, **p. 386.**

3.

(i)   a
(ii) c
(iii) b
(iv) d – This is a lateral thalamic nucleus.
(v)   b

Reference: *Psychiatry: An Evidence-Based Text*, **p. 385.**

4.

(i)   c – This is corticotrophin-releasing hormone.
(ii) d – This is cholecystokinin and is not known to be a hypothalamic hormone at the time of writing.
(iii) a
(iv) c – This is arginine vasopressin.

Reference: *Psychiatry: An Evidence-Based Text*, **p. 386.**

5. c

This is a posterior pituitary hormone.

Reference: *Psychiatry: An Evidence-Based Text*, **p. 386.**

6. c

This is not purely an exercise in memory. This correct answer can be worked out from the other parts of the question. In particular, statements 'b' and 'e', if both true, imply that statement 'c' is false; as only one statement is false overall, then clearly 'c' is false. GR stands for glucocorticoid or type 2 cortisol receptor, and MR stands for mineralocorticoid or type 1 cortisol receptor.

Reference: *Psychiatry: An Evidence-Based Text*, **pp. 386–387.**

7.

Note that the options to be chosen are those that indicate an overactive HPA axis; this is not meant to be an exercise in memory, but rather a question that tests the candidate's understanding. (It pays to read the question carefully.)
(i)   b – This is the DEX–CRH test.
(ii) b
(iii) b – As measured by CT or MRI.

Reference: *Psychiatry: An Evidence-Based Text*, **p. 387.**

8. a

T3 is the more biologically active form.

Reference: *Psychiatry: An Evidence-Based Text*, **pp. 389–390.**

9.

(i)   b – Cerebrospinal fluid levels of CRH have been reported to be elevated.
(ii) b – This is the ACTH stimulation test.
(iii) a – This is the CRH stimulation test.

Reference: *Psychiatry: An Evidence-Based Text*, **p. 387.**

10. c

The test lacks adequate specificity, with positive results also being seen in other disorders besides major depression, such as dementia, eating disorders and schizophrenia.

Reference: *Psychiatry: An Evidence-Based Text*, **pp. 387–388.**

11. e

The tonic upstream inhibition mentioned in statement 'c' conveys a unique characteristic to prolactin secretion compared with other pituitary hormones, whose secretory tone is determined largely by stimulatory agents. This discrepancy arises from prolactin's lack of a single target organ to provide a classical negative feedback loop (e.g. in contrast to ACTH). Also, lactotrophs have a much higher basal secretory activity compared with other endocrine cells and are thus more responsive to inhibition than stimulation.

Reference: *Psychiatry: An Evidence-Based Text*, **pp. 390–391.**

Chapter 28

The neurophysiology and neurochemistry of arousal and sleep

QUESTIONS

Note that for answers to extended matching items (EMIs), each option (denoted a, b, c, etc.) might be used once, more than once or not at all. For multiple-choice questions (MCQs), please select the best answer.

1. **MCQ** – Select one incorrect statement regarding the physiology of human sleep:
   (a) Both short and long sleepers have approximately the same duration of stage 3 and 4 sleep.
   (b) Cerebral cortical activity is synchronized during NREM sleep.
   (c) Hallucinations associated with delirium probably represent partial REM sleep intrusion into wakefulness.
   (d) Life expectancy is shorter in people who obtain little sleep at night.
   (e) REM sleep dominates early in the night, particularly in the deeper sleep stages, but NREM sleep becomes more prolonged later in the night.

2. **EMI** – NREM sleep
   (a) Decreased
   (b) Increased
   (c) Neither decreased nor increased

From the above list, select the option with which each of the following is best associated during NREM sleep:
   (i) Parasympathetic nervous system activity compared with sympathetic nervous system activity
   (ii) Metabolic rate
   (iii) Core body temperature
   (iv) Alveolar ventilation.

3. **MCQ** – Select the least correct statement regarding the physiology of human REM sleep:
   (a) Autonomic function is very variable.
   (b) It plays a role in memory, particularly for motor tasks.
   (c) The limbic system is inactivated.
   (d) The prefrontal cortex is inactivated.
   (e) There is intense skeletal muscle inhibition.

4. **EMI** – Neuroanatomy of sleep and wakefulness
   (a) Aminergic brainstem nuclei
   (b) Higher centres promoting wakefulness
   (c) Laterodorsal tegmental and pedunculopontine tegmental nuclei
   (d) Pathways to the cerebral cortex to enable sleep to occur
   (e) Sleep-promoting higher centres
   (f) None of the above

From the above list relating to the neuroanatomy of sleep and wakefulness, select the option with which each of the following is best associated:
   (i) Associated with the thalamus, basal forebrain and hypothalamus, these closely linked areas integrate the sleep and wakefulness drives with circadian influences.
   (ii) Include the locus coeruleus, raphe nuclei and tuberomamillary nuclei.
   (iii) These promote REM sleep when they are most active. They are inactive in NREM sleep, but activity returns during wakefulness.
   (iv) These favour wakefulness and inhibit sleep. Together they form the ascending reticular activating system.
   (v) Include the perifornical hypothalamus whose neurones release orexin.

5. **EMI** – Control of sleep and wakefulness
   (a) Circadian rhythms
   (b) Adaptive drive
   (c) Process S
   (d) None of the above

From the above list relating to processes involved in the control of sleep and wakefulness, select the option with which each of the following is best associated:
   (i) The drive to enter sleep increases, probably exponentially with the duration since the end of the previous NREM sleep episode.
   (ii) Associated with behavioural factors, such as motivation and attention, psychological factors,

such as mental activity and relaxation, and reflex factors, such as light exposure, noise and physical activity.

(iii) The suprachiasmatic nuclei are important control centres.

6. **MCQ** – Select the least correct statement regarding the neurochemistry of human sleep:

(a) Acetylcholine is associated with motor inhibition during REM sleep.

(b) Dopamine influences thoughts, emotions, behaviour and motor control.

(c) Histamine inhibits wakefulness and promotes REM sleep.

(d) Noradrenaline inhibits REM sleep and influences mood and behaviour.

(e) Serotonin promotes wakefulness.

7. **EMI** – NREM sleep

(a) Decreased

(b) Increased

(c) Neither decreased nor increased

From the above list, select the option with which each of the following is best associated during NREM sleep:

(i) Prefrontal cortical activity

(ii) Arterial P_{CO_2}

(iii) Protein synthesis

(iv) Blood pressure

(v) Cell division.

ANSWERS

1. e

NREM sleep characteristically dominates early in the night, particularly during the deeper stages, but REM sleep becomes more prolonged later in the night.

Reference: *Psychiatry: An Evidence-Based Text*, **p. 397.**

2.

(i)   b
(ii) a – The metabolic rate is typically reduced by 5 to 10 per cent.
(iii) a – The core body temperature falls as NREM sleep is entered.
(iv) a

Reference: *Psychiatry: An Evidence-Based Text*, **p. 387.**

3. c

Several areas of the limbic system are active during REM sleep.

Reference: *Psychiatry: An Evidence-Based Text*, **p. 398.**

4.

(i)   d
(ii) a
(iii) c
(iv) a
(v)   b

Reference: *Psychiatry: An Evidence-Based Text*, **pp. 398–399.**

5.

(i)   c – This is also known as the sleep homeostatic drive.
(ii) b – There are a variety of mechanisms that enable the sleep–wake cycle to adapt to environmental conditions.
(iii) a – These nuclei are in the supraoptic anterior hypothalamus and are the most important centres controlling the circadian rhythms.

Reference: *Psychiatry: An Evidence-Based Text*, **p. 398.**

6. c

Details of the effects of neurotransmitter amines on sleep and wakefulness are summarized in Table 28.1 on page 399 of the accompanying textbook.

Reference: *Psychiatry: An Evidence-Based Text*, **p. 399.**

7.

(i)   a
(ii) b – A slight increase results from a reduction in alveolar ventilation.
(iii) b – Other anabolic processes are also increased during NREM sleep.
(iv) a
(v)   b – Cell division is most rapid during NREM sleep. NREM sleep has been considered to be a restorative or a recovery phase, particularly for the brain, but probably in part for the rest of the body as well.

Reference: *Psychiatry: An Evidence-Based Text*, **p. 397–398.**

Chapter 29

The electroencephalogram and evoked potential studies

QUESTIONS

Note that for answers to extended matching items (EMIs), each option (denoted a, b, c, etc.) might be used once, more than once or not at all. For multiple-choice questions (MCQs), please select the best answer.

1. **MCQ** – Select one incorrect statement regarding the human EEG:
   (a) Currents from deep sources are less easy to detect than those from nearer the skull.
   (b) It allows absolute localization of current source.
   (c) It has higher temporal resolution than fMRI.
   (d) It particularly measures activity from cells that are aligned similarly to one another and radial to the scalp.
   (e) The limiting factor underlying recording accuracy tends to be data storage capacity.

2. **MCQ** – Select one incorrect statement regarding recording of the EEG:
   (a) Cortical electrical activity is measured using highly electrosensitive electrodes, often using a silver–silver chloride construction, with electrolyte gels.
   (b) In the international 10–20 system, CPz refers to electrodes placed between C and P locations on the longitudinal midline.
   (c) In the international 10–20 system, the numbers 10 and 20 refer to the number of scalp electrodes.
   (d) It is essential that impedance levels are reduced by as much as possible to increase the signal-to-noise ratio.
   (e) Recording systems may include montages of 32, 64, 132 or 256 electrode sites.

3. **EMI** – Generalized slow waves
   (a) Asynchronous but generalized slow waves
   (b) Focal slow waves in the delta range
   (c) Frontal intermittent rhythmical delta activity
   (d) None of the above

   From the above list relating to generalized slow waves, select the option with which each of the following is best associated:
   (i) Brainstem damage
   (ii) An organic confusional state
   (iii) A brain tumour

   (iv) A breach rhythm over a neurosurgical site
   (v) Myalgic encephalomyelitis.

4. **MCQ** – Generalized atypical spike-and-wave discharges at a frequency of around 2 or 2.5 Hz are most likely to be associated with which of the following?
   (a) Atypical antipsychotic treatment
   (b) Lennox–Gastaut syndrome
   (c) Partial epilepsy arising in the frontal lobe
   (d) Temporal lobe epilepsy
   (e) Treatment with venlafaxine.

5. **MCQ** – Select one incorrect statement regarding maturational changes of the EEG:
   (a) A picture characterized by a burst of activity and then by suppression of activity is characteristically seen in normal newborn babies.
   (b) A picture characterized by a burst of activity and then by suppression of activity is characteristically seen in premature babies.
   (c) As an individual enters old age, there tends to be a speeding up of the alpha rhythm, while if it becomes markedly slow and there is a significant increase in slow-wave activity generally, this may signify the development of a dementing disorder.
   (d) Before the age of 5 years it is very common to have a number of asymmetries of the EEG, with one hemisphere perhaps developing before the other.
   (e) During late childhood and early adolescence, the alpha rhythm begins to emerge, initially seen over central regions and gradually localizing over occipital regions.

6. **EMI** – EEG in acute organic states
   (a) Loss of the alpha rhythm and the appearance of theta waves
   (b) Lateralized triphasic complexes
   (c) Periodic high-voltage complexes

(d) Slowing of the alpha rhythm and a polymorphic picture of slower waves (theta and delta)

(e) None of the above

From the above list relating to EEG patterns that might be seen in acute organic states, select the option with which each of the following is best associated:

(i) Dementing conditions

(ii) Creutzfeldt–Jakob disease in its early stages

(iii) Herpes encephalitis

(iv) Fibromyalgia

(v) Subacute sclerosing panencephalitis.

7. **EMI** – EEG in dementia

(a) Beta activity

(b) Bifrontal triphasic waves

(c) Diffuse slowing

(d) Localized and unilateral slow-wave activity

(e) Low-amplitude EEG with relative EEG flattening

(f) None of the above

From the above list relating to EEG patterns that might typically be seen in dementias, select the option with which each of the following is best associated:

(i) Alzheimer's disease, particularly during its earlier stages

(ii) Focal dementia

(iii) Huntington's disease

(iv) Multi-infarct dementia.

8. **MCQ** – Select one incorrect statement regarding EEG beta activity:

(a) Asymmetries of induced beta activity may indicate brain pathology.

(b) It is increased by barbiturate treatment.

(c) It is increased by benzodiazepine treatment.

(d) It is increased by the use of alcohol.

(e) It is prominent in normal recordings.

9. **MCQ** – Select one correct statement regarding the N170 ERP:

(a) It is an SEP.

(b) It is derived from a waveform that has no positive components.

(c) It is found over ventral posterior regions during face-processing trials.

(d) It is so-named because of ordinal numbering, as it follows N1, N2, ... N169.

(e) It refers to a nominal auditory evoked potential.

10. **EMI** – Analytical techniques in electroencephalography

(a) Alpha

(b) Beta

(c) Gamma

(d) Lambda

(e) Mu

(f) MMN

(g) MNN

(h) None of the above

From the above list relating to analytical techniques in electroencephalography, select the option with which each of the following is best associated:

(i) Single sharp waves over the occipital pole that are associated with scanning visual scenes or pictures

(ii) Elicited by asking subjects to shut their eyes

(iii) May represent pre-attentional processes

(iv) May represent the binding mechanism within and between different populations or networks of neurones

(v) Attenuate with contralateral limb movement.

ANSWERS

1. b

This is not possible because the electrodes at the scalp are detecting the summation of electrical voltage that may be generated in many potential sites. Functional MRI does indeed have poorer temporal resolution than EEG.

Reference: *Psychiatry: An evidence-based text*, **pp. 400–401.**

2. c

These numbers refer to the fact that electrodes are placed at sites that are 10 and 20 per cent of the distances between the nasion and inion and between the pre-auricular points, as shown in Figure 29.2 on page 402 of the accompanying textbook.

Reference: *Psychiatry: An evidence-based text*, **pp. 401–402.**

3.

(i) c – Frontal intermittent rhythmical delta activity is also known as FIRDA.

(ii) a – These are slow waves that occur at a different rate and at different times in the two cerebral hemispheres. Such organic confusional states would typically arise with toxic or metabolic encephalopathies.

(iii) b

(iv) b

(v) d

Reference: *Psychiatry: An evidence-based text*, **pp. 397–398.**

4. b

This syndrome is associated with learning disabilities, multiple generalized seizure types (tonic, atonic, absence, tonic-clonic) and a poor prognosis for recovery.

Reference: *Psychiatry: An evidence-based text*, **p. 403.**

5. c

There tends to be a slight slowing of the alpha rhythm, although it should still remain above 8 Hz.

Reference: *Psychiatry: An evidence-based text*, **p. 404.**

6.

(i) d – See the previous question.

(ii) a – These are non-specific changes and may be missed. Later on in the disease, sometimes just briefly before death, the typical picture of periodic triphasic complexes is seen.

(iii) b – Note that bifrontal triphasic waves are typically seen at some stage in hepatic encephalopathy.

(iv) e

(v) c

Reference: *Psychiatry: An evidence-based text*, **pp. 404–405.**

7.

(i) c – There may also be runs of frontal delta resulting from subcortical damage. There may be a later appearance of sharper waves and sometimes of paroxysmal activity focally.

(ii) c – The EEGs are very frequently normal for the majority of the history.

(iii) e

(iv) d

Reference: *Psychiatry: An evidence-based text*, **pp. 404–405.**

8. e

It is present but scant in normal recordings. Asymmetries of induced beta activity may indicate that a brain area or side is not capable of generating faster frequencies owing to underlying pathology or damage.

Reference: *Psychiatry: An evidence-based text*, **p. 405.**

9. c

This answer can be readily derived from the fact that the other four options are incorrect statements.

Reference: *Psychiatry: An evidence-based text*, **pp. 405–406.**

10.

(i) d – It has been suggested that they represent the start of passage of information from occipital to prefrontal regions of the brain.

(ii) a – They can be seen when subjects become drowsy and over-relaxed. Conversely, they usually attenuate with eye-opening or mental exertion.

(iii) f – Mismatch negativity, or MMN, is the result of an increase in negativity following a deviant stimulus (compared with a regular stimulus).

(iv) c

(v) e – Likewise, during the imagined movement of a limb, the contralateral mu rhythm reduces.

Reference: *Psychiatry: An evidence-based text*, **pp. 406–407.**

Chapter 30

Neurochemistry

QUESTIONS

Note that for answers to extended matching items (EMIs), each option (denoted a, b, c, etc.) might be used once, more than once or not at all. For multiple-choice questions (MCQs), please select the best answer.

1. **MCQ** – Select one incorrect statement regarding astroglia:
   (a) They are involved in the decarboxylation of glutamate to glutamine and the return of the latter to neurones as the precursor of glutamate.
   (b) They are the second most common cells of the central nervous system.
   (c) They express a high density of potassium channels.
   (d) They express transporters for fast-acting neurotransmitters such as GABA and glutamate.
   (e) They provide neurones with glucose and regulate the extraneuronal environment by removing products of neuronal activity.

2. **EMI** – Neurotransmitters
   (a) Acetylcholine
   (b) Dopamine
   (c) GABA
   (d) Glutamate
   (e) Noradrenaline
   (f) Serotonin
   (g) None of the above

   From the above list of neurotransmitters, select the option with which each of the following is best associated as a major degradation enzyme:
   (i) MAO-B
   (ii) Aspartate aminotransferase
   (iii) Acetylcholinesterase.

3. **EMI** – Neurotransmitters
   (a) Acetylcholine
   (b) Dopamine
   (c) GABA
   (d) Glutamate
   (e) Noradrenaline
   (f) Serotonin
   (g) None of the above

   From the above list of neurotransmitters, select the option with which each of the following is best associated as a major synthesis enzyme:
   (i) Glutamic acid decarboxylase

   (ii) Tryptophan hydroxylase
   (iii) Choline acetyltransferase.

4. **MCQ** – Which of the following is least likely to be an effect of low doses of cannabis?
   (a) Analgesia
   (b) Calming
   (c) Euphoria
   (d) Impaired psychomotor functioning
   (e) Improved cognitive functioning.

5. **MCQ** – Select one incorrect statement regarding the cannabinoid system:
   (a) Synthetic cannabinoid ligands have potential in the treatment of pain, nausea, obesity and drug dependence.
   (b) Δ^9-Tetrahydrocannabinol is an active component of cannabis.
   (c) Δ^9-Tetrahydrocannabinol is an agonist at specific cannabinoid receptors, of which CB2 is the major brain site.
   (d) The cannabinoid system interacts with glutamate, opioid, dopamine and other neurotransmitter systems.
   (e) The naturally occurring agonists at the CB receptors, the endocannabinoids, include derivatives of arachidonic acid, anandamide and 2-arachidonylglycerol.

6. **MCQ** – Which of the following is not a monoamine neurotransmitter?
   (a) Dopamine
   (b) Glutamate
   (c) Histamine
   (d) Noradrenaline
   (e) Serotonin

7. **EMI** – Dopamine tracts
   (a) Pituitary gland
   (b) Red nucleus
   (c) Substantia nigra

(d) Ventral tegmental area

(e) None of the above

This question concerns the origins of dopamine tracts in the human brain. From the above list of brain structures, select the option with which each of the following major destinations is best associated as an origin:

(i) Limbic system

(ii) Striatum

(iii) Prefrontal cortex.

8. **EMI** – Adrenaline synthesis pathway

(a) Adrenaline-*N*-synthetase

(b) L-Aromatic amino acid decarboxylase

(c) L-Dopa

(d) Dopamine

(e) Dopamine-β-hydroxylase

(f) Noradrenaline

(g) Phenylethanolamine-*N*-methyltransferase

(h) Phenylethylamine

(i) Serotonin

(j) Serotonin hydroxylase

(k) Tyrosine

(l) Tyrosine hydroylase

(m) Tryptophan

(n) Tryptophan hydroylase

From the above list, select the option with which each label (i–viii) in the following pathway for the synthesis of adrenaline in humans is best associated:

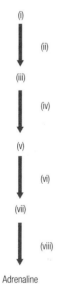

9. **MCQ** – What is the minimum number of enzyme steps from tryptophan to melatonin?

(a) 1

(b) 2

(c) 3

(d) 4

(e) Not applicable: melatonin is not a metabolite of tryptophan.

10. **EMI** – Neurotransmitters

(a) Acetylcholine

(b) Dopamine

(c) GABA

(d) Glutamate

(e) Noradrenaline

(f) Serotonin

(g) None of the above

From the above list of neurotransmitters, select the option with which each of the following is best associated as a major synthesis enzyme:

(i) Tryosine hydoxylase

(ii) Dopamine-β-hydroxylase

(iii) Glutaminase.

11. **MCQ** – Select one incorrect statement regarding acetylcholine:

(a) AChE is a glycoprotein that in one form is attached to the extracellular matrix of the cell membrane at the synapse and rapidly breaks down released acetylcholine.

(b) It has a major cell group in the basal forebrain where, from the basal nucleus of Meynert, there are projections to the cerebral cortex and parts of the amygdala, thalamus and basal ganglia.

(c) It was the first identified neurotransmitter, being detected as the substance released from the vagus nerve to increase heart rate.

(d) Its rate of synthesis is normally determined by the availability of precursors.

(e) Release-modulating autoreceptors are present on cholinergic terminals; these are primarily of the M2 subtype.

12. **EMI** – Acetylcholine synthesis pathway

(a) Acetyl-CoA

(b) AChE

(c) Choline

(d) Choline acetyltransferase

(e) Choline hydroxylase

(f) Ethanoic acid

(g) Phenylethanolamine-*N*-methyltransferase

(h) Phenylethylamine

(i) Tryptophan

(j) Tryptophan hydroylase

From the above list, select the option with which each label (i–iii) in the following pathway for the synthesis of acetylcholine in humans is best associated:

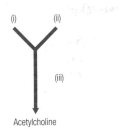

Acetylcholine

13. **EMI** – Glutamate synthesis and recycling pathway
   (a) EAAT
   (b) GABA
   (c) GABA decarboxylase
   (d) GABA synthetase
   (e) Glutamate
   (f) Glutamate decarboxylase
   (g) Glutaminase
   (h) Glutamine
   (i) Glutamine hydroxylase
   (j) Glutamine synthetase

From the above list, select the option with which each label (i–v) in the following pathway for glutamate synthesis and recycling in humans is best associated:

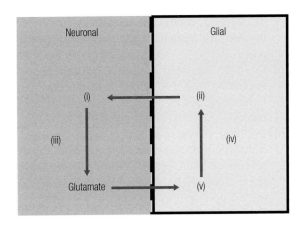

14. **MCQ** – Select one correct statement. The main inhibitory neurotransmitter in the human brain is:
   (a) Acetylcholine
   (b) Aspartate
   (c) Dopamine
   (d) GABA
   (e) Glutamate.

15. **MCQ** – Which of the following is not an ionotropic receptor?
   (a) D2 receptor
   (b) GABA$_A$ receptor
   (c) 5-HT$_3$ receptor
   (d) Nicotinic receptor
   (e) NMDA receptor.

16. **MCQ** – Select one incorrect statement regarding ionotropic receptors:
   (a) Their oligomeric proteins contain about 20 transmembrane segments arranged around a central aqueous channel.
   (b) They are large proteins generally composed of five subunits that assemble in the membrane.
   (c) They operate with a long latency.
   (d) When continuously exposed to ligand or transmitter, many of these receptors exhibit rapid desensitization, which may be an adaptive response to limit postsynaptic response under conditions of high presynaptic activity.
   (e) When open, the ion channel is usually selective to one or more ions.

17. **MCQ** – When open, which of the following ions does the ion channel of the GABA$_A$ receptor predominantly conduct?
   (a) Ca^{2+}
   (b) Cl$^-$
   (c) K$^+$
   (d) Mg^{2+}
   (e) Na$^+$

18. **MCQ** – Which of the following receptors have voltage-dependent ion channels?
   (a) AMPA receptors
   (b) 5-HT$_{2A}$ receptors
   (c) Kainate receptors
   (d) NMDA receptors
   (e) All of the above.

19. **MCQ** – Select the best correct response. Nicotinic receptors are particularly involved in which of the following functions?
   (a) Cognition
   (b) Memory
   (c) Muscle tone
   (d) Reward
   (e) All of the above.

20. **MCQ** – Which of the following is not a metabotropic receptor?
   (a) β-adrenoceptor
   (b) D1 receptor
   (c) H2 receptor
   (d) 5-HT$_3$ receptor
   (e) M2 receptor.

21. **MCQ** – Select one incorrect statement regarding metabotropic receptors:
   (a) As their action is mediated by biochemical processes, the effect of receptor stimulation is relatively long-lasting, typically seconds to minutes.
   (b) G-proteins are the transduction components that are linked to G-protein-coupled receptors and exist as a cluster of subunits.
   (c) Termination of the signal mediated by the G-protein is usually brought about by the hydrolysis of GTP

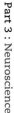

to GDP by GTPase, which the α-subunit possesses intrinsically.

(d) They are the most common class of central nervous system receptors.

(e) They have a characteristic structural design with six hydrophobic transmembrane regions.

22. **EMI** – Signalling mechanisms and metabotropic receptors
   (a) cAMP
   (b) Ca^{2+}
   (c) DAG
   (d) $G\alpha_s$
   (e) IP3
   (f) PKA
   (g) PKC
   (h) PLC

In relation to signalling mechanisms and metabotropic receptors, select the option from the above list with which each of the following is best associated:

(i) An enzyme which, when activated, cleaves PIP2.

(ii) Continuing from part (i), PIP2 is cleaved into IP3 and what else?

(iii) This triggers the release of Ca^{2+} from intracellular stores, resulting in a rise in $[Ca^{2+}]$ within the cell and activation of downstream events.

(iv) This activates PKC.

23. **MCQ** – Select the best correct option. What is the name given to the action of certain drugs in diminishing the constitutive activity of metabotropic receptors?
   (a) Agonism
   (b) Antagonism
   (c) Inverse agonism
   (d) Partial antagonism
   (e) Reciprocal antagonism.

24. **EMI** – Neurochemistry
   (a) D2R
   (b) D3R
   (c) D4R

Select the option from the above list with which each of the following is best associated:

(i) Found in substantial concentrations in the retina

(ii) Found in the highest concentrations in the striatum; also found in the pituitary gland, where it is involved in the tonic inhibition of prolactin secretion

(iii) Found in the striatum and limbic structures, and may have a particular involvement as an autoreceptor in presynaptic control of dopamine release.

25. **EMI** – Adrenoceptors
   (a) α_1
   (b) α_2
   (c) β_1
   (d) β_2
   (e) β_3

Select the option from the above list of human adrenoceptors with which each of the following is best associated:

(i) Found in high concentrations in the cerebellum; activate G_s to stimulate adenylate cyclase.

(ii) Found as autoreceptors in noradrenergic regions of the hindbrain; decrease adenylate cyclase through coupling to G_i.

(iii) Found mostly in the striatum and globus pallidus; activate G_s to stimulate adenylate cyclase.

(iv) Found in high concentrations in the locus coeruleus; activation generally results in an excitatory effect via G_q-mediated pathways.

26. **EMI** –5-HT receptors
   (a) 1A
   (b) 2A
   (c) 2C
   (d) 4
   (e) 6

Select the option from the above list of human 5-HT receptors with which each of the following is best associated:

(i) Excitatory receptors with effects mediated by stimulation of adenylate cyclase. Found in many cortical and subcortical brain regions. Closely involved in cognitive function through their ability to regulate cholinergic neurotransmission. Also involved in anxiety, affect and control of body mass.

(ii) Found in the basal ganglia and limbic regions of the brain. Appear to inhibit dopaminergic activity, influencing motor function. Have effects on food intake.

(iii) Excitatory receptors with effects mediated by stimulation of adenylate cyclase. Found in several subcortical brain regions and in the gastrointestinal tract. Have effects on learning and memory and are a drug target for the treatment of cognitive and dementing disorders.

(iv) Excitatory postsynaptic receptors which work via the stimulation of PLC. Found in many brain regions, including the cortex and basal ganglia where they influence dopaminergic neurotransmission. They are thought to be involved in some of the beneficial effects of atypical antipsychotic drugs on cognitive and negative features of psychotic illness and in minimizing extrapyramidal side-effects.

27. **MCQ** – Select the best correct option. Which of the following muscarinic receptors function as inhibitory autoreceptors in the hippocampus and cortex?
   (a) M1
   (b) M2
   (c) M3
   (d) M4
   (e) M5.

28. **EMI** – Histaminergic receptors
   (a) H1
   (b) H2
   (c) H3

Select the histaminergic receptor option from the above list with which each of the following is best associated:
   (i) Excitatory receptors found in the hypothalamus and limbic structures
   (ii) Primarily presynaptic, act as inhibitory autoreceptors
   (iii) Thought to mediate drug effects on sedation and food intake
   (iv) Primarily presynaptic, act as heteroreceptors controlling the release of other transmitters, including acetylcholine.

29. **MCQ** – Select one incorrect statement regarding mGluRs:
   (a) They are all expressed in the mammalian brain in both neuronal and glial cells.
   (b) They are dimeric GPCRs comprised of (at least) eight subtypes.
   (c) They contain a large extracellular N-terminal tail containing a glutamate binding site.
   (d) They show no sequence homology with other GPCRs.
   (e) Preclinical studies have provided evidence for the potential use of group II agonists in the treatment of schizophrenia.

30. **MCQ** – Select one incorrect statement regarding GABA$_B$ receptors:
   (a) Pharmacologically they can be distinguished from GABA$_A$ receptors by their selective affinity for baclofen and lack of affinity for muscimol and bicuculline.
   (b) They are all metabotropic receptors that belong to the GPCR family.
   (c) They are found at higher levels in the central nervous system than GABA$_A$ receptors.
   (d) They are located both pre- and postsynaptically.
   (e) Two major subunits have been identified, which form heterodimers together, whereby one subunit contains the ligand binding site and the other mediates G-protein signalling.

31. **EMI** – Pharmacology of major neurotransmitter systems
   (a) Inhibition of neurotransmitter metabolism
   (b) Inhibition of neurotransmitter reuptake
   (c) Inhibition of the vesicular monoamine transporter
   (d) ↑ Neurotransmitter synthesis

Regarding the pharmacology of major neurotransmitter systems, select the option from the above list with which the therapeutic mechanism of action of each of the following drug treatments is best associated:
   (i) Tryptophan treatment in depression
   (ii) Treatment with SSRIs in depression
   (iii) Treatment with MAOIs in depression
   (iv) The use of tetrabenazine in Huntington's disease
   (v) Treatment of Alzheimer's disease with donepezil.

32. **MCQ** – Which of the following is least likely to be true regarding the action of clozapine at therapeutic doses?
   (a) Antimuscarinic activity
   (b) D4R antagonism > D2R antagonism
   (c) GABA$_A$ receptor antagonism
   (d) 5-HT$_{1A}$ receptor partial agonism
   (e) 5-HT$_{2C}$ receptor antagonism.

33. **MCQ** – Which of the following, at 'therapeutic/physiological' dosage, is most likely to bind within the channel pore of the GABA$_A$ receptor and block ion flow?
   (a) Barbiturates
   (b) Flumazenil
   (c) Muscimol
   (d) Nitrazepam
   (e) Picrotoxin.

34. **MCQ** – Select one incorrect statement regarding neuropeptides:
   (a) A neuropeptide is a short neuroactive protein of generally fewer than 100 amino acids.
   (b) An increase in neuronal demand for peptide synthesis can usually induce a rapid response.
   (c) Neuronal release of large vesicles, containing neuropeptides, and of small vesicles, containing neurotransmitters, are regulated differently in that peptides are typically released at a high neuronal firing frequency while neurotransmitters are released at a low frequency.
   (d) Peptides bind with high specificity and high affinity to their receptors, which are generally G-protein-coupled or metabotropic receptors.
   (e) Unlike classical neurotransmitters, synaptic inactivation of neuropeptides is generally performed by enzymes and there is generally no active reuptake process.

35. **MCQ** – Select one incorrect statement regarding CCK:
   (a) It binds to two different subtypes of receptors which are both GPCRs and display approximately 50 per cent homology.
   (b) It is a peptide neurotransmitter that was originally isolated from the brain.
   (c) It is co-localized with dopamine in a significant subset of mesencephalic neurones originating within the ventral tegmental area and terminating in the nucleus accumbens.
   (d) It produces a reduction in food intake, via the hindbrain CCK$_1$ receptors, while also inhibiting expression of orexigenic peptides in the hypothalamus.
   (e) Its actions include the induction of anxiety-related behaviour in humans and experimental animals, an action via stimulation of CCK$_2$ receptors.

36. **MCQ** – Select one incorrect statement regarding NT:
   (a) It is synthesized as part of a 170-amino acid precursor protein that also contains the related hexapeptide neuromedin N.

(b) Its actions include pain, nociception, hyperthermia and the inhibition of growth hormone release.

(c) NT immunoreactive neurones and terminal systems and receptors are found in many parts of the brain, including the basal and anterior hypothalamus, nucleus accumbens and several brainstem nuclei.

(d) NTS1 regulates dopaminergic function in both the nucleus accumbens and dorsal striatum by reducing function of the D2 autoreceptor and the activity of postsynaptic D2Rs located on glutamate terminals.

(e) The NTS3 receptor is a type I amino acid receptor single-transmembrane-spanning receptor and is found in adipocytes as well as in neurones and glia.

37. **MCQ** – Select one correct option. Which of the following is not an opioid neuropeptide?
(a) Dynorphin A
(b) Met^5-encephalin
(c) α/β-Neoendorphin
(d) Nociceptin
(e) Substance P.

38. **EMI** – Feeding neuropeptides
(a) ↑ Appetite/feeding
(b) ↓ Appetite/feeding
(c) Neither of the above

Regarding feeding neuropeptides, select the option from the above list with which physiological levels of each of the following is best associated:
(i) AgRP
(ii) α-MSH
(iii) NPY
(iv) Leptin
(v) Ghrelin.

39. **MCQ** – Via which of the following types of receptor is sodium oxybate most likely to cause its therapeutic actions in narcolepsy?
(a) nAChR
(b) GABA$_A$
(c) GABA$_B$
(d) Glutamate
(e) 5-HT$_3$.

40. **MCQ** – Select one incorrect statement regarding BDNF:
(a) A functional coding region polymorphism (Met66Val) of *BDNF*, associated with smaller hippocampal volumes and poor performance on hippocampus-dependent memory tasks, has been proposed as a risk factor for the development of schizophrenia.
(b) BDNF and its receptor TrkB are expressed widely in association with glutamatergic synapses.
(c) It is involved in long-term potentiation; CREB, a transcription factor implicated in memory processing, is a major mediator of neuronal BDNF responses.
(d) It regulates synaptic plasticity, helping to support the survival of existing neurones and to encourage the growth and differentiation of new neurones and synapses.
(e) Neurotrophins are abnormally regulated in animal models of psychiatric illness and are changed after antipsychotic or antidepressant administration; altered BDNF levels in blood and cerebrospinal fluid have been reported in humans with schizophrenia.

ANSWERS

1. b

They are the most common cells of the central nervous system.

Reference: *Psychiatry: An evidence-based text*, **p. 410.**

2.

(i)   b
(ii) d
(iii) a

Reference: *Psychiatry: An evidence-based text*, **p. 413.**

3.

(i)   c
(ii) f
(iii) a

Reference: *Psychiatry: An evidence-based text*, **p. 413.**

4. e

Low doses of cannabis can cause impaired cognitive functioning.

Reference: *Psychiatry: An evidence-based text*, **p. 412.**

5. c

The major brain site is CB1.

Reference: *Psychiatry: An evidence-based text*, **p. 412.**

6. b

Reference: *Psychiatry: An evidence-based text*, **p. 413.**

7.

(i)   d – Via the mesolimbic system from the ventral tegmental area
(ii) c – Via the nigrostriatal pathway
(iii) d – Via the mesocortical system.

Reference: *Psychiatry: An evidence-based text*, **p. 413.**

8.

(i)   k
(ii)   l
(iii) c
(iv)   b
(v)   d
(vi)   e
(vii) f
(viii) g

Reference: *Psychiatry: An evidence-based text*, **p. 414.**

9. d

Tryptophan is converted into serotonin via two enzyme steps (see Figure 30.3 on page 414 of the accompanying textbook) and serotonin is converted by two enzymes to form melatonin.

Reference: *Psychiatry: An evidence-based text*, **pp. 414–415.**

10.

(i)   b
(ii) e
(iii) d

Reference: *Psychiatry: An evidence-based text*, **p. 413.**

11. c

Its release by the vagus nerve causes the cardiac rate to diminish. (Recall that this is a parasympathetic action.)

Reference: *Psychiatry: An evidence-based text*, **pp. 415–416.**

12.

(i)   a or c.
(ii) c [if 'a' was chosen for (i)] or a [if 'c' was chosen for (i)].
(iii) d

Reference: *Psychiatry: An evidence-based text*, **p. 416.**

13.

(i)   h
(ii) h
(iii) g
(iv) j
(v)   e

Reference: *Psychiatry: An evidence-based text*, **p. 417.**

14. d

Reference: *Psychiatry: An evidence-based text*, **p. 417.**

15. a

This is a metabotropic receptor.

Reference: *Psychiatry: An evidence-based text*, **pp. 417–421.**

16. c

Because of the close linkage between ligand binding and ion channel opening, ionotropic receptors operate with a very short latency (a few ms). Therefore, receptors of this type control fast synaptic transmission in the nervous system.

Reference: *Psychiatry: An evidence-based text*, **pp. 417–418.**

17. b

This leads to hyperpolarization in the postsynaptic cell.

Reference: *Psychiatry: An evidence-based text*, **p. 418.**

18. d

Note that 5-HT$_{2A}$ receptors are metabotropic.

Reference: *Psychiatry: An evidence-based text*, **pp. 418–422.**

19. e

Nicotinic receptors are involved in a wide range of physiological processes.

Reference: *Psychiatry: An evidence-based text*, **p. 419.**

20. d

Note that other subtypes of 5-HT receptors, such as 5-HT$_{2A}$ receptors, are metabotropic.

Reference: *Psychiatry: An evidence-based text*, **pp. 419–423.**

21. e

There are characteristically seven hydrophobic transmembrane regions within a single polypeptide chain such that G-protein-coupled receptors wrap back and forth through the lipid cell membrane and are exposed to both the intracellular and extracellular cell surfaces (as shown in Fig. 30.7 on page 420 of the accompanying textbook). Hence an alternative name for this group of receptors: the seven-transmembrane domain (7TM) receptors.

Reference: *Psychiatry: An evidence-based text*, **pp. 419–421.**

22.

(i) h
(ii) c
(iii) e
(iv) c

Reference: *Psychiatry: An evidence-based text*, **pp. 420–421.**

23. c

Such an effect is relatively common for drugs that are antagonists at such receptors.

Reference: *Psychiatry: An evidence-based text*, **p. 421.**

24.

(i) c
(ii) a
(iii) b

Reference: *Psychiatry: An evidence-based text*, **p. 421.**

25.

(i) d
(ii) b
(iii) c
(iv) a

Reference: *Psychiatry: An evidence-based text*, **pp. 421–422.**

26.

(i) e
(ii) c
(iii) d
(iv) b

Reference: *Psychiatry: An evidence-based text*, **p. 422.**

27. b

M2 and M4 receptors are also involved in spinal cord function, notably nociception, and are also important outside the central nervous system.

Reference: *Psychiatry: An evidence-based text*, **pp. 422–423.**

28.

(i) a
(ii) c
(iii) a
(iv) c

Reference: *Psychiatry: An evidence-based text*, **p. 423.**

29. a

mGluR$_6$ is confined to the retina.

Reference: *Psychiatry: An evidence-based text*, **p. 423.**

30. c

Reference: *Psychiatry: An evidence-based text*, **p. 423.**

31.

(i) d – This increases serotonin biosynthesis.
(ii) b – Hence the name of this group of drugs.
(iii) a
(iv) c
(v) a

Reference: *Psychiatry: An evidence-based text*, **pp. 424–425.**

32. c

Reference: *Psychiatry: An evidence-based text*, **pp. 426–427.**

33. e

This is a potent convulsant which, at a sufficiently high concentration, can cause widespread seizure activity.

Reference: *Psychiatry: An evidence-based text*, **pp. 427–428.**

34. b

Neuropeptides are synthesized from precursor proteins produced from specific genes. In most cases, these gene products give rise to a propeptide, which is then cleaved by peptidase enzymes to form the peptide neurotransmitter. This means that increases in production of neuropeptide require an increase in gene expression, a slow process that can take hours or even days. This limiting step means that an increase in neuronal demand for peptide synthesis cannot induce a rapid response.

Reference: *Psychiatry: An evidence-based text*, **pp. 428–429.**

35. b

Cholecystokinin (CCK), as implied by its name, was originally isolated from the gut. However, CCK is distributed extensively and abundantly within the central nervous system.

Reference: *Psychiatry: An evidence-based text*, **p. 429.**

36. b

The actions of NT (neurotensin) include analgesia, hypothermia and release of growth hormone and prolactin.

Reference: *Psychiatry: An evidence-based text*, **p. 429.**

37. e

Substance P is one of the tachykinin proteins, which include NKA and NKB, all synthesized from the same preprotachykinin gene.

Reference: *Psychiatry: An evidence-based text*, **pp. 429–430.**

38.

(i) a – AgRP (Agouti-related protein) is produced in the arcuate nucleus in the hypothalamus and is co-localized with NPY (neuropeptide Y) in neurones. It increases appetite and decreases metabolism and energy expenditure.

(ii) b – α-MSH (α-melanocyte stimulating hormone) is an anorectic peptide that plays an inhibitory role in feeding and energy storage.

(iii) a – NPY increases food intake. In obesity, an increase in NPY activity is thought to be brought about by high levels of glucocorticoids abolishing the negative feedback of corticotropin-releasing hormone on NPY synthesis and release.

(iv) b – Leptin is produced by adipose tissue; leptin secretion increases as fat is deposited and diminishes as the adipocyte stores of fat decrease. Leptin signals to the brain that the body has had enough to eat, by inhibiting the activity of neurones that contain NPY and AgRP and stimulating receptors containing MSH.

(v) a – Ghrelin is produced in the stomach and pancreas to stimulate appetite and increase adiposity and is thought to act in concert with leptin.

Reference: *Psychiatry: An evidence-based text*, **p. 432.**

39. c

Sodium oxybate is used for the treatment of narcolepsy with cataplexy, and is also a drug with the potential for abuse. It is thought to act via $GABA_B$ receptors. There is evidence that sodium oxybate may also be useful in the treatment of fibromyalgia.

Reference: *Psychiatry: An evidence-based text*, **pp. 427–428.**

40. a

The single nucleotide polymorphism in *BDNF* (in italics because this is referring to the gene) is the other way around, i.e. Val66Met.

Reference: *Psychiatry: An evidence-based text*, **pp. 432–433.**

Chapter 31

Neuropathology

QUESTIONS

Note that for answers to extended matching items (EMIs), each option (denoted a, b, c, etc.) might be used once, more than once or not at all. For multiple-choice questions (MCQs), please select the best answer.

1. **EMI** – Central nervous system pathological changes
   (a) Central chromatolysis
   (b) ↑ GFAP
   (c) α-Synuclein immunoreactive Papp–Lantos inclusions
   (d) None of the above

Select the option from the above list containing microscopic central nervous system pathological changes with which each of the following is best associated:
   (i) Parkinson's disease
   (ii) Neuronal cell body swelling with dispersion of the Nissl substance
   (iii) Accompanies astrocytosis
   (iv) MSA.

2. **MCQ** – Which of the following pathological changes is pathognomonic of Alzheimer's disease?
   (a) Gliosis
   (b) Hippocampal atrophy
   (c) Intracellular neurofibrillary tangles
   (d) Neuritic (senile) plaques
   (e) None of the above.

3. **EMI** – Vasculopathy-related genes
   (a) *APP*
   (b) *CST3*
   (c) *GSN*
   (d) *NOTCH3*
   (e) None of the above

Select the option from the above list containing genes with which each of the following vasculopathies is best associated:
   (i) CADASIL
   (ii) HCHWA-D
   (iii) HCHWA-I
   (iv) Familial amyloidosis, Finnish type.

4. **MCQ** – Which of the following microscopic pathological changes is least likely to be seen in Creutzfeldt–Jakob disease?
   (a) Deposition of the pathological form of the prion protein
   (b) Intranuclear cats-eye inclusions
   (c) Neuronal cell loss
   (d) Reactive astrogliosis
   (e) Spongiform changes.

5. **MCQ** – Select the best option. Which of the following pathological microscopic changes are typically seen in tangle-only frontotemporal lobar dementia?
   (a) Absence of Aβ pathology
   (b) Cortical neuronal loss
   (c) Gliosis
   (d) Numerous neurofibrillary tangles
   (e) All of the above.

6. **MCQ** – Which of the following pathological features is least likely to be typically seen in dementia pugilistica?
   (a) Absence of Aβ pathology
   (b) Fenestration of the cavum septum pellucidum
   (c) Loss of pigmented cells from the substantia nigra
   (d) Neurofibrillary tangles throughout the cerebral cortex
   (e) Scarring to the inferior surface of the cerebellum.

7. **EMI** – Movement disorders
   (a) Huntington's disease
   (b) Motor neurone disease
   (c) Multiple system atrophy
   (d) Parkinson's disease
   (e) Progressive supranuclear palsy

Select the option from the above list of movement disorders with which each of the following is best associated:
   (i) Marked atrophy of the caudate and putamen, with a corresponding increase in the size of the ventricles
   (ii) Loss of pigmented cells from the locus coeruleus
   (iii) Greenish discoloration and shrinkage of the putamen.

8. **EMI** – Common locations for neuroepithelial tumours
   (a) Cerebellum
   (b) Cerebral hemispheres

(c) Conus medullaris

(d) Lateral ventricles

Select the location from the above list with which each of the following neuroepithelial tumours is best associated:

(i) Astrocytoma

(ii) Central neurocytoma

(iii) Oligodendroglioma

(iv) Myxopapillary ependymoma.

9. **MCQ** – Which of the following is the neuropathological change most consistently observed in schizophrenia?

(a) Disruption of normal gyrification

(b) Lateral ventricular enlargement and reduced brain volume

(c) Loss of normal brain asymmetry

(d) Periventricular gliosis

(e) Reduced size of the corpus callosum.

10. **EMI** – Movement disorders

(a) Huntington's disease

(b) Motor neurone disease

(c) Multiple system atrophy

(d) Parkinson's disease

(e) Progressive supranuclear palsy

Select the option from the above list with which each of the following is best associated:

(i) Pallor of the substantia nigra but sparing of the locus coeruleus

(ii) Mild atrophy of the midbrain, superior cerebellar peduncles and discoloration of the dentate nucleus of the cerebellum

(iii) The spinal cord is thinner than normal and the anterior nerve roots appear atrophic and discoloured. The brain may appear normal macroscopically, although in some cases the precentral gyrus may be atrophic.

11. **EMI** – Common locations for neuroepithelial tumours

(a) Cauda equina

(b) Cerebellum

(c) Cerebral hemispheres

(d) Lateral ventricles

Select the location from the above list with which each of the following neuroepithelial tumours is best associated:

(i) Medulloblastoma

(ii) Glioblastoma

(iii) Paraganglioma.

ANSWERS

1.

(i) c – Parkinson's disease is an α-synucleinopathy, and immunostaining with antibodies against α-synuclein is now the method of choice for identifying the Lewy bodies that characterize the disease at the microscopic level. This is shown in Figure 31.7 on page 440 of the accompanying textbook.

(ii) a – Also, the nucleus moves to the edge of the cell.

(iii) b – Astrocytosis is accompanied by the production of large amounts of the intermediate filament protein GFAP (glial acidic fibrillary protein), immunostaining for which is used routinely to detect astrocytosis. This is shown in Figure 31.1(e) on page 435 of the accompanying textbook.

(iv) c – α-Synuclein immunoreactive Papp–Lantos inclusions are considered diagnostic for MSA (multiple system atrophy).

Reference: Psychiatry: An evidence-based text, **Ch. 31.**

2. e

Reference: Psychiatry: An evidence-based text, **Ch. 31.**

3.

(i) d – CADASIL (cerebral autosomal dominant arteriopathy with subcortical infarcts and leucoencephalopathy) is associated with mutations in the *NOTCH3* gene, resulting in multiple infarcts in the frontal white matter and basal ganglia.

(ii) a – HCHWA-D (hereditary cerebral haemorrhage with amyloidosis, Dutch type) results from a mutation in the same *APP* (amyloid precursor protein) gene that is central to the pathology of Alzheimer's disease.

(iii) b – HCHWA-I (hereditary cerebral haemorrhage with amyloidosis, Icelandic type) results from a mutation in the *CST3* gene that encodes for the cystatin C protein.

(iv) c – This gene encodes for gelsolin.

Reference: Psychiatry: An evidence-based text, **p. 439.**

4. b

Creutzfeldt–Jakob disease is the most common form of human prion disease. Intranuclear cats-eye inclusions may be seen in the frontotemporal lobar dementias (FTLDs). An example of such an inclusion in the dentate gyrus of a patient with FTLD is shown in Figure 31.4 on page 438 of the accompanying textbook.

Reference: Psychiatry: An evidence-based text, **pp. 437–439.**

5. e

Reference: Psychiatry: An evidence-based text, **p. 438.**

6. a

In the original boxer studies, carried out using silver staining techniques, no amyloid plaques were seen. However, when the cases were revisited using immunocytochemistry for the Aβ peptide, large numbers of diffuse deposits were observed. Similarly, diffuse Aβ has been observed in a proportion of patients who die soon after a single episode of severe head injury. This has prompted further investigations of possible links between trauma and the subsequent development of neurodegeneration. One possible mechanism for this is the initiation of neuroinflammation.

Reference: Psychiatry: An evidence-based text, **pp. 439–440.**

7.

(i) a – Atrophy of the caudate and putamen with lateral ventricular enlargement are evident on coronal MRI scans as well as postmortem.

(ii) d – This can be seen postmortem in sections of the pons.

(iii) c

Reference: Psychiatry: An evidence-based text, **pp. 440–441.**

8.

(i) b
(ii) d
(iii) b
(iv) c

Reference: Psychiatry: An evidence-based text, **p. 442.**

9. b

This finding is based largely on structural neuroimaging studies (MRI and CT).

Reference: Psychiatry: An evidence-based text, **pp. 442–443.**

10.

(i) e – This can be seen postmortem in sections of the mesencephalon.

(ii) e – These changes can help distinguish PSP (progressive supranuclear palsy) from Parkinson's disease.

(iii) b – The precentral gyrus may be atrophic if there has been particularly prominent upper motor neurone disturbance. Luxol-fast blue staining of the spinal cord will show pallor of the corticospinal tracts.

Reference: Psychiatry: An evidence-based text, **pp. 440–441.**

11.

(i) b
(ii) c
(iii) a

Reference: Psychiatry: An evidence-based text, **p. 442.**

Chapter 32

Neuroimaging

QUESTIONS

Note that for answers to extended matching items (EMIs), each option (denoted a, b, c, etc.) might be used once, more than once or not at all. For multiple-choice questions (MCQs), please select the best answer.

1. **EMI** – Neuroimaging techniques
   (a) Brain anatomy
   (b) Brain blood flow
   (c) Brain chemistry

Select the type of information from the above list with which each of the following neuroimaging techniques is best associated:
   (i) CT (without a contrast agent)
   (ii) fMRI
   (iii) FLAIR.

2. **EMI** – Nuclear magnetic resonance (NMR)
   (a) B_0
   (b) M
   (c) $M(t)$
   (d) M_{xy}
   (e) M_z
   (f) x,y
   (g) z

Select the symbol from the above list with which each of the following nuclear magnetic resonance parameters is best associated:
   (i) Longitudinal plane
   (ii) Sum magnetization vector
   (iii) Transverse magnetization.

3. **MCQ** – Select one incorrect statement regarding T1- and T2-weighted MRI:
   (a) At any given field structure, the T1 is shorter for cerebrospinal fluid (CSF) than for grey matter, and in turn shorter for grey matter than for white matter.
   (b) T1 is measured when the longitudinal magnetization reaches approximately 63 per cent of its maximum value after a 90° RF pulse brings it to zero.
   (c) T1 is the longitudinal time constant and indexes the rate at which the longitudinal magnetization returns to its maximum value following an RF pulse.
   (d) The T1 is particularly short for fat.
   (e) The value of T1 varies with the magnetic field strength.

4. **MCQ** – Select the best option. By what factor is the magnetic field strength inside the bore of the main magnet of a 3T MRI scanner typically likely to be greater than the strength of the earth's magnetic field at sea level?
   (a) 5–10
   (b) 50–100
   (c) 500–1000
   (d) 5000–10 000
   (e) 50 000–100 000

5. **MCQ** – The presence of which of the following in a subject is least likely to be an absolute contraindication to him having a brain scan safely in a modern 3T MRI scanner?
   (a) A haemostatic clip
   (b) A history of a small piece of metal having entered an eye some years before
   (c) A metallic hip implant
   (d) An aneurysm clip
   (e) An artificial cardiac pacemaker.

6. **MCQ** – Select the least correct statement regarding deoxyhaemoglobin:
   (a) It can be used as an endogenous contrast agent in fMRI.
   (b) It is diamagnetic.
   (c) Its concentration generally rises in a brain region with greater activation of that region.
   (d) Its measurement is fundamental to the BOLD effect.
   (e) Its molecules have unpaired electrons.

7. **EMI** – MR spectroscopy
   (a) ^{13}C
   (b) ^{1}H
   (c) ^{19}F
   (d) ^{17}O
   (e) ^{31}P
   (f) None of the above

Select the type of MR spectroscopy, if any, from the above list with which each of the following substances can best have its brain concentration measured in living humans:

(i) NAA

(ii) Pi

(iii) Na⁺.

8. **MCQ** – Select the least correct statement regarding SPECT neuroimaging:

   (a) Gamma cameras are used for detection.

   (b) The data reconstruction may reflect cerebral blood flow.

   (c) The data reconstruction may reflect cerebral tissue binding.

   (d) The radioligand emits single γ photons.

   (e) Subjects need to be in the scanner to assess the state of their brain at the time of (or very soon after) ligand administration.

9. **EMI** – PET ligands

   (a) D2R/D3R

   (b) Glucose metabolism

   (c) 5-HT1A receptors

   (d) CB1 receptors

   (e) None of the above

Select the type of *in vivo* human brain study, if any, from the above list with which each of the following PET ligands is best associated:

   (i) [¹⁸F]FDG

   (ii) [¹¹C]raclopride

   (iii) [carbonyl-¹¹C]WAY-100635

   (iv) [¹¹C]MePPEP.

10. **EMI** – Neuroimaging techniques

    (a) Brain anatomy

    (b) Brain blood flow

    (c) Brain chemistry

    (d) None of the above

Select the type of information from the above list with which each of the following neuroimaging techniques is best associated:

   (i) Proton MRS

   (ii) DTI

   (iii) ASL.

11. **EMI** – Nuclear magnetic resonance parameters

    (a) B_0

    (b) M

    (c) $M(t)$

    (d) M_{xy}

    (e) M_z

    (f) x,y

    (g) z

Select the symbol from the above list with which each of the following nuclear magnetic resonance parameters is best associated:

   (i) Static magnetic field

   (ii) Transverse plane

   (iii) Longitudinal magnetization

   (iv) The magnetization vector at a given time after the RF pulse.

12. **EMI** – MR spectroscopy

    (a) ¹³C

    (b) ¹H

    (c) ¹⁹F

    (d) ¹⁷O

    (e) ³¹P

    (f) None of the above

Select the type of MR spectroscopy, if any, from the above list with which each of the following substances can best have its brain concentration measured in living humans:

   (i) PME

   (ii) Lactate

   (iii) Cho

   (iv) Fluoxetine.

ANSWERS

1.

(i) a – CT (X-ray computed tomography), without the use of a contrast agent, is a structural imaging technique in brain studies.

(ii) b – fMRI gives an index of brain blood flow when used in brain studies. Strictly speaking, BOLD (blood oxygen level dependent) fMRI indexes the BOLD effect, but brain blood flow is the best of the three possible options given here.

(iii) a – FLAIR (fluid-attenuated inversion recovery) MRI sequences are used to produce structural brain scans in brain studies. Figure 32.18 on page 456 of the accompanying textbook shows a middle cerebral artery infarct in a FLAIR MRI scan.

Reference: Psychiatry: An evidence-based text, **Ch. 32.**

2.

(i) g

(ii) b

(iii) d

Reference: Psychiatry: An evidence-based text, **p. 448.**

3. a

If you cannot remember all the details of how the T1 is measured, then you should still be able to come to the correct answer by recalling the appearance of a T1-weighted MRI brain scan (as shown, for example, in Fig. 32.10a on page 450 of the accompanying textbook). Recall that in such a scan, CSF looks almost black, the grey matter looks relatively grey and the white matter looks relatively white. The only way to reconcile this appearance with options 'a' and 'd' is if the T1 values are in the following order: T1 (CSF) > T1 (grey matter) > T1 (white matter); in other words, option 'a' is incorrect.

Reference: Psychiatry: An evidence-based text, **pp. 449–450.**

4. e

At the surface of the earth, the earth's magnetic field strength is around 30 to 60 µT.

Reference: Psychiatry: An evidence-based text, **p. 450.**

5. c

The radiographer should be informed beforehand in such a case. It may be permissible for such a person to undergo MR neuroimaging, depending on various circumstances.

In respect of option 'b', note that any person who has such a history should not be allowed near such a scanner unless he or she has had orbital X-rays taken and cleared

by a radiologist. Just one small sliver of metal could tear through the eye while the subject is in the scanner.

Reference: Psychiatry: An evidence-based text, **pp. 450–451.**

6. b

It is paramagnetic, having unpaired electrons. In contrast, oxyhaemoglobin is diamagnetic.

Reference: Psychiatry: An evidence-based text, **p. 452.**

7.

(i) b – NAA (*N*-acetyl aspartate) is particularly prominent in proton MRS scans, as shown in Figure 32.16(a) on page 455 of the accompanying textbook.

(ii) e – Pi (inorganic phosphate) can be measured using 31-phosphorus MRS, as shown in Figure 32.17 on page 455 of the accompanying textbook.

(iii) f

Reference: Psychiatry: An evidence-based text, **pp. 452–455.**

8. e

One particular advantage of SPECT is that some 99m-technetium-based ligands can be used to determine cerebral blood flow at a time when the subject is not even in the same room as the gamma camera. There may be a window of opportunity of at least half an hour after ligand administration during which the subject can undergo scanning; such SPECT scanning will show the state of the cerebral blood flow shortly after the ligand was administered, owing to a change in the ligand from a lipophilic form (when it can readily cross the blood–brain barrier) to a hydrophilic form, as shown in Figure 32.19 on page 456 of the accompanying textbook. This property has allowed SPECT neuroimaging to be used to study cerebral blood flow during hallucinations in schizophrenia. Epilepsy studies (ictal SPECT) are similarly, therefore, also made possible.

Reference: Psychiatry: An evidence-based text, **pp. 456–457.**

9.

(i) b – This radiotracer is a marker for glucose metabolism. An example of such a PET scan is shown in Figure 32.32 on page 463 of the accompanying textbook.

(ii) a – This is a dopamine D2/D3 receptor radioligand.

(iii) c

(iv) d

Reference: Psychiatry: An evidence-based text, **pp. 458–463.**

10.

(i) c – This is a form of MRS.

(ii) a – DTI (diffusion tensor imaging) can be used to infer the location of white matter tracts in the brain.

(iii) b – ASL (arterial spin labelling) is a form of imaging in which endogenous water molecules in arterial blood are non-invasively given a special magnetization tag in the neck before entering the brain. The tagged images of the brain are then collected and allow cerebral blood flow to be determined.

Reference: *Psychiatry: An evidence-based text,* **Ch. 32.**

11.

(i) a
(ii) f
(iii) e
(iv) c – Note that RF stands for radiofrequency

Reference: *Psychiatry: An evidence-based text,* **p. 448.**

12.

(i) e – The PME (phosphomonoesters) peak indexes membrane phospholipid anabolism and can be measured using 31-phosphorus MRS, as shown in Figure 32.17 on page 455 of the accompanying textbook.

(ii) b – Lactate is not usually seen in the normal adult human brain. Its presence in the proton MRS scan from a patient with a glioblastoma is shown in Figure 32.16(c) on page 455 of the accompanying textbook; here it indicates anaerobic respiration.

(iii) b – Cho (choline) can be measured using proton MRS, as shown in Figure 32.16(a) on page 455 of the accompanying textbook.

(iv) c – Owing to the virtual absence of ^{19}F compounds usually in the body, the introduction of a therapeutic fluorine-containing drug such as the SSRI fluoxetine means that levels of this drug and its principal metabolite can be measured using ^{19}F MRS.

Reference: *Psychiatry: An evidence-based text,* **pp. 452–455.**

Chapter 33

Genetics

QUESTIONS

Note that for answers to extended matching items (EMIs), each option (denoted a, b, c, etc.) might be used once, more than once or not at all. For multiple-choice questions (MCQs), please select the best answer.

1. **MCQ** – Suppose one of your siblings suffers from an autosomal recessive disorder which first manifests in childhood, but that you and your parents do not suffer from this disease. What is the probability that you are heterozygous for this disease?
   (a) 1/2
   (b) 1/3
   (c) 1/4
   (d) 2/3
   (e) 3/4.

2. **MCQ** – We continue with the scenario described in Question 1. Suppose now that you marry someone who is unaffected by this autosomal recessive disorder and whose parents are also unaffected by it. Assume that your spouse does not carry the autosomal recessive disease allele. If the probability that you carry it as a heterozygote is x (corresponding to the answer to the previous question), what is the probability that your first son, by your unaffected spouse, is unaffected by the disease but is a carrier?
   (a) $x/2$
   (b) $x/3$
   (c) $x/4$
   (d) $2x/3$
   (e) $3x/4$.

3. **MCQ** – Referring to the scenario in Questions 1 and 2, suppose your unaffected first son, who is potentially a carrier, marries a similarly unaffected woman who is also a potential carrier. If your son and his wife each has a probability of y of being carriers for this particular autosomal recessive disease, what is the probability that their first child will be affected by this disease?
   (a) $y^2/2$
   (b) $y^2/3$
   (c) $y^2/4$
   (d) $y/2$
   (e) $y/4$.

4. **EMI** – Advances in genetics
   (a) Franklin, Rosalind
   (b) Mendel, Gregor
   (c) Mullis, Kary
   (d) Northern, Jo
   (e) Southern, Ed
   (f) None of the above

Select the person, if any, from the above list with which each of the following advances in genetics is best associated:
   (i) Structure of DNA
   (ii) PCR
   (iii) Law of independent assortment
   (iv) Northern blotting
   (v) Southern blotting.

5. **EMI** – Stages of mitosis
   (a) Anaphase
   (b) Interphase
   (c) Mesophase
   (d) Metaphase
   (e) Nanophase
   (f) Prophase
   (g) Telophase
   (h) None of the above

Select the option from the above stages of mitosis with which each of the following descriptions is best associated:
   (i) The stage during which chromosomes are duplicated
   (ii) The spindles retract, pulling a chromosome to each pole
   (iii) A spindle forms from a centriole at each cell pole to the centromere.

6. **MCQ** – Which of the following bases is found in human RNA but not usually in human DNA?
   (a) A
   (b) C
   (c) G
   (d) T
   (e) U.

7. **EMI** – Nucleic acid bases
   (a) Purine
   (b) Pyrimidine
   (c) Neither of the above

Select the class from the above list with which each of the following nucleic acid bases is best associated:

    (i)   A

    (ii) C

    (iii) G

    (iv) T

    (v) U.

8. **EMI** – Chromosomal patterns

    (a) Down syndrome

    (b) Edward syndrome

    (c) Klinefelter syndrome

    (d) Patau syndrome

    (e) Turner syndrome

    (f) None of the above

Select the option from the above list with which each of the following human chromosomal patterns is best associated:

    (i)   Trisomy 18

    (ii) Trisomy 13

    (iii) XXY

    (iv) XO.

9. **MCQ** – Select the best option. Where the mode of inheritance is known and the phenotype can be clearly defined, a LOD score of –2 implies:

    (a) Odds against linkage = 2: 1

    (b) Odds against linkage = 10: 1

    (c) Odds against linkage = 100: 1

    (d) Odds in favour of linkage = 2: 1

    (e) Odds in favour of linkage = 100: 1.

10. **MCQ** – Select one incorrect statement regarding VCFS:

    (a) Between 10 and 30 per cent are diagnosed with schizophrenia, bipolar disorder, ASD or schizoaffective disorder.

    (b) In > 90 per cent of cases it is caused by a duplication.

    (c) It occurs in around one in 4000 live births.

    (d) It is associated with a higher than expected frequency of ADHD and poor social skills.

    (e) Its phenotype is diverse but of interest to psychiatry because of the behavioural and psychiatric aspects of the condition.

11. **MCQ** – Select the best option. Molecular mechanisms that can lead to Prader–Willi syndrome and Angelman syndrome include:

    (a) Imprinting

    (b) Microdeletions

    (c) Point mutations

    (d) Uniparental disomy

    (e) All of the above.

12. **EMI** – Chromosomal abnormalities

    (a) Fragile X syndrome

    (b) Fragile X syndrome E

    (c) Friedreich's ataxia

    (d) Huntington's disease

    (e) Myotonic dystrophy

    (f) Panic disorder

    (g) Schizophrenia

Select the option from the above list with which each of the following human chromosomal abnormalities is best associated:

    (i)   Unstable CGG repeat at Xq27.3

    (ii) Unstable CAG repeat at 4p16.3

    (iii) Interstitial duplication on chromosome 15 – dup(15) (q24q26).

13. **EMI** – Heritability

    (a) < 25 per cent

    (b) 30–40 per cent

    (c) 50–60 per cent

    (d) 70–90 per cent

    (e) > 95 per cent

Select the heritability option from the above list with which each of the following diseases is best associated:

    (i)   Bipolar mood disorder

    (ii) Alzheimer's disease

    (iii) DSM-IV anorexia nervosa.

14. **MCQ** – Select the best option. APP mutations are most closely associated with which of the following diseases?

    (a) Alzheimer's disease

    (b) Autism

    (c) Bipolar mood disorder

    (d) Obsessive-compulsive disorder

    (e) Schizophrenia.

15. **EMI** – Heritability

    (a) < 25 per cent

    (b) 30–40 per cent

    (c) 50–60 per cent

    (d) 70–90 per cent

    (e) > 95 per cent

Select the option from the above list with which each of the following diseases is best associated:

    (i)   Alcohol dependence in men

    (ii) Alcohol dependence in women

    (iii) Anxiety disorders

    (iv) Schizophrenia.

16. **EMI** – Chromosomal abnormalities

    (a) Fragile X syndrome

    (b) Fragile X syndrome E

    (c) Friedreich's ataxia

    (d) Huntington's disease

    (e) Myotonic dystrophy

    (f) Panic disorder

    (g) Schizophrenia

Select the option from the above list with which each of the following human chromosomal abnormalities is best associated:

    (i)   CTG repeat in the 3′ untranslated region of DMPK

    (ii) Unstable GAA repeat

    (iii) Translocation disrupting DISC1.

ANSWERS

1. d

Your sibling must be homozygous, a/a say, because he/she suffers from the disease. Therefore each of your parents must be heterozygous with respect to this disorder, i.e. A/a, since neither of them is affected but one of their children is affected. Therefore, when your parents mate, their offspring will, on average, be in the following ratio: ¼ A/A:½ A/a:¼ a/a. You are unaffected (you are no longer a child and so you are past the age of first manifestation of this autosomal recessive disorder). Therefore you are not a/a but must be either A/A or A/a. The probability that you are heterozygous for the disorder (i.e. A/a) = P(you are A/a)/[P(you are A/A) + P(you are A/a)] = (½)/(¼ + ½) = (½)/(¾) = ½ × ⁴/3 = ²/3.

Reference: Psychiatry: An evidence-based text, **Ch. 33.**

2. a

Your unaffected spouse does not carry the autosomal recessive disease allele, and so must be A/A. If you are heterozygous (A/a), then your mating with your spouse will, on average, produce offspring in the ratio ½ A/A:½ A/a. So the probability that your first son, by your unaffected spouse, is unaffected by the disease but is a carrier, i.e. that your first son is A/a, is ½ x.

Reference: Psychiatry: An evidence-based text, **Ch. 33.**

3. c

If both your son and his wife are unaffected carriers, then they will each be heterozygous (A/a), and their mating with each other will, on average, produce offspring in the ratio ¼ A/A:½ A/a:¼ a/a. So the probability that their first child will be affected by the disease, i.e. that the child is a/a, is $y × y × ¼ = y^2/4$.

Reference: Psychiatry: An evidence-based text, **Ch. 33.**

4.

(i)   a
(ii) c – The inventor of PCR (polymerase chain reaction) was awarded the Nobel Prize for developing this technique.
(iii) b – This is Mendel's second law.
(iv) f – This refers to a method of blotting electrophoretically separated RNA from a gel to a membrane that is exposed to a labelled probe. It is a form of RNA analysis which is analogous to the use of Southern blotting for DNA analysis, but whereas Southern blotting was named after its inventor (see part v), northern blotting was named by analogy. (There is also a western blotting technique in existence.)
(v)   e

Reference: Psychiatry: An evidence-based text, **p. 465.**

5.

(i)   f – The chromosomes become distinct during early prophase. By late prophase the duplicated chromosomes are seen to be joined at the centromere.
(ii) a
(iii) d

Reference: Psychiatry: An evidence-based text, **p. 466.**

6. e

U (uracil) occurs in RNA but not usually in DNA.

Reference: Psychiatry: An evidence-based text, **pp. 466–467.**

7.

(i)   a
(ii) b
(iii) a
(iv) b
(v)   b – The pyrimidine U (uracil) in RNA usually takes the place of the pyrimidine T (thymine) found in DNA.

Reference: Psychiatry: An evidence-based text, **pp. 466–467.**

8.

(i)   b
(ii) d
(iii) c
(iv) e

Reference: Psychiatry: An evidence-based text, **p. 467.**

9. c

The LOD (logarithm of odds) score is the logarithm (to base 10) of the probability that the recombination fraction has some given value, divided by the probability that the value is 0.5.

Reference: Psychiatry: An evidence-based text, **p. 470.**

10. b

In more than 90 per cent of cases, VCFS (velocardiofacial syndrome) is caused by a hemizygous microdeletion in 22q11.2.

Reference: Psychiatry: An evidence-based text, **pp. 470–471.**

11. e

These neurogenetic disorders result from loss of expression of paternal (Prader–Willi syndrome) or maternal (Angelman syndrome) genes on 15q11–13. All four molecular mechanisms given as options can lead to the imbalance between maternal and paternal gene expression, although microdeletions are the most common cause of both of these syndromes.

Reference: *Psychiatry: An evidence-based text*, **p. 471.**

12.

(i) a

(ii) d

(iii) f

Reference: *Psychiatry: An evidence-based text*, **p. 471.**

13.

(i) d – Its heritability is high, in the region of 85 per cent.

(ii) d – Twin studies have reported an estimated heritability of up to 80 per cent.

(iii) c – The heritability of narrowly defined DSM-IV anorexia nervosa has been estimated at 56 per cent.

Reference: *Psychiatry: An evidence-based text*, **pp. 473–480.**

14. a

APP (amyloid precursor protein) mutations are associated with an autosomal-dominant, early-onset form of Alzheimer's disease. APP is a cell membrane protein cleaved by three proteolytic enzymes (secretases). Mutations in *APP* on chromosome 21 cluster near sites where the beta-amyloid peptide is cleaved from APP and also where the beta-amyloid peptide itself is cleaved.

Reference: *Psychiatry: An evidence-based text*, **p. 473.**

15.

(i) c

(ii) c

(iii) b – Anxiety disorders appear to be moderately heritable, with estimates of heritability ranging from 30 to 40 per cent.

(iv) d – The heritability of schizophrenia is estimated to be approximately 80 per cent.

Reference: *Psychiatry: An evidence-based text*, **pp. 474–481.**

16.

(i) e – In myotonic dystrophy (DM) there may be a CTG repeat in *DMPK* (myotonin protein kinase).

(ii) c

(iii) g – *DISC1* (disrupted-in-schizophrenia 1) is a gene on chromosome 1 whose mutant truncation is associated with major psychiatric illness, in particular schizophrenia. It may play a role in the regulation of cytoskeletal function.

Reference: *Psychiatry: An evidence-based text*, **p. 471.**

PART 4

Mental health problems and mental illness

Chapter 34

Classification and diagnostic systems

QUESTIONS

Note that for answers to extended matching items (EMIs), each option (denoted a, b, c, etc.) might be used once, more than once or not at all. For multiple-choice questions (MCQs), please select the best answer.

1. **MCQ** – Which of the following does not appear as a mental disorder classified in DSM-IV-TR?
   (a) Caffeine-induced sleep disorder
   (b) Drapetomania
   (c) Dyspareunia
   (d) Premature ejaculation
   (e) Sleepwalking disorder.

2. **EMI** – Classification of mental disorders
   (a) DSM-I
   (b) DSM-II
   (c) DSM-III
   (d) DSM-III-R
   (e) DSM-IV

   Select the option from the above list with which each of the following is best associated:
   (i) Introduced operationalized definitions, whereby each disorder was diagnosed by empirically determined criteria indifferent to prior ideological assumptions.
   (ii) Published in 1968, this was based upon the eighth edition of the ICD.
   (iii) Published in 1994 with almost 300 diagnoses.

3. **EMI** – DSM-IV-TR axes
   (a) Axis I
   (b) Axis II
   (c) Axis III
   (d) Axis IV
   (e) Axis V

   Select the DSM-IV-TR axis from the above list with which each of the following is best associated:
   (i) Personality disorders
   (ii) Psychosocial and environmental problems
   (iii) Other conditions that may be a focus of clinical attention.

4. **MCQ** – On which axis of DSM-IV-TR is mental retardation diagnosed?
   (a) I
   (b) II
   (c) III
   (d) IV
   (e) V

5. **EMI** – ICD-10 axes
   (a) Axis I
   (b) Axis II
   (c) Axis III
   (d) Axis IV
   (e) Axis V

   Select the ICD-10 axis from the above list with which each of the following is best associated:
   (i) Personality disorders
   (ii) Psychosocial problems
   (iii) Mental retardation.

6. **EMI** – DSM axes
   (a) DSM-I
   (b) DSM-II
   (c) DSM-III
   (d) DSM-III-R
   (e) DSM-IV
   (f) DSM-IV-TR

   Select the option from the above list with which each of the following is best associated:
   (i) Led by Robert Spitzer, this was published in 1987. Criteria were amended based on new research findings.
   (ii) Frequently carried the phrase 'reaction' as in 'schizophrenic reaction', reflecting the ideas of Adolf Meyer.
   (iii) 'Organic mental syndromes' no longer appeared, for such a term was considered to hint at an untenable distinction between brain and mind. Instead, a new section appeared for 'mental disorders due to a general medical condition'.
   (iv) Published in 2000.

7. **EMI** – DSM-IV-TR axes
   (a) Axis I
   (b) Axis II
   (c) Axis III
   (d) Axis IV
   (e) Axis V

Select the DSM-IV-TR axis from the above list with which each of the following is best associated:

(i) Global assessment of functioning

(ii) General medical conditions

(iii) Clinical disorders

(iv) Mental retardation.

ANSWERS

1. b

Drapetomania was described as a disease of the mind causing nineteenth-century slaves in the southern USA to betray their apparently naturally submissive natures by absconding to freedom.

Caffeine-induced sleep disorder is classified under 292.89 in DSM-IV-TR. Dyspareunia is classified under 302.76 in DSM-IV-TR. Premature ejaculation is classified under 302.75 in DSM-IV-TR. Sleepwalking disorder is classified under 307.46 in DSM-IV-TR.

Reference: Psychiatry: An evidence-based text, **p. 489.**

2.

(i)   c
(ii) b
(iii) e

Reference: Psychiatry: An evidence-based text, **pp. 492–493.**

3.

(i)   b
(ii) d
(iii) a

Reference: Psychiatry: An evidence-based text, **pp. 493–494.**

4. b

Personality disorders are also diagnosed on axis II.

Reference: Psychiatry: An evidence-based text, **p. 493.**

5.

(i)   a
(ii) c – This corresponds to axis IV of DSM-IV-TR.
(iii) a

Reference: Psychiatry: An evidence-based text, **p. 497.**

6.

(i)   d
(ii) a – The term 'reaction' was no longer used in this way in DSM-II.
(iii) e
(iv) f – Compared with DSM-IV it included revisions of the supporting information (e.g. clinical course) but not of the diagnostic criteria.

Reference: Psychiatry: An evidence-based text, **pp. 492–495.**

7.

(i)   e
(ii) c
(iii) a
(iv) b

Reference: Psychiatry: An evidence-based text, **pp. 493–494.**

Chapter 35

Cognitive assessment

QUESTIONS

Note that for answers to extended matching items (EMIs), each option (denoted a, b, c, etc.) might be used once, more than once or not at all. For multiple-choice questions (MCQs), please select the best answer.

1. **MCQ** – Select the correct option. Which of the following contributes to the GCS?
   (a) EEG activity
   (b) Diastolic blood pressure
   (c) Respiratory function
   (d) Systolic blood pressure
   (e) Verbal response.

2. **EMI** – States of impaired awareness
   (a) Coma
   (b) Death confirmed by brainstem tests
   (c) Locked-in syndrome
   (d) Minimally conscious state
   (e) Vegetative state

Select the state of impaired awareness from the above list with which each of the following is best associated:
   (i) Awareness: absent; sleep–wake cycle: present; GCS score: E4, M4, V2; motor function: no purposeful movement; respiratory function: preserved; EEG activity: slow-wave activity; cerebral metabolism: severely reduced.
   (ii) Awareness: present; sleep–wake cycle: present; response to pain: present in eyes only; GCS score: E4, M1, V1; motor function: volitional vertical movements preserved; respiratory function: preserved; EEG activity: normal; cerebral metabolism: mildly reduced.

   (iii) Awareness: present; sleep–wake cycle: present; GCS score: E4, M3, V3; motor function: some consistent verbal and purposeful movement; respiratory function: preserved.

3. **MCQ** – Select one incorrect option. Balint's syndrome characteristically involves:
   (a) Bilateral damage to the dorsal stream of visual perceptual processing
   (b) Optic ataxia
   (c) Oculomotor dyspraxia
   (d) Prosopagnosia
   (e) Simultanagnosia.

4. **EMI** – Taxonomy of memory
   (a) Conditioning
   (b) Episodic
   (c) Explicit
   (d) Implicit
   (e) Long-term
   (f) Motor skills
   (g) Priming
   (h) Semantic
   (i) Short-term
   (j) Spatial

From the above list, select the option with which each label (i–x) in the following taxonomy of memory is best associated:

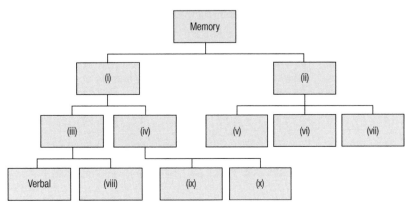

5. **MCQ** – Select one incorrect statement regarding memory:
   (a) A transient amnesic syndrome can occur in disorders such as concussion and epilepsy.
   (b) An example of a sufferer from amnesic syndrome is patient HM, whose anterior medial temporal lobes were surgically removed as a treatment for epilepsy.
   (c) In right-handed people, memory impairment following damage to the temporal neocortex tends to affect knowledge of objects and language if the left temporal lobe is principally affected, and knowledge of people if the right temporal lobe is principally affected.
   (d) Severe damage along the course of the circuit of Papez causes an amnesic syndrome – an inability to acquire long-term procedural memories, associated with some degree of retrograde amnesia.
   (e) The existence of focal retrograde amnesia as a result of brain damage is controversial, and such cases often turn out to have a psychiatric or forensic explanation.

6. **MCQ** – Select the best option. In which of the following dysphasias is naming not affected?
   (a) Broca's
   (b) Conduction
   (c) Global
   (d) Transcortical motor
   (e) None of the above.

7. **EMI** – Types of dysphasia
   (a) Broca's
   (b) Conduction
   (c) Global
   (d) Transcortical motor
   (e) Transcortical sensory
   (f) Wernicke's

Select the type of dysphasia from the above list with which each of the following is best associated:
   (i) Fluency: unaffected; comprehension: affected; repetition: affected.
   (ii) Fluency: unaffected; comprehension: unaffected; repetition: affected.
   (iii) Fluency: unaffected; comprehension: affected; repetition: unaffected.
   (iv) Fluency: affected; comprehension: unaffected; repetition: affected.

8. **MCQ** – Select one incorrect statement regarding language and its disorders:
   (a) An example of Broca's dysphasia is: 'Cinderella... poor...um...'dopted her...scrubbed floor...um...tidy... poor...um...'dopted...si-sisters and mother... ball... Ball... prince...um...shoe...'.
   (b) An example of Wernicke's dysphasia is: 'I can't tell you what that is, but I know what it is, but I don't know where it is. But I don't know what it's under. I know it's... you couldn't say it's... I couldn't say what it is...'.
   (c) Dysgraphia is particularly associated with damage to the angular gyrus.
   (d) In surface dyslexia the ability to read letter by letter is lost, whereas in deep dyslexia there is a dependency on letter-by-letter reading with difficulty in reading irregular words.
   (e) Language is predominantly represented in the left hemisphere in the majority of left-handed people.

9. **MCQ** – Which of the following parts of the frontal lobe is most likely to be associated with the control of behaviour, especially social behaviour, under guidance by emotion, empathy and theory of mind?
   (a) Anterior cingulate
   (b) Lateral prefrontal cortex
   (c) M1
   (d) Supplementary motor area
   (e) Ventromedial cortex.

10. **MCQ** – Which of the following tests is least likely to diagnose dysexecutive syndromes?
   (a) Go–no go task
   (b) Luria's alternating bimanual sequence test
   (c) Luria's fist-side-palm sequence test
   (d) Mini-Mental State Examination
   (e) Verbal fluency.

11. **MCQ** – Select one incorrect statement regarding praxis:
   (a) Limb kinetic dyspraxia refers to a type of dyspraxia in which movements are performed adequately but dysfluently
   (b) Oral apraxia may accompany Broca's aphasia.
   (c) Pout and palmomental reflexes can occur in association with dyspraxia and with dysexecutive syndromes, as they reflect a loss of the motor inhibition normally exercised by the frontal lobes.
   (d) Praxis is associated with the dominant hemisphere, which controls the more skilled hand and language.
   (e) Skilled actions may be intransitive, involving another object such as a piano, or transitive, such as waving.

ANSWERS

1. e

The best verbal response is recorded on the following scale: 5 = oriented; 2 = confused; 3 = inappropriate words; 4 = incomprehensible sounds; 5 = none. In the case of the presence of an endotracheal tube or a tracheostomy, the letter T is recorded.

Reference: *Psychiatry: An evidence-based text*, **p. 500.**

2.

(i)   e
(ii) c
(iii) d

Reference: *Psychiatry: An evidence-based text*, **pp. 500–501.**

3. d

This syndrome was first described in 1907 by the Hungarian neurologist Rezso Balint. It follows bilateral damage to the dorsal stream of visual perceptual processing, whereas prosopagnosia is more likely to be associated with damage to the ventral stream of visual processing.

Reference: *Psychiatry: An evidence-based text*, **p. 504.**

4.

(i)   c – Declarative memory. (We cannot swap the labels of i and ii because of the location of verbal memory in the given taxonomy.)
(ii) d – Procedural memory.
(iii) i – Working memory.
(iv) e
(v, vi, vii) These are a, f and g (in any order)
(viii) j
(ix, x) These are b and h (in either order).

Reference: *Psychiatry: An evidence-based text*, **pp. 504–505.**

5. d

There is an inability to acquire new long-term declarative memories. Coronal MRI scans are shown on p. 506 of the accompanying textbook.

Reference: *Psychiatry: An evidence-based text*, **p. 505–507.**

6. e

Reference: *Psychiatry: An evidence-based text*, **p. 508.**

7.

(i)   f
(ii) b
(iii) e
(iv) a

Reference: *Psychiatry: An evidence-based text*, **pp. 508–509.**

8. d

In surface dyslexia, patients become dependent on letter-by-letter reading with resulting difficulty in reading irregular words such as 'pint', which are read to rhyme with 'mint'. In deep dyslexia, the ability to read letter by letter is lost, with a resulting inability to read nonsense words such as 'proke', and semantic reading errors, such as 'sister' for 'brother'.

Reference: *Psychiatry: An evidence-based text*, **pp. 508–509.**

9. e

This is the orbitofrontal cortex. Theory of mind refers to our ability to impute mental states such as desires and beliefs to others.

Reference: *Psychiatry: An evidence-based text*, **pp. 509–510.**

10. d

Executive function is difficult to test in the clinic. Patients with dysexecutive syndromes severe enough to cause major disruption to long-term decision-making can score full marks on standard cognitive tests such as the MMSE. The Luria tests are illustrated in Figure 35.15 on page 511 of the accompanying textbook.

Reference: *Psychiatry: An evidence-based text*, **pp. 510–511.**

11. e

Transitive skilled actions involve another object, while waving is an example of an intransitive skilled action.

Reference: *Psychiatry: An evidence-based text*, **p. 511.**

Chapter 36

Neurology for psychiatrists

QUESTIONS

Note that for answers to extended matching items (EMIs), each option (denoted a, b, c, etc.) might be used once, more than once or not at all. For multiple-choice questions (MCQs), please select the best answer.

1. **EMI** – Types of headache
   (a) Cervicogenic tension headache
   (b) Cluster headache
   (c) Migraine

   Select the type of headache from the above list with which each of the following is best associated:
   (i) Presentation in middle age and more common in men
   (ii) Preceding aura in around 10 per cent of cases; a slow build-up usually occurs (lasting between, say, 30 min and several hours)
   (iii) The quality of the headache is often described as being 'tight', 'squeezing', 'like a tight band around my head'.

2. **EMI** – Symptoms of diplopia
   (a) A problem at the neuromuscular junction
   (b) An infiltrative cause
   (c) Isolated fourth cranial nerve palsy
   (d) Limitation of ocular abduction or adduction
   (e) None of the above

   Select the aetiology from the above list with which each of the following symptoms of diplopia is best associated:
   (i) Diplopia that is fatiguable or variable
   (ii) Horizontally spaced images
   (iii) Progressive diplopia
   (iv) Vertical diplopia maximal on down-gaze
   (v) Painful diplopia.

3. **MCQ** – Select one incorrect statement:
   (a) Damage to the visual system posterior to the chiasm results in homonymous hemianopia.
   (b) In patients over the age of 60 years, jaw claudication and a significantly raised erythrocyte sedimentation rate may be secondary to giant cell arteritis.
   (c) Oscillopsia is a common symptom of loss of oculomotor control at the level of the cerebellum or its connections with the oculomotor centres of the brainstem; it is not usually associated with other complaints of cerebellar dysfunction.

   (d) Pain of neuropathic origin is usually described as having a 'burning', 'electric' or 'tingling' quality and can be aggravated by superficial stimulation (e.g. contact with bedclothes).
   (e) Trigeminal neuralgia is diagnosed on the strength of a classic history of paroxysmal, shooting discomfort in the distribution of one or more divisions of the fifth cranial nerve, typically in response to local stimulation (touching, shaving, eating or teeth-cleaning); attacks occur in clusters punctuated by periods of spontaneous remission.

4. **EMI** – Abnormal movements
   (a) Chorea
   (b) Hemiballismus
   (c) Myoclonus
   (d) Tic
   (e) Tremor

   Select the abnormal movement from the above list with which each of the following is best associated:
   (i) Occurs following injury to the contralateral subthalamic nucleus, typically ischaemic or haemorrhagic, and usually self-limiting within a period of weeks
   (ii) A recognized feature of autoimmune disease, including systemic lupus erythematosus and the antiphospholipid syndrome
   (iii) Many cases, particularly in patients under the age of 40 years, represent a benign physiological phenomenon
   (iv) A willed movement, executed in response to an irresistible impulse.

5. **MCQ** – Select one incorrect statement:
   (a) Down-beating nystagmus suggests a cerebellar lesion.
   (b) Optic disc swelling is a sign of an acute and active process and should never be ignored.
   (c) Partial ptosis, together with miosis in the same eye, form the defining features of Horner's syndrome.

(d) Shaking movements, even a brief convulsion, may be described during a faint.

(e) Urinary incontinence during a disturbance of consciousness does not exclude a haemodynamic cause.

6. **MCQ** – Select one incorrect statement regarding the cranial nerves:
   (a) A lesion of the glossopharyngeal nerve causes loss of sensation over the posterior tongue and palatal regions.
   (b) A patient with tenth nerve dysfunction may complain of hoarseness, swallowing difficulty and a tendency to aspirate, owing to muscular weakness in the palate and vocal folds and loss of the efferent arm of the gag reflex.
   (c) An upper motor neurone seventh nerve palsy only affects the muscles of the lower face.
   (d) Damage to the accessory nerve produces weakness of shoulder-shrugging and head-turning towards the side of the lesion.
   (e) The most common cause of an isolated global or lower motor neurone facial weakness is Bell's palsy.

7. **EMI** – Spinal roots and reflexes
   (a) C2
   (b) C3
   (c) C4
   (d) C5
   (e) C6
   (f) C7
   (g) C8
   (h) T1
   (i) T2
   (j) T3
   (k) T4
   (l) T5
   (m) T6
   (n) T7
   (o) T8
   (p) T9
   (q) T10
   (r) T11
   (s) T12
   (t) L1
   (u) L2
   (v) L3
   (w) L4
   (x) L5
   (y) S1
   (z) S2
   (aa) S3

Select the spinal root from the above list with which each of the following reflexes is usually transmitted:
   (i) Supinator
   (ii) Triceps
   (iii) Knee
   (iv) Finger
   (v) Ankle.

8. **MCQ** – Select one incorrect statement:
   (a) A patient with a spastic paraparesis probably has a lesion in the spinal cord between T1 and L1 - so you should examine for a sensory level.
   (b) CADASIL is an inherited disorder.
   (c) Exaggerated (brisk) reflexes indicate loss of central modulation and thus indicate a central lesion at a level higher than the reflex being tested.
   (d) The inherited spinocerebellar ataxias are autosomal recessive.
   (e) Ubiquitin inclusions are found in the brain of a subset of patients with frontotemporal dementia and of patients with motor neurone disease.

9. **MCQ** – Which of the following signs is least likely to be associated with MS?
   (a) Cerebellar ataxia
   (b) Disorders of eye-movement control
   (c) Monocular visual loss
   (d) Spastic paraparesis
   (e) Tabes dorsalis.

10. **MCQ** – Select one incorrect statement regarding the early stages of Lyme disease:
    (a) It is caused by a spirochaete.
    (b) It is difficult to treat.
    (c) It manifests dermatologically.
    (d) It manifests systemically.
    (e) The causative organism is transmitted by tick bites.

11. **MCQ** – Select one incorrect statement regarding Wernicke's encephalopathy:
    (a) In its classic form the syndrome comprises acute confusion, eye-movement abnormalities and ataxia.
    (b) It is a common complication of alcoholism.
    (c) It is associated with anorexia nervosa.
    (d) It is associated with hyperemesis of pregnancy.
    (e) It is caused by vitamin B12 deficiency

12. **MCQ** – Select the best option. If a young patient suffers from a movement disorder, psychiatric symptoms (ranging from anxiety and depression to psychosis) and hepatic dysfunction, which of the following is an autosomal recessive inherited disorder that should be considered in the differential diagnosis of this case?
    (a) Guillain–Barré syndrome
    (b) Huntington's disease
    (c) Korsakoff's syndrome
    (d) Multiple sclerosis
    (e) Wilson's disease.

13. **EMI** – Types of stroke
    (a) Anterior cerebral artery
    (b) Carotid dissection
    (c) Middle cerebral artery
    (d) Posterior cerebral artery

Select the type of stroke from the above list with which each of the following is best associated:

(i) Horner's syndrome on the side opposite the hemiparesis
(ii) A hemiparesis that is worse in the arm and a homonymous quadrantanopia
(iii) Homonymous hemianopia
(iv) Leg weakness and disinhibition.

14. **MCQ** – Which of the following antiepileptic drugs does not induce the metabolism of hormonal contraception?

(a) Carbamazepine
(b) Levetiracetam
(c) Phenytoin
(d) Topiramate
(e) None of the above.

15. **MCQ** – Select one incorrect statement regarding meningitis:

(a) A patient with meningitis will be severely unwell, irritable and sometimes drowsy, delirious or fitting.
(b) A rapidly spreading purple and red rash over the trunk, limbs and mucous membranes accompanies, and may precede, meningococcal infection, while encephalitis may present similarly but usually manifests as mild to moderate confusion, pyrexia and headache.
(c) Before the administration of an antibiotic, it should be confirmed that the meningitis is bacterial rather than viral and the sensitivity of the bacteria should be established.
(d) Symptoms (if they can be reported) are dominated by intense photophobic headache, nausea, vomiting and neck stiffness; meningeal pain results in severe restriction of movement in adjacent structures, which may result in Kernig's sign.
(e) There may be signs of cardiovascular instability owing to haematogenous infection.

16. **EMI** – Causes of meningitis and encephalitis

(a) Bacterial (non-tuberculous)
(b) Tuberculous
(c) Viral
(d) None of the above

Select the type of infectious cause in the assessment of meningitis and encephalitis from the above list with which each of the following cerebrospinal fluid appearances is best associated:

(i) Fibrin web
(ii) Clear
(iii) Turbid, syrup-like.

17. **EMI** – Causes of meningitis and encephalitis

(a) Bacterial (non-tuberculous)
(b) Tuberculous
(c) Viral
(d) None of the above

Select the type of infectious cause from the above list with which each of the following cerebrospinal fluid findings is best associated:

(i) Mild to moderate elevation of protein level and a glucose concentration < 60 per cent of its plasma value
(ii) Protein level: normal range to mild elevation; glucose concentration: 60–80 per cent of the plasma level
(iii) Moderate to marked elevation of the protein level with a glucose concentration that is markedly lower than its plasma level.

18. **EMI** – Subtests of the WAIS

(a) Verbal scale
(b) Performance scale
(c) Not a WAIS subtest

Select the scale from the above list with which each of the following is best associated:

(i) Digit span
(ii) Comprehension
(iii) Block design
(iv) Stroop.

19. **MCQ** – Select one incorrect statement regarding neuropsychiatric investigations:

(a) A number of important laboratory measurements can be made on cerebrospinal fluid; suspected bacterial, mycobacterial or fungal infection may be confirmed by immediate microscopy.
(b) CT angiography is the favoured imaging modality for non-invasive investigation of intracranial vascular disease.
(c) Differences of 20 or more IQ points between verbal and performance subscores, or between full-scale score and premorbid estimates, give rise to concern.
(d) EEG periodic bi- or triphasic discharges are typical of sporadic sCJD and vCJD.
(e) Nerve biopsies are typically taken from the ankle or wrist, since at these sites the nerve bundles consist of sensory fibres; nerve histology enables a firm diagnosis of vasculitic neuropathy to be established or excluded.

20. **EMI** – Anti-epileptic drugs (AEDs)

(a) Carbamazepine
(b) Lacosamide
(c) Lamotrigine
(d) Levetiracetam
(e) Phenytoin
(f) Sodium valproate
(g) Topiramate

Select the AED from the above list with which each of the following is best associated:

(i) A 27-year-old woman has been successfully treated with this AED since her teenage years, but she has developed gum hypertrophy and slight coarsening of her facial features.

(ii) A 39-year-old man is on monotherapy with this AED for generalized tonic-clonic seizures. Recently a speech disorder has been noted, and he has now been referred to a psychiatrist because of suicidal ideation.

(iii) This AED is particularly associated with serious skin reactions including Stevens–Johnson syndrome.

21. **MCQ** – Which of the following drugs is used in the treatment of MS and is an mAChR antagonist?
(a) Baclofen
(b) Interferon beta
(c) Interferon gamma
(d) Methylprednisolone
(e) Oxybutynin.

22. **EMI** – Treatment of headache
(a) Acetazolamide
(b) Amitriptyline
(c) Beta-blocker
(d) Indometacin
(e) Triptan group
(f) Topiramate

From the above list, select the drug or drug group, used for the treatment of headache, with which each of the following is most closely associated:
(i) Side-effects include depression, fatigue, bradycardia and arterial insufficiency.
(ii) Serotonin receptor agonist.
(iii) Indicated in idiopathic intracranial hypertension, it may cause tingling in the peripheries, altered taste sensation and visual blurring.
(iv) Used for the acute treatment of paroxysmal hemicrania, its mode of action is prostaglandin inhibition.

23. **EMI** – WAIS subtests
(a) Verbal scale
(b) Performance scale
(c) Not a WAIS subtest

Select the scale from the above list with which each of the following is best associated:
(i) Digit symbol
(ii) Go–no go
(iii) Information
(iv) Similarities.

ANSWERS

1.

(i)   b
(ii) c
(iii) a

Reference: *Psychiatry: An evidence-based text*, **pp. 519–520.**

2.

(i)   a
(ii) d
(iii) b
(iv) c
(v)   b

Reference: *Psychiatry: An evidence-based text*, **p. 521.**

3. c

Oscillopsia is an inability to maintain stable fixation on the visual environment. It is usually accompanied by the other cardinal complaints of cerebellar dysfunction (walking and balance difficulties, clumsiness and slurring of speech), and nystagmus is an expected finding on examination.

Reference: *Psychiatry: An evidence-based text*, **pp. 520–521.**

4.

(i)   b
(ii) a
(iii) e – This is essential tremor.
(iv) d

Reference: *Psychiatry: An evidence-based text*, **pp. 522–523.**

5. a

The direction of oscillation in nystagmus is diagnostically important. Horizontal nystagmus is caused by a lesion to the cerebellar circuitry on the side to which it is maximal. Down-beating nystagmus suggests a lesion at the base of the brainstem.

Reference: *Psychiatry: An evidence-based text*, **pp. 524–526.**

6. d

Damage to XI produces weakness of shoulder-shrugging and head-turning away from the side of the lesion.

Reference: *Psychiatry: An evidence-based text*, **pp. 526–527.**

7.

(i)   f
(ii) e
(iii) w
(iv) g
(v)   y

Reference: *Psychiatry: An evidence-based text*, **p. 528.**

8. d

They are autosomal dominant disorders. An alternative name for spinocerebellar ataxia is autosomal dominant cerebellar ataxia.

Reference: *Psychiatry: An evidence-based text*, **pp. 528–529.**

9. e

Reference: *Psychiatry: An evidence-based text*, **p. 530.**

10. b

The early stages of Lyme disease are responsive to treatment with antibacterials such as doxycycline, amoxicillin, cefuroxime axetil and erythromycin.

Reference: *Psychiatry: An evidence-based text*, **pp. 530–531.**

11. e

The cause is vitamin B1 (thiamine) deficiency, leading to an acute syndrome of midbrain and brainstem dysfunction.

Reference: *Psychiatry: An evidence-based text*, **p. 531.**

12. e

This is a recessively inherited disorder of copper metabolism. Unbound circulating copper is deposited in the liver, cornea and brain (particularly the basal ganglia), giving rise to the major clinical features: liver dysfunction, corneal discoloration, movement disorders and psychiatric symptoms. Wilson's disease should be considered in all young patients with a movement disorder and in patients with psychiatric symptoms together with liver dysfunction.

Reference: *Psychiatry: An evidence-based text*, **p. 531.**

13.

(i)   b – This is caused by disruption of the carotid sympathetic plexus.
(ii) c – Dysphasia may also occur if the dominant hemisphere is involved.
(iii) d – Brainstem-related and cerebellar signs may occur.
(iv) a – Isolated anterior cerebral artery territory infarction is rare but is associated predominantly with contralateral leg weakness and personality change (disinhibition).

Reference: *Psychiatry: An evidence-based text*, **p. 531.**

14. b

Reference: *Psychiatry: An evidence-based text*, **p. 532.**

15. c

Management of suspected meningitis or encephalitis should begin with prompt administration of broad-spectrum intravenous antibiotics or acyclovir, or both. Delaying to wait for the results of diagnostic tests may prove fatal.

Reference: *Psychiatry: An evidence-based text*, **pp. 532–533.**

16.

(i) b
(ii) c
(iii) a

Reference: *Psychiatry: An evidence-based text*, **p. 533.**

17.

(a) a
(b) c
(c) b

Reference: *Psychiatry: An evidence-based text*, **p. 533.**

18.

(i) a – The ability to repeat a lengthening sequence of digits, first forwards and then backwards.
(ii) a – A test of practical reasoning.
(iii) b – A test of visuospatial and constructional abilities.
(iv) c

Reference: *Psychiatry: An evidence-based text*, **p. 535.**

19. d

Periodic bi- or triphasic discharges are typical of the later stages of sCJD (sporadic Creutzfeld–Jacob disease) but are not seen in vCJD (variant Creutzfeld–Jacob disease), so this finding can have important diagnostic implications.

Reference: *Psychiatry: An evidence-based text*, **pp. 534–537.**

20.

(i) e
(ii) g – Speech and language difficulties and weight loss are among the principal side-effects and disadvantages of this AED. It may also cause anxiety and depression as side-effects and, less commonly, suicidal ideation.
(iii) c

Reference: *Psychiatry: An evidence-based text*, **p. 538.**

21. e

This mAChR (muscarinic acetylcholine receptor) antagonist is used for the symptomatic treatment of urinary frequency and nocturia in MS.

Reference: *Psychiatry: An evidence-based text*, **p. 538.**

22.

(i) c
(ii) e – Used for the acute treatment of migraine.
(iii) a
(iv) d

Reference: *Psychiatry: An evidence-based text*, **p. 539.**

23.

(i) b – This is a test of visuomotor coordination and of motor and mental processing speed.
(ii) c
(iii) a – This is a graded test of culturally specific general knowledge.
(iv) a – This is a graded test of concept formation requiring the subject to explain what two items have in common.

Reference: *Psychiatry: An evidence-based text*, **p. 535.**

Chapter 37

Organic disorders

QUESTIONS

Note that for answers to extended matching items (EMIs), each option (denoted a, b, c, etc.) might be used once, more than once or not at all. For multiple-choice questions (MCQs), please select the best answer.

1. **MCQ** – Which of the following is most likely to occur as a result of cerebral involvement following vitamin B12 deficiency?
   - (a) Dementia
   - (b) Depression
   - (c) Mania
   - (d) Megaloblastic madness
   - (e) Personality change.

2. **MCQ** – Which one of the following postmortem signs is particularly associated with delayed post-anoxic leucoencephalopathy?
   - (a) Basal ganglia spongiform change
   - (b) Bilateral internuclear ophthalmoplegia
   - (c) Cerebellar atrophy
   - (d) Diffuse white matter demyelination
   - (e) Systemic, segmental panarteritis.

3. **EMI** – Immune-related disorders
   - (a) Hashimoto's encephalopathy
   - (b) Limbic encephalitis
   - (c) Multiple sclerosis
   - (d) Sarcoidosis
   - (e) Susac's syndrome
   - (f) Sydenham's chorea
   - (g) Systemic lupus erythematosus.

Which of the above immune-related disorders is most likely to be the cause in the following vignettes?
   - (i) A 38-year-old man who has started to develop some psychiatric symptoms, mainly delusions and 'occasional forgetfulness'. In spite of being a non-smoker all his life, he has a long history of having gradually developed chest problems, including coughing and dyspnoea.
   - (ii) A 24-year-old female postgraduate student who has gradually been becoming more tired presents with depression. Her mother relates that a few years ago the patient suffered from a marked facial rash. The patient is currently photosensitive and shows evidence of weight loss and some thinning of her scalp hair. Routine urinalysis shows proteinuria.
   - (iii) A 26-year-old female patient is admitted to hospital with delirium. She had been complaining of headache

and hearing loss. Cerebral MRI shows multiple areas of increased signal intensity on FLAIR, scattered throughout the white matter and grey matter, with a predilection for the corpus callosum.
   - (iv) A 26-year-old African-American female patient has gradually developed increasing somnolence. A routine blood test shows hypercalcaemia.

4. **MCQ** – Which of the following types of hallucination is particularly common with prolonged levodopa or dopamine agonist treatment of Parkinson's disease?
   - (a) Auditory hallucinations
   - (b) Gustatory hallucinations
   - (c) Olfactory hallucinations
   - (d) Visual hallucinations
   - (e) Hallucinations are uncommon.

5. **MCQ** – Which of the following is the most common cause of ALS?
   - (a) Autosomal dominant inheritance, secondary to a mutation in a gene different from superoxide dismutase (*SOD*)
   - (b) Autosomal dominant inheritance, secondary to a mutation in *SOD*
   - (c) Autosomal recessive inheritance
   - (d) Sporadic
   - (e) X-linked inheritance.

6. **EMI** – Case vignettes
   - (a) ALS
   - (b) Choreoacanthocytosis
   - (c) DRPLA
   - (d) Huntington's disease
   - (e) Myotonic dystrophy type 1
   - (f) Parkinson's disease
   - (g) Progressive supranuclear palsy
   - (h) Spinocerebellar ataxia

Which of the above disorders is most likely to be the cause in the following vignettes?
   - (i) A 54-year-old teetotal man who feels depressed is referred to you. The referral letter notes that a few months ago he developed a tremor in his hands (R

> L). When he walks into your outpatient clinic you notice a reduced arm swing and that his steps are relatively small and shuffling.

(ii) A 44-year-old man has been referred with 'emotional incontinence'. When getting dressed he has been finding it necessary to ask his wife to help him to button up his shirt.

(iii) A 58-year-old woman, who very occasionally is becoming forgetful, has frequent falls because of postural instability.

(iv) A 28-year-old man, who was adopted and does not know his biological family, has developed a marked change in his personality; he occasionally becomes irritable and impulsive, which is out of character with his previous personality. Indeed, when taking a history from his wife you discover that he seems to suffer from apparently poor judgement and occasional aggressiveness, again out of character compared with how she remembers him from five years before when they first met. Also, he is becoming increasingly clumsy and has started dropping things.

7. **MCQ** – Which type of movement abnormality is usually the first to appear in Tourette's syndrome?
   (a) Cervical dystonic movements
   (b) Facial dystonic movements
   (c) Motor tics
   (d) Sensory tics
   (e) Vocal tics.

8. **MCQ** – In which of the following movement disorders are you most likely to see a fixed, vacuous, wide-mouthed dystonic smile, discoloration of the corneal limbus and the 'face of the giant panda' sign on a T2-weighted MRI scan of the midbrain?
   (a) Choreoacanthocytosis
   (b) DRPLA
   (c) Huntington's disease
   (d) Spinocerebellar ataxia
   (e) Wilson's disease.

9. **EMI** – Genetic causes of movement disorders
   (a) Autosomal dominant inheritance
   (b) Autosomal recessive inheritance
   (c) X-linked inheritance
   (d) Not inherited

Select the option from the above list with which each of the following is best associated:
   (i) PARK1
   (ii) PARK2
   (iii) DRPLA
   (iv) SCA19.

10. **MCQ** – Which of the following vascular disorders usually has the earliest age of onset?
   (a) Behçet's disease
   (b) Binswanger's disease

(c) Cranial arteritis
(d) Cerebral amyloid angiopathy
(e) Transient global amnesia.

11. **MCQ** – Select one incorrect statement regarding CADASIL:
   (a) It is an autosomal dominant disorder in which mutations are found in *Notch3* on chromosome 19.
   (b) Its early course is characterized by the onset of recurrent migraine headaches, typically with aura, in the first or second decade.
   (c) Skin biopsy may commonly give false-negative results.
   (d) The associated strokes are typically of the lacunar type, reflecting infarcts that occur primarily in the basal ganglia.
   (e) Two unusual manifestations are intracerebral haemorrhage and reversible delirium.

12. **EMI** – Traumatic causes of organic disorders
   (a) Chronic subdural haematoma
   (b) Dementia pugilistica
   (c) Diffuse axonal injury
   (d) Subacute subdural haematoma

Select the option from the above list of organic disorders with which each of the following is best associated:
   (i) Tends to present with drowsiness and delirium, and symptoms may fluctuate for days.
   (ii) Many patients may not recall any head trauma. After a latent interval of months to years, patients gradually develop dementia, often accompanied by headache; personality change may occur; rarely, it may present with depression.
   (iii) Typically, patients are rendered immediately unconscious at the moment of injury. Some may never regain consciousness. Those that do may develop a persistent vegetative state or may emerge into delirium.

13. **MCQ** – Select one incorrect statement regarding carbon monoxide poisoning:
   (a) At carboxyhaemoglobin levels of 40–50 per cent, stupor and ataxia appear.
   (b) Cherry-red discoloration of the lips, nails and skin is usually seen in white Caucasian patients.
   (c) Headache and delirium appear at a carboxyhaemoglobin level of 10–30 per cent.
   (d) In survivors, characteristic CT/MRI changes may be seen in the globus pallidus.
   (e) When the carboxyhaemoglobin level rises above 50 per cent, coma and convulsions appear.

14. **EMI** – Clinical features of pellagra
   (a) Acute pellagra
   (b) Chronic pellagra
   (c) Neither of the above

Select the option from the above list with which each of the following clinical features is best associated:

(i) Dysarthria
(ii) Diarrhoea
(iii) Cogwheel rigidity.

15. **MCQ** – Select the best correct option. Chronic poisoning with which metal is most likely to lead to personality change or parkinsonism (or both), with the parkinsonism including 'cock-walk'?
(a) Hg
(b) K
(c) Mn
(d) Pb
(e) Sn.

16. **MCQ** – Which of the following is least likely to be seen with chronic arsenic intoxication?
(a) Alopecia
(b) Dementia
(c) Erethism
(d) Hyperkeratosis
(e) Mees' lines.

17. **EMI** – Toxic and metabolic disorders
(a) Acquired hepatocerebral degeneration
(b) Arsenic intoxication
(c) Bismuth intoxication
(d) Central pontine myelinolysis
(e) Dialysis dementia
(f) Fahr's syndrome
(g) Hepatic encephalopathy
(h) Hepatic porphyria
(i) Hypoglycaemia
(j) Lead encephalopathy
(k) Manganism
(l) Mercury intoxication
(m) Thallium intoxication
(n) Tin intoxication
(o) Uraemia

Select the option from the above list with which each of the following clinical features is best associated:
(i) Flaccid quadriplegia with delirium occurring soon after correcting chronic hyponatraemia.
(ii) Patients may initially experience some lassitude or a mild degree of somnolence; however, eventually delirium appears that is often marked by visual hallucinations. Asterixis and multifocal myoclonus are common.
(iii) Episodes occur of abdominal pain with vomiting, constipation or diarrhoea, often accompanied by delirium, which is often marked by affective lability, delusions of persecution and visual hallucinations.
(iv) Anxiety, palpitations, tremulousness and diaphoresis occur. Patients may also complain of hunger, nausea, headache and generalized weakness.
(v) Delirium occurs, which may be accompanied by excitation, hallucinations, delusions, ataxia and seizures. Patients also complain of a metallic taste in the mouth.

18. **EMI** – Infectious and related diseases
(a) Bacterial
(b) Protozoan
(c) Viral
(d) None of the above

Select the option from the above list with which the causative organism of each of the following diseases is best associated:
(i) Progressive multifocal leucoencephalopathy
(ii) Infectious mononucleosis
(iii) SSPE
(iv) Whipple's disease
(v) Malaria.

19. **MCQ** – With which of the following diseases are cat faeces particularly associated?
(a) Encephalitis lethargica
(b) GPI
(c) Herpes simplex encephalitis
(d) Malaria
(e) Toxoplasmosis.

20. **MCQ** – Select one incorrect statement regarding Creutzfeldt–Jakob disease:
(a) About 85 per cent of cases occur on a sporadic basis, about 10 per cent are inherited on an autosomal dominant basis, and the remainder represent iatrogenic infections.
(b) The cerebrospinal fluid is acellular with a normal glucose.
(c) The cerebrospinal fluid total protein level is usually highly elevated.
(d) The presentation may be the alien hand sign.
(e) With progression, almost all patients become profoundly demented, and the dementia is accompanied by myoclonus in almost 90 per cent of cases.

21. **MCQ** – Which of the following is the commonest neuropsychiatric feature of Cushing's syndrome?
(a) Anxiety of pathological degree (on its own)
(b) Delirium
(c) Depression
(d) Mania
(e) Schizophreniform psychosis.

22. **MCQ** – Which of the following causes of primary adrenocortical insufficiency is least likely to cause a chronic presentation?
(a) Adrenoleucodystrophy
(b) Haemorrhagic infarction
(c) Metastatic disease
(d) Sarcoidosis
(e) Tuberculosis.

23. **EMI** – Biochemical test results
(a) ↑ T4, ↑ TSH
(b) ↑ T4, ↓ TSH

(c) T4 in the normal range
(d) ↓ T4, ↑ TSH
(e) ↓ T4, ↓ TSH

Select the biochemical test result from the above list with which each of the following diseases is most likely to be associated:
(i) Graves' disease
(ii) Tri-iodothyronine thyrotoxicosis
(iii) Hypothalamic tumour secreting TRH
(iv) Pituitary adenoma secreting TSH
(v) Primary hypothyroidism.

24. **EMI** – Forms of hypothyroidism
(a) Primary
(b) Secondary
(c) Tertiary

Select the form of hypothyroidism from the above list that is most likely to be caused by each of the following:
(i) Lithium treatment
(ii) Carbamazepine treatment
(iii) Infarction of the hypothalamus.

25. **MCQ** – Which of the following is likely to be the first clinical presentation of normal-pressure hydrocephalus?
(a) Aggressiveness
(b) Akinetic mutism

(c) Gait disturbance
(d) Mania
(e) Urinary incontinence.

26. **EMI** – Genetic causes of movement disorders
(a) Autosomal dominant inheritance
(b) Autosomal recessive inheritance
(c) X-linked inheritance
(d) Not inherited

Select the inheritance option from the above list with which each of the following is best associated:
(i) Choreoacanthocytosis
(ii) Wilson's disease
(iii) DM1
(iv) FXTAS.

27. **EMI** – Forms of hypothyroidism
(a) Primary
(b) Secondary
(c) Tertiary

Which of the above forms of hypothyroidism is most likely to be caused by each of the following?
(i) Amiodarone treatment
(ii) Granulomatous disease
(iii) Infarction of the pituitary gland
(iv) Iodine deficiency.

ANSWERS

1. a

Symptoms of vitamin B12 deficiency referable to the cerebrum or spinal cord tend to appear subacutely over weeks or months. Cerebral involvement manifests most commonly with dementia (which may be marked by hallucinations and delusions). Personality change may also occur and, rarely, depression or mania. Another rare manifestation is megaloblastic madness.

Reference: *Psychiatry: An evidence-based text*, **p. 589.**

2. d

Delayed post-anoxic leucoencephalopathy may occur in a small minority of those patients who make a more or less complete recovery after emerging from coma following a global hypoxic or ischaemic insult. At postmortem, there is a massive, symmetrical, diffuse demyelination of the white matter, with variable involvement of the basal ganglia.

Bilateral internuclear ophthalmoplegia is not a postmortem sign, but rather a clinical ocular sign that is pathognomonic of multiple sclerosis. Systemic, segmental panarteritis affecting medium and small arteries, with, at times, extension into arterioles, is seen on postmortem in polyarteritis nodosa. Basal ganglia spongiform change may be seen, for example, in acquired hepatocerebral degeneration.

Reference: *Psychiatry: An evidence-based text*, **pp. 564, 568–569 and 575.**

3.

(i) d – Although onset in adolescence or the middle or later years may occur, most patients fall ill in their 20s or 30s. The onset is often gradual, and many cases are discovered serendipitously on chest radiography. Perhaps 90 per cent of patients have pulmonary involvement, which may manifest with symptoms such as cough or dyspnoea. Dementia may occur and may be accompanied by a frontal lobe syndrome or by delusions and hallucinations. Cognitive deficits may occur in close to 50 per cent of patients with neurosarcoidosis. Delirium has been noted but appears to be rare.

(ii) g – This is far more common in females than in males and the majority of patients fall ill between puberty and 40 years of age. It is a systemic disease and in most cases cerebral lupus occurs in the setting of other symptoms, including constitutional symptoms (fatigue, fever, weight loss) and those referable to other organ systems. Cutaneous manifestations include photosensitivity, rashes (especially a malar rash) and alopecia. Renal involvement may manifest initially with proteinuria and cellular casts; over time, renal failure may occur. Cerebral lupus may manifest with

depression, mania, psychosis, delirium or dementia, seizures, chorea or focal signs.

(iii) e – This immune-related disorder is also known as retinocochleocerebral vasculopathy and is typically seen in young adult females. Classically one sees the subacute onset of delirium, often accompanied by headache, in the setting of sensorineuronal hearing loss and visual disturbances. The MRI lesions described are typical; the multiple areas of increased signal intensity are also seen on T2-weighted images, which should also be requested. (In some cases, these lesions may demonstrate contrast enhancement.) There is a widespread cerebral microangiopathy.

(iv) d – As mentioned in (i), most affected patients fall ill in their 20s or 30s. In the United States, sarcoidosis is far more common in black people than in white people. Hypercalcaemia occurs in a majority of patients. Cerebral involvement may be characterized by multiple granulomas or by relatively few large lesions, or even by a solitary lesion. The clinical vignette is consistent with a hypothalamic granuloma; besides somnolence, other manifestations of hypothalamic involvement include appetite disturbance and, rarely, symptomatic narcolepsy. Cerebral MRI typically reveals any macroscopic parenchymal granulomas.

Reference: *Psychiatry: An evidence-based text*, **pp. 586–590.**

4. d

Visual hallucinations are very common with prolonged treatment with either levodopa or dopamine agonists. The hallucinations are typically complex, involving scenes, animals or people, and may last from minutes to hours or even days. Importantly, early on, patients retain insight into the hallucinatory nature of these experiences and recognize that they are not real. Auditory hallucinations, or even olfactory or gustatory hallucinations, may also occur, but these are much less common.

Reference: *Psychiatry: An evidence-based text*, **p. 542.**

5. d

Approximately 90 per cent of cases of ALS (amyotrophic lateral sclerosis) are sporadic. Around 10 per cent are inherited in an autosomal dominant fashion, secondary to mutations in *SOD* (superoxide dismutase) on chromosome 21. There are very rare cases of inheritance on a recessive basis.

Reference: *Psychiatry: An evidence-based text*, **p. 544.**

6.

(i) f – While walking there is reduced arm swing, and patients often display *marche à petit pas*, wherein they take small shuffling steps.

(ii) a – Classically, patients present with weakness in one of the upper extremities, often in the hand, and there may be difficulty buttoning clothes or using small tools; over time, other limbs become involved.

(iii) g – The onset is insidious and generally occurs in the sixth decade. The disease typically presents with frequency unexplained falls owing to postural instability. An atypical parkinsonism then gradually appears. Dementia occurs in about one-half of all patients, generally well after the parkinsonism has become established. Rarely, dementia may constitute the presenting symptom.

(iv) d – Although this is an autosomal dominant disorder, and therefore in theory a positive family history should be found, exceptions may occur secondary to uncertain parentage (in this case the patient was adopted) or, more rarely, to spontaneous mutations.

Reference: *Psychiatry: An evidence-based text*, pp. 541–552.

7. c

Motor tics are usually the first to appear. Simple motor tics include blinking, brow-wrinkling, grimacing and shoulder-shrugging; complex motor tics may include touching, smelling, hopping, throwing, clapping, bending over, squatting or even such very complex acts as echopraxia or copropraxia.

Reference: *Psychiatry: An evidence-based text*, p. 550.

8. e

Reference: *Psychiatry: An evidence-based text*, p. 548.

9.

(i) a – This is a familial form of Parkinson's disease (4q21).
(ii) b – This is a familial form of Parkinson's disease (6q25–27).
(iii) a – DRPLA (dentatorubralpallidoluysian atrophy) is a gradually progressive autosomal dominantly inherited disorder: mutations exist in the gene for atrophin-1 on chromosome 12, which consists of an expansion of a normally occurring CAG repeat.
(iv) a – Spinocerebellar ataxia (SCA) is an autosomal dominantly inherited syndrome. SCA19 (genetic locus 1p21-q21) is associated with cognitive impairment.

Reference: *Psychiatry: An evidence-based text*, p. 543, 548–549.

10. a

This typically presents in the 20s or 30s.

Reference: *Psychiatry: An evidence-based text*, pp. 552–557.

11. b

The onset of migraine headaches tends to occur in the third or fourth decade. This is followed by recurrent strokes or transient ischaemic attacks (TIAs) in the fourth or fifth decade, and dementia in the sixth or seventh decade.

Reference: *Psychiatry: An evidence-based text*, p. 554.

12.

(i) d
(ii) a
(iii) d

Reference: *Psychiatry: An evidence-based text*, p. 557–559.

13. b

Contrary to popular belief, such discoloration is in fact rare; if anything, most patients display a degree of cyanosis.

Reference: *Psychiatry: An evidence-based text*, p. 560.

14.

(i) a – This is a characteristic feature of encephalopathic (acute) pellagra.
(ii) b
(iii) a

Reference: *Psychiatry: An evidence-based text*, p. 561.

15. c

Chronic Mn (manganese) poisoning can cause these clinical features. The most characteristic feature of the parkinsonism is the distinctive dystonic gait abnormality known as 'cock-walk', whereby patients walk on their metatarsophalangeal joints as if they were wearing high heels; at times, the elbows may be flexed, creating the overall impression of the walk of a rooster.

Reference: *Psychiatry: An evidence-based text*, p. 562.

16. c

This personality change is associated with mercury intoxication and is classically characterized by emotional lability, shyness and anxiety, all of which may be accompanied by insomnia.

Reference: *Psychiatry: An evidence-based text*, pp. 563–564.

17.

(i) d – This disorder is classically characterized clinically by the development of a combination of flaccid quadriplegia and delirium, and pathologically by demyelination in the central portion of the pons, all occurring within 2–3 days of overly rapid correction of chronic hyponatraemia.
(ii) o – In some cases one might see diffuse multifocal muscle twitching; dysarthria may also occur. In a minority of patients, seizures, typically grand mal, may appear.
(iii) h – Delirium occurs in about half of cases. In some cases, stupor or coma may supervene.

(iv) i – The autonomic symptoms appear fairly promptly as the blood glucose level falls below 2.5 mM (45 mg/dL).

(v) j – The delirium and metallic taste are features of the full syndrome and may occur in both children and adults.

Reference: *Psychiatry: An evidence-based text*, **pp. 563–566.**

18.

(i) c – This disorder occurs secondary to a central nervous system opportunistic infection by the JC virus.

(ii) c – This disorder is caused by the Epstein–Barr virus.

(iii) c – SSPE (subacute sclerosing panencephalitis) occurs secondary to a reactivation of a dormant measles virus that lacks a normal M-protein.

(iv) a – This disorder occurs secondary to infection with the bacillus *Tropheryma whippelii*.

(v) b – This disorder occurs secondary to infection with the protozoon *Plasmodium*.

Reference: *Psychiatry: An evidence-based text*, **pp. 567–571.**

19. e

Infection by *Toxoplasma gondii* is common in birds and mammals; cats serve as the definitive hosts and oocysts found in cat faeces may remain viable for up to a year. Primary infection in humans occurs secondary to eating contaminated food or undercooked lamb, pork or beef from infected animals and is common.

Reference: *Psychiatry: An evidence-based text*, **pp. 571.**

20. c

In a very small minority of patients, the cerebrospinal fluid total protein level may show a mild elevation. The 14-3-3 protein is found in 50–95 per cent of cases.

Reference: *Psychiatry: An evidence-based text*, **pp. 571–572.**

21. c

Depression is the most prominent neuropsychiatric feature and occurs in 50–75 per cent of patients with Cushing's syndrome and may be the presenting feature. Anxiety commonly accompanies the depression, as agitated depression. The depression at times may be severe, with psychotic features. Both suicide attempts and completed suicides may occur.

Anxiety of pathological degree has been noted in about 10 per cent of patients but is most often seen in the context of depression.

Reference: *Psychiatry: An evidence-based text*, **pp. 573–574.**

22. b

Reference: *Psychiatry: An evidence-based text*, **p. 575.**

23.

(i) b
(ii) c

(iii) a
(iv) a
(v) d

Reference: *Psychiatry: An evidence-based text*, **pp. 575–577.**

24.

(i) a
(ii) c
(iii) c

Reference: *Psychiatry: An evidence-based text*, **p. 577.**

25. c

Patients may walk with short steps on a somewhat widened base, and sometimes there is a degree of shuffling, but the distinctive feature is a 'magnetic' gait; some may complain that it feels as if their feet are 'glued to the floor'.

Reference: *Psychiatry: An evidence-based text*, **pp. 583.**

26.

(i) b – This is neuroacanthocytosis, which is an autosomal recessive condition occurring secondary to mutations in *VPS13A* at 9q21 (formerly known as *CHAC*), which codes for chorein. There may be considerable phenotypic heterogeneity in the same family.

(ii) b – This is an autosomal recessive disorder resulting from mutations in *ATP7B* on chromosome 13 which codes for the copper-binding ATPase ATP7B; multiple different mutations have been identified.

(iii) a – DM1 (myotonic dystrophy type 1) is inherited in an autosomal dominant fashion with almost 100 per cent penetrance but variable expressivity, even within the same family. Mutations consist of an expansion of a normally occurring CTG triplet in *DMPK* (myotonic dystrophy protein kinase) on 19q13.3. 'Anticipation' may occur, in which, in succeeding generations, and with expansion of the triplet repeat, the disease becomes more severe and has an earlier onset. Anticipation is more likely with maternal transmission than paternal cases.

(iv) c – Like fragile X syndrome, FXTAS (fragile X-associated tremor/ataxia syndrome) occurs as a result of a mutation in *FMR1* (fragile X mental retardation) on the long arm of the X chromosome, with an increase in the number of CGG repeats up into the permutation range of from 55 to 200.

Reference: *Psychiatry: An evidence-based text*, **p. 547–551.**

27.

(i) a
(ii) c
(iii) b
(iv) a

Reference: *Psychiatry: An evidence-based text*, **p. 577.**

Chapter 38

Schizophrenia and paranoid psychoses

QUESTIONS

Note that for answers to extended matching items (EMIs), each option (denoted a, b, c, etc.) might be used once, more than once or not at all. For multiple-choice questions (MCQs), please select the best answer.

1. **MCQ** – Of the following, with whom are the 'four As' of schizophrenia most closely associated?
   (a) Emil Kraeplin
   (b) Eugen Bleuler
   (c) Karl Jaspers
   (d) Karl Schneider
   (e) Kurt Schneider.

2. **MCQ** – During which quarter of the year are northern hemisphere patients with schizophrenia most likely to have been born?
   (a) First 3 months
   (b) Second 3 months
   (c) Third 3 months
   (d) Last 3 months
   (e) There is no season of birth effect.

3. **EMI** – Risk for developing schizophrenia
   (a) The risk of schizophrenia is raised at least twofold.
   (b) There is not believed to be a significantly increased risk.

   Select the option from the above list with which each of the following is best associated:
   (i) Being male
   (ii) Being black Afro-Caribbean in the UK
   (iii) Having a schizophrenogenic mother.

4. **EMI** – Antipsychotic medication
   (a) < 10 per cent
   (b) 10–25 per cent
   (c) 25–70 per cent
   (d) 70–90 per cent
   (e) > 90 per cent

   Select the option from the above list with which each of the following is best associated:
   (i) The risk of relapse of schizophrenia over 1 year when patients with schizophrenia stop their antipsychotic medication

   (ii) The level of D2R occupancy by first-generation antipsychotics at which extrapyramidal side-effects appear clinically
   (iii) The level of D2R occupancy at therapeutic doses of aripiprazole
   (iv) The level of D2R occupancy of clozapine at therapeutic doses.

5. **MCQ** – Select one incorrect statement regarding trials of antipsychotics in schizophrenia:
   (a) CUtLASS 1 showed a significant benefit in terms of quality of life of being randomized to a second-generation antipsychotic compared with a first-generation antipsychotic.
   (b) In CATIE phase II, clozapine stood out as the most effective drug for treatment-resistant schizophrenia.
   (c) In CUtLASS 2, clozapine stood out as the most effective drug for treatment-resistant schizophrenia.
   (d) The 18-month CATIE found that on the primary measure the second-generation antipsychotics risperidone, quetiapine and ziprasidone were similar to perphenazine.
   (e) The TEOSS study showed that olanzapine, risperidone and molindone were generally of similar efficacy in childhood schizophrenia.

6. **MCQ** – Which of the following treatments currently appears to be the least helpful for patients with schizophrenia?
   (a) Assertive community therapy
   (b) Compliance therapy
   (c) Psychoeducation
   (d) Psychoanalytically oriented group therapy
   (e) Social skills training.

7. **EMI** – Risk for developing schizophrenia
   (a) The risk of schizophrenia is raised at least twofold.
   (b) There is not believed to be a significantly increased risk.

Select the option from the above list with which each of the following is best associated:

(i) Having middle-ear disease

(ii) Regular exposure to double-bind situations while growing up, i.e. having parents who communicate with the child in abnormal ways leading to feelings of ambivalence and ambiguity, with messages that are typically vague, ambiguous and confusing

(iii) Regular cannabis abuse.

ANSWERS

1. b

Bleuler's fundamental symptoms became known as the 'four As': ambivalence, loosening of associations, affective incongruity and blunting, and autism, by which he meant emotional withdrawal.

Reference: *Psychiatry: An evidence-based text*, **p. 593.**

2. a

One of the most reproducible findings in schizophrenia is that affected patients are far more likely to have been born in the first 3 months of the year; this is the 'season of birth' effect.

Reference: *Psychiatry: An evidence-based text*, **p. 597.**

3.

(i)   b
(ii)   a
(iii) b

Reference: *Psychiatry: An evidence-based text*, **pp. 598–599.**

4.

(i)   b – There is approximately a one in five risk of relapse under these circumstances.
(ii) d – This level has been variously estimated as 70–78 per cent.

(iii) e
(iv) c

Reference: *Psychiatry: An evidence-based text*, **pp. 600–601.**

5. a

There was definitely no benefit in this respect of second-generation antipsychotics compared with first-generation antipsychotics. This is shown in Figure 38.3 on page 602 of the accompanying textbook.

Reference: *Psychiatry: An evidence-based text*, **pp. 602–603.**

6. d

This is not an appropriate approach for patients with schizophrenia.

Reference: *Psychiatry: An evidence-based text*, **pp. 604–605.**

7.

(i)   a – One study suggested that schizophrenia might be caused by irritation of the brain that could occur from middle-ear disease. The study determined that people who had middle-ear disease were over 3.6 times more likely to have a later diagnosis of schizophrenia (or over four times more likely if the middle-ear disease was on the left side).
(ii) b – It is no longer believed that parents can cause schizophrenia through their communication styles.
(iii) a – Cannabis abuse raises the risk for schizophrenia by 2- to 4.5-fold.

Reference: *Psychiatry: An evidence-based text*, **pp. 596–599.**

Chapter 39

Mood disorders/affective psychoses

QUESTIONS

Note that for answers to extended matching items (EMIs), each option (denoted a, b, c, etc.) might be used once, more than once or not at all. For multiple-choice questions (MCQs), please select the best answer.

1. **EMI** – Bipolar diagnoses
   (a) DSM-IV-TR bipolar I disorder
   (b) DSM-IV-TR bipolar II disorder
   (c) ICD-10 bipolar affective disorder
   (d) None of the above

   Select the option from the above list with which each of the following is best associated (note that depressive episode can include major depressive episode in this question):
   (i) Requires at least two episodes of mood disturbance, one of which must be hypomanic, manic or mixed.
   (ii) Requires at least one depressive episode and at least one hypomanic episode but the absence of any manic episodes.
   (iii) Diagnosed following the occurrence of at least one manic episode or mixed episode, with or without depressive episodes.

2. **MCQ** – Select one incorrect statement regarding drugs used in the treatment of affective disorders:
   (a) Antidepressants reduce the level of CRP.
   (b) Antidepressants reduce the levels of pro-inflammatory cytokines.
   (c) Anti-manic medications tend to block the effects of dopamine.
   (d) Patients with uncorrected hypothyroidism have a good response to antidepressants.
   (e) Prodopaminergic stimulants can trigger mania.

3. **EMI** – Psychological aetiological factors in mood disorders
   (a) Cognitive distortions
   (b) Cognitive triad
   (c) Psychodynamic theory
   (d) None of the above

   Select the option from the above list with which each of the following concepts is best associated:
   (i) Mania as a defence against depression
   (ii) Personalization
   (iii) Learned helplessness
   (iv) Arbitrary inference
   (v) Depression as a reaction to loss.

4. **MCQ** – Select one incorrect statement regarding affective disorders:
   (a) Brown and Harris' study of the social origins of depression in women identified a lack of a confiding relationship as a risk factor for depression.
   (b) In the 6 months following a life event, the risk for depression and deliberate self-harm is markedly increased.
   (c) Patients with depression have elevated standardized mortality ratios compared with the general population.
   (d) The average length of a single depressive episode is about 4 weeks.
   (e) Women are around twice as likely as men to suffer from depression.

5. **EMI** – Diagnosis of depression in ICD-10
   (a) Common (but non-core) symptoms
   (b) Core symptoms
   (c) Neither of the above

   Select the option from the above list with which each of the following symptoms is best associated:
   (i) Pessimistic thoughts
   (ii) Diminished appetite
   (iii) Depressed mood.

6. **MCQ** – For diagnosing a major depressive episode, DSM-IV-TR requires the presence of five or more of nine symptoms during the same 2-week period, and these should represent a change from previous functioning. Which of the following is not one of these nine symptoms?
   (a) Diminished ability to think or concentrate, or indecisiveness, nearly every day
   (b) Diurnal variation of mood nearly every day
   (c) Insomnia or hypersomnia nearly every day
   (d) Markedly diminished interest or pleasure, in all or almost all activities most of the day, nearly every day
   (e) Recurrent thoughts of death or recurrent suicidal ideation.

7. **MCQ** – Which of the following medications is least likely to cause depression?
   (a) Chloramphenicol
   (b) Isradipine
   (c) Orphenadrine
   (d) Prednisolone
   (e) Sodium oxybate.

8. **EMI** – NICE stepped-care model for depression
   (a) Step 1
   (b) Step 2
   (c) Step 3
   (d) Step 4
   (e) Step 5
   (f) None of the above

Select the option from the steps in the NICE stepped-care model with which each of the following aspects of management is best associated:
   (i) Assessment only
   (ii) ECT
   (iii) Complex psychological interventions
   (iv) Watchful waiting
   (v) Computerized CBT.

9. **MCQ** – Select one incorrect statement regarding rapid-cycling bipolar disorder:
   (a) A rapid-cycling pattern is seen predominantly in men.
   (b) In some individuals it can be associated with antidepressant use.
   (c) Of patients with bipolar disorder seen in mood clinics, it is estimated that 10–20 per cent will have rapid cycling.
   (d) The pattern can occur at any time during the course of bipolar disorder and is associated with a poorer long-term prognosis.
   (e) The term 'rapid cycling' is applied to bipolar disorder when four or more separate mood episodes occur within a 12-month period.

10. **MCQ** – Which of the following is not a diagnostic or severity rating scale for bipolar disorder?
    (a) CARS-M
    (b) HAD
    (c) MDQ
    (d) MINI
    (e) PSQ.

11. **MCQ** – Which of the following medications is least likely to induce symptoms of mania?
    (a) Amitriptyline
    (b) Atomoxetine
    (c) Chloroquine
    (d) Glibenclamide
    (e) Vigabatrin.

12. **EMI** – Historical developments
    (a) Beck
    (b) Freud, Sigmund
    (c) Kendler
    (d) Klein
    (e) Paykel

Select the person from the above list with whom each of the following concepts or historical developments is best associated:
    (i) Depressive position
    (ii) Influential twin study of depression
    (iii) Cognitive triad.

13. **EMI** – Historical developments
    (a) Abramson
    (b) Brown and Harris
    (c) Cade
    (d) Harris and Barraclough
    (e) Rosenthal

Select the person or persons from the above list with whom each of the following historical developments is best associated:
    (i) Therapeutic use of lithium in mania
    (ii) Meta-analysis of suicide in bipolar disorder
    (iii) SAD.

14. **EMI** – Diagnosis of depression in ICD-10
    (a) Common (but non-core) symptoms
    (b) Core symptoms
    (c) Neither of the above

Select the option from the above list with which each of the following symptoms is best associated:
    (i) Ideas or acts of self-harm or suicide
    (ii) Comfort eating
    (iii) Reduced concentration and attention
    (iv) Loss of interest and enjoyment.

ANSWERS

1.

(i)   c
(ii) b
(iii) a

Reference: *Psychiatry: An evidence-based text*, **p. 610.**

2. d

Such patients tend to have a poor response.

Reference: *Psychiatry: An evidence-based text*, **pp. 611–612.**

3.

(i)   c
(ii) a
(iii) d
(iv) a
(v)   c

Reference: *Psychiatry: An evidence-based text*, **pp. 613–614.**

4. d

The average length is closer to 6 months.

Reference: *Psychiatry: An evidence-based text*, **pp. 614–616.**

5.

(i)   a
(ii) a
(iii) b

Reference: *Psychiatry: An evidence-based text*, **p. 617.**

6. b

Reference: *Psychiatry: An evidence-based text*, **pp. 617–618.**

7. c

This antimuscarinic drug is much more likely to cause euphoria as a side-effect.

Reference: *Psychiatry: An evidence-based text*, **p. 619.**

8.

(i)   a
(ii) e
(iii) d

(iv) b
(v)   b

Reference: *Psychiatry: An evidence-based text*, **p. 622.**

9. a

It is seen predominantly in women.

Reference: *Psychiatry: An evidence-based text*, **p. 625.**

10. b

HADS = Hospital Anxiety and Depression Scale; CARS-M = Clinician-Administered Rating Scale for Mania; MDQ = Mood Disorder Questionnaire; MINI = Mini International Neuropsychiatric Inventory; PSQ = Psychosis Screening Questionnaire.

Reference: *Psychiatry: An evidence-based text*, **pp. 628, 786.**

11. d

This is a sulphonylurea anti-diabetic drug.

Reference: *Psychiatry: An evidence-based text*, **pp. 628.**

12.

(i)   d
(ii) c
(iii) a

Reference: *Psychiatry: An evidence-based text*, **Ch. 39.**

13.

(i)   c
(ii) d
(iii) e

Reference: *Psychiatry: An evidence-based text*, **Ch. 39.**

14.

(i)   a
(ii) c – In ICD-10, this does not appear as either one of the three core symptoms or the seven sets of common symptoms.
(iii) a
(iv) b

Reference: *Psychiatry: An evidence-based text*, **p. 617.**

Chapter 40

Neurotic and stress-related disorders

QUESTIONS

Note that for answers to extended matching items (EMIs), each option (denoted a, b, c, etc.) might be used once, more than once or not at all. For multiple-choice questions (MCQs), please select the best answer.

1. **MCQ** – Which of the following neurotic conditions occurs most frequently?
   (a) Generalized anxiety disorder
   (b) Mixed anxiety and depression
   (c) Obsessive-compulsive disorder
   (d) Panic disorder
   (e) Phobia.

2. **MCQ** – Which of the following are features of generalized anxiety disorder?
   (a) Derealization
   (b) Feeling keyed up
   (c) Lability of mood
   (d) Perceptual distortion
   (e) All of the above.

3. **MCQ** – Which of the following is least likely to be a symptom of anxiety?
   (a) Dysphagia
   (b) Muscle tension
   (c) Rotational vertigo
   (d) Tachycardia
   (e) Tension headache.

4. **EMI** – Characteristic features of neurotic and stress-related disorders
   (a) Agoraphobia
   (b) Generalized anxiety disorder
   (c) Mixed anxiety and depressive disorder
   (d) Panic disorder
   (e) Social phobias
   (f) Specific (isolated) phobias

Select the diagnostic option from the above list with which each of the following sets of features is best associated:
   (i) Persistent 'free-floating' anxiety symptoms involving elements of apprehension, motor tension and autonomic overactivity

(ii) Recurrent attacks of severe anxiety not restricted to any particular situation or set of circumstances, and therefore unpredicable
(iii) Fear of scrutiny by other people in comparatively small groups.

5. **EMI** – Historical concepts/developments
   (a) Cullen
   (b) Freud, Sigmund
   (c) Hebb
   (d) Watson
   (e) Whyth
   (f) Wolpe

Select the person from the above list with which each of the following is best associated:
   (i) Systematic desensitization was first described by him.
   (ii) Little Albert.
   (iii) The concept of 'neurosis' was first used by him for disorders of the nervous system for which there appeared to be no physical cause.

6. **EMI** – Gender ratios of neurotic and stress-related disorders
   (a) Male (M) significantly greater than female (F)
   (b) M approximately equal to F
   (c) M significantly less than F

Select the option from the above list with which each of the following is best associated:
   (i) Specific phobias
   (ii) Agoraphobia
   (iii) Social phobia
   (iv) Generalized anxiety disorder
   (v) Panic disorder.

7. **MCQ** – Select one incorrect statement regarding panic disorder:
   (a) An association with benign joint laxity has been described, with a very high increase in incidence.
   (b) Patients may experience angor animus.

(c) The lifetime prevalence is around 4 per cent, compared with 8 per cent for panic attacks alone.

(d) There is good evidence of a genetic inherited predisposition.

(e) With treatment, 20-year follow-up shows that most patients remain entirely panic-free.

8. **EMI** – Differential diagnosis of generalized anxiety disorder and depressive disorder

(a) Depressive disorder

(b) Generalized anxiety disorder

Select the diagnosis from the above list with which each of the following features is better associated:

(i) More frequency in people with premorbid anxious personality

(ii) Panic attacks are comparatively rare

(iii) Anhedonia

(iv) No diurnal variation of mood

(v) Early-morning wakening.

9. **MCQ** – Select one incorrect statement regarding obsessive-compulsive disorder:

(a) Insight is characteristically not maintained.

(b) Males have an earlier onset than females.

(c) Most individuals have an age of onset in the early 20s.

(d) Obsessional symptoms may be seen in up to 20–30 per cent of patients with depressive disorder.

(e) Rituals may arise from *folie de doute.*

10. **MCQ** – Select one correct statement regarding the aetiology of obsessive-compulsive disorder:

(a) A premorbid anankastic personality disorder does not predispose to the subsequent development of obsessive-compulsive disorder.

(b) Cerebral blood flow studies have tended not to show any significant changes in obsessive-compulsive disorder.

(c) Some children and adolescents develop obsessive-compulsive disorder and motor tics after beta-haemolytic streptococcal infections.

(d) There is no increased incidence of obsessive-compulsive disorder in people with brain injury.

(e) There is poor evidence for a genetic component.

11. **EMI** – Phobias

(a) Agoraphobia

(b) Specific phobia

(c) Social phobia

Select the diagnosis from the above list with which each of the following features is best associated:

(i) Poor response to MAOI treatment

(ii) Feared objects include public transport

(iii) Feared objects include eating in public.

12. **MCQ** – Select one incorrect statement regarding post-traumatic stress disorder:

(a) Characteristically there is increased arousal and hypervigilance.

(b) Characteristically there are intrusive recollections in the form of thoughts, nightmares and flashbacks.

(c) Man-made disasters are more likely to cause it than natural disasters.

(d) Onset characteristically follows trauma without a latency period.

(e) Reduced hippocampal volume has been reported in American Vietnam veteran sufferers.

13. **EMI** – Historical concepts/developments

(a) Cullen

(b) Freud, Anna

(c) Freud, Sigmund

(d) Hebb

(e) Watson

(f) Whytt

(g) Wolpe

Select the person from the above list with which each of the following is best associated:

(i) Little Hans

(ii) The term 'illness of the nerves'

(iii) The development and application of an inverted-U shaped curve to the relationship between performance and anxiety.

14. **EMI** – Phobias

(a) Agoraphobia

(b) Specific phobia

(c) Social phobia

Select the diagnosis from the above list with which each of the following features is best associated:

(i) Acrophobia

(ii) The age of onset is usually between 3 and 8 years

(iii) Two peaks of onset: at 5 years and between 11 and 15 years

(iv) Poor response to SSRI treatment.

ANSWERS

1. b

It has a frequency of around 48 per cent.
                    Reference: *Psychiatry: An evidence-based text*, **p. 644.**

2. e

                    Reference: *Psychiatry: An evidence-based text*, **p. 645.**

3. c

This is not a feature of anxiety.
                    Reference: *Psychiatry: An evidence-based text*, **pp. 645–646.**

4.

(i)   b
(ii) d
(iii) e
                    Reference: *Psychiatry: An evidence-based text*, **p. 643.**

5.

(i)   f
(ii) d – Watson's experiment on Little Albert took place in 1920.
(iii) a – Used by William Cullen in 1784.
                    Reference: *Psychiatry: An evidence-based text*, **Ch. 40.**

6.

(i)   c
(ii) c – The ratio of females to males is around 2.5:1.
(iii) c – The ratio of females to males is around 2.5:1 (although it may be approximately equal in those seeking treatment).
(iv) c – The ratio of females to males is around 2:1.
(v)   c – It is two to three times more common in females than in males.
                    Reference: *Psychiatry: An evidence-based text*, **pp. 645, 649, 653.**

7. e

Follow-up over 20 years shows that fewer than 50 per cent of treated patients remain entirely panic-free.
                    Reference: *Psychiatry: An evidence-based text*, **pp. 649–651.**

8.

(i)   b
(ii) a
(iii) a
(iv) b
(v)   a
                    Reference: *Psychiatry: An evidence-based text*, **p. 651.**

9. a

Insight is maintained.
                    Reference: *Psychiatry: An evidence-based text*, **pp. 656–657.**

10. c

This finding may suggest a cell-mediated autoimmune aetiology.
                    Reference: *Psychiatry: An evidence-based text*, **p. 657.**

11.

(i)   b
(ii) a
(iii) c
                    Reference: *Psychiatry: An evidence-based text*, **p. 653.**

12. d

Onset follows trauma with a latency period of a few weeks to months.
                    Reference: *Psychiatry: An evidence-based text*, **p. 660.**

13.

(i)   c – In 1909, Sigmund Freud described the development of a phobia of horses in a 5-year-old child called 'Little Hans'.
(ii) f – This term was used by Whytt in 1768, superseding the term 'vapours', and preceding the use of the term 'neurosis'.
(iii) d – Hebb developed this Yerkes–Dodson relationship and applied it to the relationship between performance and anxiety.
                    Reference: *Psychiatry: An evidence-based text*, **Ch. 40.**

14.

(i)   b – This is a fear of heights.
(ii) b
(iii) c
(iv) b
                    Reference: *Psychiatry: An evidence-based text*, **p. 653.**

Chapter 41

Dissociative (conversion), hypochondriasis and other somatoform disorders

QUESTIONS

Note that for answers to extended matching items (EMIs), each option (denoted a, b, c, etc.) might be used once, more than once or not at all. For multiple-choice questions (MCQs), please select the best answer.

1. **MCQ** – Select one correct characteristic feature of dissociative fugue:
   (a) Activities of daily living are usually not preserved.
   (b) Basic self-care is usually not preserved.
   (c) Simple social interactions with strangers are usually preserved.
   (d) There is usually an absence of current stressors.
   (e) Travel is usually without purpose.

2. **MCQ** – Select one incorrect statement regarding St Louis hysteria:
   (a) It is a psychoanalytic term for phobic anxiety.
   (b) It is also known as Briquet's syndrome.
   (c) It is also known as somatization disorder.
   (d) It refers to individuals with recurrent and multiple unexplained physical symptoms commencing before the age of 30 years.
   (e) It refers to individuals with recurrent and multiple unexplained physical symptoms of chronic duration.

3. **MCQ** – Select one incorrect statement regarding conversion disorder:
   (a) A premorbid histrionic, dependent, passive-aggressive or antisocial personality disorder may be present in up to one-fifth of cases.
   (b) Precipitating factors include severe stress, such as the recent death of a close relative whose physical symptoms may be modelled by the patient.
   (c) Symptoms suggestive of it occurring in middle age or beyond are very likely the result of organic illness.
   (d) The age of onset is usually in adolescence or early adulthood.
   (e) There is good evidence in favour of a genetic predisposition.

4. **EMI** – Somatoform disorders
   (a) Body dysmorphic disorder
   (b) Hypochondriacal disorder
   (c) Persistent somatoform pain disorder
   (d) Somatization disorder

Select the diagnosis from the above list with which each of the following sets of features is best associated:
   (i) Symptoms begin in the teenage years or, rarely, in the 20s, usually before the age of 30 years. Prevalence rates of up to 2 per cent have been found in females. Patients have long and complicated medical histories.
   (ii) Onset can occur at any age but is most frequent in the 30s and 40s. The disorder is considered to be common in general medical practice. Although many patients may have a past history of injuries, they often show no current evidence of tissue or nerve damage.
   (iii) The most common age of onset is from adolescence through to the third decade. Patients are more likely to present to a plastic surgeon or dermatologist than to a psychiatrist.

5. **MCQ** – Which of the following somatoform disorders is not more common in women than in men?
   (a) Body dysmorphic disorder
   (b) Hypochondriacal disorder
   (c) Persistent somatoform pain disorder
   (d) Somatization disorder
   (e) None of the above.

6. **MCQ** – Pimozide has been found to be especially effective in the treatment of which of the following?
   (a) Hypochondriacal disorder
   (b) Dysmorphophobia
   (c) Monosymptomatic hypochondriacal psychosis
   (d) Münchausen syndrome
   (e) Myalgic encephalomyelitis.

7. **EMI** –Differential diagnosis of dissociative and other somatoform disorders
   (a) Dissociative disorders
   (b) Factitious disorders

(c) Malingering

(d) Somatoform disorders

Select the option from the above list with which each of the following sets of symptoms is best associated:

(i) Physical and psychological symptoms are present and there is unconscious motivation.

(ii) Unconscious motivation is present but psychological symptoms are absent.

(iii) There is conscious motivation and the voluntary production of symptoms.

ANSWERS

1. c

The differential diagnosis includes organic fugue, where basic self-care and activities of daily living are not characteristically preserved, and postictal states, where there is an absence of current stressors and travel is without purpose.

Reference: *Psychiatry: An evidence-based text,* **pp. 667–668.**

2. a

Anxiety hysteria is a psychoanalytic term for phobic anxiety.

Reference: *Psychiatry: An evidence-based text,* **p. 666.**

3. e

There is little such evidence.

Reference: *Psychiatry: An evidence-based text,* **pp. 669–670.**

4.

(i) d
(ii) c
(iii) a

Reference: *Psychiatry: An evidence-based text,* **pp. 671–677.**

5. b

It is slightly more common in males, or at least with the same frequency as females, in contrast to other somatoform disorders, which are more common in women.

Reference: *Psychiatry: An evidence-based text,* **pp. 671–677.**

6. c

Reference: *Psychiatry: An evidence-based text,* **p. 682.**

7.

(i) b
(ii) d
(iii) c – Note that in factitious disorders there is an absence of conscious motivation.

Reference: *Psychiatry: An evidence-based text,* **p. 683.**

Chapter 42

Eating disorders

QUESTIONS

Note that for answers to extended matching items (EMIs), each option (denoted a, b, c, etc.) might be used once, more than once or not at all. For multiple-choice questions (MCQs), please select the best answer.

1. **MCQ** – Which of the following is a pathognomonic feature of anorexia nervosa?
   (a) A problem with being able to eat
   (b) A wish to look attractive
   (c) Anorexia
   (d) Attempting to avoid being fat
   (e) None of the above.

2. **EMI** – Eating disorders
   (a) Anorexia nervosa
   (b) Bulimia nervosa
   (c) Eating disorder not otherwise specified

This question concerns the above DSM-IV-TR diagnoses of eating disorders. Select the option from the above list with which each of the following is best associated:
   (i) DSM-IV-TR includes restrictive and binge-eating/purging subtypes of this diagnosis.
   (ii) The incidence is around eight per 100000 per year.
   (iii) The most common eating disorder in the outpatient setting.
   (iv) The prevalence is around 1 per cent.
   (v) The average age of onset is 19 years.

3. **MCQ** – Select one incorrect statement regarding eating disorders:
   (a) Cluster C personality disorders are the most common personality disorder cluster among those with eating disorders.
   (b) In anorexia nervosa the concordance rate is higher for monozygotic twins than for dizygotic twins.
   (c) Obsessive-compulsive personality disorder is a risk factor for anorexia nervosa and bulimia nervosa.

   (d) Perfectionism is a risk factor for anorexia nervosa and bulimia nervosa.
   (e) The ICD-10 criteria for anorexia nervosa include weight loss to Quetelet's body mass index (BMI) of 17.5 kg/m^2 or less, used for age 16 years and over.

4. **MCQ** – Which of the following is the first-line treatment of choice for bulimia nervosa?
   (a) A second-generation antipsychotic
   (b) A tricyclic antidepressant
   (c) An SSRI
   (d) Cognitive-behaviour therapy
   (e) Family therapy.

5. **MCQ** – Which of the following is the best predictor of death in anorexia nervosa?
   (a) Hypocalcaemia
   (b) Hypophosphataemia
   (c) Low serum albumin
   (d) Low serum urea
   (e) Low TSH.

6. **MCQ** – Select one incorrect statement regarding eating disorders:
   (a) Bisphosphonates should not be used in young women.
   (b) Fluoxetine has been licensed for the treatment of bulimia nervosa.
   (c) In general, antipsychotics are safe to use in eating disorders.
   (d) It is particularly concerning if the pulse rate is less than 40 beats/min in anorexia nervosa.
   (e) The common thyroid function test pattern in anorexia nervosa includes low T3 and normal TSH.

ANSWERS

1. e

People with eating disorders do not have a problem with their eating. Anorexia nervosa does not develop because people want to look attractive. They do not have anorexia; indeed they are usually ravenous. It is a common clinical mistake to believe that patients with anorexia nervosa are attempting to avoid 'being fat'; rather, they have a phobia of being at a normal weight.

Reference: *Psychiatry: An evidence-based text*, **pp. 687.**

2.

(i)   a
(ii) a
(iii) c
(iv) b
(v) b –This is slightly older than in anorexia nervosa.

Reference: *Psychiatry: An evidence-based text*, **pp. 688–689.**

3. d

It has been found to be a risk factor for anorexia nervosa only.

Reference: *Psychiatry: An evidence-based text*, **pp. 688–690.**

4. d

There is general agreement in the field, supported by The National Institute for Health and Clinical Excellence (NICE), that cognitive-behaviour therapy is the treatment of choice for bulimia nervosa, delivered in group or individual format.

Reference: *Psychiatry: An evidence-based text*, **p. 693.**

5. c

Together with severity of weight loss, low serum albumin (resulting from starvation or severe infection) is a predictor of death in anorexia nervosa.

Reference: *Psychiatry: An evidence-based text*, **pp. 695.**

6. c

Prolongation of the QTc interval and QT variability are good predictors of life-threatening ventricular arrhythmias. Prolonged starvation with a low BMI, causing atrophy and histological changes in cardiac muscle and collagen fibres, and purging behaviours, resulting in hypokalaemia and hypomagnesaemia, may be directly arrhythmogenic or may prolong the QTc interval in patients with eating disorders. A genetic or medication-related prolonged QTc interval may increase this risk, and medications (many psychotropic) should be used with caution in patients with eating disorders.

Bisphosphonates should not be used in young women because of the potential for serious side-effects such as teratogenicity. It is particularly concerning if the pulse rate is less than 40 beats/min in anorexia nervosa, owing to the consequent risk of arrhythmias.

Reference: *Psychiatry: An evidence-based text*, **Ch. 42.**

Chapter 43

Personality disorders

QUESTIONS

Note that for answers to extended matching items (EMIs), each option (denoted a, b, c, etc.) might be used once, more than once or not at all. For multiple-choice questions (MCQs), please select the best answer.

1. **EMI** – Classification of personality disorders by clusters
   (a) Cluster A
   (b) Cluster B
   (c) Cluster C
   (d) Cluster D

   Select the cluster from the above list with which each of the following DSM-IV-TR personality disorders is best associated:
   (i) Antisocial personality disorder
   (ii) Schizotypal personality disorder
   (iii) Avoidant
   (iv) Obsessive-compulsive disorder.

2. **MCQ** – Select one incorrect statement regarding personality disorders:
   (a) They affect around 7–10 per cent of the population.
   (b) They are associated with poor interpersonal relationships.
   (c) They are primarily disturbances of behaviour, not symptoms.
   (d) They can only formally be diagnosed in ICD-10 and DSM-IV-TR from the age of 16 years onwards.
   (e) They tend to be persistent.

3. **EMI** – Classification of personality disorders by clusters
   (a) Cluster A
   (b) Cluster B
   (c) Cluster C
   (d) Cluster D

   Select the option from the above list with which each of the following ICD-10 personality disorders is best associated:
   (i) Dependent
   (ii) Anankastic
   (iii) Paranoid
   (iv) Histrionic.

4. **EMI** – Types of personality disorder
   (a) Intermediate
   (b) Type R
   (c) Type S
   (d) None of the above

   Select the option from the above list with which each of the following is best associated:
   (i) Borderline
   (ii) Paranoid
   (iii) Anankastic
   (iv) Impulsive.

5. **EMI** – Treatments for personality disorders
   (a) Bateman and Fonagy
   (b) Beck
   (c) Freud, Sigmund
   (d) Klein
   (e) Malan and Storr
   (f) Ryle
   (g) Tyrer, Peter

   Select the person or people from the above list with which the development of each of the following treatments for personality disorders is best associated:
   (i) CAT
   (ii) MBT
   (iii) Nidotherapy.

6. **EMI** – Treatments for personality disorders
   (a) Anxious personality disorder
   (b) Borderline personality disorder
   (c) Histrionic personality disorder
   (d) Impulsive personality disorder
   (e) Paranoid personality disorder

   Select the option from the above list with which each of the following treatments is most likely to be useful:
   (i) MBT
   (ii) Social problem-solving
   (iii) Nidotherapy.

ANSWERS

1.

(i) b
(ii) a
(iii) c
(iv) d

Reference: *Psychiatry: An evidence-based text*, **p. 705.**

2. d

A formal diagnosis of personality disorder cannot be made before the age of 18 years.

Reference: *Psychiatry: An evidence-based text*, **p. 704.**

3.

(i) c
(ii) d
(iii) a
(iv) b

Reference: *Psychiatry: An evidence-based text*, **p. 705.**

4.

(i) c – Type S are treatment-seeking.
(ii) b – Type R are treatment-resisting.
(iii) a
(iv) a

Reference: *Psychiatry: An evidence-based text*, **p. 709.**

5.

(i) f – This treatment was introduced by Anthony Ryle.
(ii) a – MBT (mentalization-based treatment) was introduced by Bateman and Fonagy.
(iii) g – This treatment, named after the Latin *nidus*, or 'nest', was introduced by Peter Tyrer.

Reference: *Psychiatry: An evidence-based text*, **pp. 709–710.**

6.

(i) b
(ii) d
(iii) e

Reference: *Psychiatry: An evidence-based text*, **pp. 709–710.**

Chapter 44

Perinatal psychiatry

QUESTIONS

Note that for answers to extended matching items (EMIs), each option (denoted a, b, c, etc.) might be used once, more than once or not at all. For multiple-choice questions (MCQs), please select the best answer.

1. **MCQ** – Select one incorrect statement regarding pseudocyesis:
   (a) Amenorrhoea is a feature.
   (b) An illusion of fetal movements is a clinical feature.
   (c) It occurs only in humans.
   (d) There is enlargement of the uterus.
   (e) Clinical features include enlargement of the breasts and nipples and a discharge of colostrum.

2. **EMI** – Medical complications of pregnancy
   (a) Delirium
   (b) Iron-deficiency anaemia
   (c) Obstructive sleep apnoea
   (d) Wernicke's encephalopathy
   (e) None of the above

Select the medical complication from the above list with which each of the following is most likely to be associated:
   (i) Pica
   (ii) Hyperemesis gravidarum
   (iii) Late pregnancy
   (iv) Chorea gravidarum.

3. **MCQ** – Select one incorrect statement regarding pregnancy:
   (a) A poor mother–fetus relationship is a predictor of impaired mother–infant bonding.
   (b) Benzodiazepines carry the risk of floppy infant syndrome.
   (c) Beta-blockers carry the risk of neonatal hypoglycaemia.
   (d) Prepartum anxiety is an independent predictor of postpartum depression.
   (e) Tocophobia is not an indication for elective Caesarean section.

4. **MCQ** – Which of the following is not a characteristic feature of fetal alcohol syndrome?
   (a) Growth retardation
   (b) Microcephaly
   (c) Short palpebral fissures
   (d) Short philtrum
   (e) Thick vermilion border

5. **EMI** – Treatments for prepartum depression
   (a) Increased risk of congenital cardiac lesions
   (b) Increased risk of preterm birth, respiratory distress and neonatal convulsions
   (c) Premature uterine contractions
   (d) Toxic effects on the newborn, including agitation, altered muscle tone, problems with breathing and sucking and neonatal pulmonary hypertension
   (e) None of the above

Select the side-effects from the above list with which each of the following treatments for prepartum depression is best associated:
   (i) ECT
   (ii) Treatment with paroxetine during the first trimester
   (iii) SSRI use during the third trimester
   (iv) Tricyclic antidepressants.

6. **MCQ** – Select the statement most likely to be incorrect regarding substance misuse during pregnancy:
   (a) Hair and meconium analysis improves the diagnosis of opiate and cocaine abuse in mothers who present unexpectedly in labour.
   (b) If it is decided to withdraw heroin, this should be done in the second trimester, replacing it with methadone.
   (c) Methadone maintenance improves the birth weight, but it may depress respiration in the newborn and lead to a more severe and prolonged withdrawal syndrome.
   (d) Narcotics are teratogenic.
   (e) Newborn infants of mothers who have been abusing narcotics during pregnancy should be kept in hospital for at least 14 days; in the baby, respiratory depression can be treated by naloxone, and seizures and withdrawal symptoms can be treated by sedatives such as diazepam or by morphine itself.

7. **MCQ** – Which of the following psychotropic drugs, when taken at therapeutic doses by pregnant mothers during the key period of fetal cardiac development, is most likely to cause Ebstein's anomaly?
    (a) Clozapine
    (b) Haloperidol
    (c) Lamotrigine
    (d) Lithium
    (e) Olanzapine.

8. **MCQ** – Select one incorrect statement regarding perinatal psychiatry:
    (a) Often, between the third and fifth days postpartum, mothers experience a sudden, fleeting and unexpected period of sensitivity and uncharacteristic weeping.
    (b) Pregnancy often worsens chronic delusional states and bipolar and cycloid psychoses.
    (c) Querulent reactions may follow a severe labour experience.
    (d) Secondary tocophobia may result from an excessively painful labour.
    (e) The incidence of depression in women following spontaneous abortion or ectopic pregnancy is much higher than that in the general population, rising to a higher level still in such women who are also childless.

9. **MCQ** – Select one correct statement regarding postnatal depression:
    (a) It has a characteristic clinical picture.
    (b) Patients presenting with postpartum depression rarely have co-morbid disorders.
    (c) Postpartum depression is a homogeneous disorder.
    (d) The incidence of depression is raised in the puerperium.
    (e) The suicide rate is below the female rate in the general population.

10. **MCQ** – Which of the following is most likely to be the commonest cause of postpartum delirium in the Western world?
    (a) Cerebral venous thrombosis
    (b) Eclampsia
    (c) Postpartum cerebral angiopathy
    (d) Sheehan's syndrome
    (e) Subdural haemorrhage.

ANSWERS

1. c

It occurs in several other mammalian species.

Reference: *Psychiatry: An evidence-based text*, **p. 715.**

2.

(i) b – Pica is common in pregnancy, especially geophagia and amylophagia, which can lead to iron-deficiency anaemia, bowel obstruction and worm infections.

(ii) d – Although thiamine treatment has been readily available since 1936, hyperemesis gravidarum still causes Wernicke's encephalopathy.

(iii) c

(iv) a

Reference: *Psychiatry: An evidence-based text*, **p. 716.**

3. e

Tocophobia (fear of parturition) may be a reason for elective Caesarean section.

Reference: *Psychiatry: An evidence-based text*, **p. 716.**

4. e

The vermilion border is characteristically thin in fetal alcohol syndrome.

Reference: *Psychiatry: An evidence-based text*, **p. 717.**

5.

(i) c

(ii) a

(iii) d

(iv) b

Reference: *Psychiatry: An evidence-based text*, **pp. 716–717.**

6. d

They are not teratogenic, but a high proportion of the infants of narcotic addicts are of low birth weight, explained partly by prematurity and partly by intrauterine growth retardation. A withdrawal syndrome develops in most such babies.

Reference: *Psychiatry: An evidence-based text*, **p. 717.**

7. d

Reference: *Psychiatry: An evidence-based text*, **p. 718.**

8. b

Pregnancy has no effect on chronic delusional states and may have a beneficial effect on menstrual, bipolar and cycloid (acute polymorphic) psychoses.

Reference: *Psychiatry: An evidence-based text*, **pp. 718–721.**

9. e

Reference: *Psychiatry: An evidence-based text*, **p. 722.**

10. b

Infection is another relatively common important cause in the Western world.

Reference: *Psychiatry: An evidence-based text*, **p. 725.**

Chapter 45

Psychosexual medicine

QUESTIONS

Note that for answers to extended matching items (EMIs), each option (denoted a, b, c, etc.) might be used once, more than once or not at all. For multiple-choice questions (MCQs), please select the best answer.

1. **EMI** – Writers on sexuality
   (a) Alfred Kinsey
   (b) Henry Havelock Ellis
   (c) Shere Hite
   (d) Sigmund Freud
   (e) Von Krafft Ebing
   (f) Wilhelm Reich
   (g) William Masters and Virginia Johnson
   (h) None of the above

Select the authors, if any, from the above list who wrote each of the following works:
   (i) *Psychopathia Sexualis*
   (ii) *Three Essays on the Theory of Sexuality*
   (iii) *The Hite Report on Female Sexuality*
   (iv) *Human Sexual Inadequacy.*

2. **EMI** – Psychosexual researchers
   (a) Alfred Kinsey
   (b) Henry Havelock Ellis
   (c) Shere Hite
   (d) Wilhelm Reich
   (e) William Masters and Virginia Johnson
   (f) None of the above

Select the people, if any, from the above list who are best associated with each of the following methodologies in the field of psychosexual research:
   (i) Individualistic, large-scale, questionnaire-based research
   (ii) Direct observation of sexual acts in the laboratory, sometimes using 'assigned partners'
   (iii) Personal interview and filming of sexual acts, with a focus on counting the frequency of sexual events rather than focusing on the whole experience. Presented data that could probably not have been obtained without observation of child sexual abuse or through collaborations with child molesters.

3. **EMI** – Contributions to psychosexual medicine
   (a) Alfred Kinsey
   (b) Henry Havelock Ellis

   (c) Shere Hite
   (d) Von Krafft Ebing
   (e) Wilhelm Reich
   (f) William Masters and Virginia Johnson

Who from the above list is best associated with each of the following key contributions in the field of psychosexual medicine?
   (i) Elaborated the psychosomatic mechanisms connecting blocked sexual energy and neurosis, and developed a theory of character based on these blocks.
   (ii) Showed that around 70 per cent of women do not have orgasms through in–out thrusting intercourse but are able to achieve orgasm easily by masturbation or other direct clitoral stimulation.
   (iii) Coined the term 'necrophilia'.

4. **MCQ** – During which of the Masters and Johnson stages of female sexual arousal does the vagina lengthen and distend, with ballooning or tenting at the proximal end, and the uterus elevate?
   (a) Excitement
   (b) Orgasm
   (c) Plateau
   (d) Resolution
   (e) None of the above.

5. **MCQ** – Select one correct statement regarding the frequency of myotonic contractions of the pelvic floor during orgasm:
   (a) It is approximately the same in males and females and occurs at a rate of approximately one every 0.8 s.
   (b) It is approximately the same in males and females and occurs at a rate of approximately one every 2 s.
   (c) It is higher in males than in females.
   (d) It is lower in males than in females.
   (e) Male orgasm does not usually involve myotonic contractions of the pelvic floor.

6. **MCQ** – Which, if any, of the following is not a cause of erectile dysfunction?
   (a) Alprostadil

(b) Cardiovascular disease
(c) Diabetes mellitus
(d) Rectal cancer
(e) None of the above.

7. **MCQ** – Select one incorrect statement regarding PDE5 inhibitors used to treat erectile dysfunction:
   (a) They allow GMP to accumulate.
   (b) They are generally ineffective without sexual stimulation.
   (c) They increase penile blood flow.
   (d) They inhibit the action of phosphodiesterase type 5.
   (e) They promote smooth muscle relaxation.

8. **MCQ** – Select one incorrect statement regarding ejaculatory problems:
   (a) Men suffering from delayed ejaculation often come from families in which the showing of emotion was not encouraged.
   (b) The most common one is premature ejaculation.
   (c) The squeeze technique may help some men to delay orgasm.
   (d) The stop–start technique may help some men to delay orgasm.
   (e) They tend to have an organic cause.

9. **EMI** – Psychosexual medicine
   (a) Anorgasmia
   (b) Erectile dysfunction
   (c) Premature ejaculation
   (d) Vaginismus
   (e) None of the above

Select the option from the above list which is best associated with each of the following:
   (i) Often a transient problem in adolescence
   (ii) May result from treatment with SSRIs.
   (iii) Treatment with graded dilators may be helpful.

10. **EMI** – Psychosexual medicine
    (a) Bestiality
    (b) Erotophonia
    (c) Exhibitionism
    (d) Frotteurism
    (e) Sadomasochism
    (f) Voyeurism

Select the option from the above list with which each of the following is best associated:
   (i) Sexual arousal or activity where the infliction of pain, humiliation or bondage plays a key role.
   (ii) A disorder of sexual preference involving sexualized telephone calls to strangers.
   (iii) A consistent sexual drive towards watching others engaged in sexual activity, or in other intimate activities.

11. **EMI** – Writers on sexuality
    (a) Alfred Kinsey
    (b) Henry Havelock Ellis
    (c) Shere Hite
    (d) Sigmund Freud
    (e) Von Krafft Ebing
    (f) Wilhelm Reich
    (g) William Masters and Virginia Johnson
    (h) None of the above

Select the authors, if any, from the above list who wrote each of the following works:
   (i) *Human Sexual Response*
   (ii) *The Function of the Orgasm*
   (iii) *Sexual Behavior in the Human Female*
   (iv) *Studies in the Psychology of Sex.*

12. **EMI** – Psychosexual medicine
    (a) Alfred Kinsey
    (b) Henry Havelock Ellis
    (c) Shere Hite
    (d) Von Krafft Ebing
    (e) Sigmund Freud
    (f) William Masters and Virginia Johnson

Who from the above list is best associated with each of the following key contributions in the field of psychosexual medicine?
   (i) First statistical reports of childhood masturbation
   (ii) Developed a theory of childhood sexuality, including a stage model of psychosexual development
   (iii) Coined the term 'autoerotic'
   (iv) Coined the term 'masochism'.

13. **EMI** – Psychosexual medicine
    (a) Bestiality
    (b) Erotophonia
    (c) Exhibitionism
    (d) Frotteurism
    (e) Paedophilia
    (f) Sexual sadism
    (g) Voyeurism

Select the option from the above list with which each of the following is best associated:
   (i) The continual or repetitive desire to expose one's genitals to strangers, usually of the opposite gender, without seeking or desiring any further contact.
   (ii) A disorder of sexual preference involving pressing or rubbing oneself against the bodies of strangers in pursuit of sexual arousal.
   (iii) A disorder of sexual preference involving sexual activity with animals.

ANSWERS

1.

(i)   e – First published in 1886.
(ii) d – Published in 1905.
(iii) c – First published in 1976.
(iv) g – Published in 1970.

Reference: *Psychiatry: An evidence-based text*, **pp. 734–735.**

2.

(i)   c
(ii) e
(iii) a

Reference: *Psychiatry: An evidence-based text*, **pp. 734–735.**

3.

(i)   e
(ii) c
(iii) d

Reference: *Psychiatry: An evidence-based text*, **pp. 734–735.**

4. c

Also during this stage, the turgid cuff at the distal end of the vagina increases and the clitoris retracts.

Reference: *Psychiatry: An evidence-based text*, **p. 736.**

5. a

In both males and females the release of genital vasocongestion also occurs during orgasm.

Reference: *Psychiatry: An evidence-based text*, **p. 736.**

6. a

Alprostadil (prostaglandin E_1) may be used for treating erectile dysfunction; it is administered by intracavernosal injection or intraurethral application. (Its use as a treatment should only be considered after excluding treatable medical causes of the erectile dysfunction.) It may also be used as a diagnostic test.

Reference: *Psychiatry: An evidence-based text*, **pp. 743–744.**

7. a

They allow cyclic GMP to accumulate. This is illustrated in Figure 45.5 on page 744 of the accompanying textbook.

Reference: *Psychiatry: An evidence-based text*, **pp. 743–744.**

8. e

Ejaculatory problems are predominantly psychogenic, with only a minority being caused by organic disease.

Reference: *Psychiatry: An evidence-based text*, **pp. 744–745.**

9.

(i)   c
(ii) a
(iii) d

Reference: *Psychiatry: An evidence-based text*, **Ch. 45.**

10.

(i)   e – Sadism is arousal in association with inflicting pain, while masochism is arousal in association with having pain or humiliation inflicted. Affected individuals often feel arousal in both situations.
(ii) b
(iii) f – Other intimate activities, in this context, may include, for example, the victim undressing.

Reference: *Psychiatry: An evidence-based text*, **pp. 748–749.**

11.

(i)   g – Published in 1966.
(ii) f – Published in 1927.
(iii) a – Published in 1953.
(iv) b – This seven-volume work was published between 1897 and 1928.

Reference: *Psychiatry: An evidence-based text*, **pp. 734–735.**

12.

(i)   a
(ii) e
(iii) b
(iv) d

Reference: *Psychiatry: An evidence-based text*, **pp. 734–735.**

13.

(i)   c
(ii) d
(iii) a

Reference: *Psychiatry: An evidence-based text*, **pp. 748–749.**

Chapter 46

Gender identity disorders

QUESTIONS

Note that for answers to extended matching items (EMIs), each option (denoted a, b, c, etc.) might be used once, more than once or not at all. For multiple-choice questions (MCQs), please select the best answer.

1. **MCQ** – Which of the following is not classified as a disorder of gender identity in the ICD-10?
   (a) Autogynaephilia
   (b) Dual-role transvestism
   (c) Gender identity disorder of childhood
   (d) Transsexualism
   (e) Other gender identity disorders.

2. **EMI** – ICD-10 diagnoses and definitions
   (a) Dual-role transvestism
   (b) Egodystonic sexual orientation
   (c) Fetishistic transvestism
   (d) Gender identity disorder of childhood
   (e) Sexual maturation disorder
   (f) Transsexualism
   (g) None of the above

Select the option from the above list with which each of the following is best associated:
   (i) The individual suffers from uncertainty about his or her gender identity or sexual orientation, which causes anxiety or depression.
   (ii) The wearing of clothes of the opposite sex for part of the individual's existence in order to enjoy the temporary experience of membership of the opposite sex, but without any desire for a more permanent sex change or associated surgical reassignment. No sexual excitement accompanies the cross-dressing.
   (iii) A desire to live and be accepted as a member of the opposite sex, usually accompanied by a sense of discomfort with, or inappropriateness of, one's anatomical sex and a wish to have hormonal treatment and surgery to make one's body as congruent as possible with the preferred sex.

3. **MCQ** – Select one incorrect statement regarding the transsexual identity in the ICD-10 definition of transsexualism:
   (a) It must not be a symptom of another mental disorder, such as schizophrenia.
   (b) It must not be associated with any genetic abnormality.
   (c) It must not be associated with any intersex abnormality.
   (d) It must not be associated with any sex chromosome abnormality.
   (e) It should have been present persistently for at least 1 year.

4. **MCQ** – Select the best option. Which of the following are associated with regrets regarding gender reassignment surgery?
   (a) Lack of an earlier history of childhood gender identity disorder
   (b) Personality disorder
   (c) Poor family support
   (d) Poor support from friends
   (e) All of the above.

ANSWERS

1. a

In ICD-10, disorders of gender identity are classified as disorders of adult personality and behaviour. Autogynaephilia is the state of being sexually aroused by the idea of having both male and female sexual attributes.

Reference: *Psychiatry: An evidence-based text*, **pp. 754–755.**

2.

(i)   e – This is ICD-10 F66.0.
(ii) c – This is ICD-10 F64.2. That no sexual excitement accompanies the cross-dressing distinguishes this disorder from fetishistic transvestism (ICD-10 F65.1).
(iii) f – This is ICD-10 F64.0.

Reference: *Psychiatry: An evidence-based text*, **pp. 754–755.**

3. e

It should have been present persistently for at least 2 years.

Reference: *Psychiatry: An evidence-based text*, **p. 754.**

4. e

Reference: *Psychiatry: An evidence-based text*, **p. 758.**

Chapter 47

Paraphilias and sexual offenders

QUESTIONS

Note that for answers to extended matching items (EMIs), each option (denoted a, b, c, etc.) might be used once, more than once or not at all. For multiple-choice questions (MCQs), please select the best answer.

1. **MCQ** – Select one incorrect statement regarding the findings of Kinsey in *Sexual Behavior in the Human Male* (1948) and *Sexual Behavior in the Human Female* (1953):
   (a) Almost three-quarters of males had engaged in premarital sexual intercourse before the age of 20 years.
   (b) Around one-fifth of females had engaged in premarital sexual intercourse before the age of 20 years.
   (c) Around one-half of males had been unfaithful to their wives during marriage.
   (d) Females reached a sexual peak during their 30s.
   (e) Males reached a sexual peak during their mid-20s.

2. **EMI** – Paraphilias: Scott's analogy
   (a) Crash through by force
   (b) Peek over
   (c) Reach over and touch
   (d) Stand on the wall
   (e) Turn away
   (f) None of the above

Sexual behaviour is motivated by a desire for affection and a need to belong, and not merely by a desire for orgasm. A useful analogy by Scott relating to paraphilias is that of a barrier or wall resulting from anxiety in forming adult relationships. If the wall is too big, then the individual may engage in one of the above options. Select the option from the above list which is most closely associated with each of the following:
   (i) Indecent assault
   (ii) Voyeurism
   (iii) Fetishism.

3. **MCQ** – Select one incorrect statement regarding sexual disorders and paraphilias:
   (a) Androgen-insensitivity syndrome results in a male appearing female.
   (b) Between the ages of 1 and 5 years, gender role is established by cultural expectation whatever the genetic sex.

   (c) Congenital adrenal hyperplasia leads to increased levels of testosterone, resulting in a female appearing male.
   (d) Latent perversion represents a fixed, as opposed to regressed, deviation.
   (e) Paraphilias should be distinguished from facultative deviation resulting from the unavailability, usually transiently, of normal sexual contacts.

4. **MCQ** – Select one incorrect statement regarding human sexuality and its disorders:
   (a) Human fetuses do not masturbate.
   (b) Klinefelter's syndrome has been associated with psychosexual infantilism and paedophilia.
   (c) Paraphilias are often experienced as insistent, demanded and fixated.
   (d) Those with paraphilias often describe an inability to stop the paraphilic behaviour, unless someone externally intervenes, and also a feeling of altered consciousness at the time.
   (e) US students were experimentally conditioned to develop a foot fetish.

5. **EMI** – Transgenderism
   (a) Transsexualism
   (b) Transvestism
   (c) Neither of the above

Select the option from the above list which is best associated with each of the following:
   (i) In the toilet there is repulsion at one's own genitalia.
   (ii) Biological males use female communal toilets only when cross-dressing.
   (iii) If cross-dressing is stopped, then the individual becomes anxious; this is relieved by cross-dressing and by masturbation.

6. **EMI** – Classification of exhibitionism by Rooth
   (a) Type 1
   (b) Type 2
   (c) Both of the above approximately equally
   (d) Neither of the above

Select the option from the above classifications of exhibitionism that is most closely associated with each of the following features of exhibitionism:
- (i) The offender tends to expose a flaccid penis and does not masturbate.
- (ii) Accounts for about one-fifth of cases.
- (iii) The offender tends to feel anxious, guilty and humiliated because of it.

7. **MCQ** – Select one incorrect statement regarding sexual offenders:
- (a) Hebephilia refers to a sexual preference for prepubertal children or children under 13 years of age.
- (b) Most male rapists in the Western world are under 25 years of age, single and not mentally ill.
- (c) Rape is not confined to humans, with examples in nature including ducks, gorillas, scorpions and bees.
- (d) Recidivism in paedophilia is associated with early onset, offending against both sexes and deviant arousal to paedophile images on penile plethysmography.
- (e) To meet the DSM-IV-TR diagnostic criteria for paedophilia, the offender must be at least 16 years of age and at least 5 years older than the victim.

8. **EMI** – Paraphilias/disorders of sexual preference
- (a) Apotemnophilia
- (b) Asphyxiophilia
- (c) Biastophilia
- (d) Chrematistophilia
- (e) Hybristophilia
- (f) Infundibulation
- (g) Klismaphilia
- (h) Masochism
- (i) Narratophilia
- (j) Necrophilia
- (k) Sadism
- (l) Scataphilia
- (m) Scotophilia
- (n) Teledildonics
- (o) Zoophilia

Select the option from the above list that is most closely associated with each of the following objects of deviant sexual desire and/or preference:
- (i) Observing an unsuspecting person who is naked
- (ii) Rape
- (iii) Being an amputee
- (iv) Listening to accounts of sexual activity.

9. **EMI** – Paraphilias/disorders of sexual preference
- (a) Asphyxiophilia
- (b) Chrematistophilia
- (c) Hybristophilia
- (d) Infundibulation
- (e) Klismaphilia
- (f) Masochism
- (g) Necrophilia
- (h) Pygmalionism
- (i) Sadism
- (j) Scataphilia
- (k) Scotophilia
- (l) Urethralism
- (m) Urophilia
- (n) Vampirism
- (o) Teledildonics
- (p) Zoophilia

Select the option from the above list which is most closely associated with each of the following objects of deviant sexual desire and/or preference:
- (i) A person which has committed a crime
- (ii) Being robbed by the sexual partner
- (iii) Use of a noose around the neck (to enhance orgasm)
- (iv) Rectal enemas.

10. **MCQ** – Select one incorrect statement regarding serial killers in the Western world:
- (a) They tend to be aged 20–30 years.
- (b) They tend to be from lower socioeconomic groups.
- (c) They tend to be psychotic.
- (d) They tend to be white Caucasian.
- (e) They tend to have a history of using firearms and dramatic scenarios to express resentment and anger.

11. **MCQ** – Which of the following is not an instrument specifically for assessing risk in sex offenders?
- (a) RSVP
- (b) SARN
- (c) SNAP-20
- (d) STATIC-99
- (e) SVR-20.

12. **EMI** – Legislation relevant to sexual offenders in England and Wales
- (a) Crime and Disorder Act 1998
- (b) Crime (Sentences) Act 1997
- (c) Criminal Justice Act 1991
- (d) Criminal Justice Act 2003
- (e) Criminal Justice and Court Services Act 2000
- (f) Sex Offenders Act 1997

Select the Act from the above list that is most closely associated with each of the following:
- (i) This Act has placed a legal responsibility on the police and probation services to assess and manage those at risk of serious harm to others, including sex offenders, through MAPPAs.
- (ii) Under this Act, a defendant can face trial for a sexual offence even if the offence occurred abroad.
- (iii) This Act introduced 'indeterminate sentences for public protection' in respect of high-risk offenders, a measure equivalent to a life sentence.

13. **EMI** – Paraphilias: Scott's analogy

   (a) Crash through by force
   (b) Peek over
   (c) Reach over and touch
   (d) Stand on the wall
   (e) Turn away
   (f) None of the above

Select the option from the above list relating to Scott's 'wall' analogy for paraphilias (see Question 2) that is most closely associated with each of the following:

   (i)   Paedophilia
   (ii) Rape
   (iii) Exhibitionism
   (iv) Frotteurism.

ANSWERS

1. e

It was reached during late adolescence.

Reference: *Psychiatry: An evidence-based text*, **p. 761.**

2.

(i) c
(ii) b
(iii) e

Reference: *Psychiatry: An evidence-based text*, **p. 762.**

3. d

Latent perversion is generally well compensated for and becomes apparent only under stress, mental illnes (e.g. depression) and/or substance abuse. Latent perversion represents regressed, as opposed to a fixed, deviation.

Reference: *Psychiatry: An evidence-based text*, **p. 762.**

4. a

They have been observed engaging in such behaviour *in utero.*

Reference: *Psychiatry: An evidence-based text*, **pp. 762–764.**

5.

(i) a
(ii) b
(iii) b

Reference: *Psychiatry: An evidence-based text*, **p. 765.**

6.

(i) a
(ii) b
(iii) a

Reference: *Psychiatry: An evidence-based text*, **p. 766.**

7. a

It refers to a sexual preference for young people of adolescent age.

Reference: *Psychiatry: An evidence-based text*, **pp. 767–770.**

8.

(i) m
(ii) c – Also known as raptophilia.

(iii) a – It may lead to individuals, known as 'wannabes', disabling or injuring themselves.
(iv) i

Reference: *Psychiatry: An evidence-based text*, **pp. 771–772.**

9.

(i) c
(ii) b – Also applies to being charged or forced to pay for sexual intercourse.
(iii) a – Also known as autoerotic asphyxia or hypoxyphilia.
(iv) e

Reference: *Psychiatry: An evidence-based text*, **pp. 771–772.**

10. c

They tend to be non-psychotic.

Reference: *Psychiatry: An evidence-based text*, **p. 772.**

11. c

SNAP-20 = synaptosomal associated protein; RSVP = Risk of Sexual Violence Protocol; SARN = Sexual Assessment of Risk and Need; STATIC-99 = (static factors); SVR-20 = Sexual Violence Risk-20.

Reference: *Psychiatry: An evidence-based text*, **p. 774.**

12.

(i) e – Following the Criminal Justice and Court Services Act 2000, under Sections 67 and 68, a legal responsibility has been placed on the police and probation services to assess and manage those at risk of serious harm to others, including sex offenders, through MAPPAs (multi-agency public protection arrangements) which place a duty on psychiatrists to co-operate with this.
(ii) f
(iii) d

Reference: *Psychiatry: An evidence-based text*, **p. 776.**

13.

(i) e
(ii) a
(iii) d
(iv) c

Reference: *Psychiatry: An evidence-based text*, **p. 762.**

Chapter 48

Psychiatric assessment of physical illness

QUESTIONS

Note that for answers to extended matching items (EMIs), each option (denoted a, b, c, etc.) might be used once, more than once or not at all. For multiple-choice questions (MCQs), please select the best answer.

1. **EMI** – Blood test results
   (a) Addison's disease
   (b) Dehydration
   (c) Excessive alcohol intake
   (d) Hepatocellular disease
   (e) Renal failure
   (f) None of the above

   Select the option from the above list that is most closely associated with each of the following sets of laboratory blood test results:
   (i) $\uparrow K^+$, $\downarrow Na^+$.
   (ii) $\uparrow$ γ-glutamyltransferase (γGT), $\uparrow$ mean corpuscular volume (MCV).
   (iii) $\uparrow$ aspartate aminotransferase (AST), $\uparrow$ bilirubin.
   (iv) $\uparrow$ albumin, $\uparrow$ haematocrit, $\uparrow$ urea, $\uparrow$ creatinine.

2. **MCQ** – Select one incorrect statement regarding aspects of history-taking to be borne in mind when interviewing a patient with a physical illness:
   (a) A tactful enquiry about childhood abuse should be made; childhood sexual abuse is a predisposing factor for several psychiatric disorders in adult life, including the functional somatic syndromes that are commonly seen in medical practice.
   (b) For patients with visual impairment, the interviewer should avoid sitting with a source of light behind them; the source of light should be on the interviewer's face.
   (c) Frequent attendance at a GP's surgery for minor or unexplained symptoms raises the possibility of a somatization syndrome.
   (d) Post-traumatic stress disorder is most likely as a response to medical illness.
   (e) Speech is impossible for patients who are being treated in an intensive care (ICU) or high-dependency unit (HDU) and who are being ventilated via endotracheal intubation; only a limited assessment can be undertaken, and it is necessary to used closed rather than open-ended questions, with printed cards usefully giving the patient the opportunity to give affirmative and negative answers.

3. **MCQ** – The development of psychotic symptoms in an adult during the course of a medical illness is most likely to indicate the onset of which of the following?
   (a) Delirium
   (b) Depression
   (c) Mania
   (d) Post-traumatic stress disorder
   (e) Schizophrenia.

4. **MCQ** – Select one incorrect statement regarding mental capacity in relation to a treatment decision a patient is required to make, under the law in England and Wales:
   (a) In most cases in medical practice, lack of capacity results from cognitive impairment.
   (b) Lack of capacity exists if patients are unable to communicate a decision.
   (c) Lack of capacity exists if patients are unable to retain the information given to them.
   (d) Lack of capacity exists if patients are unable to understand information relevant to the decision.
   (e) The law assumes that people have the capacity to make decisions about their own treatment unless refusing treatment may lead to permanent damage and premature death.

5. **EMI** – Questions in the assessment of medically ill patients
   (a) AUDIT
   (b) BDI
   (c) BMI
   (d) CAGE
   (e) GCHQ
   (f) GHQ
   (g) HADS
   (h) MMSE
   (i) PANSS

(j) SANS

(k) SAPS

(l) VNR

(m) None of the above

Select the option from the above list with which each of the following is best associated:

(i) A 21-item depression questionnaire which has been widely used with medical patients. It contains somatic questions and so it could lead to false-positive results.

(ii) This brief screening test is used to detect severely affected problem drinkers. It asks four questions.

(iii) Suitable for the detection of hazardous drinking.

ANSWERS

1.

(i)   a

(ii) c – These results may be the first indicators of hazardous alcohol consumption. The blood alcohol level may be raised before lunch. With increasingly high intake of alcohol, there will be increasing evidence of hepatocellular disease.

(iii) d

(iv) b – These results are consistent with dehydration; further evidence can be gleaned by physical examination and by measuring the urine output (which will be reduced).

References: Longmore M, Wilkinson I, Török E (2001) *Oxford Handbook of Clinical Medicine*, 5th edn. Oxford: Oxford University Press, **pp. 678–679**; *Psychiatry: An evidence-based text*, **p. 779**.

2. d

It is most likely to be diagnosed in patients admitted following road traffic and other major accidents and following serious assault.

Reference: *Psychiatry: An evidence-based text*, **pp. 780–781**.

3. a

Visual or tactile hallucinations are the most common sensory disturbances. Secondary delusions may be superimposed on these false perceptions. The level of consciousness is impaired, but the symptoms fluctuate, and so a history from nursing staff is essential to chart the course of the delirium.

Reference: *Psychiatry: An evidence-based text*, **pp. 781, 785**.

4. e

The law assumes that people have the capacity to make decisions about their own treatment, even if refusing treatment may lead to permanent damage and premature death.

Reference: *Psychiatry: An evidence-based text*, **p. 785**.

5.

(i)   b – The BDI (Beck Depression Inventory) was one of the earliest structured questionnaires.

(ii) d – It does not detect hazardous drinking and can seem too confrontational for use with this group.

(iii) a – The AUDIT (Alcohol Use Disorders Inventory) is more suitable than the CAGE questionnaire for the detection of hazardous drinking.

Reference: *Psychiatry: An evidence-based text*, **p. 786**.

Part 4 : Mental health problems and mental illness

Chapter 49

Overlapping multi-system, multi-organ illnesses/syndromes

QUESTIONS

Note that for answers to extended matching items (EMIs), each option (denoted a, b, c, etc.) might be used once, more than once or not at all. For multiple-choice questions (MCQs), please select the best answer.

1. **MCQ** – Select the best correct option. Which of the following is correct regarding Gulf War illness?
   (a) It is causally associated with exposure to organophosphate pesticides.
   (b) It is causally associated with pyridostigmine bromide given prophylactically to protect against soman.
   (c) There are changes in normalized blood flow to deep brain structures.
   (d) Differential pathology has been reported in neutrophils (mainly necrotic).
   (e) All of the above.

2. **MCQ** – Select the best correct option. Historically, which of the following has been attributed to somatization as an explanation of previously 'unexplained' symptoms?
   (a) Diabetes mellitus
   (b) Graves' disease
   (c) Multiple sclerosis
   (d) Parkinson's disease
   (e) All of the above.

ANSWERS

1. e

Reference: *Psychiatry: An evidence-based text*, **pp. 788–791.**

2. e

Somatization could be said to have a poor track record, having been offered as an explanation of all these medical conditions in the past.

Reference: *Psychiatry: An evidence-based text*, **pp. 790, 798.**

Chapter 50

Multiple chemical sensitivity

QUESTIONS

Note that for answers to extended matching items (EMIs), each option (denoted a, b, c, etc.) might be used once, more than once or not at all. For multiple-choice questions (MCQs), please select the best answer.

1. **MCQ** – For which of the following chemicals does ICD-10 not have a specific code?
   (a) Disinfectants
   (b) Halogenated insecticides
   (c) Herbicides
   (d) Organophosphate insecticides
   (e) Rodenticides.

2. **MCQ** – Select one incorrect statement regarding multiple chemical sensitivity:
   (a) American studies suggest that up to around one-third of people are sensitive to everyday chemicals.
   (b) In the USA it is more common in lower socioeconomic groups.
   (c) In the USA it is more common in women than in men.
   (d) It is associated with impaired cardiac function.
   (e) It is associated with neurocognitive deficits.

3. **EMI** – Multiple chemical sensitivity
   (a) Heavy metals (mercury, lead, cadmium, arsenic, organometallics, tributyltin)
   (b) Highly substituted, poly- or per-halogenated organic compounds with chlorine, bromine or fluorine (e.g. DDT, DDE, lindane, hexachlorobenzene, hexachlorocyclohexanes, PCBs, aldrin, dieldrin, PBDEs, perfluoro-octanoic acid polymers and derivatives)
   (c) Organophosphates, nerve agents
   (d) PAHs
   (e) Phthalates, nonylphenol, bisphenol A and B
   (f) VOCs, aliphatic and aromatic compounds, formaldehyde, aldehydes, esters, ketones, toluene
   (g) None of the above

Select the chemical class, if any, from the above list which is most closely associated with each of the following sets of known biological activities:
   (i)   Nerve toxins
   (ii) Disruption of brain function, nerve damage, carcinogenic

   (iii) Carcinogenic, mutagenic, kidney and liver damage, endocrine disruption.

4. **EMI** – Multiple chemical sensitivity
   (a) Heavy metals (mercury, lead, cadmium, arsenic, organometallics, tributyltin)
   (b) Highly substituted, poly- or per-halogenated organic compounds with chlorine, bromine or fluorine (e.g. DDT, DDE, lindane, hexachlorobenzene, hexachlorocyclohexanes, PCBs, aldrin, dieldrin, PBDEs, perfluoro-octanoic acid polymers and derivatives)
   (c) Organophosphates, nerve agents
   (d) PAHs
   (e) Phthalates, nonylphenol, bisphenol A and B
   (f) VOCs, aliphatic and aromatic compounds, formaldehyde, aldehydes, esters, ketones, toluene
   (g) None of the above

Select the chemical class, if any, from the above list which is most closely associated, as a cause of multiple chemical sensitivity, with each of the following sets of common sources or uses:
   (i)   Flame-retardants
   (ii) Burning fuels
   (iii) Fragrances and perfumes
   (iv) Exhaust fumes
   (v)   Non-stick kitchen utensils.

5. **MCQ** – Which of the following molecules is the most important cause of hepatocellular toxicity in paracetamol overdose?
   (a) Acetaminophen
   (b) Glucuronide metabolite
   (c) Quinoneimine metabolite
   (d) Sulphate (sulfate) metabolite
   (e) None of the above.

6. **EMI** – Multiple chemical sensitivity
   (a) Diethylstilboestrol
   (b) Methoxychlor
   (c) Paraquat
   (d) Phthalates

(e) Tributyltin

(f) None of the above

Select the chemical from the above list exposure to which is most closely associated with each of the following diseases:

(i) Vaginal adenocarcinoma

(ii) Cervical adenocarcinoma

(iii) Early-onset parkinsonism.

7. **MCQ** – Select one incorrect statement regarding the NO/ONOO hypothesis:

(a) Nitric oxide and water combine to form ONOO, which is a very potent oxidizing molecule.

(b) Oxidative stress and superoxide stimulate VR1.

(c) Prior brain injury or damage followed by a modest systemic infection leads to a massive inflammatory response in the central nervous system in experimental animals.

(d) The vanilloid receptor and NO evoke stimulation of excitatory NMDA glutamate receptors.

(e) VR1 is a promiscuous chemoreceptor found on C-nerve fibres.

8. **EMI** – Developmental effects of environmental exposures

(a) Anophthalmia

(b) Attention deficit hyperactivity disorder

(c) Learning and development disabilities

(d) Obesity

(e) Schizophrenia

Select the condition from the above list that is most closely associated with exposure to each of the following:

(i) Food colorants

(ii) Benlate (a fungicide, withdrawn from the market in 2001)

(iii) Phthalates.

ANSWERS

1. a

ICD-10 does not have specific codes for disinfectants.

Reference: Psychiatry: An evidence-based text, **p. 795.**

2. b

Reference: Psychiatry: An evidence-based text, **pp. 795–796.**

3.

(i)   c
(ii) f
(iii) b

Reference: Psychiatry: An evidence-based text, **p. 797.**

4.

(i)   b
(ii) d – PAHs are polyaromatic hydrocarbons
(iii) f
(iv) d
(v)   b

Reference: Psychiatry: An evidence-based text, **p. 797.**

5. c

N-acetyl-*p*-benzoquinoneimine is a highly reactive metabolite which can be formed once the metabolic pathways of paracetamol (acetaminophen) by conjugation with sulphate (sulfate) or glucuronyl groups have become exhausted, as may occur following overdose.

Reference: Psychiatry: An evidence-based text, **p. 805.**

6.

(i)   a – An increased incidence has been reported in the daughters of mothers who took diethylstilboestrol during the first trimester.
(ii) a – As in (i).
(iii) c – This herbicide is also associated with pulmonary injury. Its reduction is coupled with formation of toxic reaction oxygen species (ROS).

Reference: Psychiatry: An evidence-based text, **p. 806.**

7. a

Nitric oxide and superoxide combine to form ONOO (peroxynitrite), which is indeed a very potent oxidizing molecule.

Reference: Psychiatry: An evidence-based text, **p. 807.**

8.

(i)   b
(ii) a – A ruling by the USA high court awarded damages to John Castillo who was born without eyes, following his mother's exposure to benlate on a single day when she was accidentally sprayed with the fungicide while 6–7 weeks' pregnant with John. A rat study showed that benlate is concentrated in the eyes.
(iii) d – The phthalates were banned in some countries from 1977, but in the USA the toy industry launched strong resistance to a ban in America. A positive association has been reported between urinary phthalate metabolites and adult male obesity (aged 20–59 years).

Reference: Psychiatry: An evidence-based text, **pp. 810–813.**

Chapter 51

Mental health problems in patients with myalgic encephalomyelitis

QUESTIONS

For multiple-choice questions (MCQs), please select the best answer.

1. **MCQ** – Select one incorrect statement regarding myalgic encephalomyelitis (ME):
   (a) Between 1934 and 2010 fewer than 10 ME-type epidemics occurred worldwide.
   (b) In 1934 there was a major ME-like epidemic in Los Angeles.
   (c) The Nightingale Research Foundation study of around 2000 sufferers during 1984–1992 found that nurses and physicians comprised one of the highest proportions of sufferers by occupation.
   (d) The Nightingale Research Foundation study of around 2000 sufferers during 1984–1992 showed a marked fall in the number of cases of female sufferers from the time of menopause.
   (e) The Nightingale Research Foundation study of around 2000 sufferers during 1984–1992 showed a marked increase in the number of cases of female sufferers compared with males from the time of puberty.

2. **MCQ** – Select one correct statement. Which of the following was the trigger most frequently ascribed by patients as a possible cause of their present illness in the Nightingale Research Foundation study of around 2000 sufferers during 1984–1992?
   (a) Foreign travel
   (b) Immunization
   (c) Post-infection
   (d) Post-surgery
   (e) Post-trauma.

ANSWERS

1. a

During this period there have been at least 70 such epidemics around the world. Note that the occurrence of the words 'The Nightingale Research Foundation study of around 2000 sufferers during 1984–1992' in more than one of the options means that clearly such a study has indeed taken place. Also, options 'e' and 'd' are consistent with each other, making it less likely that either of these is incorrect.

Option 'c' is consistent with an infectious nature to the aetiology of ME.

Reference: *Psychiatry: An evidence-based text*, **pp. 821–823.**

2. c

As shown in Figure 51.5 on page 824 of the accompanying textbook, this was by far the most common cause (53 per cent).

Reference: *Psychiatry: An evidence-based text*, **p. 824.**

Chapter 52

Pain and psychiatry

QUESTIONS

Note that for answers to extended matching items (EMIs), each option (denoted a, b, c, etc.) might be used once, more than once or not at all. For multiple-choice questions (MCQs), please select the best answer.

1. **EMI** – Historical developments in the field of pain
   (a) Breuer and Freud
   (b) Descartes
   (c) Engel
   (d) Melzack and Wall
   (e) Stengel
   (f) None of the above

From the above list, select the people with whom each of the following historical developments is best associated:
   (i) Believed that, although pain may originally develop from an external source, it often becomes a psychological phenomenon. Described risk factors for developing chronic pain, including a history of defeat, significant guilt, unsatisfied aggressive impulses and a history of real or imagined loss
   (ii) The gate theory
   (iii) Wrote *Meditations on First Philosophy* and showed that the experience of pain depends upon the integrity of the sensory nerve pathway from the periphery to the brain.

2. **EMI** – Mechanisms for experiencing pain
   (a) Delusional pain
   (b) Dissociative conditions
   (c) Exaggeration of an existing trivial painful condition
   (d) Fear of pain
   (e) Hypochondriacal disorder
   (f) Identification with the sufferer
   (g) Pain arising because of muscle tension, which may be concerned directly with worries about pain
   (h) Painful conditions of debatable origin because of difficulty in diagnosis
   (i) Undiagnosed medical condition

From the above list of conditions, select the option with which each of the following mechanisms by which pain is experienced despite apparent insufficient sensory stimuli is best associated:

   (i) The disease may be at an early stage or the biochemical or radiological markers may not show abnormality.
   (ii) Patients believe that they have a serious or progressive physical disorder that persists despite negative investigations and reassurance; this may occur in patients who have previously experienced an organic pain but who have had apparently successful treatment.
   (iii) This is frequent and occurs in people who are worried about what the pain means and its impact; these individuals tend to have a low pain threshold.

3. **MCQ** – Which of the following is the commonest associated psychiatric diagnosis found in patients with chronic pain?
   (a) Depression
   (b) Panic disorder
   (c) Personality disorder
   (d) Phobia
   (e) Stress disorder.

4. **MCQ** – Of the following, which is least likely to be a risk factor for suicide in patients with chronic pain?
   (a) Comfort eating
   (b) Desire for escape from pain
   (c) Hopelessness about pain
   (d) Pain catastrophizing
   (e) Sleep-onset insomnia co-occurring with pain.

5. **MCQ** – Select one incorrect statement regarding pain and psychiatry:
   (a) In a World Health Organization survey, people with back and neck pain were over 2.5 times more likely to have generalized anxiety disorder than controls without such pain.
   (b) It is frequently found that people with chronic pain have relatives with a similar condition.
   (c) Serotonin and noradrenaline reuptake inhibitors

are more effective than selective serotonin reuptake inhibitors (SSRIs) in reducing neuropathic pain.

(d) Spinal cord dorsal horn G cells are activated by branches from large myelinated fibres concerned with touch and proprioception and are inhibited by the action of C fibres.

(e) The pain sensitivity of patients with panic disorder is significantly higher than that of controls, and patients with chronic painful conditions are more likely than average to have panic.

6. **MCQ** – Which of the following treatments for post-traumatic stress disorder has not been shown to be effective?

(a) Amitriptyline

(b) Cognitive-behaviour therapy

(c) Debriefing

(d) Eye movement desensitization and reprocessing (EMDR)

(e) Mirtazapine.

7. **MCQ** – Select one incorrect statement regarding pain and psychiatry:

(a) Cognitive-behaviour therapy has been shown to be of definite value in patients with persistent somatoform pain disorder who have reached the stage of accepting that medical or surgical interventions are not indicated.

(b) Most people encountered in clinical practice with factitious disorder are healthcare professionals, with a considerable female preponderance.

(c) Personality disorders, particularly of the passive-dependent and histrionic types, are considerably overrepresented among patients with somatization disorder compared with control subjects with anxiety and depression.

(d) SSRIs are more effective than amitriptyline in the treatment of persistent somatoform pain disorder.

(e) There is a higher rate of alcohol and analgesic misuse in patients with chronic pain.

ANSWERS

1.

(i) c

(ii) d – A circuit diagram of the gate-control theory of pain perception proposed by Melzack and Wall in 1965 is shown in Figure 52.1 on page 836 of the accompanying textbook.

(iii) b – This book (*Meditations Touchant la Première Philosophie*) was published in the 1640s.

Reference: *Psychiatry: An evidence-based text*, **pp. 835–836.**

2.

(i) i

(ii) e

(iii) c

Reference: *Psychiatry: An evidence-based text*, **p. 837.**

3. a

According to standard psychiatric schedules, depressive illness is the most common associated psychiatric disorder found in patients with chronic pain. Between 20 and 50 per cent of patients attending chronic pain clinics fulfil the criteria for this diagnosis.

Reference: *Psychiatry: An evidence-based text*, **pp. 838–839.**

4. a

Reference: *Psychiatry: An evidence-based text*, **p. 838.**

5. e

The pain sensitivity of patients with panic disorder has been reported to be no different from that of controls.

Reference: *Psychiatry: An evidence-based text*, **pp. 836–839.**

6. c

Psychological debriefing and superficial treatments of this type are not valuable and have been found to worsen the prognosis in patients with more intense symptoms. Mayou *et al.* (2000) conducted a 3-year follow-up of a randomized controlled trial of psychological debriefing for road traffic accident victims, having previously concluded that at 4 months it was ineffective. The intervention group had a significantly worse outcome at 3 years in terms of general psychiatric symptoms, travel anxiety when being a passenger, pain, physical problems, overall level of functioning and financial problems. Patients who initially had high intrusion and avoidance symptoms remained symptomatic if they had received the intervention, but recovered if they did not receive the intervention. Thus, in such patients, psychological debriefing appears to be ineffective and has adverse long-term effects.

References: Mayou RA, Ehlers A, Hobbs M (2000) Psychological debriefing for road traffic accident victims. Three-year follow-up of a randomised controlled trial. *British Journal of Psychiatry* **176: 589–93;** *Psychiatry: An evidence-based text*, **p. 839.**

7. d

There are two established treatments for persistent somatoform pain disorder, namely antidepressants and cognitive-behaviour therapy. Antidepressants that inhibit both serotonin and noradrenaline uptake, such as amitriptyline and venlafaxine, are more effective than the SSRIs.

Reference: *Psychiatry: An evidence-based text*, **pp. 840–841.**

Chapter 53

Sleep disorders

QUESTIONS

Note that for answers to extended matching items (EMIs), each option (denoted a, b, c, etc.) might be used once, more than once or not at all. For multiple-choice questions (MCQs), please select the best answer.

1. **MCQ** – Select one incorrect statement. The multiple sleep latency test:
   (a) Involves asking the subject to try to fall asleep in a darkened room four times during the day
   (b) Is an objective test of daytime sleepiness
   (c) Requires ECG
   (d) Requires EEG
   (e) Requires EMG.

2. **MCQ** – Select the best correct option. Which of the following drugs has a hypnotic action related to direct gamma-aminobutyric acid-A (GABA$_A$) receptor action?
   (a) Eszopiclone
   (b) Indiplon
   (c) Nitrazepam
   (d) Zolpidem
   (e) All of the above.

3. **EMI** – Sleep disorders
   (a) Antidepressants
   (b) Antipsychotics
   (c) Lithium
   (d) None of the above

From the above list select the option with which each of the following is best associated:
   (i) ↑ total sleep time
   (ii) ↓ sleep latency
   (iii) ↑ sleep latency
   (iv) ↓ stage 1 NREM sleep.

4. **MCQ** – Select the best correct option regarding the effects of cholinesterase inhibitors on sleep:
   (a) They increase the duration of REM sleep
   (b) They often cause insomnia
   (c) They often cause intense dreams
   (d) They often cause nightmares
   (e) All of the above.

5. **EMI** – Effects of social and 'recreational' drugs
   (a) Alcohol
   (b) Amphetamine
   (c) Caffeine
   (d) Cannabinoid
   (e) Nicotine

From the above list of social and 'recreational' drugs, select the option with which each of the following is best associated:
   (i) Has a similar effect on GABA receptors as the hypnotics, but it also has its own receptor and acts as a glutamate inhibitor. Low doses increase sleep time, reduce sleep latency, reduce latency before stages 3 and 4 of NREM sleep, and suppress REM sleep
   (ii) Acts as an antagonist at adenosine receptors and tends to increase wakefulness
   (iii) Increases activity at dopamine, noradrenaline and 5-HT synapses, particularly in the brainstem and cerebral cortex. Has an alerting effect, reduces total sleep time and reduces the duration of stages 3 and 4 of NREM sleep and of REM sleep.

6. **MCQ** – Select one incorrect statement regarding sleepiness:
   (a) In children, excessive daytime sleepiness often leads to poor school performance and impaired concentration, which may be interpreted as attention-deficit hyperactivity disorder.
   (b) It is associated with deterioration in physical performance, particularly for prolonged or monotonous tasks, with a sense of fatigue and even episodes of automatic behaviour, in which inappropriate actions are carried out with reduced vigilance and subsequent amnesia.
   (c) Pre-accident driving behaviour tends to include maintaining almost constant speed owing to automatic-pilot driving.
   (d) Sleep-related driving accidents occur particularly between 2 am and 6 am.
   (e) Sleep-related driving accidents occur particularly between 2 pm and 4 pm.

7. **EMI** – Sleep disorders
   (a) Antidepressants
   (b) First-generation antipsychotics
   (c) Lithium salts

From the above list select the option with which each of the following is most consistently associated:
   (i) Do not significantly increase REM sleep latency
   (ii) Increase REM sleep
   (iii) Reduce REM sleep.

8. **EMI** – Effects of social and 'recreational' drugs
   (a) Alcohol
   (b) Amphetamine
   (c) Caffeine
   (d) Cannabinoid
   (e) Cocaine
   (f) Nicotine
   (g) None of the above

From the above list of drugs, select the option with which each of the following is best associated:
   (i) It reduces total sleep time, increases the sleep latency and reduces the duration of stages 3 and 4 of NREM sleep and of REM sleep. It commonly causes insomnia if taken in large doses.
   (ii) After large doses, stages 3 and 4 of NREM sleep are reduced. Chronic intake can severely disrupt the sleep–wake cycle, and even after stopping regular use abnormal sleep architecture often persists for a prolonged period.
   (iii) Acts at cholinergic receptors. In low doses it is excitatory, but in high doses it is inhibitory. It appears to reduce the total sleep time, increase sleep latency and reduce the duration of REM sleep in higher doses.

9. **MCQ** – Select one incorrect statement regarding narcolepsy:
   (a) Lack of functioning of orexin-producing neurones in the perifornical hypothalamus appears to be a common factor in classical narcolepsy.
   (b) Nocturnal sleep tends to occur without awakenings.
   (c) The intensity of dream mentation is increased, with hypnagogic and hypnopompic hallucinations and vivid dreams at night.
   (d) The physiological loss of muscle tone in REM sleep is manifested as cataplexy, a loss of muscle tone in response to sudden or intense emotion, usually laughter.
   (e) The physiological loss of muscle tone in REM sleep is manifested as sleep paralysis, often at the onset of sleep.

10. **EMI** – Sleep disorders
   (a) Dexamphetamine
   (b) First-generation antipsychotic
   (c) Modafinil
   (d) Second-generation antipsychotic

   (e) Sodium oxybate
   (f) None of the above

From the above list select the most appropriate treatment option for each of the following:
   (i) First-line drug treatment for excessive daytime sleepiness
   (ii) Second-line drug treatment for excessive daytime sleepiness
   (iii) Drug treatment for cataplexy that does not respond to venlafaxine.

11. **MCQ** – Which of the following is characteristically seen in idiopathic hypersomnia?
   (a) Cataplexy
   (b) Frequent nocturnal awakenings
   (c) Hypnagogic hallucinations
   (d) Sleep paralysis
   (e) None of the above.

12. **MCQ** – Select one incorrect statement regarding insomnia:
   (a) It is associated with a faster cardiac rate during all stages of sleep.
   (b) It is associated with a higher delta power on the EEG during sleep.
   (c) It is associated with intrusion of alpha waves on the EEG.
   (d) It is more common in females and in older people.
   (e) It is the most common sleep disorder, and at any one time 10–15 per cent of the population is affected.

13. **EMI** – Clinical types of primary insomnia
   (a) Anxiety states
   (b) Chronic fatigue syndrome (myalgic encephalomyelitis)
   (c) Psychophysiological (conditioned) insomnia
   (d) Sleep state misperception

From the above list of clinical types of primary insomnia, select the option with which each of the following is best associated:
   (i) There is often hypersomnia initially, followed by a prolonged period of insomnia, which is usually related to poor sleep hygiene associated with anxiety about obtaining sufficient sleep.
   (ii) An apprehensive concern about difficulties in sleeping, which perpetuates insomnia. The sleep difficulty may become a major concern during wakefulness.
   (iii) Often associated with poor sleep at night and waking with panic attacks.

14. **EMI** – Sleep control in depression
   (a) Strong
   (b) Weak
   (c) Neither of the above

From the above list select the option which best describes the change, if any, of each of the following aspects of sleep control in depression:

(i) REM sleep drive
(ii) NREM sleep drive.

15. **EMI** – Sleep control in depression
    (a) Increased
    (b) Decreased
    (c) Neither of the above

From the above list select the option that best describes the change, if any, of each of the following aspects of sleep control in depression:
    (i)   REM sleep latency
    (ii) Stages 3 and 4 NREM sleep
    (iii) REM sleep
    (iv) Total sleep time.

16. **EMI** – Sleep in depression
    (a) Increased/elevated
    (b) Decreased
    (c) Neither of the above

From the above list select the option that best describes the change, if any, of each of the following aspects of sleep in depression:
    (i)   Effect on mood of sleep deprivation
    (ii) Effect on the drive to NREM of sleep deprivation
    (iii) Effect on the duration of REM sleep of sleep deprivation
    (iv) Effect on the duration of REM sleep of most antidepressant drugs.

17. **MCQ** – Select one incorrect statement regarding post-traumatic stress disorder and sleep:
    (a) As with usual nightmares, the associated nightmares arise from stages 1 and 2 of NREM sleep as well as from REM sleep.
    (b) The associated nightmares and motor abnormalities often respond to prazosin.
    (c) The associated nightmares occur especially between midnight and 3 am.
    (d) The content of the associated nightmares tends to relate to the precipitating event, although it may be generalized and hardly recognizable.
    (e) There tends to be a hyperarousal state both while awake and while asleep.

18. **MCQ** – Select one incorrect statement regarding sleep in dementia, particularly Alzheimer's disease:
    (a) Sundowning is a problem particularly with Alzheimer's disease.
    (b) The duration of stage 3 of NREM sleep tends to be shortened.

(c) The duration of stage 4 of NREM sleep tends to be shortened.
(d) The normal sleep architecture tends to be maintained.
(e) There tends to be an increase in REM sleep latency and a shorter duration of REM sleep.

19. **MCQ** – Select the best option. Which of the following is not an NREM sleep disorder?
    (a) Sexual activity in sleep
    (b) Sleep-eating
    (c) Sleep terrors
    (d) Sleeptalking
    (e) None of the above (i.e. they are all NREM sleep disorders).

20. **MCQ** – Select one incorrect statement regarding REM sleep behaviour disorder:
    (a) Clonazepam is usually effective.
    (b) Melatonin is usually effective.
    (c) It is characterized by dreams with an aggressive content.
    (d) It usually occurs in young adults.
    (e) There is usually retention of muscle tone during REM sleep.

21. **MCQ** – Which of the following is least likely to be an effective treatment of Ekbom's syndrome?
    (a) Clonazepam
    (b) Gabapentin
    (c) Oxycodone
    (d) Paroxetine
    (e) Ropinirole.

22. **MCQ** – Which of the following is least likely to be a cause of restless legs syndrome?
    (a) Familial
    (b) Iron overload
    (c) Lithium
    (d) Pregnancy
    (e) Renal failure.

23. **EMI** – Types of dream
    (a) NREM sleep dreams
    (b) REM sleep dreams

From the above list select the type of dream with which each of the following is better associated.
    (i)   Involve problem-solving
    (ii) More emotional content
    (iii) Simpler content.

ANSWERS

1. c

The ECG (electrocardiogram) will not give signals that allow you to assess whether the subject is awake or asleep. Instead, EOG (electro-oculography) signals are required.

Reference: *Psychiatry: An evidence-based text*, **p. 845.**

2. e

Reference: *Psychiatry: An evidence-based text*, **p. 845.**

3.

(i) b
(ii) b
(iii) d
(iv) d

Reference: *Psychiatry: An evidence-based text*, **p. 846.**

4. e

Reference: *Psychiatry: An evidence-based text*, **p. 846.**

5.

(i) a
(ii) c
(iii) b

Reference: *Psychiatry: An evidence-based text*, **p. 846.**

6. c

Pre-accident behaviour includes fluctuating vehicle speed owing to intermittent loss of muscle activity in the leg controlling the accelerator at the transition into sleep, shunting accidents at traffic lights and roundabouts, and weaving from lane to lane. At the time of the accident, there is often no evidence of braking or having taken avoiding action.

Reference: *Psychiatry: An evidence-based text*, **pp. 846–847.**

7.

(i) b
(ii) a – Note that the effects of antipsychotics on REM sleep are variable; the question uses the words 'most consistently' and so the correct answer here is 'a'. This also applies to part (iii) of this question.
(iii) c

Reference: *Psychiatry: An evidence-based text*, **p. 846.**

8.

(i) c
(ii) a – Large intakes of alcohol can also have a diuretic effect which can cause awakenings from sleep.
(iii) f

Reference: *Psychiatry: An evidence-based text*, **p. 846.**

9. b

In narcolepsy, sleep itself is destabilized, with frequent nocturnal awakenings.

Reference: *Psychiatry: An evidence-based text*, **p. 847.**

10.

(i) c
(ii) a – An alternative is methylphenidate.
(iii) e

Reference: *Psychiatry: An evidence-based text*, **p. 848.**

11. e

This condition usually affects young adults and is characterized by prolonged unrefreshing sleep, difficulty in waking in the mornings, and prolonged unrefreshing naps. None of the other features of narcolepsy are present.

Reference: *Psychiatry: An evidence-based text*, **p. 848.**

12. b

Reference: *Psychiatry: An evidence-based text*, **p. 848.**

13.

(i) b – The poor sleep hygiene is secondary to the fatigue.
(ii) c
(iii) a

Reference: *Psychiatry: An evidence-based text*, **pp. 848–849.**

14.

(i) a – This and the other answers are illustrated in Figure 53.1 on page 849 of the accompanying textbook.
(ii) b

Reference: *Psychiatry: An evidence-based text*, **p. 849.**

15.

(i) b – This and the other answers are illustrated in Figure 53.1 on page 849 of the accompanying textbook.
(ii) b
(iii) a
(iv) b

Reference: *Psychiatry: An evidence-based text*, **p. 849.**

16.

(i) a – Sleep deprivation may elevate the mood in depression, and indeed may even lead to mania in bipolar disorder.

(ii) a

(iii) b – This is particularly the case if sleep is lost during the latter part of the night.

(iv) b

Reference: Psychiatry: An evidence-based text, **p. 849.**

17. a

Reference: Psychiatry: An evidence-based text, **p. 849.**

18. d

The normal sleep architecture disintegrates, with loss of sleep cycles of NREM and REM sleep.

Reference: Psychiatry: An evidence-based text, **pp. 849–850.**

19. e

Reference: Psychiatry: An evidence-based text, **p. 850.**

20. d

It typically occurs in elderly males and is often the first feature of degenerative neurological conditions, particularly parkinsonism, but also multiple system atrophy and Lewy body disease.

Reference: Psychiatry: An evidence-based text, **p. 850.**

21. d

The most effective treatment for Ekbom's syndrome (restless legs syndrome) is a dopaminergic agent such as ropinirole or pramipexole, but benzodiazepines, opiates and anti-epileptic drugs such as gabapentin may be useful. SSRIs such as citalopram and paroxetine may worsen symptoms.

Reference: Psychiatry: An evidence-based text, **p. 850.**

22. b

It may be secondary to iron deficiency.

Reference: Psychiatry: An evidence-based text, **p. 850.**

23.

(i) a

(ii) b

(iii) a

Reference: Psychiatry: An evidence-based text, **p. 851.**

Chapter 54

Suicide and deliberate self-harm

QUESTIONS

Note that for answers to extended matching items (EMIs), each option (denoted a, b, c, etc.) might be used once, more than once or not at all. For multiple-choice questions (MCQs), please select the best answer.

1. **MCQ** – Select the best answer. Durkheim viewed suicide as a social phenomenon occurring under which of the following conditions?
   (a) Altruistic
   (b) Anomic
   (c) Egoistic
   (d) Fatalistic
   (e) All of the above.

2. **EMI** – Suicide rates
   (a) High (≥ 21 per 100 000 population)
   (b) Low (0–3 per 100 000 population)

   From the above list select the suicide rate with which each of the following countries is better associated:
   (i) Russia
   (ii) Kazakhstan
   (iii) Bahamas
   (iv) Lithuania
   (v) Paraguay.

3. **MCQ** – Select one incorrect statement regarding methods of suicide:
   (a) Drowning is the preferred method of suicide by young people in the Western world.
   (b) From 1998, the size of packets of analgesics that can be sold over the counter at retail outlets was restricted by English law to 32 tablets; subsequently, suicide rates from paracetamol and salicylates declined by over 20 per cent.
   (c) In Asia, ingestion of pesticides in rural areas is common, and self-immolation is commonly observed in women.
   (d) In England, from 1993 onwards, it was required that new cars be fitted with catalytic converters; suicide by exhaust inhalation, once the most popular male method, declined by 90 per cent over the ensuing decade.
   (e) In North America, firearms are involved in around 60 per cent of male suicides and 30 per cent of female suicides.

4. **MCQ** – Select one incorrect statement regarding the epidemiology of suicide:
   (a) Annual suicide rates are higher for men than for women in all major countries.
   (b) From the age of 15 years, the suicide rate approximates that of the adult population.
   (c) In 10- to 14-year-olds, the suicide rate is approximately one per 100 000 of the population per year.
   (d) In adults, there is not a consistent association between suicide rate and age.
   (e) In children under the age of 10 years the suicide rate is near zero.

5. **EMI** – Epidemiology of suicide
   (a) Higher
   (b) Approximately the same
   (c) Lower

   From the above list select the option that best corresponds to each of the following:
   (i) In the UK, the SMR for suicide in men from social class V compared with men from social class I
   (ii) In the UK and Japan, the suicide rate on Tuesdays compared with Mondays
   (iii) In Swedish male conscripts, the risk of suicide in those with low vs high logic test performance scores.

6. **MCQ** – Which of the following groups has not been found to have an especially high risk of suicide in the UK?
   (a) Dentists
   (b) Doctors
   (c) Pharmacists
   (d) Publicans
   (e) Students.

7. **MCQ** – Select the commonest method of suicide found in male prisoners in England and Wales:
   (a) Drowning
   (b) Hanging
   (c) Jumping or falling from a high place

(d) Poisoning
(e) Sharp objects.

8. **EMI** – Neurobiology of suicide
   (a) Higher
   (b) Approximately the same
   (c) Lower

From the above list select the option which best corresponds to each of the following:
   (i) The CSF 5-HIAA levels in suicide attempters compared with controls
   (ii) The CSF 5-HIAA levels in high-lethality compared with low-lethality attempters
   (iii) The likelihood of being a carrier of the 779C allele for *TPH* in impulsive offenders with a suicidal history compared with controls.

9. **EMI** – Suicide
   (a) Anxiety disorder
   (b) Bipolar disorder
   (c) Depressive disorder
   (d) Substance-related disorder

From the above list select the option which best corresponds to each of the following:
   (i) Which of these is the commonest diagnosis in cases of suicide?
   (ii) Which of these is the second most common diagnosis in cases of suicide?
   (iii) Which of these is the least common diagnosis in cases of suicide?

10. **MCQ** – In schizophrenia, which of the following shows the strongest association with suicide?
    (a) Alcohol misuse
    (b) Family history of suicide
    (c) Fear of mental disintegration
    (d) Gender
    (e) Living alone.

11. **MCQ** – Which of the following groups of patients with personality disorder has the highest association with suicidal behaviour?
    (a) Cluster A personality disorders
    (b) Cluster B personality disorders
    (c) Cluster C personality disorders
    (d) Older people with personality disorder
    (e) There is no particular association between personality disorder and suicidal behaviour.

12. **EMI** – Epidemiology of suicide
    (a) Higher
    (b) Approximately the same
    (c) Lower

From the above list select the option that best corresponds to each of the following:
   (i) In the UK, the rate of suicide in unemployed men compared their employed counterparts

(ii) The rate of suicide in winter months compared with the rest of the year
(iii) The SMR for suicide in male prisoners aged between 15 and 17 years in England and Wales compared with that in matched non-prisoners.

13. **EMI** – Neurobiology of suicide
    (a) ↑
    (b) Approximately the same/no change
    (c) ↓

From the above list select the option which best corresponds to each of the following:
   (i) The prolactin response to fenfluramine in suicide attempters
   (ii) 5-HTT sites in the platelets of suicide attempters
   (iii) The density of 5-HT2A receptors in the platelets of suicide attempters.

14. **EMI** – Pro-suicidal or anti-suicidal actions of medication
    (a) ↑
    (b) Approximately the same/no change
    (c) ↓

From the above list select the option which best corresponds to each of the following:
   (i) Suicide attempts in children and young people aged 6–18 years receiving selective serotonin reuptake inhibitors (SSRIs)
   (ii) Suicide deaths in children and young people aged 6–18 years receiving SSRIs
   (iii) Suicide deaths in adults with bipolar disorder receiving lithium.

15. **MCQ** – Select one incorrect statement regarding suicide:
    (a) About a third of UK prisoner suicide cases have a past psychiatric history.
    (b) Clozapine may be anti-suicidal in schizophrenia.
    (c) Epilepsy confers a threefold increase in the probability for suicide over the population base rate.
    (d) In the UK, until 1965, poisoning with domestic coal gas accounted for about half of all suicides; in the years following the introduction of natural gas in 1965 there was almost no change in the suicide rate, suggesting method substitution.
    (e) There are no positive meta-analyses showing an association between *DRD4* (locus 11p15.5) and suicide or suicidal behaviour.

16. **EMI** – Epidemiology of parasuicide
    (a) 15–24 years
    (b) 25–34 years
    (c) 45–54 years

From the above list of age ranges, select the option which best corresponds to each of the following:
   (i) This age group accounts for about 40 per cent of cases of parasuicide

(ii) This age group accounts for about 25 per cent of cases of parasuicide

(iii) This age group accounts for about 10 per cent of cases of parasuicide.

17. **MCQ** – Select one incorrect statement regarding parasuicide (particularly in the UK):

(a) About 85 per cent of parasuicide cases are male.

(b) In the general population, 3–5 per cent of people have had some degree of suicidal thinking in the past year and 1 per cent in the past week.

(c) Of self-injury cases, around three-quarters involve cutting to the arm or wrist.

(d) Self-poisoning accounts for 80–90 per cent of presentations.

(e) There is an association with social deprivation and average income; in England, for example, the rate of parasuicide in the most disadvantaged quintile of the population has been reported to be three to four times that of the least disadvantaged quintile.

18. **EMI** – Neurobiology of suicide

(a) ↑

(b) Approximately the same/no change

(c) ↓

From the above list select the option which best corresponds to each of the following findings from postmortem brain studies of suicide cases:

(i) Gene expression of 5-HT2A receptors

(ii) CRH binding sites

(iii) Presynaptic serotonergic binding sites

(iv) Binding of [^{3}H]phorbal dibutyrate to protein kinase C.

19. **MCQ** – Select one incorrect statement regarding parasuicide:

(a) Completed suicide occurs in 1–2 per cent of cases in the first year after parasuicide.

(b) Completed suicide occurs in 3–9 per cent over 10–20 years after parasuicide in the most disturbed cases, such as people with schizophrenia or severe borderline personality disorder.

(c) Haw and colleagues reported that almost half of cases have personality disorder and an additional third have accentuated personality traits.

(d) In clinical populations, 16 per cent of parasuicide cases repeat self-harm within 6 months and a quarter over 10 years.

(e) Personality traits with which parasuicide has been reported to have a strong association include aggression, anxiety, neuroticism, impulsivity, hostility and psychoticism.

20. **EMI** – Risk factors for repetition of non-fatal self-harm and for completed suicide

(a) Completed suicide

(b) Non-fatal repetition of self-harm

(c) Both of the above

This question concerns NICE guidelines regarding risk factors for repetition of non-fatal self-harm and for completed suicide. From the above list select the best option for which each of the following is a risk factor:

(i) Male

(ii) Living alone

(iii) High suicidal intent

(iv) Unemployment

(v) Alcohol problems.

21. **EMI** – NICE guidelines on risk factors for repetition of non-fatal self-harm and for completed suicide

(a) Completed suicide

(b) Non-fatal repetition of self-harm

(c) Both of the above

From the above list select the best option for which each of the following is a risk factor:

(i) Older age

(ii) Hopelessness

(iii) Poor physical health

(iv) Antisocial personality

(v) Psychiatric history, especially as an in-patient.

22. **EMI** – Suicide rates

(a) High (≥ 21 per 100 000 population)

(b) Low (0–3 per 100 000 population)

From the above list select the suicide rate with which each of the following countries is better associated:

(i) Egypt

(ii) Azerbaijan

(iii) Belarus

(iv) Finland

(v) Japan.

ANSWERS

1. e

Reference: *Psychiatry: An evidence-based text*, **p. 854.**

2.

(i)   a
(ii) a
(iii) b
(iv) a
(v)   b

Reference: *Psychiatry: An evidence-based text*, **p. 855.**

3. a

Jumping from high places is preferred by young people, compared with drowning, which is a choice of older people.

Reference: *Psychiatry: An evidence-based text*, **p. 855.**

4 a

In China, the annual suicide rate is higher in women than in men.

Reference: *Psychiatry: An evidence-based text*, **pp. 855–856.**

5.

(i)   a – Four times higher. This is illustrated in the graph of Figure 54.3 on page 856 of the accompanying textbook.
(ii) c – More suicides were found to occur on Mondays, in the UK and Japan, than on the other days of the week.
(iii) a – The level of performance on the logic test was inversely correlated with the suicide rate; the risk of suicide was three times higher in those with low than in those with high logic test performance. These data, published in 2005, are illustrated in the graph of Figure 54.4 on page 857 in the accompanying textbook.

Reference: *Psychiatry: An evidence-based text*, **pp. 856–857.**

6. e

Other groups with a high risk include veterinarians, salesmen, farmers, drivers and nurses. Access to means may be a relevant factor, e.g. drugs for healthcare practitioners and pesticides and guns for farmers. Students are not at special risk of suicide.

Reference: *Psychiatry: An evidence-based text*, **p. 856.**

7. b

Ninety per cent of prisoner suicides are by hanging.

Reference: *Psychiatry: An evidence-based text*, **p. 856.**

8.

(i)   c – 5-HIAA is a major metabolite of serotonin.
(ii) c
(iii) a – This *TPH* genotype finding was reported in 1998 in a sample of Finnish offenders.

Reference: *Psychiatry: An evidence-based text*, **p. 857.**

9.

(i)   c
(ii) d
(iii) b

Reference: *Psychiatry: An evidence-based text*, **p. 858.**

10. c

The associations of suicide with schizophrenia are different from those that apply to the general population. For example, options 'a', 'b', 'd' and 'e' show a weak or absent association in schizophrenia in contrast to suicides generally. The relative risk for option 'c', on the other hand, is approximately six.

Reference: *Psychiatry: An evidence-based text*, **p. 858.**

11. b

Reference: *Psychiatry: An evidence-based text*, **p. 859.**

12.

(i)   a – Two to three times higher.
(ii) c – In both hemispheres, the rate in winter months is about half that of the rest of the year, but such seasonal variations are now diminishing.
(iii) a – In a 2005 study the SMR for suicide in prison inmates was five, with a particular excess in boys aged 15–17 years (SMR = 18).

Reference: *Psychiatry: An evidence-based text*, **p. 856.**

13.

(i)   c – This is blunted in suicide attempters.
(ii) c – There are fewer 5-HTT sites in platelets of suicide attempters.
(iii) a

Reference: *Psychiatry: An evidence-based text*, **p. 857.**

14.

(i)   a – The odds ratio (OR) is 1.52.
(ii) a – The OR is 15.62.
(iii) c – The current data support the view that lithium is specifically anti-suicidal in comparison with placebo and other mood stabilizers in bipolar disorder, and its

use would be associated with 50 per cent fewer suicides than might otherwise be the case.

Reference: *Psychiatry: An evidence-based text*, **p. 859.**

15. d

In the years following 1965 the suicide rate declined without any evidence of method substitution.

Reference: *Psychiatry: An evidence-based text*, **pp. 855–860.**

16.

(i)   a
(ii) b
(iii) c

Reference: *Psychiatry: An evidence-based text*, **p. 862.**

17. a

The rate in females is greater than that in males; some 60 per cent of parasuicide cases are female.

Reference: *Psychiatry: An evidence-based text*, **p. 862.**

18.

(i)   a
(ii) c
(iii) c
(iv) c – This study was carried out in teenage suicide victims.

Reference: *Psychiatry: An evidence-based text*, **pp. 857–858.**

19. b

The correct range is a lot higher, at 10–15 per cent.

Reference: *Psychiatry: An evidence-based text*, **pp. 862–863.**

20.

(i)   a
(ii) a
(iii) c
(iv) c
(v)   b

Reference: *Psychiatry: An evidence-based text*, **p. 863.**

21.

(i)   a
(ii) c
(iii) a
(iv) b
(v)   c

Reference: *Psychiatry: An evidence-based text*, **p. 863.**

22.

(i)   b
(ii) b
(iii) a
(iv) a
(v)   a

Reference: *Psychiatry: An evidence-based text*, **p. 855.**

Emergency psychiatry

QUESTIONS

Note that for answers to extended matching items (EMIs), each option (denoted a, b, c, etc.) might be used once, more than once or not at all. For multiple-choice questions (MCQs), please select the best answer.

1. **MCQ** – In an elderly patient with an acute behavioural disturbance in whom dementia with Lewy bodies is present or cannot be ruled out, if non-drug approaches are insufficient, which of the following is the first pharmacological treatment recommended by the Royal College of Psychiatrists?
   (a) Intramuscular haloperidol
   (b) Intramuscular lorazepam
   (c) Oral haloperidol
   (d) Oral lorazepam
   (e) Oral olanzapine.

2. **MCQ** – The Royal College of Psychiatrists recommends a monitoring schedule be put in place after a patient has been injected with a medication for acute behavioural disturbance. Which of the following recordings is not a recommended component of a typical schedule?
   (a) Blood pressure at 30 min after injection
   (b) Blood pressure at 60 min after injection
   (c) Monitor for signs of neurological reactions such as acute dystonia and acute parkinsonism
   (d) Pulse and respiration as soon as possible after injection, then every 15 min for 1 hour
   (e) Temperature, using Tempadots, as soon as possible after injection, then at 5, 10, 15 and 60 min.

3. **MCQ** – Of the following, which is the least common feature of acute dystonic reactions?
   (a) Grimacing
   (b) Oculogyric crisis
   (c) Opisthotonos
   (d) Retrocollis
   (e) Tongue protrusion.

4. **MCQ** – Select the best option. With which of the following drugs is oculogyric crisis associated?
   (a) Benzodiazepines

   (b) Cisplatin
   (c) Lithium
   (d) Metoclopramide
   (e) All of the above.

5. **MCQ** – Which of the following is least likely to be a feature of neuroleptic malignant syndrome?
   (a) Altered consciousness
   (b) Hypothermia
   (c) Labile blood pressure
   (d) Muscular rigidity
   (e) Tachycardia.

6. **MCQ** – Select one correct option. Characteristic features of neuroleptic malignant syndrome include:
   (a) Flaccidity
   (b) Leucopenia
   (c) Reduced serum creatine kinase
   (d) Reduced urinary myoglobin
   (e) Urinary incontinence.

7. **MCQ** – Which of the following is not usually a life-threatening side-effect of clozapine?
   (a) Agranulocytosis
   (b) Constipation
   (c) Myocarditis
   (d) Parotid enlargement
   (e) Pulmonary embolism.

8. **MCQ** – Which of the following drugs is least likely to cause serotonin syndrome?
   (a) Cyproheptadine
   (b) Fluoxetine
   (c) Fluvoxamine
   (d) Lithium
   (e) Paroxetine.

ANSWERS

1. d

The Royal College recommends that haloperidol should be used for sedation in elderly patients only if dementia with Lewy bodies has been ruled out. The Royal College sedation guidelines for elderly patients are shown in Figure 55.2 on page 872 of the accompanying textbook.

Reference: *Psychiatry: An evidence-based text*, **p. 872.**

2. d

It is recommended that the pulse and respiration should be measured as soon as possible after injection and then every 5 min for 1 hour.

Reference: *Psychiatry: An evidence-based text*, **p. 872.**

3. d

Reference: *Psychiatry: An evidence-based text*, **p. 873.**

4. e

Reference: *Psychiatry: An evidence-based text*, **p. 873.**

5. b

Hyperthermia (or hyperpyrexia) is a characteristic feature of neuroleptic malignant syndrome.

Reference: *Psychiatry: An evidence-based text*, **p. 874.**

6. e

Reference: *Psychiatry: An evidence-based text*, **p. 874.**

7. d

Reference: *Psychiatry: An evidence-based text*, **p. 874.**

8. a

Cyproheptadine, which is an antihistaminic, antiserotonin and anticholinergic medication, has been used as a treatment for serotonin syndrome.

Reference: *Psychiatry: An evidence-based text*, **pp. 874–875.**

Chapter 56

Care of the dying and bereaved

QUESTIONS

Note that for answers to extended matching items (EMIs), each option (denoted a, b, c, etc.) might be used once, more than once or not at all. For multiple-choice questions (MCQs), please select the best answer.

1. **MCQ** – Which of the following drugs is solely a component of Step 3 of the World Health Organization (WHO) analgesic ladder?
   (a) Aspirin
   (b) Codeine
   (c) Morphine
   (d) Nefopam
   (e) Paracetamol.

2. **EMI** – Relative strengths of opioids
   (a) Codeine
   (b) Diamorphine
   (c) Fentanyl
   (d) Methadone

   From the above list select the opioid that best corresponds to each of the following potency ratios (where morphine has a potency of one):
   (i)   0.1
   (ii) 2–3
   (iii) 5–10
   (iv) 100–150.

3. **MCQ** – Side-effects that may occur when opioids are initially taken by opioid-naïve patients or when the opioid dose is escalated rapidly are least likely to include:
   (a) Confusion and hallucinations
   (b) Diarrhoea
   (c) Myoclonus
   (d) Nausea and vomiting
   (e) Sedation.

4. **MCQ** – Select one incorrect statement regarding palliative care:
   (a) A review of the psychomotor skills of patients taking long-term opioids concluded that the evidence supported no impairment of driving-related skills and that patients taking opioids were no more likely to be involved in motor accidents.
   (b) During the dying phase, anticipatory drugs are typically prescribed subcutaneously for ease of administration.
   (c) In order to help a patient achieve a 'good death', the recognition of impending death is important.
   (d) In the Kübler–Ross stage 3, patients may typically make promises with themselves, their doctors or God.
   (e) Many patients with cancer and with pain, without a previous history of addiction, become addicted to opioids prescribed for pain control.

5. **EMI** – Phases of normal adjustment after diagnosis of life-threatening illness
   (a) Phase 1
   (b) Phase 2
   (c) Phase 3

   This question concerns the phases of normal adjustment a patient is likely to experience after a diagnosis of a life-threatening illness, as described by Massie and Holland. From the above list select the option which best corresponds to each of the following:
   (i)   Adaptation
   (ii) Disbelief and denial
   (iii) Dysphoria
   (iv) A temporary emotional distancing from the crisis.

6. **EMI** – Kübler-Ross stages, from diagnosis to death
   (a) Stage 1
   (b) Stage 2
   (c) Stage 3
   (d) Stage 4
   (e) Stage 5
   (f) Stage 6
   (g) Stage 7

   This question concerns the stages through which patients may pass from diagnosis to death, as described by Kübler-Ross. From the above list select the option that best corresponds to each of the following characteristic features:
   (i) Family members may find the patient's emotions difficult to cope with and require support themselves.
   (ii) When the impact of the diagnosis has subsided, the patient then has to face the losses, whether real or imaginary, ahead.

(iii) This is the stage of bargaining.

(iv) There may be fear of disfigurement, abandonment and uncontrolled symptoms such as pain.

7. **EMI** – Anticipatory drugs
   (a) Cyclizine
   (b) Hyoscine butylbromide
   (c) Midazolam
   (d) Morphine
   (e) Paroxetine

From the above list select the anticipatory drug that best corresponds to each of the following indications in palliative care:
   (i) As an anti-emetic
   (ii) Agitation
   (iii) Pain
   (iv) Noisy respiratory tract secretions.

8. **EMI** – Care of the bereaved
   (a) Anticipatory grief
   (b) Bereavement
   (c) Grief
   (d) Mourning
   (e) None of the above

From the above list select the option that best corresponds to each of the following:
   (i) The primarily emotional (affective) reaction to the loss of a loved one through death
   (ii) The social expressions or acts expressive of grief that are shaped by the practices of a given social or cultural group
   (iii) The psychological and emotional reaction to anticipation of bereavement
   (iv) The objective situation of having lost someone significant.

9. **EMI** – Researchers on loss and bereavement
   (a) Bowlby, Robertson and Ainsworth
   (b) Freud
   (c) Klass
   (d) Lindemann
   (e) Parkes
   (f) Rubin
   (g) Stroebe and Schut
   (h) Worden

From the above list select those people who are best associated with each of the following studies or theoretical developments in our understanding of loss and bereavement:
   (i) The dual-process model of coping with bereavement
   (ii) Wrote *Mourning and Melancholia*
   (iii) Developed a theory of bereavement as a psychosocial transition
   (iv) Described the Two-Track Model of Bereavement, in which the loss is conceptualized as two interactive axes or tracks.

10. **MCQ** – Select one incorrect statement regarding bereavement:
    (a) Anniversaries are often times of renewed grieving.
    (b) Lindemann studied the bereaved survivors of a nightclub fire.
    (c) Stroebe and Strauss argue the need for 'dosage' of grieving when respite is taken from either loss- or restoration-oriented coping activities as an adaptive means of coping.
    (d) Track I in the Two-Track Model of Bereavement is concerned with biopsychosocial functioning.
    (e) There is no increase in the suicide risk in men or women who have been newly widowed.

11. **EMI** – Parkes and Bowlby's four-phase model of bereavement
    (a) Phase of disorganization and despair
    (b) Phase of numbness
    (c) Phase of pining
    (d) Phase of reorganization and recovery

From the above phases in Parkes and Bowlby's four-phase model of bereavement, select the option that best corresponds to each of the following:
   (i) The pangs of grief reduce in intensity, interspersed with longer periods of apathy.
   (ii) This is the immediate reaction to the shock of death.
   (iii) A sense of the presence of the dead person, illusions, misinterpretations and hypnogogic hallucinations may occur.
   (iv) The second phase.

12. **EMI** – Bereavement outcomes
    (a) Poor bereavement outcome
    (b) Protective factor in terms of bereavement outcome
    (c) Neither of the above

From the above list select the option that best corresponds to each of the following factors in terms of the effect of each factor on bereavement outcome:
   (i) Perceived control by the grieving person over daily activities
   (ii) The death was a stigmatized one, such as suicide
   (iii) The grieving person is socially isolated.

13. **EMI** – Researchers on loss and bereavement
    (a) Bowlby, Robertson and Ainsworth
    (b) Freud
    (c) Klass
    (d) Lindemann
    (e) Parkes
    (f) Rubin
    (g) Stroebe and Schut
    (h) Worden

From the above list select those people who are best associated with each of the following studies or theoretical developments in our understanding of loss and bereavement:
   (i) Carried out the first systematic study of acute grief, in 1944

(ii) In the 1980s, proposed a model of grieving in which the grieving person must accomplish four tasks before mourning can be completed and a healthy adjustment made

(iii) Early work focused on the behaviour and attachments of children separated from their mothers under traumatic conditions

(iv) Proposed a 'continuing bonds model of grief'; bereaved people are said to remain involved and connected to the deceased and they actively construct an inner representation of the deceased that is part of the grieving.

14. **MCQ** – Which of the following is least likely to be a risk factor for complicated grief disorder?
(a) A death over several months
(b) A dependent relationship with the deceased person
(c) Childhood abuse and serious neglect
(d) Childhood separation anxiety
(e) Lack of support after the death.

ANSWERS

1. c

This is the strong opioid of choice in the UK. Figure 56.2 on page 877 of the accompanying textbook depicts the WHO analgesic ladder.

Reference: *Psychiatry: An evidence-based text*, **p. 877.**

2.

(i) a
(ii) b
(iii) d
(iv) c

Reference: *Psychiatry: An evidence-based text*, **p. 877.**

3. b

Constipation is a likely side-effect under these circumstances. It should be pre-empted and laxatives prescribed.

Reference: *Psychiatry: An evidence-based text*, **pp. 877–878.**

4. e

Very few such patients become addicted.

Reference: *Psychiatry: An evidence-based text*, **pp. 878–891.**

5.

(i) c – The third phase is that of adaptation.
(ii) a
(iii) b – The patient may exhibit anxiety, depression and poor concentration.
(iv) a

Reference: *Psychiatry: An evidence-based text*, **p. 880.**

6.

(i) b – The patient may express feelings of resentment and frustration may be directed in all directions, towards family and friends, healthcare professionals, or even to God.
(ii) d – It may be the loss of health and independence or the loss of role in society and among peers and family.
(iii) c
(iv) d

Reference: *Psychiatry: An evidence-based text*, **p. 880.**

7.

(i) a – An alternative is haloperidol.
(ii) c
(iii) d
(iv) c

Reference: *Psychiatry: An evidence-based text*, **p. 881.**

8.

(i) c
(ii) d
(iii) a
(iv) b

Reference: *Psychiatry: An evidence-based text*, **p. 881.**

9.

(i) g
(ii) b
(iii) e
(iv) f

Reference: *Psychiatry: An evidence-based text*, **p. 882.**

10. e

The suicide risk of widows and widowers is increased, particularly in the first week after bereavement, but falls in the first month.

Reference: *Psychiatry: An evidence-based text*, **pp. 881–885.**

11.

(i) a
(ii) b
(iii) a
(iv) c

Reference: *Psychiatry: An evidence-based text*, **pp. 882–883.**

12.

(i) b
(ii) a
(iii) a
(iv) a

Reference: *Psychiatry: An evidence-based text*, **pp. 883–884.**

13.

(i) d
(ii) h – These tasks are as follows: to accept the reality of the loss; to work through the pain of grief; to adjust to an environment in which the deceased is missing; and emotionally to relocate the deceased and move on with life.
(iii) a
(iv) c – Klass and colleagues suggested that, although the intensity of the relationship may diminish with time, the relationship does not disappear and can help to inform the grieving person's future. This model is supported by some eastern cultures and the grief process of children.

Reference: *Psychiatry: An evidence-based text*, **p. 882.**

14. a

A sudden unexpected death is a particular risk factor for complicated grief disorder, as is lack of preparation before the death.

Reference: *Psychiatry: An evidence-based text*, **p. 886.**

PART 5

Approaches to treatment

Chapter 57

Clinical psychopharmacology

QUESTIONS

Note that for answers to extended matching items (EMIs), each option (denoted a, b, c, etc.) might be used once, more than once or not at all. For multiple-choice questions (MCQs), please select the best answer.

1. **EMI** – Clinical psychopharmacology
   (a) Oral solution
   (b) Oral tablet
   (c) Intramuscular
   (d) Intravenous

From the above list, select the option with which each label (i–iv) in the following graph of plasma concentration vs time is best associated:

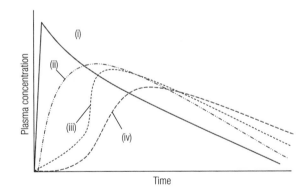

2. **MCQ** – What is the apparent volume of distribution for a drug with 50 per cent bioavailability when a dose of 1 g results in a plasma concentration of 80 mg/L?
   (a) 12.5 L
   (b) 6.25 L
   (c) 1.25 L
   (d) 0.16 L
   (e) 0.08 L.

3. **MCQ** – Select one incorrect statement regarding pharmacokinetics:
   (a) Phase I metabolism generally involves minor chemical reactions such as hydroxylation and demethylation.
   (b) Phase I metabolism is catalysed by cytochrome P450 and other enzymes in the liver and sometimes in the gut and elsewhere.
   (c) Phase II reactions involve the conjugation of the drug or primary metabolite with another molecule to form a complex.

   (d) Psychoactive drugs are usually highly lipid-soluble and show a small volume of distribution.
   (e) Sublingual administration avoids first-pass metabolism.

4. **EMI** – Psychotropic drugs
   (a) CYP1A2
   (b) CYP2C19
   (c) CYP2C9
   (d) CYP2D6
   (e) CYP3A4
   (f) None of the above

From the above list select the best option for which each of the following psychotropic drugs is a substrate:
   (i) Risperidone
   (ii) Zolpidem
   (iii) Caffeine
   (iv) Amphetamine.

5. **MCQ** – Select the best answer. For which of the following is amitriptyline not usually a substrate?
   (a) CYP1A2
   (b) CYP2C19
   (c) CYP2D6
   (d) CYP3A4
   (e) None of the above (i.e. amitriptyline is a substrate for all of the above options).

6. **EMI** – Psychotropic drugs
   (a) CYP1A2
   (b) CYP2C19
   (c) CYP2C9
   (d) CYP2D6
   (e) CYP3A4
   (f) None of the above

From the above list select the best option for which each of the following psychotropic drugs is an inhibitor:
   (i) Duloxetine
   (ii) Modafinil
   (iii) Paroxetine.

7. **MCQ** – Select the best answer. Which of the following is not usually significantly inhibited by fluvoxamine?
   (a) CYP1A2
   (b) CYP2C19
   (c) CYP2D6
   (d) CYP3A4
   (e) None of the above (that is, fluvoxamine usually inhibits all of the above options).

8. **EMI** – Psychotropic drugs
   (a) CYP1A2
   (b) CYP2C19
   (c) CYP2C9
   (d) CYP2D6
   (e) CYP3A4
   (f) None of the above

From the above list select the best option for which each of the following psychotropic drugs is a substrate.
   (i) Citalpram
   (ii) Atomoxetine
   (iii) Zaleplon
   (iv) Clozapine.

9. **EMI** – Enzyme inducers
   (a) CYP1A2
   (b) CYP2C19
   (c) CYP2C9
   (d) CYP2D6
   (e) CYP3A4
   (f) None of the above

From the above list select the best option for which each of the following is usually an enzyme inducer.
   (i) Dexamethasone
   (ii) Cigarette smoke
   (iii) Barbiturates
   (iv) St John's wort.

10. **MCQ** – Select the correct option. The volume of distribution is given by:
   (a) Clearance + elimination rate constant
   (b) Clearance × elimination rate constant
   (c) Clearance/(elimination rate constant)
   (d) (Elimination rate constant)/clearance
   (e) (Elimination rate constant)/(square root of the clearance).

11. **MCQ** – Select the least correct statement regarding pharmacokinetics:
   (a) Amisulpride is excreted unchanged.
   (b) Attainment of plasma steady state usually takes about two half-lives to achieve in regular drug dosing.
   (c) Lithium is excreted unchanged.
   (d) Sulpiride is excreted unchanged.
   (e) The action of drugs is dependent on their concentration at the site of action, which, in turn, is proportional to drug plasma level.

12. **EMI** – Enzyme inducers
   (a) CYP1A2
   (b) CYP2C19
   (c) CYP2C9
   (d) CYP2D6
   (e) CYP3A4
   (f) None of the above

From the above list select the best option for which each of the following is usually an enzyme inducer:
   (i) Modafinil
   (ii) Secobarbital
   (iii) Chargrilled meat.

13. **MCQ** – Select the best option. For which of the following psychotropic drugs is therapeutic drug monitoring very useful?
   (a) Citalopram
   (b) Clozapine
   (c) Diazepam
   (d) Fluoxetine
   (e) All of the above.

14. **EMI** – Precursors
   (a) ACh
   (b) Dopamine
   (c) GABA
   (d) Serotonin

From the above list select the best option for which each of the following is a precursor:
   (i) Choline
   (ii) Glutamate
   (iii) L-Tryptophan
   (iv) L-Tyrosine.

15. **EMI** – Clinical psychopharmacology
   (a) ACh
   (b) Dopamine
   (c) GABA
   (d) Serotonin

From the above list select the best option for which each of the following is a metabolite:
   (i) Choline
   (ii) 5-HIAA
   (iii) Melatonin.

16. **EMI** – Clinical psychopharmacology
   (a) Ach
   (b) Dopamine
   (c) GABA
   (d) Glutamate
   (e) Serotonin

From the above list select the option the interaction with which is considered the most important for the therapeutic action of each of the following psychotropic drugs:
   (i) Amitriptyline
   (ii) MAOI
   (iii) Nitrazepam

(iv) Lamotrigine

(v) Baclofen.

17. **MCQ** – Select the best option. Which of the following is an atypical antipsychotic drug that has a similar chemical structure to that of clozapine?

(a) Amisulpride

(b) Aripiprazole

(c) Quetiapine

(d) Risperidone

(e) All of the above.

18. **EMI** – Psychotropic drugs

(a) Aliphatic phenothiazine

(b) Butyrophenone

(c) Diphenylbutylpiperidine

(d) Piperazine phenothiazine

(e) Piperidine phenothiazine

(f) Substituted benzamide

(g) Thioxanthine

(h) None of the above

From the above list select the group in which each of the following psychotropic drugs best belongs:

(i) Chlorpromazine

(ii) Fluphenazine

(iii) Olanzapine

(iv) Sulpiride.

19. **EMI** – Psychotropic drugs

(a) Aliphatic phenothiazine

(b) Butyrophenone

(c) Diphenylbutylpiperidine

(d) Piperazine phenothiazine

(e) Piperidine phenothiazine

(f) Substituted benzamide

(g) Thioxanthine

(h) None of the above

From the above list select the group in which each of the following psychotropic drugs best belongs:

(i) Amisulpride

(ii) Flupentixol

(iii) Pimozide

(iv) Zuclopenthixol.

20. **MCQ** – Which of the following antipsychotics are usually associated with the highest rate of extrapyramidal side-effects at therapeutic dosage?

(a) Aripiprazole

(b) Piperazine phenothiazines

(c) Piperidine phenothiazines

(d) Risperidone

(e) Substituted benzamides.

21. **MCQ** – The use of which of the following antipsychotics carries the lowest risk of weight gain at therapeutic dosage?

(a) Aripiprazole

(b) Clozapine

(c) Olanzapine

(d) Quetiapine

(e) Risperidone.

22. **MCQ** – Which of the following antipsychotics tends to be the least sedative at therapeutic dosage?

(a) Aripiprazole

(b) Chlorpromazine

(c) Clozapine

(d) Olanzapine

(e) Quetiapine.

23. **MCQ** – Select one incorrect statement regarding anticonvulsant drugs:

(a) Glass syringes should be used with paraldehyde, as it dissolves some plastics.

(b) Most benzodiazepines have anticonvulsant properties, as they enhance GABA activity.

(c) Tiagabine is a fatty acid.

(d) Valproate is a fatty acid.

(e) Weight gain is a common side-effect of topiramate.

24. **MCQ** – Select one incorrect statement regarding anticonvulsant drugs:

(a) Paraldehyde undergoes significant pulmonary excretion.

(b) Phenytoin shows first-order metabolism.

(c) Topiramate is a fructose derivative.

(d) Vigabatrin is a fatty acid.

(e) Vigabatrin is a GABA analogue.

25. **MCQ** – Select one incorrect statement regarding drugs for Alzheimer's disease:

(a) Common side-effects of donepezil include nausea and diarrhoea.

(b) Donepezil is subject to hepatic metabolism catalysed by CYP2D6 and CYP3A4.

(c) Galantamine is derived from the bulbs and flowers of snowdrops and related species.

(d) Memantine is subject to hepatic metabolism catalysed by CYP2D6.

(e) Rivastigmine causes pseudo-irreversible inhibition of acetylcholinesterase.

26. **MCQ** – Which of the following drugs is an MAOI closely related to the amphetamines and sharing their stimulant properties?

(a) Isocarboxazid

(b) Levetiracetam

(c) Phenelzine

(d) Tranylcypromine

(e) None of the above.

27. **MCQ** – Which of the following foods does not, in general, need to be avoided while taking MAOI medication?

(a) Cottage cheese

(b) Fermented soya bean extract

(c) Mature cheddar

(d) Pickled herring

(e) Yeast extract.

28. **MCQ** – The antihistaminergic action of tricyclic antidepressants accounts mainly for which of the following side-effects?
(a) Dry mouth
(b) Hypotension
(c) Priapism
(d) Sedation
(e) Urinary retention.

29. **MCQ** – Which of the following antipsychotics is a D_2R partial agonist?
(a) Amisulpride
(b) Aripiprazole
(c) Clozapine
(d) Olanzapine
(e) Quetiapine.

30. **MCQ** – Which of the following antidepressants most markedly inhibits the reuptake of both serotonin and noradrenaline?
(a) Citalopram
(b) Duloxetine
(c) Escitalopram
(d) Reboxetine
(e) L-Tryptophan.

31. **MCQ** – Select one incorrect statement regarding treatment with lithium salts:
(a) Adverse effects are related to bodily levels and increase rapidly above a plasma level of 1 mM; the most common milder symptoms include thirst, polyuria day and night, and fine hand tremor.
(b) In bipolar disorder treated with lithium, abrupt reductions in plasma lithium levels are associated with increased frequency of relapse.
(c) In the UK, NICE recommends that a mood stabilizer such as lithium should be prescribed prophylactically in bipolar disorder only after two or more severe manic episodes, or in recurrent hypomania characterized by significant risk of suicide, functional impairment or high rate of relapse.

(d) Hyperparathyroidism is a side-effect of long-term use, so that monitoring of calcium is advisable in such cases.
(e) Studies suggest that an appropriate target plasma lithium level range for bipolar disorder prophylaxis is 0.8–1.2 mM at 12 hours post-dose sampling.

32. **MCQ** – On a flight, a male passenger who has no previous history of acting aggressively, and who is taking benzodiazepine medication, engages in 'air rage'. Which of the following is the most likely cause of this (assuming that it applies to this passenger)?
(a) Alcohol beverages
(b) Dehydration
(c) Feeling cold
(d) Hunger
(e) Hypoxia.

33. **MCQ** – Select one incorrect statement regarding drugs and dependency:
(a) Acamprosate is a taurine derivative that interacts with GABA systems; it somewhat reduces relapse to alcohol reuse.
(b) Amphetamines such as dexamfetamine can cause dependence and psychoses.
(c) At the time of writing, zopiclone has not been found to be addictive.
(d) Caffeine is a weak stimulant that is an ingredient of many analgesic preparations; withdrawal can be followed by a headache, which can be severe.
(e) Disulfiram is indicated as an adjunct in the treatment of chronic alcohol dependence; it inhibits aldehyde dehydrogenase, leading to interruption of alcohol metabolism at the acetaldehyde stage, causing unpleasant symptoms.

34. **MCQ** – Type A adverse drug reactions do not include which of the following?
(a) Agranulocytosis with clozapine
(b) Extrapyramidal reactions to haloperidol
(c) Nausea and diarrhoea with donepezil
(d) Sedation with a benzodiazepine
(e) Sedation with some antipsychotics.

ANSWERS

1.

(i)   d – The plasma concentration reaches a peak faster than with the other three options.
(ii) c
(iii) a
(iv) b

Reference: *Psychiatry: An evidence-based text*, **p. 895.**

2. b

Fifty per cent bioavailability gives 1 g × 50 per cent = 1000 mg × 50 per cent = 500 mg. So the apparent volume of distribution = (500 mg)/(80 mg/L) = 6.25 L.

Reference: *Psychiatry: An evidence-based text*, **p. 896.**

3. d

This option contradicts itself; if these drugs are highly lipid-soluble, then they are likely to show a large or very large volume of distribution. Thus it should be possible to work out the answer to this question from an understanding of the concept of the volume of distribution.

Reference: *Psychiatry: An evidence-based text*, **pp. 895–896.**

4.

(i)   e
(ii) e
(iii) a
(iv) d

Reference: *Psychiatry: An evidence-based text*, **p. 897.**

5. d

Reference: *Psychiatry: An evidence-based text*, **p. 897.**

6.

(i)   d
(ii) b
(iii) d

Reference: *Psychiatry: An evidence-based text*, **p. 897.**

7. c

Reference: *Psychiatry: An evidence-based text*, **p. 897.**

8.

(i)   b
(ii) d
(iii) e
(iv) a

Reference: *Psychiatry: An evidence-based text*, **p. 897.**

9.

(i)   d
(ii) a
(iii) e
(iv) e

Reference: *Psychiatry: An evidence-based text*, **p. 897.**

10. c

The clearance of a drug is the rate of elimination of the drug and is equal to the product of the elimination rate constant and the volume of distribution. The correct result follows.

Reference: *Psychiatry: An evidence-based text*, **p. 897.**

11. b

Attainment of steady state usually takes four to five half-lives to achieve in regular dosing. Steady state is achieved when the rate of drug availability equals the rate of drug removal.

Reference: *Psychiatry: An evidence-based text*, **pp. 896–897.**

12.

(i)   a
(ii) c
(iii) a

Reference: *Psychiatry: An evidence-based text*, **p. 897.**

13. b

With clozapine, therapeutic drug monitoring is useful principally because the plasma level attained varies considerably in individuals given the same dose (gender and smoking status have a profound influence on clozapine metabolism).

Reference: *Psychiatry: An evidence-based text*, **p. 898–899.**

14.

(i)   a
(ii) c
(iii) d
(iv) b

Reference: *Psychiatry: An evidence-based text*, **p. 900.**

15.

(i)   a
(ii) d
(iii) d – In the pineal gland.

Reference: *Psychiatry: An evidence-based text*, **p. 900.**

16.

(i) e
(ii) e
(iii) c
(iv) d
(v) c

Reference: Psychiatry: An evidence-based text, p. 900.

17. c

Like clozapine, quetiapine is a dibenzodiazepine derivative.

Reference: Psychiatry: An evidence-based text, p. 904.

18.

(i) a
(ii) d
(iii) h – The groups given as options (apart from 'h') are all subgroups of typical antipsychotics; olanzapine is an atypical antipsychotic and is, in fact, a thienobenzodiazepine.
(iv) f

Reference: Psychiatry: An evidence-based text, p. 904.

19.

(i) f – Like sulpiride, amisulpride is a substituted benzamide. Amisulpride is usually classified as an atypical antipsychotic, whereas sulpiride is usually classified as a typical antipsychotic.
(ii) g
(iii) c
(iv) g – As for flupentixol.

Reference: Psychiatry: An evidence-based text, p. 904.

20. b

For example, fluphenazine and trifluoperazine.

Reference: Psychiatry: An evidence-based text, p. 904.

21. a

Reference: Psychiatry: An evidence-based text, p. 904.

22. a.

Reference: Psychiatry: An evidence-based text, p. 904.

23. e

Topiramate is one of the few drugs used in psychiatry that reliably causes weight loss.

Reference: Psychiatry: An evidence-based text, p. 905.

24. b

It shows capacity-limited or zero-order metabolism.

Reference: Psychiatry: An evidence-based text, pp. 905–906.

25. d

Memantine is indeed metabolized in the liver, to inactive compounds. However, cytochrome P450 enzymes are not involved.

Reference: Psychiatry: An evidence-based text, p. 906.

26. d

Reference: Psychiatry: An evidence-based text, p. 907.

27. a

The well-known interactions with other amines and similar substances result from the monoamine oxidase inhibition that prevents the breakdown of tyramine in ingested tyramine-rich foods.

Reference: Psychiatry: An evidence-based text, p. 907.

28. d

The sedation is sometimes profound, as is an antihistaminergic effect. Dry mouth and urinary retention are anticholinergic side-effects. Hypotension and priapism are alpha-adrenergic blocking effects.

Reference: Psychiatry: An evidence-based text, p. 907.

29. b

Aripiprazole is also a partial agonist at serotonergic 5-hydroxytryptamine-1A (5-HT1A) receptors.

Reference: Psychiatry: An evidence-based text, p. 904.

30. b

The serotonin noradrenaline reuptake inhibitors (SNRIs), which include venlafaxine and duloxetine, were developed with a similar rationale to the selective serotonin reuptake inhibitors (SSRIs), but with an additional claim that, as they acted selectively on two neurotransmitters (noradrenaline as well as serotonin), they would prove more effective than the SSRIs. This claim is still debated.

Reference: Psychiatry: An evidence-based text, p. 907.

31. c

NICE recommends that a mood stabilizer should be prescribed prophylactically in bipolar disorder:

• After a single severe manic episode
• After two or more episodes of mania
• In recurrent hypomania characterized by significant risk of suicide, functional impairment or high rate of relapse.

Reference: Psychiatry: An evidence-based text, pp. 898, 909–910.

32. a

The combination of a benzodiazepine and alcohol is particularly prone to lead to paradoxical reactions.

Reference: *Psychiatry: An evidence-based text,* **p. 911.**

33. c

Addiction has been documented with zopiclone.

Reference: *Psychiatry: An evidence-based text,* **pp. 912–913.**

34. a

This is a type B reaction. Such reactions cannot, at least initially, be predicted from a drug's known pharmacological actions.

Reference: *Psychiatry: An evidence-based text,* **p. 913.**

Chapter 58

Electroconvulsive therapy

QUESTIONS

Note that for answers to extended matching items (EMIs), each option (denoted a, b, c, etc.) might be used once, more than once or not at all. For multiple-choice questions (MCQs), please select the best answer.

1. **MCQ** – Select the best option. Modern electroconvulsive therapy (ECT) is the electrical induction of a generalized cerebral seizure of which of the following types?
   (a) Akinetic
   (b) Atonic
   (c) Absences
   (d) Myoclonic jerk
   (e) Tonic–clonic.

2. **MCQ** – The series of studies of ECT at the New York State Psychiatric Institute from 1987, which led to a refinement of the original theory relating to its mode of action, were led by:
   (a) Bini
   (b) Cerletti
   (c) Kendell
   (d) Ottosson
   (e) Sackeim.

3. **MCQ** – Select the least correct statement regarding the effects of ECT:
   (a) Bilateral ECT causes symmetrical increases in blood flow in the cortex.
   (b) Bilateral ECT causes symmetrical increases in blood flow in subcortical networks.
   (c) Right unilateral ECT causes asymmetrical increases in cortical blood flow.
   (d) Right unilateral ECT causes asymmetrical increases in subcortical blood flow.
   (e) Right unilateral ECT causes increases in blood flow in the left temporal lobe and left thalamus.

4. **MCQ** – Select the least correct statement. Repeated electroconvulsive shock to laboratory animals has been shown to:
   (a) Down-regulate the number of beta-adrenoceptors in the cortex and hippocampus.
   (b) Increase functional measures of acetylcholine.
   (c) Increase functional measures of dopamine.
   (d) Increase functional measures of noradrenaline.
   (e) Increase functional measures of serotonin.

5. **MCQ** – Select the best option. According to the Royal College of Psychiatrists, ECT is the potential treatment of choice in which of the following?
   (a) Acute schizophrenia
   (b) Catatonia
   (c) Mania
   (d) Severe depressive illness associated with attempted suicide
   (e) All of the above.

6. **EMI** – Electroconvulsive therapy
   (a) Higher
   (b) Approximately the same
   (c) Lower

From the above list select the option with which each of the following findings from research into ECT is best associated:
   (i) The dose of electricity for right unilateral ECT compared with that for bilateral ECT to give an approximately equal clinical efficacy for both
   (ii) The acute cognitive adverse effects of right unilateral ECT compared with bilateral ECT
   (iii) The possibility of enduring retrograde amnesia following right unilateral ECT compared with bilateral ECT.

ANSWERS

1. e

This is the grand mal type of seizure.

Reference: *Psychiatry: An evidence-based text,* **p. 922.**

2. e

Reference: *Psychiatry: An evidence-based text,* **p. 922.**

3. e

There is relative sparing of the left temporal lobe and the left medial thalamus.

Reference: *Psychiatry: An evidence-based text,* **p. 923.**

4. b

Functional measures of acetylcholine decrease, which is one plausible explanation for some of the cognitive adverse effects of ECT.

Reference: *Psychiatry: An evidence-based text,* **p. 923.**

5. d

Reference: *Psychiatry: An evidence-based text,* **pp. 924–925.**

6.

(i) a
(ii) c
(iii) c

Reference: *Psychiatry: An evidence-based text,* **Ch. 58.**

Chapter 59

Transcranial magnetic stimulation and vagus nerve stimulation

QUESTIONS

Note that for answers to extended matching items (EMIs), each option (denoted a, b, c, etc.) might be used once, more than once or not at all. For multiple-choice questions (MCQs), please select the best answer.

1. **MCQ** – Select the best option. Which of the following is a major side-effect of rTMS in humans?
   (a) Cognitive impairment
   (b) Headache
   (c) Neuroendocrine effects
   (d) Neuropathological change
   (e) None of the above.

2. **MCQ** – Select one incorrect statement regarding TMS and VNS:
   (a) In electroconvulsive therapy a seizure is the goal of electrical stimulation, whereas in rTMS a seizure is a side-effect.
   (b) Once implanted, VNS, used to treat depression, remains on continuously, but clinical relief of depression is often slow.
   (c) Response rates and remission rates with rTMS for depression are approximately equal to those with electroconvulsive therapy.
   (d) Side-effects of VNS for the treatment of depression are few but may particularly include hoarseness.
   (e) The vagus nerve has numerous afferent fibres that are enteroreceptive

ANSWERS

1. b

This probably results from the muscle contraction under the site of the TMS electrode.

Reference: *Psychiatry: An evidence-based text*, **p. 932.**

2. c

Response rates and remission rates with rTMS are far below those of electroconvulsive therapy. Hoarseness may result from VNS owing to stimulation of the recurrent laryngeal nerve.

Reference: *Psychiatry: An evidence-based text*, **Ch. 59.**

Chapter 60

Psychotherapy: an introduction

QUESTIONS

Note that for answers to extended matching items (EMIs), each option (denoted a, b, c, etc.) might be used once, more than once or not at all. For multiple-choice questions (MCQs), please select the best answer.

1. **EMI** – Psychological treatments
   (a) Arts therapies
   (b) Family therapy
   (c) Group analysis
   (d) Interpersonal therapy
   (e) Psychodynamic long-term therapy

From the above list select the best psychological treatment option for which each of the following is an indication:
   (i) Alcoholism
   (ii) Capacity to tolerate frustration
   (iii) Social phobia
   (iv) Family has suffered a life-event
   (v) Learning disability.

2. **EMI** – Psychological treatments
   (a) Cognitive-behavioural therapy
   (b) Family therapy
   (c) Group analysis
   (d) Psychodynamic long-term therapy
   (e) Short-term dynamic psychotherapy

From the above list select the most appropriate psychological treatment option for which each of the following is a contraindication:
   (i) Severe obsessional states
   (ii) Major problems with self-disclosure
   (iii) Patients with positive beliefs about dysfunctional aspects of their behaviour.

3. **MCQ** – Select the best option. For which of the following conditions is there clear evidence of the effectiveness of DBT?
   (a) Cocaine misuse
   (b) Childhood disorders
   (c) Depression
   (d) Obsessive-compulsive disorder
   (e) Personality disorder.

4. **MCQ** – Select the best option. For which of the following conditions is there clear evidence of the effectiveness of community reinforcement approaches?
   (a) Cocaine misuse
   (b) Childhood disorders
   (c) Depression
   (d) Obsessive-compulsive disorder
   (e) Personality disorder.

5. **MCQ** – Select the best option. For which of the following conditions is there clear evidence of the effectiveness of cognitive-behavioural therapy?
   (a) Bulimia nervosa
   (b) Childhood disorders
   (c) Depression
   (d) Post-traumatic stress disorder
   (e) All of the above.

6. **MCQ** – Select the best option. Which of the following is true regarding the integrated practice of psychotherapy with medication, managed by the same practitioner?
   (a) Medication issues can usefully be addressed at the beginning of the session.
   (b) Medication issues can usefully be addressed at the end of the session.
   (c) Giving extra medication is not likely to be helpful with dealing with symptoms that occur as a result of therapy.
   (d) Symptoms are likely to increase at the end of therapy.
   (e) All of the above.

7. **MCQ** – Choose the best option. Select one incorrect statement regarding the triangle of person:
   (a) It includes future goals.
   (b) It includes infantile object relations/history.
   (c) It includes transference.
   (d) It was described by Malan.
   (e) All of the above.

8. **EMI** – Psychological defences
   (a) Alcohol dependency
   (b) Anorexia nervosa
   (c) Anxiety disorder
   (d) Depression
   (e) Obsessive-compulsive disorder

From the above list select the diagnosis with which each of the following defences is best associated:

(i)   Body is unconsciously perceived as occupied by introject of 'intrusive' mother

(ii) Identification with lost object

(iii) Magical thinking.

9. **MCQ** – Select an incorrect statement regarding the study of unconscious processes in groups by Sigmund Freud:

(a) Freud described a process in which the crowd follows the leader who personifies their own ideals.

(b) Freud described these unconscious processes in *Group Psychology and the Analysis of the Ego*.

(c) Freud's work was the start of the study of unconscious processes in groups.

(d) When a group becomes pathologically dependent on the leader, Freud described how the group is highly likely, nevertheless, to be critical of the leader.

(e) When a group follows a leader, Freud described how the capacity for thinking and decision-making is projected into the leader.

10. **MCQ** – Select the best option. Wilfred Bion defined the unconscious tendency of a group to avoid work on the primary task as being which of the following?

(a) Basic assumption mentality

(b) Regression of the group

(c) Obsessive work avoidance

(d) Workgroup

(e) Workgroup regression.

11. **EMI** – Psychological defences

(a) Alcohol dependency

(b) Anorexia nervosa

(c) Anxiety disorder

(d) Depression

(e) Obsessive-compulsive disorder

From the above list select the diagnosis with which each of the following defences is best associated:

(i)   Object losses in remote or recent past

(ii) Defences of isolation, undoing and reaction formation

(iii) Difficulty separating from mother.

12. **EMI** – Basic assumptions (Bion)

(a) Death wish

(b) Dependency

(c) Fight/flight

(d) Pairing

From the above list select the basic assumption described by Bion with which each of the following group phenomena is best associated:

(i)   The group behaves as if there is a danger or enemy.

(ii) The group follows the leader who is its most paranoid member.

(iii) The group functions in the grip of a phantasy that a future event will solve whatever the group's problem is.

ANSWERS

1.

(i) c
(ii) e
(iii) d
(iv) b
(v) a

Reference: *Psychiatry: An evidence-based text*, **pp. 936–937.**

2.

(i) d
(ii) c
(iii) a

Reference: *Psychiatry: An evidence-based text*, **pp. 936–937.**

3. e

DBT can be effective in the treatment of self-harm in borderline personality disorder.

Reference: *Psychiatry: An evidence-based text*, **pp. 938–939.**

4. a

Reference: *Psychiatry: An evidence-based text*, **pp. 938–939.**

5. e

Reference: *Psychiatry: An evidence-based text*, **pp. 938–939.**

6. e

Reference: *Psychiatry: An evidence-based text*, **p. 941.**

7. a

The triangle of person includes options 'b' and 'c' and also the current life situation/symptom. It is illustrated in Figure 60.2 on page 942 of the accompanying textbook.

Reference: *Psychiatry: An evidence-based text*, **pp. 942–943.**

8.

(i) b
(ii) d
(iii) e

Reference: *Psychiatry: An evidence-based text*, **p. 943.**

9. d

Freud described a process in which the crowd follows the leader who personifies their own ideals. In doing so, the capacity for thinking and decision-making is projected into the leader, on whom the group becomes pathologically dependent; at this point, criticizing the leader becomes impossible.

Reference: *Psychiatry: An evidence-based text*, **p. 944.**

10. a

Reference: *Psychiatry: An evidence-based text*, **p. 944.**

11.

(i) d
(ii) e
(iii) b

Reference: *Psychiatry: An evidence-based text*, **p. 943.**

12.

(i) c – The danger or enemy should either be attacked or fled from.
(ii) c
(iii) d – Some imagined coupling will bring about salvation.

Reference: *Psychiatry: An evidence-based text*, **p. 944.**

Chapter 61

Dynamic psychotherapy

QUESTIONS

Note that for answers to extended matching items (EMIs), each option (denoted a, b, c, etc.) might be used once, more than once or not at all. For multiple-choice questions (MCQs), please select the best answer.

1. **MCQ** – Select one incorrect statement regarding dynamic psychotherapy:
   (a) Countertransference refers to responses that an analyst can have to a patient that appear to be irrational or exaggerated and that may also carry a strong emotional charge.
   (b) It is possible to enact distress, rather than articulating it, during therapeutic sessions, behaviour that is sometimes referred to as acting out.
   (c) The defence of denial compromises the individual's ability to discern what is external reality.
   (d) The defence of splitting disrupts the experienced self's internal cohesion.
   (e) The three components of the working alliance are agreement on the goals of treatment, agreement on the method of treatment, and the empathic bond between therapists and their patients.

2. **EMI** – Dynamic psychotherapy innovators
   (a) Bowlby, Sir John
   (b) Freud, Sigmund
   (c) Jung, Carl
   (d) Klein, Melanie
   (e) Kohut, Heinz
   (f) Lacan, Jacques
   (g) Winnicott, Donald

From the above list select the innovator with whom the development of each of the following in dynamic psychotherapy is best associated.
   (i) Collective unconscious
   (ii) Depressive position
   (iii) Transitional object.

3. **EMI** – Dynamic psychotherapy innovators
   (a) Bowlby, Sir John
   (b) Freud, Sigmund
   (c) Jung, Carl
   (d) Klein, Melanie
   (e) Kohut, Heinz
   (f) Lacan, Jacques
   (g) Winnicott, Donald

From the above list select the innovator with whom the development of each of the following in dynamic psychotherapy is best associated:
   (i) Good-enough mother
   (ii) Mirror phase of development
   (iii) Rebalancing of the personality through individuation.

4. **EMI** – Dynamic psychotherapy innovators
   (a) Bowlby, Sir John
   (b) Freud, Sigmund
   (c) Jung, Carl
   (d) Klein, Melanie
   (e) Kohut, Heinz
   (f) Lacan, Jacques
   (g) Winnicott, Donald

From the above list select the innovator with whom the development of each of the following in dynamic psychotherapy is best associated:
   (i) Paranoid schizoid position
   (ii) The concepts of the complex and the archetype
   (iii) Attachment theory.

5. **EMI** – Group dynamic psychotherapy
   (a) Bion, Wilfrid
   (b) Freud, Anna
   (c) Foulkes, S.H.
   (d) Yalom, Irving

From the above list select the innovator with whom the development of each of the following in group dynamic psychotherapy is best associated:
   (i) Instillation of hope as a therapeutic factor in groups
   (ii) Founded group analysis
   (iii) Emphasized the importance of cohesion to a group's success.

ANSWERS

1. b

This is referred to as 'acting in'.

Reference: *Psychiatry: An evidence-based text*, **pp. 948–949.**

2.

(i)   c
(ii) d
(iii) g

Reference: *Psychiatry: An evidence-based text*, **pp. 949–951.**

3.

(i)   g
(ii) f
(iii) c

Reference: *Psychiatry: An evidence-based text*, **pp. 949–951.**

4.

(i)   d
(ii) c
(iii) a

Reference: *Psychiatry: An evidence-based text*, **pp. 949–951.**

5.

(i)   d
(ii) c
(iii) d

Reference: *Psychiatry: An evidence-based text*, **pp. 951–952.**

Chapter 62

Family therapy

QUESTIONS

Note that for answers to extended matching items (EMIs), each option (denoted a, b, c, etc.) might be used once, more than once or not at all. For multiple-choice questions (MCQs), please select the best answer.

1. **MCQ** – Select one incorrect statement regarding family therapy:
   (a) In problem-oriented versions of family therapy, the therapist and the team start with an exploration of the problems – what is going wrong and what the underlying cause may be.
   (b) Later waves of family therapy that advocate more narrative, collaborative and non-directive approaches were developed by social workers.
   (c) Many of the pioneers of family therapy were medically trained and specialists in psychiatry.
   (d) Minuchin and colleagues studied the effects of family therapy by measuring levels of free fatty acids in family members.
   (e) Regarding systemic family therapy, the word systemic derives from systemic risk.

2. **EMI** – Innovators in family therapy
   (a) Bateson *et al.*
   (b) Brown and Birley
   (c) Fromm-Reichman
   (d) Haley
   (e) Jackson
   (f) Lacan
   (g) Lidz *et al.*
   (h) The Milan group
   (i) Vaughn and Leff
   (j) Watzlawick *et al.*
   (k) Weakland
   (l) Winnicott
   (m) Yalom

From the above list select those people with whom the introduction of each of the following concepts in family therapy is best associated:
   (i) Family homeostasis
   (ii) Viewing the double-bind as a three-person process
   (iii) The double-bind theory.

3. **EMI** – Family therapy theory
   (a) Circularities
   (b) Double-bind communications
   (c) Family genograms
   (d) Pathological triangles
   (e) Solution-focus approaches

From the above list select the concept from family therapy theory with which each of the following is best associated:
   (i) Were considered, in the past, to be a cause of schizophrenia
   (ii) Essentially repetitive patterns of interaction. The question of looking for a starting point in relationship difficulties is therefore seen as unproductive
   (iii) An example of these would be how a grandparent could seriously undermine and disempower their child (parent) by giving contradictory instructions to their grandchild.

4. **MCQ** – In the practice of family therapy, a problem may be cast in a less negative and destructive light, and the actions of the family members as having positive intent, even if the outcomes appear to be problematic. What is this process best termed?
   (a) Externalization
   (b) Narrative therapy
   (c) Punctuation
   (d) Reframing
   (e) Storying.

5. **EMI** – Innovators in family therapy
   (a) Brown and Birley
   (b) Fromm-Reichman
   (c) Haley
   (d) Jackson
   (e) Lacan
   (f) Leff and Isaacs
   (g) Lidz *et al.*
   (h) The Milan group
   (i) Vaughn and Leff
   (j) Watzlawick *et al.*
   (k) Weakland
   (l) Winnicott
   (m) Yalom

From the above list select those people with whom the introduction of each of the following concepts in family therapy is best associated:

(i) Circularities

(ii) Pathological triangles

(iii) Circular questioning.

6. **MCQ** – Select one incorrect statement regarding family therapy:

(a) A family therapist may ask the parents, say, to discuss issues of conflict; this is a structural technique called intensification.

(b) During the 1980s, there was a gradual shift from an emphasis on patterns of actions to an emphasis on the construction of meanings and their creation in families and between the family and the therapist.

(c) Family genograms are rarely used nowadays.

(d) Jackson suggested that families act as if they are regulated by a set of largely unconscious rules.

(e) Parents may pull one of their ill children into their own conflict; this is an example of the concept of triangulation.

ANSWERS

1. e

The word 'systemic' in this context derives from general systems theory, which became one of the guiding conceptual frameworks for family therapy.

Reference: *Psychiatry: An evidence-based text*, **pp. 955–956.**

2.

(i) e – This term was introduced by Jackson to suggest that a symptom in one or more of the family members develops and functions as a response to the actions of the others in a family and becomes part of the patterning of the system.

(ii) k

(iii) a – This concept was put forward by Bateson and colleagues in 1956. Schizophrenia was said to develop as a result of exposure to double-bind situations. Bateson subsequently revised the double-bind theory to suggest that the process is a reciprocal one, with the child also engaged in double-binding communication.

Reference: *Psychiatry: An evidence-based text*, **Ch. 62.**

3.

(i) b

(ii) a

(iii) d

Reference: *Psychiatry: An evidence-based text*, **Ch. 62.**

4. d

From the outset, family therapists employed the technique of reframing (or re-storying), which attempted to offer a new or different way of seeing a problem as an intervention. For example, conflict in a couple could be discussed as showing a fiery passion and as something that could eventually make their relationship stronger.

Reference: *Psychiatry: An evidence-based text*, **p. 962.**

5.

(i) j – Systems theory stresses the interdependence of action in families and other relationships. Each person is seen as influencing the others, and their responses in turn influence them, which influences the first person's responses, and so on. Any action is therefore also seen as a response, and a response also as an action. Paul Watzlawick and colleagues coined the term 'circularities' to capture these essentially repetitive patterns of interaction. Even if we can identify who appeared to start a particular family sequence, such as an argument, this may in turn have been a response to a previous episode; therefore the question of looking for a starting point in relationship difficulties – who started it – is seen as unproductive.

(ii) c – Haley made the observation that humans, unlike other species, have in-laws. An example is given in Question 3.

(iii) h – A family therapy team of psychiatrists in Milan produced the idea that family therapy should proceed on the basis of the therapist asking the family questions in order both to explore their understanding and to trigger new ways of thinking through the questions that are asked. The questions were not predetermined but were shaped in a circular way by what and how the family had previously responded.

Reference: *Psychiatry: An evidence-based text*, **Ch. 62.**

6. c

Currently, they are one of the most frequently used and powerful techniques in family therapy.

Reference: *Psychiatry: An evidence-based text*, **Ch. 62.**

Chapter 63

Marital therapy

QUESTIONS

Note that for answers to extended matching items (EMIs), each option (denoted a, b, c, etc.) might be used once, more than once or not at all. For multiple-choice questions (MCQs), please select the best answer.

1. **MCQ** – The least common psychotherapeutic method of conducting marital therapy is:
   (a) Cognitive-behaviour marital therapy
   (b) Emotionally focused marital therapy
   (c) Mentalization-based marital therapy
   (d) Psychodynamic/psychoanalytical marital therapy
   (e) Systemic marital therapy.

2. **EMI** – Marital therapy techniques
   (a) Cognitive-behaviour marital therapy
   (b) Emotionally focused marital therapy
   (c) Mentalization-based marital therapy
   (d) Psychodynamic/psychoanalytical marital therapy
   (e) Systemic marital therapy

   From the above list select the marital therapy technique with which each of the following sets of characteristics is best associated:
   (i) This marital therapy has its roots in attachment theory.
   (ii) Key to this understanding of the couple relationship is the idea that it is a 'phantasy' relationship.
   (iii) In this form of marital therapy, attention is paid to the use of language by the couple – both at the level of specific content, including the kinds of words chosen, and at the level of process or what the language is meant to do in the couple. Attention is also paid to the use of power. Therapists assume that any behaviour has a role and a meaning – there is a purpose to a behaviour, no matter how reactive it appears.
   (iv) Therapists are active and assertive, on the basis that changing a destructive relationship requires greater energy than exists to maintain it. Therapists can take up different roles at different times – guide, teacher, confronter, referee, empathizer – and they may set homework to be done by a couple between sessions. Their aim, however, is to ensure that the couple take more and more responsibility for the quality of their relationship. Attention is paid to the balance of the therapy.

3. **EMI** – Marital therapy techniques
   (a) Cognitive-behaviour marital therapy
   (b) Emotionally focused marital therapy
   (c) Mentalization-based marital therapy
   (d) Psychodynamic/psychoanalytical marital therapy
   (e) Systemic marital therapy

   From the above list select the marital therapy technique with which each of the following indications is best associated:
   (i) There are clear patterns of relationship stemming from families of origin perceptible in the couple.
   (ii) A couple have a particular interest in the meaning of their relationship – why it is like it is – and want to change it.
   (iii) Neither partner is suffering from overwhelming individual difficulties stemming from their own psychopathology.
   (iv) There is a clear communication problem within the couple.

4. **EMI** – Marital therapy techniques
   (a) Cognitive-behaviour marital therapy
   (b) Emotionally focused marital therapy
   (c) Mentalization-based marital therapy
   (d) Psychodynamic/psychoanalytical marital therapy
   (e) Systemic marital therapy

   From the above list select the marital therapy technique with which each of the following sets of techniques is best associated:
   (i) One of the main tasks of this type of marital therapy is to create and actively maintain a positive therapeutic alliance by the use of acceptance and empathy, together with a willingness to demonstrate engagement with the couple through actively validating each partner's experience.
   (ii) This is a short-term therapy of up to 25 sessions, which may begin weekly and then reduce in frequency once the therapist has understood the nature of the maladaptive interactions and goals have been set for change. It tends to be

highly structured, with therapists taking the role of collaborator, seeking the couple's agreement with their evaluation of the nature of the couple relationship and the steps that will be taken to bring about change.

(iii) There are regular weekly sessions of 50–60 min, generally on an open-ended basis. The sessions require strict technical handling: informal interactions are kept to a minimum and the sessions are deliberately unstructured with no teaching or guiding. The therapist creates a neutrally expectant space for the couple to use in whatever way they will.

5. **EMI** – Marital therapy techniques
   (a) Cognitive-behaviour marital therapy
   (b) Emotionally focused marital therapy
   (c) Mentalization-based marital therapy
   (d) Psychodynamic/psychoanalytical marital therapy
   (e) Systemic marital therapy

From the above list select the marital therapy technique with which each of the following indications is best associated:
   (i) A couple can make use of symbolism and are not excessively concrete in their thinking.
   (ii) There is not an ongoing affair and there is not simultaneous substance abuse.

(iii) The couple want to rebuild the relationship despite the difficulties between them.
(iv) Where one partner will need active and effective engagement to join the couple therapy.

6. **EMI** – Marital therapy techniques
   (a) Cognitive-behaviour marital therapy
   (b) Emotionally focused marital therapy
   (c) Mentalization-based marital therapy
   (d) Psychodynamic/psychoanalytical marital therapy
   (e) Systemic marital therapy

From the above list select the marital therapy technique with which each of the following indications is best associated:
   (i) One of the couple has a narcissistic personality disorder.
   (ii) There are complexities and confusions stemming from multiple sources of input into the couple situation.
   (iii) The couple have a clear attachment system pattern going on.
   (iv) Dysfunctional patterns of relating have proved unshiftable through other means, including other therapies, and the couple are prepared to engage in potentially long-term work.

ANSWERS

1. c

At present, in the UK, options 'a', 'b', 'd' and 'e' are the most common ways of treating the couple relationship psychotherapeutically.

Reference: *Psychiatry: An evidence-based text*, **pp. 938–939, 967.**

2.

(i) **b** – Attachment theory has investigated the kinds of attachment relationship that infants and children make and has shown how they lead to either secure or insecure dependency on another.

(ii) **d** – The relationship is considered to be permeated with unconscious projections on to, and in part accepted by, each other. This means that one partner will manifest emotions, thoughts and behaviours that actually belong to the other partner, forming a complex interlocking system of experience that can be very difficult to unravel.

(iii) **e**

(iv) **e** – Attention is paid to the balance of the therapy: the amount of attention paid to each partner, the degree of intensity of confrontation with each, the assumption that both partners are involved in the problem, the equal treatment of both in terms of any individual session, and so on.

Reference: *Psychiatry: An evidence-based text*, **Ch. 63.**

3.

(i) **e**

(ii) **d**

(iii) **a** – If a partner is suffering from his/her own psychopathology, then some cognitive-behaviour work

may help his/her partner to cope with them, e.g. in maintaining social skills.

(iv) **a**

Reference: *Psychiatry: An evidence-based text*, **Ch. 63.**

4.

(i) **b** – Each partner's experience is seen in the context of attachment reactions.

(ii) **a**

(iii) **e** – Characteristically, the couple will experience this emptiness as though it were full of demands, expectations, prohibitions and punishments, so revealing their unconscious relating.

Reference: *Psychiatry: An evidence-based text*, **Ch. 63.**

5.

(i) **d**

(ii) **a**

(iii) **b**

(iv) **e**

Reference: *Psychiatry: An evidence-based text*, **Ch. 63.**

6.

(i) **d**

(ii) **e** – These sources of input into the couple system may, for example, be from social services, schools and other extended family members.

(iii) **b** – An example would be one partner pursuing/attacking and the other withdrawing/avoiding.

(iv) **d**

Reference: *Psychiatry: An evidence-based text*, **Ch. 63.**

Chapter 64

Group therapy

QUESTIONS

Note that for answers to extended matching items (EMIs), each option (denoted a, b, c, etc.) might be used once, more than once or not at all. For multiple-choice questions (MCQs), please select the best answer.

1. **MCQ** – Select one incorrect statement regarding group dynamics:
   (a) According to Mills, group norms exist in symbolic form in the mind, and are elements of group culture.
   (b) Group interaction sustained over time tends to become highly flexible and unpredictable.
   (c) Hare studied the process of interaction in small groups and found that much human behaviour in groups is directed to solving problems.
   (d) Mills considers group norms as a set of statements about feelings and behaviour; they are cognitive and moral statements.
   (e) Mills considers that, as statements, group norms are distinct from feelings and from behaviour.

2. **EMI** – Concepts in group psychotherapy
   (a) Balint group
   (b) Group cohesion
   (c) Group norm
   (d) None of the above

From the above list, select the option with which each of the following concepts in group psychotherapy is best associated:
   (i) Considered by Yalom to be the group counterpart to the therapeutic relationship in individual psychotherapy.
   (ii) A force, pressure or interpersonal glue that attracts individuals to, and involves and maintains them in, the group.
   (iii) A naïve subject placed in a group situation was asked to match the perceived length of a line, drawn on a piece of paper in front of him, to one of three other lines drawn on another piece of paper. The other group members were confederates of the experimenter and gave the wrong answer. There is pressure on the subject to answer incorrectly.
   (iv) A group of junior doctors meets weekly during their psychiatry rotation with a senior consultant psychiatrist in psychotherapy. The task of the group is to give the doctors an opportunity to present case material in order to reflect on their interactions with their patients and other staff from a psychodynamic perspective.

3. **EMI** – Developments in group psychotherapy
   (a) Bion
   (b) Foulkes
   (c) Freud
   (d) Pratt
   (e) Yalom

From the above list, select the person with whom each of the following historical developments in group psychotherapy is best associated:
   (i) Conducted thought-action clinics in which he lectured groups of patients with tuberculosis
   (ii) Wrote *The Theory and Practice of Group Psychotherapy*
   (iii) Wrote *Experiences in Groups*.

4. **MCQ** – Select the best option. Which of the following is not one of Yalom's therapeutic factors in group psychotherapy?
   (a) Altruism
   (b) Catharsis
   (c) Differential behaviour
   (d) Instillation of hope
   (e) Interpersonal learning.

5. **EMI** – Phenomena experienced during group psychotherapy
   (a) Altruism
   (b) Catharsis
   (c) Differential behaviour
   (d) Existential factors
   (e) Instillation of hope
   (f) Interpersonal learning
   (g) Universality

From the above list, select the concept with which each of the following phenomena experienced by patients during group psychotherapy is best associated:
   (i) The experience of finding that one is not a

unique, irreparably damaged, repulsive or unworthy individual

(ii) The shared experience of deep feeling

(iii) The experience of finding that, however low one's self-esteem, something one says to another group member is perceived as extremely valuable by the recipient.

ANSWERS

1. b

Group interaction sustained over time becomes highly structured and predictable.

Reference: Psychiatry: An evidence-based text, **pp. 974–975.**

2.

(i)   b
(ii) b
(iii) c – Asch studied the effects of group (normative) pressure on members' perceptions of an obvious, clearly visible situation, such as this one.
(iv) a

Reference: Psychiatry: An evidence-based text, **pp. 975–976.**

3.

(i)   d – Through his charismatic leadership, Pratt taught the patients how to deal with their sputum and he attempted to inspire them to live with their illness. He observed the powerful impact of mutual encouragement and learning that developed among the group members.
(ii) e – The first edition was published in 1970.
(iii) a – This was first published in 1961.

Reference: Psychiatry: An evidence-based text, **pp. 977–979.**

4. c

Imitative behaviour is one of Yalom's therapeutic factors.

Reference: Psychiatry: An evidence-based text, **pp. 951, 978.**

5.

(i)   g
(ii) b
(iii) a

Reference: Psychiatry: An evidence-based text, **p. 978.**

Chapter 65

Cognitive-behavioural therapy

QUESTIONS

Note that for answers to extended matching items (EMIs), each option (denoted a, b, c, etc.) might be used once, more than once or not at all. For multiple-choice questions (MCQs), please select the best answer.

1. **MCQ** – Which of the following is not part of the five-areas assessment model used in cognitive-behavioural therapy?
   (a) Altered behaviour
   (b) Altered memory
   (c) Altered physical symptoms
   (d) Altered thinking
   (e) Life situation, relationships and practical problems.

2. **EMI** – Changes in thinking
   (a) Anxiety disorders
   (b) Depression
   (c) Neither of the above

From the above list, select the diagnosis, if any, with which each of the following characteristic changes in thinking of patients, from a cognitive-behavioural therapy perspective, is best associated:
   (i) Negative view of the world
   (ii) Decreased perception of their ability to cope with perceived danger
   (iii) Increased perception of danger and threat
   (iv) Negative view of self.

3. **EMI** – Cognitive processes
   (a) Anxiety disorders
   (b) Depression
   (c) Neither of the above

From the above list, select the diagnosis, if any, with which each of the following characteristic cognitive processes in patients, from a cognitive-behavioural therapy perspective, is best associated:
   (i) Impaired problem-solving skills.
   (ii) They take longer to retrieve positive memories and are more readily able to access negative memories.
   (iii) They are more prone to scan for potential threats.
   (iv) They are more prone to have lower thresholds for noticing potential threats.

4. **MCQ** – Select one incorrect statement regarding cognitive-behavioural therapy:
   (a) An example of a core belief is: 'If you don't please everyone, then they will be upset with you.'

   (b) Beck's seminal book on this subject was *Cognitive Therapy and the Emotional Disorders*.
   (c) It was developed by Aaron Beck in the 1960s.
   (d) Psychological patterns may be tackled by noticing thought patterns, correcting misconceptions and learning more helpful attitudes through processes such as reality-testing, introspection and learning.
   (e) The cognitive model states that it is our interpretation of a particular situation, rather than the situation itself, that may lead to distress.

5. **EMI** – Cognitive distortions
   (a) All-or-nothing thinking
   (b) Catastrophizing
   (c) Discounting the positive
   (d) Emotional reasoning
   (e) Labelling
   (f) Magnification
   (g) Mind-reading
   (h) Minimization
   (i) Over-generalization
   (j) Personalization
   (k) Selective abstraction

From the above list, select the cognitive distortion, associated with cognitive-behavioural therapy, with which each of the following examples is best associated:
   (i) 'Anyone can get a first-class honours degree in mathematics.'
   (ii) 'I did well in my last examination, but that was just luck.'
   (iii) 'They think that I can't do anything right.'

6. **EMI** – Cognitive distortions
   (a) All-or-nothing thinking
   (b) Catastrophizing
   (c) Discounting the positive
   (d) Emotional reasoning
   (e) Labelling
   (f) Magnification
   (g) Mind-reading
   (h) Minimization

(i) Over-generalization
(j) Personalization
(k) Selective abstraction

From the above list select the cognitive distortion, associated with cognitive-behavioural therapy, with which each of the following examples is best associated:

(i) 'Unless I do everything right, I am a failure.'
(ii) 'I can never do anything right.'
(iii) Giving a global description to oneself, such as 'I am an idiot.'

7. **EMI** – Cognitive distortions
(a) Black-and-white thinking
(b) Catastrophizing
(c) Discounting the positive
(d) Emotional reasoning
(e) Labelling
(f) Magnification
(g) Mind-reading
(h) Minimization
(i) Over-generalization
(j) Personalization
(k) Selective abstraction

From the above list, select the cognitive distortion, associated with cognitive-behavioural therapy, with which each of the following examples is best associated:

(i) Having made just one mistake, thinking 'That [one] arithmetical mistake in my maths paper means that I am a bad student.'
(ii) 'My colleague didn't stop to talk to me – maybe I've done something wrong.'
(iii) 'If I fail this exam, I'll never get a job.'
(iv) Thinking that something is true just because it 'feels' true.

ANSWERS

1. b

The missing area is altered feelings (or emotions or mood). These are illustrated in Figure 65.1 on page 985 of the accompanying textbook.

Reference: Psychiatry: An evidence-based text, **p. 985.**

2.

(i)   b
(ii) a
(iii) a
(iv) b

Reference: Psychiatry: An evidence-based text, **p. 985.**

3.

(i)   b
(ii) b
(iii) a
(iv) a

Reference: Psychiatry: An evidence-based text, **p. 985.**

4. a

Core beliefs are said to be beliefs and statements that the individual makes about the self or the world. They tend to be global, over-generalized and absolute. In contrast, the example given falls into the category of conditional assumptions/dysfunctional assumptions/beliefs/rules; these are deeper-seated than automatic thoughts and are 'understandings about how the world works'.

Reference: Psychiatry: An evidence-based text, **Ch. 65.**

5.

(i)   h – A way of manipulating the evidence by minimizing the positives about a given situation.
(ii) c – Positive experiences or qualities are frequently discounted.
(iii) g – Believing that you know what other people are thinking.

Reference: Psychiatry: An evidence-based text, **p. 987.**

6.

(i)   a – A situation is viewed under only two categories rather than on a continuum.
(ii) i – Assuming that, because something has happened once, it will happen again.
(iii) e

Reference: Psychiatry: An evidence-based text, **p. 987.**

7.

(i)   k – Being unable to see the whole picture, and instead focusing on one particular detail ('mental filter').
(ii) j – Believing that other people's actions are because of you or something that you have done.
(iii) b – Predicting the worst possible consequences without considering other possible outcomes.
(iv) d

Reference: Psychiatry: An evidence-based text, **p. 987.**

Chapter 66

Other individual psychotherapies

QUESTIONS

Note that for answers to extended matching items (EMIs), each option (denoted a, b, c, etc.) might be used once, more than once or not at all. For multiple-choice questions (MCQs), please select the best answer.

1. **MCQ** – Select the best option. Which of the following is not conventionally considered to be one of the arts therapies?
   (a) Art therapy
   (b) Dance therapy
   (c) Music therapy
   (d) Psychodrama
   (e) None of the above (i.e. all of the above are arts therapies).

2. **MCQ** – Which of the following is not a stage of a separation differentiation that is common in art therapy?
   (a) Acknowledgement
   (b) Assimilation
   (c) Familiarization
   (d) Isolation
   (e) Repetition.

3. **MCQ** – Select one incorrect statement regarding art therapy and music therapy:
   (a) Art therapy can involve sculpture.
   (b) In image art psychotherapy, free expression, spontaneous expression and thematic drawings are utilized simultaneously.
   (c) In music therapy, live music-making requires the use of a musical instrument or tuned/untuned percussion.
   (d) Music and musical pauses induce cardiovascular and respiratory changes in the listener.
   (e) The Conversational Model may be applied to art therapy; it is a developmental model in which what is said and done in therapy is aimed at promoting understanding.

4. **MCQ** – Blood and Zatorre used PET to investigate the neural correlates of responses to listening to 'shivers-down-the-spine' ('chills')-inducing music. Select one incorrect statement regarding this work:
   (a) An example of the type of music was Barber's *Adagio for Strings*.
   (b) As the intensity of 'chills' increased, cerebral blood flow changes occurred in brain regions thought to be involved in reward/motivation, emotion and arousal.
   (c) There was an associated increase in cardiac rate.
   (d) There was an associated reduction in depth of respiration.
   (e) There were associated electromyographic changes.

5. **MCQ** – Unless otherwise stated, the following options refer to humans. Select one incorrect statement regarding the Mozart effect:
   (a) EEG studies have shown that the Mozart effect is associated with right frontal and left temporoparietal coherent activity.
   (b) In pre-school children, extended exposure to learning and playing music by Mozart and Beethoven has been found to be associated with improved spatiotemporal reasoning that was still present 24 hours later.
   (c) Listening to Mozart's K448 has been found to be associated with better scores on IQ spatial reasoning tasks.
   (d) Patients with seizures have not been found to show a significant reduction in epileptiform activity in association with listening to Mozart.
   (e) The Mozart effect has been found to occur in rats.

6. **EMI** – Psychotherapies
   (a) Gestalt therapy
   (b) Narrative therapy
   (c) Person-centred therapy
   (d) Personal construct therapy

From the above list, select the individual therapy with the development of which each of the following is best associated:
   (i) Carl Rogers
   (ii) George Kelly
   (iii) Michael White and David Epson
   (iv) Fritz Perls and colleagues.

7. **EMI** – Theoretical aspects
   (a) Gestalt therapy
   (b) Narrative therapy
   (c) Person-centred therapy
   (d) Personal construct therapy

From the above list, select the individual therapy that is best associated with each of the following theoretical aspects:

    (i) Includes the notion of dental/oral aggression

    (ii) Emphasizes the internal world of the client, who has lost touch with his actualizing tendency

    (iii) A person's processes are considered to be psychologically channelized by the ways in which he or she anticipates events.

8. **EMI** – Key concepts

    (a) Gestalt therapy

    (b) Narrative therapy

    (c) Person-centred therapy

    (d) Personal construct therapy

From the above list, select the individual therapy with which each of the following sets of key concepts is best associated:

    (i) We view the world via our construing 'goggles'.

    (ii) 'Self-stories' involve selective memory and are multi-stranded and often inconsistent.

    (iii) Clients are encouraged to 'taste' their experience.

9. **EMI** – Theoretical foundations

    (a) Gestalt therapy

    (b) Narrative therapy

    (c) Person-centred therapy

    (d) Personal construct therapy

From the above list, select the individual therapy that is best associated with each of the following theoretical foundations:

    (i) Based on constructive alternativism

    (ii) Roots in psychoanalysis

    (iii) Roots in family therapy and counselling

10. **EMI** – Key concepts

    (a) Gestalt therapy

    (b) Narrative therapy

    (c) Person-centred therapy

    (d) Personal construct therapy

From the above list, select the individual therapy with which each of the following sets of key concepts is best associated:

    (i) Four 'load-bearing walls'

    (ii) Cycle of experience

    (iii) Modulation corollary

    (iv) Unconditional positive regard is required for change to occur.

11. **MCQ** – Which of the following is least likely to be a key concept of personal construct theory?

    (a) Decision-making cycle

    (b) Fixed role therapy

    (c) Repertory grid technique

    (d) Re-storying conceptually to reorient

    (e) The ABC model.

ANSWERS

1. d

Reference: *Psychiatry: An evidence-based text*, **pp. 994.**

2. e

The final stage is disposal (of the artwork).

Reference: *Psychiatry: An evidence-based text*, **p. 995.**

3. d

Live music-making in music therapy can involve the subject's voice without a musical instrument.

Reference: *Psychiatry: An evidence-based text*, **pp. 994–996.**

4. d

There was an associated increase in depth of respiration.

Reference: *Psychiatry: An evidence-based text*, **p. 998.**

5. d

In a study by Hughes *et al.* (1998), in 23 out of 29 instances of being exposed to Mozart's K448, significant decreases in epileptiform activity were noted from patients, even in coma.

References: Hughes JR, Daaboul Y, Fino JJ, Shaw GL (1998) The 'Mozart effect' on epileptiform activity. *Clinical EEG* **29**: 109–19; *Psychiatry: An evidence-based text*, **pp. 998–999.**

6.

(i)   c
(ii) d
(iii) b
(iv) a – Other founders were Laura Perls, Ralph Hefferline and Paul Goodman.

Reference: *Psychiatry: An evidence-based text*, **p. 1001.**

7.

(i)   a
(ii) c
(iii) d

Reference: *Psychiatry: An evidence-based text*, **p. 1001.**

8.

(i)   c
(ii) b – Narratives are 'self-stories'.
(iii) a

Reference: *Psychiatry: An evidence-based text*, **p. 1001.**

9.

(i)   d – In this, humans are considered to act on the world rather than to respond to it.
(ii) a
(iii) b

Reference: *Psychiatry: An evidence-based text*, **p. 1001.**

10.

(i)   a – These are phenomenological method, dialogical relationship, field-theoretical strategies and experimental freedom.
(ii) d
(iii) d
(iv) c

Reference: *Psychiatry: An evidence-based text*, **p. 1001.**

11. d

This is associated with narrative therapy.

Reference: *Psychiatry: An evidence-based text*, **p. 1001.**

Chapter 67

Therapeutic communities

QUESTION

For multiple-choice questions (MCQs), please select the best answer.

1. **MCQ** – Select one incorrect statement regarding therapeutic communities:
   (a) Patients are not viewed as experts in their own condition.
   (b) Research evidence shows their health economic benefits.
   (c) There is a body of research evidence regarding their effectiveness, particularly for personality disorder.
   (d) They are set up to maximize feedback, particularly from the peer group.
   (e) Working at Northfield Hospital, Birmingham, Tom Main coined the term therapeutic community.

ANSWER

1. a

Therapeutic communities have for a long time viewed their patients as 'expert' in their own condition, a view increasingly recognized as important by health systems.

Reference: *Psychiatry: An evidence-based text*, **Ch. 67.**

Chapter 68

Effectiveness of psychotherapy

QUESTIONS

Note that for answers to extended matching items (EMIs), each option (denoted a, b, c, etc.) might be used once, more than once or not at all. For multiple-choice questions (MCQs), please select the best answer.

1. **MCQ** – Select one incorrect statement regarding the effectiveness of psychotherapy:
   (a) Dialectical behavioural therapy (DBT) has been shown to be highly efficacious in treating depression.
   (b) DBT has been shown to be highly efficacious in treating suicidality and self-harm in borderline women.
   (c) Meta-analyses entered the medical field via the psychotherapies.
   (d) The literature on randomized controlled trials clearly identifies behavioural and cognitive-behavioural treatments as highly efficacious in the treatment of anxiety disorders.
   (e) There appears to be a bias against publishing negative studies; the effect sizes associated with published studies are significantly larger than those of unpublished investigations in psychotherapy.

2. **MCQ** – Select the correct option. The National Institute of Mental Health (NIMH) Treatment of Depression Collaborative Research Program randomized moderately to severely depressed patients to receive cognitive-behavioural psychotherapy, interpersonal psychotherapy, imipramine plus clinical management, or placebo plus clinical management. Clinical management consisted of a weekly meeting of 20–30 min to discuss medication, side-effects and the patient's clinical status. What was the overall outcome post-therapy?
   (a) The cognitive-behavioural psychotherapy group showed significantly more improvement than the interpersonal psychotherapy group, which in turn was not significantly different from the imipramine plus clinical management group.
   (b) The interpersonal psychotherapy group showed significantly more improvement than the cognitive-behavioural psychotherapy group, which in turn was not significantly different from the imipramine plus clinical management group.
   (c) The cognitive-behavioural psychotherapy group showed significantly more improvement than the interpersonal psychotherapy group, which in turn showed significantly more improvement than the imipramine plus clinical management group.
   (d) There were no significant differences between the two psychotherapy groups or between the psychotherapy groups and the imipramine plus clinical management group.
   (e) There were no significant differences between all four groups.

3. **MCQ** – Which of the following therapist factors has a significant effect on patient outcome following psychotherapy when the patient is not disturbed?
   (a) Age
   (b) Ethnicity
   (c) Experience
   (d) Gender
   (e) None of the above.

ANSWERS

1. a

DBT has not been shown to be highly efficacious in the treatment of depression.

Reference: *Psychiatry: An evidence-based text,* **pp. 1010–1012.**

2. d

Reference: *Psychiatry: An evidence-based text,* **p. 1011.**

3. e

None of these four therapist factors leads to a significant difference in patient outcome. Research findings suggest that the therapist's age, gender and ethnicity appear to have little or no impact on results, and nor are there significant differences in outcome when therapist and client are matched on these variables. A meta-analysis of 125 studies found that there was no correlation between dropout rate and the therapist's experience in years or professional qualifications – although there is some evidence that experience becomes a more important predictor of outcome with patients who are more disturbed.

Reference: *Psychiatry: An evidence-based text,* **p. 1013.**

PART 6

Clinical specialities

Chapter 69

Addiction psychiatry

QUESTIONS

Note that for answers to extended matching items (EMIs), each option (denoted a, b, c, etc.) might be used once, more than once or not at all. For multiple-choice questions (MCQs), please select the best answer.

1. **EMI** – Binding sites in substance misuse
   (a) Bind to G-protein-coupled receptors
   (b) Interact with ionotropic receptors or ion channels
   (c) Target monoamine transporters
   (d) None of the above

   From the above list, select the binding site with which each of the following misused substances is best associated:
   (i) Alcohol
   (ii) Cannabinoids
   (iii) Cocaine
   (iv) GBH.

2. **MCQ** – Substance misuse in personality disorder is not associated with which of the following?
   (a) Dropout from treatment
   (b) Increased HIV-risk behaviours
   (c) Increased infection rates
   (d) No change in social functioning
   (e) Psychiatric problems.

3. **EMI** – Legal classification of drugs
   (a) Class A
   (b) Class B
   (c) Class C
   (d) Class D
   (e) Class E
   (f) None of the above

   From the above list, select the class, if any, under the British Misuse of Drugs Regulations (2001), in which each of the following drugs is found:
   (i) Codeine
   (ii) Anabolic steroids
   (iii) Cocaine
   (iv) Ecstasy.

4. **EMI** – Legal classification of drugs
   (a) Schedule 1
   (b) Schedule 2
   (c) Schedule 3
   (d) Schedule 4, part I
   (e) Schedule 4, part II

   (f) Schedule 5
   (g) None of the above

   From the above list, select the schedule, if any, under the British Misuse of Drugs Regulations (2001) in which each of the following drugs is found:
   (i) Cannabis
   (ii) Anabolic steroids
   (iii) Cocaine
   (iv) Zolpidem.

5. **EMI** – Binding sites in substance misuse
   (a) Bind to G-protein-coupled receptors
   (b) Interact with ionotropic receptors or ion channels
   (c) Target monoamine transporters
   (d) None of the above

   From the above list, select the binding site with which each of the following misused substances is best associated:
   (i) Amphetamines
   (ii) Benzodiazepines
   (iii) MDMA
   (iv) Nicotine
   (v) Opioids.

6. **MCQ** – Select one incorrect statement. The ICD-10 criteria for 'F10.0 Acute intoxication due to use of alcohol' require the presence of at least one of the following features of dysfunctional behaviour:
   (a) Aggression
   (b) Argumentativeness
   (c) Depressed mood
   (d) Impaired attention
   (e) Interference with personal functioning.

7. **MCQ** – Select one incorrect statement. The ICD-10 criteria for 'F10.0 Acute intoxication due to use of alcohol' require the presence of at least one of the following signs:
   (a) Conjunctival injection
   (b) Nystagmus
   (c) Slurred speech
   (d) Tremor
   (e) Unsteady gait.

8. **MCQ** – Select one incorrect option. To make a diagnosis of substance abuse, DSM-IV-TR requires that at least one of the following should occur within a 12-month period:
   (a) Continued substance abuse despite having persistent or recurrent social or interpersonal problems caused or exacerbated by the effects of the substance
   (b) Recurrent substance-related financial difficulties
   (c) Recurrent substance-related legal problems
   (d) Recurrent substance use resulting in a failure to fulfil major role obligations at work, school, or home
   (e) Recurrent substance use resulting in situations in which it is physically hazardous.

9. **MCQ** – Select one incorrect option. To make a diagnosis of substance dependence, DSM-IV-TR requires that at least three of the following should have been experienced or exhibited at any time in the same 12-month period:
   (a) A great deal of time is spent in activities necessary to obtain the substance, use the substance, or recover from its effects.
   (b) The substance is often taken in larger amounts over a longer period than was intended.
   (c) There is a persistent desire or unsuccessful efforts to cut down or control substance use.
   (d) Tolerance defined by either a need for markedly increased amounts of the substance to achieve intoxication or desired effect, or markedly diminished effect with continued use of the same amount of the substance.
   (e) Withdrawal as manifested by the characteristic withdrawal syndrome for the substance and the same (or closely related) substance being taken to relieve or avoid withdrawal symptoms.

10. **MCQ** – Select one incorrect option. To make a diagnosis of alcohol withdrawal, DSM-IV-TR requires that at least two of the following should develop within several hours to a few days after cessation of (or reduction in) alcohol use that has been heavy and prolonged:
    (a) Autonomic hyperactivity
    (b) Increased hand tremor
    (c) Insomnia
    (d) Nausea or vomiting
    (e) Slurred speech.

11. **EMI** – Alcohol withdrawal syndrome
    (a) Mild alcohol withdrawal
    (b) Moderate alcohol withdrawal
    (c) Severe alcohol withdrawal
    (d) None of the above

From the above list, select the severity, if any, of alcohol withdrawal syndrome with which each of the following is best associated:
   (i) Hallucinosis but an otherwise clear sensorium
   (ii) Disorientation, agitation, hallucinations and autonomic derangement
   (iii) Tremulousness, anxiety, nausea, vomiting, sweating, hyper-reflexia and autonomic hyperactivity.

12. **MCQ** – Select the best option. Which of the following is true of Wernicke's encephalopathy?
    (a) A global confusional state is a characteristic feature.
    (b) Ataxia is a characteristic feature.
    (c) It is a medical emergency.
    (d) Ocular abnormalities are a characteristic feature.
    (e) All of the above.

13. **MCQ** – Select one incorrect statement regarding alcoholic liver disease:
    (a) Alcoholic fatty liver may be asymptomatic or can present with right abdominal pain, nausea and vomiting, which resolve on abstinence.
    (b) AST activity is typically lower than that of ALT in alcoholic hepatitis.
    (c) In patients with poor liver function and a prothrombin time prolonged to a degree that precludes liver biopsy, the prognosis is poor.
    (d) Liver function tests may be normal in cirrhosis until the process is advanced; the diagnosis is confirmed by biopsy.
    (e) The early stages of alcoholic fatty liver characteristically produce no changes in liver function tests, other than those related to the direct effect of alcohol on liver function.

14. **MCQ** – Select one incorrect statement. Signs of opiate withdrawal typically include:
    (a) Constipation
    (b) Goose flesh, recurrent chills
    (c) Pupillary dilation
    (d) Restless sleep
    (e) Sneezing, yawning, runny eyes.

15. **MCQ** – Select one incorrect statement. Signs of cannabis intoxication typically include:
    (a) Conjunctival injection
    (b) Decreased appetite
    (c) Impaired judgement and attention
    (d) Impaired reaction time
    (e) Suspiciousness and paranoid ideation.

16. **MCQ** – Which of the following drugs is least appropriate for clinical use in opiate withdrawal?
    (a) A benzodiazepine
    (b) Buprenorphine
    (c) Clonidine
    (d) Lofexidine
    (e) Methadone.

17. **EMI** – Legal classification of drugs
    (a) Schedule 1
    (b) Schedule 2
    (c) Schedule 3
    (d) Schedule 4, part I

(e) Schedule 4, part II
(f) Schedule 5
(g) None of the above

From the above list select the Schedule, if any, under the British Misuse of Drugs Regulations (2001) in which each of the following drugs is found:

(i) Buprenorphine
(ii) Lysergide
(iii) Diamorphine
(iv) Temazepam.

18. **MCQ** – The key characteristics of the psychological intervention for the management of drug and alcohol misuse, known by the FRAMES acronym, do not include:

(a) Altered behaviour
(b) Empathy
(c) Feedback
(d) Menu
(e) Responsibility.

ANSWERS

1.

(i) b
(ii) a
(iii) c
(iv) a – GBH is gamma-hydroxybutyrate.

Reference: Psychiatry: An evidence-based text, **p. 1021.**

2. d

A review of the relationship between personality disorder and substance misuse concluded that approximately two-thirds of drug users in treatment have a personality disorder, with antisocial personality disorder being the most common.

Reference: Psychiatry: An evidence-based text, **p. 1023.**

3.

(i) b
(ii) c
(iii) a
(iv) a

Reference: Psychiatry: An evidence-based text, **p. 1024.**

4.

(i) a
(ii) e
(iii) b
(iv) d

Reference: Psychiatry: An evidence-based text, **p. 1024.**

5.

(i) c
(ii) b
(iii) c – MDMA (methylenedioxymethamphetamine) is ecstasy.
(iv) b
(v) a

Reference: Psychiatry: An evidence-based text, **p. 1021.**

6. c

The mood criterion is that of lability of mood. The other potential features include disinhibition and impaired judgement.

Reference: Psychiatry: An evidence-based text, **p. 1025.**

7. d

The other signs are difficulty in standing, decreased level of consciousness (e.g. stupor, coma) and flushed face.

Reference: Psychiatry: An evidence-based text, **p. 1025.**

8. b

Reference: Psychiatry: An evidence-based text, **p. 1026.**

9. e

This criterion is as follows. Withdrawal is manifested by either of the following:

- The characteristic withdrawal syndrome for the substance
- The same (or closely related) substance is taken to relieve or avoid withdrawal symptoms.

Reference: Psychiatry: An evidence-based text, **p. 1027.**

10. e

This criterion is a sign of alcohol intoxication. Other signs of alcohol withdrawal for this DSM-IV-TR criterion are as follows:

- Transient visual, tactile or auditory hallucinations or illusions
- Psychomotor agitation
- Anxiety
- Grand mal seizures.

Reference: Psychiatry: An evidence-based text, **pp. 1025–1028.**

11.

(i) b
(ii) c – Severe alcohol withdrawal takes place more than 24 hours and up to 5 days after stopping or decreasing alcohol intake. The autonomic derangement is typically severe.
(iii) b – Mild alcohol withdrawal occurs less than 24 hours after stopping or decreasing alcohol intake. The autonomic hyperactivity is typically minor.

Reference: Psychiatry: An evidence-based text, **p. 1028.**

12. e

Reference: Psychiatry: An evidence-based text, **p. 1028.**

13. b

AST (aspartate aminotransferase) activity is typically higher than that of ALT (alanine aminotransferase) in alcoholic hepatitis and Reye's syndrome, in contrast to most types of liver disease.

Reference: Psychiatry: An evidence-based text, **pp. 1028–1029.**

14. a

Diarrhoea, rather than constipation, is a typical feature of opiate withdrawal.

Reference: *Psychiatry: An evidence-based text*, **p. 1031.**

15. b

A typical feature of cannabis intoxication is increased appetite.

Reference: *Psychiatry: An evidence-based text*, **p. 1031.**

16. a

Benzodiazepines are not recommended by the British Association of Psychopharmacology or by The National Institute for Health and Clinical Excellence (NICE). In their 2007 clinical guidance (number 52) NICE do recommend, however, that:

If a person presenting for opioid detoxification is also benzodiazepine dependent, healthcare professionals should consider benzodiazepine detoxification. When deciding whether this should be carried out concurrently with, or separately from, opioid detoxification, healthcare professionals should take into account the person's preference and the severity of dependence for both substances.

NICE recommends that methadone or buprenorphine should be offered as the first-line treatment in opioid detoxification, while clonidine should not be used routinely in opioid detoxification. Lofexidine may be considered for people:

- who have made an informed and clinically appropriate decision not to use methadone or buprenorphine for detoxification
- who have made an informed and clinically appropriate decision to detoxify within a short time period
- with mild or uncertain dependence (including young people).

References: National Institute for Health and Clinical Excellence (2007) *Drug Misuse: Opioid Detoxification. NICE Clinical Guideline 52.* **London: NICE;** *Psychiatry: An evidence-based text,* **p. 1037.**

17.

(i) c
(ii) a – Schedule 1 includes drugs such as cannabis and lysergide which are not used medicinally.
(iii) b
(iv) c

Reference: *Psychiatry: An evidence-based text,* **p. 1024.**

18. a

The 'A' stands for advice, as in giving advice on how to change.

Reference: *Psychiatry: An evidence-based text,* **p. 1038.**

Chapter 70

Child and adolescent psychiatry

QUESTIONS

Note that for answers to extended matching items (EMIs), each option (denoted a, b, c, etc.) might be used once, more than once or not at all. For multiple-choice questions (MCQs), please select the best answer.

1. **MCQ** – Select one incorrect option. The following factors are associated with an increased risk of postnatal depression:
   (a) Having a sick baby
   (b) Maternal isolation and lack of social support during or after pregnancy
   (c) Older mothers compared with teenage mothers
   (d) Women who have experienced a low level of maternal care
   (e) Women who have experienced early maternal separation.

2. **EMI** – Rates of psychiatric disorders
   (a) 7 per cent
   (b) 12 per cent
   (c) 29 per cent
   (d) 44 per cent

This question concerns the classic Isle of Wight neuropsychiatric study published in book form by Rutter, Graham and Yule in 1970. From the above list, select the rate of psychiatric disorder with which each of the following groups was associated:
   (i) Children with idiopathic epilepsy
   (ii) Children with structural brain disorders
   (iii) Children free from physical disorders
   (iv) Children with non-cerebral physical disorders.

3. **EMI** – ICD-10 multi-axial framework for child and adolescent psychiatry
   (a) Axis I
   (b) Axis II
   (c) Axis III
   (d) Axis IV
   (e) Axis V
   (f) Axis VI
   (g) None of the above

From the above list, select the ICD-10 axis for child and adolescent psychiatry with which each of the following is best associated:
   (i) Clinical psychiatric disorders
   (ii) Medical conditions
   (iii) Intellectual level.

4. **EMI** – DSM-IV-TR multi-axial framework for child and adolescent psychiatry
   (a) Axis I
   (b) Axis II
   (c) Axis III
   (d) Axis IV
   (e) Axis V
   (f) Axis VI
   (g) None of the above

From the above list, select the DSM-IV-TR axis with which each of the following is best associated:
   (i) Developmental disorders
   (ii) Mental retardation
   (iii) Psychosocial and environmental factors.

5. **MCQ** – Select one incorrect statement regarding the Isle of Wight study of 10- and 11-year-olds by Rutter and colleagues:
   (a) 2.5 per cent had an emotional disorder.
   (b) 4 per cent had a conduct disorder.
   (c) 5.7 per cent had a physical disorder, with higher rates of psychiatric disorder being found in those with a physical disorder.
   (d) 6.8 per cent had a diagnosable psychiatric disorder.
   (e) The ratio of boys to girls among those with a psychiatric disorder was nearly 1:2.

6. **MCQ** – Select one incorrect statement regarding child protection:
   (a) One study found that Indian social work professionals did not consider physical 'maltreatment' to be as seriously abusive as did their American counterparts.
   (b) One study found that Indian social work professionals, more than American social work professionals, considered a wider range of adult sexual behaviours to be seriously abusive to children.
   (c) One study found that Indian social work professionals, more than American social work professionals, considered a wider range of media images to be seriously abusive to children.

(d) Sweden has outlawed all forms of corporal punishment of children.

(e) The rates of death from child maltreatment in Sweden are lower than those in Spain, Greece and Italy.

7. **MCQ** – Select one incorrect statement regarding common pre-school problems:

(a) Behavioural problems such as temper tantrums and sleeping and feeding difficulties are very common in pre-school children.

(b) Behavioural problems such as temper tantrums and sleeping and feeding in pre-school children are usually considered, not as psychiatric disorders, but rather as part of normal developmental variation.

(c) Childhood conduct disorder has a very good outcome; in the classic study by Robins, 5 per cent went on to develop an antisocial personality disorder.

(d) Conduct disorder is more common in boys than in girls.

(e) The three most significant associated factors in conduct disorder found in the Ontario Child Health Survey were family dysfunction, parental psychopathology and low income.

8. **MCQ** – Select one incorrect statement regarding attention-deficit hyperactivity disorder:

(a) Co-morbidity is high.

(b) Hyperactivity is a cardinal feature.

(c) Impulsiveness is a cardinal feature.

(d) Poor concentration is a cardinal feature.

(e) The DSM criteria are more stringent than the ICD criteria.

9. **MCQ** – Select one incorrect statement regarding school attendance problems:

(a) In the UK, the three main peaks for school refusal are at ages 5 years, 11 years and 14–16 years.

(b) School refusal is often associated with an emotional disorder.

(c) School refusal is significantly more common in girls than in boys.

(d) Truancy is often associated with a conduct disorder.

(e) Truants are significantly more commonly male.

10. **MCQ** – Select one incorrect statement. Common features of separation anxiety disorder in childhood include:

(a) Anxiety disorders are more commonly treated among children in lower-class families.

(b) It is commonly associated with social withdrawal.

(c) It presents as a preoccupying worry that something may happen to the principal attachment figure(s) or that something may lead to the child being traumatically separated from them.

(d) Nightmares are common associated symptoms.

(e) Unexplained physical symptoms are common.

11. **MCQ** – Select one incorrect statement regarding childhood and adolescent depression:

(a) It is considered amenable to treatment with antidepressants.

(b) It may affect 8–20 per cent of children and adolescents.

(c) It resembles adult depression.

(d) Its diagnostic criteria are the same as those for adults.

(e) SSRIs are a first-line treatment.

12. **MCQ** – Select one incorrect statement regarding childhood obsessive-compulsive disorder:

(a) First-line treatment is psychological and involves behavioural techniques such as exposure and response prevention.

(b) It is extremely rare in young children.

(c) Its point prevalence rises to approximately 0.6 per cent in 13- to 15-year-olds.

(d) When it presents in adolescence, boys predominate.

(e) When it presents in the early school years, boys predominate.

13. **MCQ** – Select one incorrect statement regarding childhood schizophrenia:

(a) After the age of 13 years, the incidence rises rapidly during adolescence; the teenage prevalence is around two to three per 1000.

(b) Developmental abnormalities, dyspraxia, dyslexia and speech and language disorders are more common in people who subsequently develop early-onset schizophrenia.

(c) In children and adolescents, scholastic ability and self-care may be affected and could be the first signs of a developing psychosis.

(d) Most studies have found that 80–90 per cent of adolescents diagnosed with schizophrenia still had the diagnosis several years later.

(e) Negative symptoms may be present but are rarer in younger patients.

14. **MCQ** – DSM-IV-TR pervasive developmental disorders do not include which of the following subcategories?

(a) Asperger's syndrome

(b) Autistic disorder

(c) Childhood disintegrative disorder

(d) Rett's disorder

(e) Specific developmental disorders.

15. **MCQ** – Select one incorrect statement regarding enuresis:

(a) A behavioural programme should be tried first in childhood enuresis.

(b) At the age of 7 years, nocturnal enuresis is more common in boys.

(c) By the age of 18 years, around 1 per cent of males and a lower proportion of females have nocturnal enuresis.

(d) Childhood and adolescence nocturnal enuresis rarely leads to any lasting problems and is not considered an indicator for mental health problems in later life.

(e) Nocturnal enuresis is about twice as common in monozygotic twins as in dizygotic twins.

16. **MCQ** – Select one incorrect statement regarding child and adolescent psychiatry:

(a) Adolescent depression is associated with a high risk of depressive relapse extending into the third decade.

(b) At 10–12 years of age, faecal incontinence is much commoner in boys.

(c) Overall, the history of any anxiety disorder in childhood or adolescence is associated with a significant increase in risk for an anxiety disorder occurring in adult life, with the specificity for the same condition recurring in adulthood being high.

(d) Tourette's syndrome has a high co-morbidity, particularly with attention-deficit hyperactivity disorder and obsessive-compulsive disorder.

(e) Tourette's syndrome is rare, with a prevalence rate of about 4.5 per 10 000 among 16- and 17-year-olds.

17. **EMI** – ICD-10 multi-axial framework for child and adolescent psychiatry

(a) Axis I
(b) Axis II
(c) Axis III
(d) Axis IV
(e) Axis V
(f) Axis VI
(g) None of the above

From the above list, select the ICD-10 axis with which each of the following is best associated:

(i) Abnormal psychosocial conditions
(ii) Specific disorders of development
(iii) Global social functioning.

ANSWERS

1. c

Teenage mothers are more likely than older women to have an insecure attachment and are more likely to experience postnatal depression.

Reference: *Psychiatry: An evidence-based text*, **p. 1049**.

2.

(i)   c
(ii) d
(iii) a
(iv) b

Reference: *Psychiatry: An evidence-based text*, **p. 1052**.

3.

(i)   a
(ii) d
(iii) c

Reference: *Psychiatry: An evidence-based text*, **p. 1053**.

4.

(i)   a – Axis I also includes clinical disorders and learning disorders.
(ii) b
(iii) d

Reference: *Psychiatry: An evidence-based text*, **pp. 1053–1054**.

5. e

This ratio was approximately 2:1.

Reference: *Psychiatry: An evidence-based text*, **p. 1054**.

6. e

In spite of the truth of option 'd', rate of death from child maltreatment in Sweden is much higher than those in Spain, Greece and Italy; the last three countries have not outlawed corporal punishment but do have family-oriented cultures.

Reference: *Psychiatry: An evidence-based text*, **p. 1056**.

7. c

In this study, 45 per cent of children with conduct disorder went on to develop an antisocial personality disorder. Disturbance of conduct is a significant risk factor for substance abuse. Those individuals who manifest disturbances of conduct earlier in life go on to commit more severe criminal offences.

Reference: *Psychiatry: An evidence-based text*, **pp. 1058–1059**.

8. e

It is the other way around.

Reference: *Psychiatry: An evidence-based text*, **p. 1059**.

9. c

School refusal is approximately equally common in boys and girls.

Reference: *Psychiatry: An evidence-based text*, **p. 1060**.

10. a

In spite of being more common in lower social classes, anxiety disorders are more commonly treated among children in middle- and upper-class families.

Reference: *Psychiatry: An evidence-based text*, **pp. 1060–1061**.

11. e

SSRIs confer little, if any, benefit in under-18s with depression, while exposing them to small but significant risks, in particular of precipitating suicidal ideation.

Reference: *Psychiatry: An evidence-based text*, **pp. 1061–1062**.

12. d

Obsessive-compulsive disorder seems to present at two stages; in adolescence, girls predominate.

Reference: *Psychiatry: An evidence-based text*, **p. 1062**.

13. d

The majority of studies have found that 50 per cent or more of adolescents diagnosed with schizophrenia are found to have no illness or a different, less severe, diagnosis on follow-up.

Reference: *Psychiatry: An evidence-based text*, **pp. 1062–1063**.

14. e

Specific developmental disorders are differentiated from pervasive developmental disorders and general learning difficulties.

Reference: *Psychiatry: An evidence-based text*, **pp. 1066–1067**.

15. a

Prior to treatment, the management should include the exclusion of physical causes.

Reference: *Psychiatry: An evidence-based text*, **p. 1067**.

16. c

The specificity of the same condition recurring in adulthood is low.

Reference: *Psychiatry: An evidence-based text*, **pp. 1067–1069**.

17.

(i) e
(ii) b
(iii) f

Reference: *Psychiatry: An evidence-based text*, p. 1053.

Chapter 71

Learning disability psychiatry

QUESTIONS

Note that for answers to extended matching items (EMIs), each option (denoted a, b, c, etc.) might be used once, more than once or not at all. For multiple-choice questions (MCQs), please select the best answer.

1. **MCQ** – Select one correct statement regarding moderate learning disability:
   (a) A person with moderate learning disability might be expected to have minimal or no physical or sensory problems, to hold down sheltered employment and to survive with limited support.
   (b) It corresponds to an approximate mental age of 6–9 years in adulthood.
   (c) It corresponds to an IQ range of 20–34.
   (d) It represents approximately 80 per cent of people with learning disability.
   (e) None of the above.

2. **MCQ** – Select the best statement regarding the IQ distribution of a human population:
   (a) It follows a binomial distribution.
   (b) It follows a normal distribution.
   (c) It follows a normal distribution with bulges in both the upper and lower ranges.
   (d) It follows a normal distribution with a bulge in the lower range.
   (e) It follows a normal distribution with a bulge in the upper range.

3. **EMI** – Genetic causes of learning disability
   (a) Autosomal dominant
   (b) Autosomal recessive
   (c) Trisomy
   (d) None of the above

   From the above list select the genetic cause, if any, with which each of the following potential causes of learning disability is best associated:
   (i) Down syndrome
   (ii) Sanfilippo syndrome
   (iii) Tuberose sclerosis
   (iv) Phenylketonuria
   (v) Aspartylglycosaminuria.

4. **MCQ** – Select one incorrect statement regarding learning disability psychiatry:
   (a) Alcohol abuse is less common in people with learning disability than in the non-learning-disabled population.
   (b) Drug abuse is less common in people with learning disability than in the non-learning-disabled population.
   (c) Epilepsy is much more common in those with learning disability than in the non-learning-disabled population.
   (d) In the West, there is a much higher level of divorce in families where there is a child with Down syndrome than in families with other birth defects and in those of children with no identifiable disability.
   (e) Suicide is relatively rare among adults with learning disability.

5. **MCQ** – In the Neuroleptics in Adults with Aggressive Challenging Behaviour and Intellectual Disability study by Tyrer *et al.*, published in 2008, a randomized controlled trial compared risperidone, haloperidol and placebo in the treatment of aggressive challenging behaviour in people with intellectual disability. Which treatment group showed the significantly best response at a 4-week follow-up?
   (a) Haloperidol
   (b) Placebo
   (c) Risperidone
   (d) Risperidone and haloperidol were approximately equally significantly better than placebo
   (e) There was no significant advantage in any of the three treatment groups.

6. **EMI** – Conditions associated with learning disability
   (a) Autism
   (b) Down syndrome
   (c) Fetal alcohol syndrome
   (d) Fragile X syndrome
   (e) None of the above

From the above list of specific conditions associated with learning disability, select the option with which each of the following sets of physical signs is best associated:

(i) Short stature, a single palmar crease, congenital heart abnormalities and a characteristic facial appearance

(ii) Narrow receding forehead and 'rail track' ears

(iii) Long thin face and large ears, with large testicles after puberty. There may be a wider connective tissue disorder, with lax joints, flat feet and mitral valve prolapse.

7. **EMI** – Conditions associated with learning disability
   (a) Autism
   (b) Down syndrome
   (c) Fetal alcohol syndrome
   (d) Fragile X syndrome
   (e) None of the above

Select the option from the above list with which each of the following features is best associated:

(i) First described in 1973. May be seen in about one in 500 births in the USA

(ii) Originally described by Kanner in 1943

(iii) Perhaps the most common cause of inherited mental handicap. It affects one in 4000 males and one in 8000 females and is associated with a wide range of learning disability

(iv) The risk increases dramatically with increasing maternal age, rising from about one in 1000 in a 20-year-old mother to about 40 times this rate for a 45-year-old mother.

8. **MCQ** – Which of the following is specifically a tool to look at daily living skills and which can be used with learning disability subjects?
   (a) ABAS
   (b) ARNSMR
   (c) DASH
   (d) PAS ADD
   (e) PIMRA.

9. **EMI** – Disorders associated with learning disability
   (a) Down syndrome
   (b) Fragile X syndrome
   (c) Prader–Willi syndrome
   (d) Smith–Magenis syndrome
   (e) None of the above

From the above list of disorders associated with learning disability, select the option with which each of the following behavioural phenotypes is best associated:

(i) Very demanding behaviour, severe temper tantrums, hyperactivity, aggression, self-injurious behaviour, sleeping problems, head-banging and finger-biting

(ii) Excessive eating, short stature and neonatal hypotonia

(iii) Autistic features, rapid and dysrhythmic speech, anxiety, hand-flapping or hand-biting, shyness and avoidance of eye contact.

10. **EMI** – Disorders associated with learning disability
    (a) Cornelia de Lange syndrome
    (b) Down syndrome
    (c) Fragile X syndrome
    (d) Lesch-Nyan syndrome
    (e) Tuberose sclerosis

From the above list of disorders associated with learning disability, select the option with which each of the following behavioural phenotypes is best associated:

(i) Self-mutilation following spasticity and choreoathetosis

(ii) Sleep problems, hyperactivity and non-compliant obsessiveness

(iii) Hyperactivity, anxiety, compulsions, self-injurious behaviour and autistic features.

ANSWERS

1. b

Reference: *Psychiatry: An evidence-based text*, Ch. 71.

2. d

IQ is normally distributed, but with a slight bulge in the lower IQ range, as shown in Figure 71.1 on page 1081 of the accompanying textbook.

Reference: *Psychiatry: An evidence-based text*, pp. 1080–1081.

3.

(i) c – Trisomy 21 is the most common cause.
(ii) b
(iii) a
(iv) b
(v) b

Reference: *Psychiatry: An evidence-based text*, p. 1082.

4. d

Recent research has reported lower levels of divorce in families where there is a child with Down syndrome than in families with other birth defects and those of children with no identifiable disability.

Reference: *Psychiatry: An evidence-based text*, pp. 1080–1083.

5. e

The authors concluded that the routine prescription of antipsychotic drugs early in the management of aggressive challenging behaviour, even in low doses, should no longer by regarded as a satisfactory form of care.

Reference: *Psychiatry: An evidence-based text*, p. 1085.

6.

(i) b – A photograph of a woman with Down syndrome is shown in Figure 71.4 on page 1087 of the accompanying textbook.
(ii) c – Photographs of boys with fetal alcohol syndrome are shown in Figures 71.2 and 71.3 on pages 1086 and 1087, respectively, of the accompanying textbook.
(iii) d – A photograph of an affected boy and girl is shown in Figure 71.5 on page 1088 of the accompanying textbook.

Reference: *Psychiatry: An evidence-based text*, pp. 1086–1089.

7.

(i) c
(ii) a
(iii) d
(iv) b

Reference: *Psychiatry: An evidence-based text*, pp. 1086–1089.

8. a

This is the Adaptive Behaviour Assessment System.

Reference: *Psychiatry: An evidence-based text*, Ch. 71.

9.

(i) d
(ii) c
(iii) b

Reference: *Psychiatry: An evidence-based text*, p. 1091.

10.

(i) d
(ii) e
(iii) a

Reference: *Psychiatry: An evidence-based text*, p. 1091.

Chapter 72

Old-age psychiatry

QUESTIONS

Note that for answers to extended matching items (EMIs), each option (denoted a, b, c, etc.) might be used once, more than once or not at all. For multiple-choice questions (MCQs), please select the best answer.

1. **MCQ** – Of the following, which is the most common cause of dementia in elderly people in the Western world?
   (a) Creutzfeldt–Jakob disease
   (b) Huntington's disease
   (c) Lewy body disease
   (d) Normal-pressure hydrocephalus
   (e) Parkinson's disease.

2. **EMI** – Causes of dementia
   (a) Creutzfeldt–Jakob disease
   (b) Frontotemporal dementia
   (c) Huntington's disease
   (d) Lewy body disease
   (e) Vascular dementia

   From the above list, select the cause of dementia with which each of the following early neurological features is best associated:
   (i)   Parkinsonism
   (ii) Focal neurological signs
   (iii) Primitive reflexes
   (iv) Myoclonus
   (v)   Choreoathetoid movement.

3. **MCQ** – Deficiency of which of the following vitamins is most likely to be associated with dementia?
   (a) A
   (b) B6
   (c) C
   (d) Folate
   (e) K.

4. **MCQ** – In the UK, which of the following blood tests is not recommended as a routine screen by The National Institute for Health and Clinical Excellence (NICE) to identify any treatable causes or co-morbid conditions in a dementia, unless the history or clinical picture is of relevance?
   (a) Calcium level
   (b) Glucose level
   (c) Routine electrolyte screening
   (d) Syphilis screening
   (e) Thyroid function tests.

5. **MCQ** – Which of the following causes of dementia is most likely to have a similar presentation to delirium?
   (a) Alzheimer's disease
   (b) Creutzfeldt–Jakob disease
   (c) Down syndrome
   (d) Huntington's disease
   (e) Lewy body dementia.

6. **MCQ** – The criteria for mild cognitive impairment by Peterson and colleagues (published in 2001) do not include which of the following?
   (a) 1.5 standard deviations below age-appropriate norms on memory tests or memory component of other cognitive tests
   (b) ADLs not significantly affected
   (c) Cognitive complaint, usually of memory
   (d) Not meeting DSM dementia criteria
   (e) Reduced general cognitive function (e.g. on the MMSE).

7. **MCQ** – Select one incorrect statement regarding dementia in the elderly:
   (a) Nearly one in four people over the age of 85 years in the UK have Alzheimer's disease
   (b) The AMTS can be used in the acute medical setting as a quick screening test for cognitive difficulties; it includes a list of 10 items
   (c) The number of people with Alzheimer's disease in the UK in 2007 was estimated to be around 417 000
   (d) The prevalence of dementia in adults increases with age, roughly doubling with every five-year increase over the entire age range from 30 years to over 95 years
   (e) Visual hallucinations should raise the suspicion of a delirium or Lewy body disease.

8. **MCQ** – Which of the following is the best for making a diagnosis of Alzheimer's disease?
   (a) ATMS
   (b) ICD-10 criteria

(c) MMSE

(d) NINCDS-ADRDA

(e) PET brain scan.

9. **MCQ** – Select one incorrect statement regarding dementia with Lewy bodies:

   (a) Alzheimer-type plaques are present in a similar density and distribution to those seen in Alzheimer's disease, but neurofibrillary tangles are less common.

   (b) Neuroleptic sensitivity may occur in around a third of cases.

   (c) Parkinsonism is present in up to 70 per cent of patients.

   (d) Patients tend to have less visuospatial impairment in the early stages than patients with Alzheimer's disease.

   (e) Visual hallucinations may occur and tend to be complex, often of people or animals.

10. **MCQ** – Which of the following is not a core component required to be present in the Lund–Manchester criteria for frontotemporal dementia?

    (a) Decline in personal hygiene and grooming

    (b) Early decline in social interpersonal conduct

    (c) Early impairment in regulation of personal conduct

    (d) Early loss of insight

    (e) Insidious onset and gradual progression.

11. **MCQ** – Select one incorrect statement regarding old-age psychiatry:

    (a) Drivers over the age of 70 years, in the UK, have the highest crash risk.

    (b) Frontotemporal dementia is the second commonest cause of early-onset dementia (< 65 years) after Alzheimer's disease.

    (c) Monitoring of electrolytes is advisable when treating the elderly with SSRIs owing to the risk of SIADH leading to hyponatraemia.

    (d) Partition delusions may occur in around two-thirds of patients with very-late-onset schizophrenia-like illness.

    (e) Space phobia is a relatively common type of phobia in elderly people.

ANSWERS

1. c

Reference: *Psychiatry: An evidence-based text*, **p. 1100.**

2.

(i)   d
(ii) e
(iii) b
(iv) a
(v)   c

Reference: *Psychiatry: An evidence-based text*, **p. 1101.**

3. d

Reference: *Psychiatry: An evidence-based text*, **p. 1100.**

4. d

Although this was routine in the past, the latest guidelines suggest doing this only if the history or clinical picture is of relevance.

Reference: *Psychiatry: An evidence-based text*, **p. 1101.**

5. e

There may be fluctuations in the level of consciousness and cognition.

Reference: *Psychiatry: An evidence-based text*, **p. 1102.**

6. e

Their criterion for this is normal general cognitive function (i.e. cognitive screening test), which should be in the normal range for the subject's age.

Reference: *Psychiatry: An evidence-based text*, **p. 1103.**

7. a

The actual proportion is nearly a half.

Reference: *Psychiatry: An evidence-based text*, **pp. 1100–1104.**

8. d

The NINCDS-ADRDA (National Institute of Neurological and Communicative Disorders and Stroke – Alzheimer's Disease and Related Disorders Association) criteria are the gold standard for the diagnosis of Alzheimer's disease. These criteria are summarized in Box 72.1 on page 1104 of the accompanying textbook.

Reference: *Psychiatry: An evidence-based text*, **p. 1104.**

9. d

They tend to have more visuospatial impairment and less memory impairment in the early stages than patients with Alzheimer's disease.

Reference: *Psychiatry: An evidence-based text*, **p. 1106.**

10. a

This is a supportive diagnostic feature. The missing core component criterion in the above list of options is early emotional blunting.

Reference: *Psychiatry: An evidence-based text*, **p. 1108.**

11. a

There is a slight increase in the crash risk in people over 70 years; the highest risk is in males aged 16–24 years.

Reference: *Psychiatry: An evidence-based text*, **Ch. 72.**

Chapter 73

Rehabilitation psychiatry

QUESTIONS

Note that for answers to extended matching items (EMIs), each option (denoted a, b, c, etc.) might be used once, more than once or not at all. For multiple-choice questions (MCQs), please select the best answer.

1. **EMI** – Development of rehabilitation psychiatry
   (a) Goffman, Erving
   (b) Leff, Julian
   (c) Mental After Care Association
   (d) Powell, Enoch
   (e) Tuke, William
   (f) None of the above

   From the above list, select the person or organization, if any, with which each of the following historical developments of rehabilitation psychiatry is best associated:
   (i) Opening of the Retreat in York
   (ii) The TAPS study
   (iii) Moral treatment
   (iv) Laid the foundations in the UK of organized aftercare for people discharged from a mental hospital.

2. **EMI** – Social inclusion in rehabilitation psychiatry
   (a) ↑
   (b) About the same
   (c) ↓

   From the above list, select the option with which each of the following is best associated in people with severe mental illness, compared with their peers:
   (i) Size of social networks
   (ii) Likelihood of being married
   (iii) Physical morbidity
   (iv) Likelihood of being the victims of crime.

3. **MCQ** – Select one incorrect statement regarding rehabilitation psychiatry:
   (a) Psychiatric rehabilitation focuses on strengths rather than weaknesses.
   (b) Psychiatric rehabilitation focuses on symptoms rather than function.
   (c) Rehabilitation can involve changing the environment in order to decrease the impact of illness at both the individual and the societal level.
   (d) Rehabilitation is an active process for the individual in acquiring attitudes and skills that allow the person to overcome the effects of an illness or disorder.

   (e) Stigma and discrimination refer to the effects of societal views towards mental illness and, according to John Wing, they can, in part, help us to understand the effects of mental illness on an individual.

4. **EMI** – Assessment tools in rehabilitation psychiatry
   (a) Camberwell Assessment of Need – Clinical Version
   (b) Health of the Nation Outcome Scale
   (c) Manchester Short Assessment of Quality of Life
   (d) Social Functioning Questionnaire
   (e) None of the above

   From the above list of assessment tools, select the option with which each of the following is best associated:
   (i) Covers 22 life domains and can incorporate the views of the assessor, user and carer. It identifies serious need and also incorporates the view of users as to what they would find useful support
   (ii) A summary outcome measure that focuses mainly on symptoms
   (iii) Composed of five eight-item scales, which assess a person's level of competence in a particular area.

5. **MCQ** – The pharmacological treatment of choice for treatment-resistant psychosis is:
   (a) Aripiprazole
   (b) Clozapine
   (c) ECT
   (d) Flupentixol decanoate (depot)
   (e) Risperidone (depot).

6. **EMI** – Stages of evaluation in a rehabilitation service
   (a) Audit of standards
   (b) Confirmation of efficacy in practice
   (c) Enquiry
   (d) Feasibility and acceptability
   (e) International dissemination
   (f) Intervention dissection
   (g) Outcome

   From the above list of evaluation stages (after Tyrer, 2006), select the option with which each of the following sets of tasks to be completed is best associated:

(i) Simple audit studies

(ii) Large randomized controlled trial

(iii) Exploratory trials (case–control and randomized).

7. **EMI** – Social inclusion in rehabilitation psychiatry

(a) ↑

(b) About the same

(c) ↓

From the above list select the option with which each of the following is best associated in people with severe mental illness, compared with their peers:

(i) Reciprocity of social networks

(ii) Likelihood of ending up in prison

(iii) Likelihood of cohabiting

(iv) Life expectancy.

8. **EMI** – Stages of evaluation in a rehabilitation service

(a) Audit of standards

(b) Confirmation of efficacy in practice

(c) Enquiry

(d) International dissemination

(e) Intervention dissection

(f) Outcome

(g) None of the above

From the above list of evaluation stages (after Tyrer, 2006), select the option with which each of the following sets of tasks to be completed is best associated:

(i) Constant monitoring

(ii) Follow-up of cohorts

(iii) Qualitative and observational studies

(iv) Policy and promotion.

ANSWERS

1.

(i) e – This was in 1796; William Tuke was a Quaker merchant.

(ii) b – The large-scale TAPS (Team for the Assessment of Psychiatric Services) study, led by Julian Leff, into the closure of Friern Hospital in north London, has confirmed that people do well with adequate support, even if discharged after decades of living in a hospital.

(iii) e

(iv) c – This was in 1869, 'to facilitate the readmission of the poor friendless convalescent from Lunatic Asylums into social life'. Almost a century later, as part of the UK government, Enoch Powell also dealt with provisions for the aftercare of patients with the large-scale closure of asylums.

Reference: *Psychiatry: An evidence-based text*, **p. 1120.**

2.

(i) c – i.e. on average their social networks are smaller.

(ii) c

(iii) a

(iv) a

Reference: *Psychiatry: An evidence-based text*, **p. 1120.**

3. b

It focuses on function rather than symptoms.

Reference: *Psychiatry: An evidence-based text*, **pp. 1121–1122.**

4.

(i) a

(ii) b

(iii) d – It assesses a person's level of competence in an area of social functioning.

Reference: *Psychiatry: An evidence-based text*, **p. 1124.**

5. b

The key to its successful use is management of its many side-effects.

Reference: *Psychiatry: An evidence-based text*, **p. 1124.**

6.

(i) d

(ii) b

(iii) f

Reference: *Psychiatry: An evidence-based text*, **p. 1129.**

7.

(i) c – i.e. on average their social networks are less reciprocal compared with the general population.

(ii) a

(iii) c

(iv) c

Reference: *Psychiatry: An evidence-based text*, **p. 1120.**

8.

(i) a

(ii) f

(iii) c

(iv) d

Reference: *Psychiatry: An evidence-based text*, **p. 1129.**

PART 7

Mental health service provision

Management of psychiatric services

QUESTION

Note that for answers to extended matching items (EMIs), each option (denoted a, b, c, etc.) might be used once, more than once or not at all.

1. **EMI** – Management of psychiatric services in the UK
   (a) NHS Plan
   (b) NSF
   (c) Neither of the above

From the above list select the option with which each of the following is better associated:
   (i) A strategic document for the development of adult mental health services; published in 1999
   (ii) Promoted new models of care and contained key targets and core standards for the health and social care sectors.

ANSWER

1.

(i) b

(ii) a – Published in 2000.

Reference: *Psychiatry: An evidence-based text*, **p. 1137**.

Chapter 75

Advice to special medical services

QUESTIONS

For multiple-choice questions (MCQs), please select the best answer.

1. **MCQ** – Select one incorrect statement regarding psychiatric advice to special medical services:
   (a) A survey by Canning and colleagues (1999) found that, of the 6 per cent of medical in-patients identified as dependent on illicit drugs, the great majority were taking cocaine.
   (b) Hazardous drinking is equivalent to 'at risk' drinking and is usually defined as an average daily consumption of over five units of alcohol for men and over 2.5 units for women.
   (c) Salkovskis and colleagues (1990) reported that around one-third of attendees at a hospital emergency department had scores on a self-report questionnaire indicative of psychiatric disorder.
   (d) Surgeons refer fewer patients for psychiatric assessment than do their physician colleagues.
   (e) The prevalence of problem drinking among male hospital in-patients is around 25 per cent.

2. **MCQ** – Select the best option. Cosmetic surgery is generally contraindicated in which of the following disorders?
   (a) Body dysmorphic disorder
   (b) Eating disorders, where abdominoplasty is desired
   (c) Mania
   (d) Schizophrenia
   (e) All of the above.

3. **MCQ** – Which of the following is the least common plastic/aesthetic surgery request for cosmetic reasons in the West?
   (a) Breast augmentation
   (b) Fasciectomy
   (c) Pinnaplasty
   (d) Reduction mammaplasty
   (e) Rhinoplasty.

4. **MCQ** – What is the most likely diagnosis in the case of a patient who requests amputation of a perfectly healthy digit or limb?
   (a) Amputee identity disorder
   (b) Anorexia nervosa
   (c) Major depression
   (d) Mania
   (e) Schizophrenia.

ANSWERS

1. a

The great majority were taking cannabis.

Reference: *Psychiatry: An evidence-based text,* pp. 1143–1145.

2. e

Reference: *Psychiatry: An evidence-based text,* p. 1146.

3. a

This can be used in the treatment of Dupuytren's disease. Reduction mammaplasty refers to breast reduction. Preoperative psychiatric assessment may be requested if there is doubt about a patient's capacity to consent to surgery. Preoperative assessment is also requested for some patients who seek plastic surgery for cosmetic reasons, a rapidly growing population in the USA and the UK.

Reference: *Psychiatry: An evidence-based text,* p. 1146.

4. a

Reference: *Psychiatry: An evidence-based text,* p. 1146.

PART 8

Legal and ethical aspects of psychiatry

Chapter 76

Forensic psychiatry

QUESTIONS

Note that for answers to extended matching items (EMIs), each option (denoted a, b, c, etc.) might be used once, more than once or not at all. For multiple-choice questions (MCQs), please select the best answer.

1. **EMI** – Admissions to special hospitals in the UK
   (a) ↑
   (b) About the same
   (c) ↓

   From the above list, select the option concerning the ratio of female:male admissions to special hospitals with respect to each of the following:
   (i) Overall admissions
   (ii) Civilly detained
   (iii) Have a personality disorder
   (iv) Be suicidal.

2. **MCQ** – Select one incorrect statement regarding forensic psychiatry:
   (a) In women, crime in general decreases with age.
   (b) Penrose's law states that the national homicide rate correlates negatively with the national number of psychiatric beds; it was based on a 1936 study of different European countries.
   (c) The peak age of offending in the UK is 14 years for females.
   (d) The peak age of offending in the UK is 17–18 years for males
   (e) The term 'forensic' is derived from the Roman forum, where offenders were tried.

3. **MCQ** – Select one incorrect statement regarding aspects of criminology, particularly in relation to the UK:
   (a) Convicted males have consistently outnumbered females by around five to one since 1980.
   (b) Half the indictable crimes are committed by people under the age of 21 years.
   (c) Women are more likely to be violent premenstrually in an institution compared with other times during the menstrual cycle.
   (d) Women are more likely to harm themselves premenstrually compared with other times during the menstrual cycle.
   (e) Women are more likely to offend premenstrually compared with other times during the menstrual cycle.

4. **MCQ** – Select one incorrect statement regarding juvenile delinquency, particularly in relation to the UK and USA:
   (a) A good predictor of future criminality is the extent of previous delinquency.
   (b) Around 4 per cent of children with a neurotic disorder grow up to be psychopathic adults.
   (c) Around 2 per cent of children without a psychiatric disorder grow up to be psychopathic adults.
   (d) Around 68 per cent of children with conduct disorder grow up to be psychopathic adults.
   (e) The majority of boys under the age of 17 years may commit a delinquent act.

5. **EMI** – Dunedin Multi-Disciplinary Health and Development Study
   (a) Adolescent limited offenders
   (b) Life course persistent offenders
   (c) Neither of the above

   This question concerns the results of the 32-year follow-up of a birth cohort of 1000 New Zelanders (Dunedin Multi-Disciplinary Health and Development Study by Moffitt and colleagues). From the above list, select the option with which each of the following is best associated:
   (i) Poor physical, sexual and psychiatric health (especially depression)
   (ii) Rare
   (iii) Good neurodevelopment and good social and academic skills.

6. **MCQ** – Select one incorrect statement regarding mentally abnormal offenders in the West:
   (i) In the UK, male prisoners are more likely than female prisoners to suffer from mental and physical disorders.
   (ii) In the UK, men outnumber women in prison by around 30 to one.
   (iii) There is an over-representation in prison of people with functional mental illnesses.
   (iv) There is an over-representation in prison of people with learning disabilities.
   (v) There is an over-representation in prison of people with organic mental illnesses.

7. **MCQ** – Select one incorrect statement regarding the mentally abnormal offender:
   (a) For those with a psychiatric disorder, being male is associated with an increased chance of committing an offence.
   (b) For those with a psychiatric disorder, being young is associated with an increased chance of committing an offence.
   (c) Overall, acutely mentally ill people are more likely to commit offences than those who are chronically ill.
   (d) People whose mental illness has relapsed and who are not compliant with treatment are more likely to commit offences.
   (e) The motivation for crime for those with a psychiatric disorder may be the same as for those who are not mentally ill, but it may also result from delusions, hallucinations or a deterioration in social functioning and personality owing to mental illness.

8. **MCQ** – Select one incorrect statement regarding the association of mental disorders with offending:
   (a) Homicides associated with depressive disorder are more likely to occur in the morning.
   (b) Homicides associated with depressive disorder usually involve family members.
   (c) People with mood disorders are over-represented in forensic psychiatry populations.
   (d) Schizophrenia is over-represented among offenders.
   (e) The onset of minor offending at a late age, such as shoplifting, minor sex offences and fraud, may result from dementia.

9. **EMI** – Age of criminal responsibility
   (a) < 7 years
   (b) 7 years
   (c) 8 years
   (d) 9 years
   (e) 10 years
   (f) 11 years
   (g) 12 years
   (h) 13 years
   (i) 14 years
   (j) 15 years
   (k) > 15 years

From the above list select the age at which criminal responsibility begins in each of the following countries:
   (i) England
   (ii) Scotland
   (iii) Republic of Ireland
   (iv) Wales
   (v) Northern Ireland.

10. **EMI** – Forensic psychiatry and the law
   (a) Actus rea
   (b) Doli incapax
   (c) Indictable
   (d) Mens rea
   (e) Mental capacity

From the above list select the option with which each of the following legal concepts used in forensic psychiatry is best associated:
   (i) Not legally responsible for committing a serious offence before the age of criminal responsibility
   (ii) Guilty intent
   (iii) Unlawful act
   (iv) An offence eligible for trial by jury.

11. **MCQ** – Select one incorrect statement regarding homicide by mentally disordered offenders in England and Wales between 1996 and 2010:
   (a) Around a third of all victims are female.
   (b) Around half of the female victims were killed by their partners.
   (c) Between 1996 and 1999, the three occupational groups most at risk of being homicide victims were security staff, medical staff and social workers (in order, from highest to lowest).
   (d) Homicide is necessarily unlawful.
   (e) There were around 500–600 homicides each year in these countries during the first decade of the twenty-first century.

12. **EMI** – Perpetrators of homicide
   (a) Femicide
   (b) Filicide
   (c) Internet homicide
   (d) Mass killing
   (e) Matricide
   (f) Patricide
   (g) Serial killing
   (h) Spree killings
   (i) Suicide
   (j) Uxoricide

From the above list select the type of homicide with which the killing of each of the following is best associated:
   (i) One's father
   (ii) One's wife
   (iii) One's child
   (iv) Multiple individuals at the same time and in the same location.

13. **EMI** – Types of manslaughter
   (a) Corporate liability
   (b) Involuntary manslaughter
   (c) Voluntary manslaughter
   (d) None of the above

From the above list select the type of manslaughter, if any, with which each of the following is best associated:
   (i) The defendant would be guilty of murder if it were not for the availability of the partial defence of provocation.

(ii) Homicide without malice aforethought.

(iii) The defendant would be guilty of murder if it were not for the availability of the partial defence of diminished responsibility.

14. **MCQ** – Select one incorrect statement regarding forensic psychiatry:

(a) Automatism has been successfully pleaded for an offence occurring during a hypoglycaemic attack.

(b) Automatism has been successfully pleaded for an offence occurring during sleep.

(c) Automatism has been successfully pleaded for an offence occurring during somnambulism.

(d) In cases of possible suggestibility and false confessions, the Gudjonnson Suggestibility Scale should be used.

(e) In England and Wales, developing a mental illness as a result of the ingestion of a drug or alcohol cannot be used as a defence.

15. **EMI** – Mental Health Act 1983

(a) Section 35
(b) Section 36
(c) Section 37
(d) Section 38
(e) Section 39
(f) Section 40
(g) Section 41
(h) Section 42
(i) Section 43
(j) Section 44
(k) Section 45
(l) Section 46
(m) Section 47
(n) Section 48

From the above list select the Section of the Mental Health Act 1983 with which each of the following procedures before trial for mentally disordered offenders in England and Wales is best associated:

(i) Remand to hospital for treatment
(ii) Remand to hospital for report
(iii) Remand to hospital of other prisoners (including those on remand in custody).

16. **EMI** – Mental Health Act 1983

(a) Section 35
(b) Section 36
(c) Section 37
(d) Section 38
(e) Section 39
(f) Section 40
(g) Section 41
(h) Section 42
(i) Section 43
(j) Section 44
(k) Section 45

(l) Section 46
(m) Section 47
(n) Section 48

From the above list, select the Section of the Mental Health Act 1983 with which each of the following options for sentencing for mentally disordered offenders in England and Wales is best associated:

(i) Guardianship order
(ii) Interim hospital order
(iii) Restriction order.

17. **EMI** – Mental Health Act 1983

(a) Section 35
(b) Section 36
(c) Section 37
(d) Section 38
(e) Section 39
(f) Section 40
(g) Section 41
(h) Section 42
(i) Section 43
(j) Section 44
(k) Section 45
(l) Section 46
(m) Section 47
(n) Section 48

From the above list, select the section of the Mental Health Act 1983 with which each of the following options after sentencing for mentally disordered offenders in England and Wales is best associated:

(i) Transfer direction from prison
(ii) Transfer of individuals kept in custody during Her Majesty's pleasure.

18. **EMI** – Habit and impulse-control disorders and related offences

(a) Esquirol
(b) Marc
(c) Pinel
(d) Rush
(e) Topp

This question concerns the historical development of concepts relating to habit and impulse-control disorders and related offences. From the above list select the person with whom each of the following developments is best associated.

(i) In 1833, first used the term kleptomania when describing a number of wealthy individuals who carried out bizarre, worthless thefts in which they had little intrinsic interest and to which they readily confessed when challenged.

(ii) In the eighteenth century, he referred to 'mania without delirium' as being a disease of the willpower.

(iii) Referred in 1885 to instinctive monomanias, where the individual acts 'without passion or motive but only under involuntary instinctive impulse'.

19. **MCQ** – Which of the following is true of the difference between impulse-control disorders and obsessive-compulsive disorder?
  (a) In obsessive-compulsive disorder the thought of carrying out the act is egodystonic whereas the impulses in impulse-control disorders are egosyntonic.
  (b) Only impulse-control disorders lead to relief of tension.
  (c) Only obsessive-compulsive disorder leads to relief of anxiety.
  (d) Patients never act on their obsessions in obsessive-compulsive disorder.
  (e) None of the above.

20. **MCQ** – Select one incorrect statement regarding the epidemiology of pathological gambling:
  (a) It is associated with tolerance and withdrawal phenomena.
  (b) It is more common in criminals.
  (c) It is more common in men.
  (d) It is more common in people with a past history of psychiatric disorder.
  (e) The lifetime prevalence rate is estimated to be around 0.1 per cent.

21. **MCQ** – Select one incorrect statement. Risk factors for pathological gambling include:
  (a) Alcohol abuse
  (b) Age < 45 years
  (c) Being male
  (d) Cigarette-smoking
  (e) Having debts.

22. **MCQ** – Select one incorrect statement regarding the aetiology of pathological gambling:
  (a) It is associated with low central dopamine levels.
  (b) It is associated with low central serotonin levels.
  (c) It is associated with the treatment of Parkinson's disease.
  (d) Learning theory has suggested that the pattern of intermittent (variable ratio) reinforcement, the most potent schedule for conditioning, particularly applies to gambling.
  (e) The predominant motivation is financial, with sufferers experiencing little pleasure from this activity.

23. **MCQ** – Which of the following is not an assessment tool for gambling?
  (a) BGA
  (b) CPGI
  (c) NODS
  (d) PG-YBOCS
  (e) SOGS.

24. **MCQ** – Select one incorrect statement regarding the epidemiology of arson:
  (a) Approximately 40 per cent of all serious fires in the UK are started deliberately.
  (b) The peak age for arson is 17 years for men in the UK.
  (c) The peak age for arson is 45 years for women in the UK.
  (d) There is a decreased incidence of arson among people with learning disability.
  (e) There is an increased incidence of arson among people with alcohol dependence syndrome.

25. **MCQ** – Select one incorrect statement regarding pathological stealing:
  (a) A psychodynamic theory of its aetiology includes loss substitution, in which the offence provides symbolic compensation for threatened or actual loss.
  (b) Cognitive-behavioural therapy has been found to be an effective treatment.
  (c) In ICD-10, it is defined as repeated failure to resist impulses to steal objects that are not required for personal use or monetary gain.
  (d) It is more prevalent in males.
  (e) It often responds well to antidepressant medication, especially SSRIs such as fluoxetine.

26. **EMI** – Psychodynamic theories of kleptomania
  (a) Defensive strategy
  (b) Drive theory
  (c) Loss substitution
  (d) Perversion
  (e) Self-psychological theory

From the above list select the option with which each of the following is best associated:
  (i) A means to counter fragmentation of self.
  (ii) A forbidden activity, engaged in secret.
  (iii) Engaged in by females to acquire symbolic male genitalia.
  (iv) Stolen objects represent fetishes.
  (v) A response to narcissistic injuries.

27. **MCQ** – Select one incorrect statement regarding non-accidental injury of children:
  (a) In the UK, in about 10 per cent of cases the mother's partner is not the biological father of the injured child.
  (b) In the UK, the majority of murdered children are killed by their parents.
  (c) The mother's partner competes for attention with the injured child, whom he rejects.
  (d) This term has replaced the term 'baby battering', which was coined by Kempe and Kempe in 1961.
  (e) Victims are usually children under the age of 3 years.

28. **MCQ** – Select one incorrect statement regarding partner abuse:
  (a) In England and Wales, this category of abuse results in around one female homicide per month.
  (b) In England and Wales, under the Matrimonial Causes Act 1878, a husband could forcibly return his wife to their home.

(c) In the eighteenth century, the 'rule of thumb' applied in England, whereby a man was not legally allowed to beat his wife with an implement wider than a thumb.

(d) In the USA, it has been estimated that in 25–30 per cent of marriages, one partner will push, shove or grab the other at some point.

(e) The term 'spouse abuse' has replaced 'wife battering'.

29. **EMI** – Special syndromes in forensic psychiatry
(a) De Clérambault's syndrome
(b) Munchausen syndrome
(c) Munchausen's syndrome by proxy
(d) Othello syndrome
(e) Stalking

From the above list, select the option with which each of the following is best associated:
(i) The intentional production or feigning of illness to bring about repeated hospital admissions, investigations or operations
(ii) Typologies include incompetent and resentful
(iii) Delusions of infidelity about a sexual partner can lead an individual to examine, for example, the partner's underwear and sexual organs, in an attempt to find proof of unfaithfulness.

30. **MCQ** – Select one incorrect statement regarding the representation of Afro-Caribbean people in the psychiatric and criminal justice systems in the England and Wales:
(a) They are less likely to be the victims of murder.
(b) There is an excess of women normally resident in West Africa serving sentences in England and Wales for drug smuggling.
(c) They are over-represented in locked psychiatric wards.
(d) They are over-represented in medium secure units.
(e) They are over-represented in special hospitals.

31. **EMI** – Nomenclature of psychopathic personality disorder
(a) Character neurosis
(b) Manie sans delire
(c) Moral imbecile
(d) Moral insanity
(e) Sociopathy
(f) Psychopathic inferiority
(g) Psychopathic personalities
(h) Psychopathic traits
(i) Psychopathy

From the above list, select the term with which each of the following is best associated as having introduced:
(i) Koch in 1891
(ii) Pinel in 1801
(iii) Kraeplin in 1909
(iv) Alexander.

32. **EMI** – Cleckley's differentiation of primary from secondary psychopaths
(a) Primary psychopaths
(b) Secondary psychopaths
(c) Neither of the above

From the above list, select the option with which each of the following is best associated:
(i) High anxiety/tension
(ii) Hidden guilt
(iii) Articulate (charming) qualities
(iv) Do not seek assistance.

33. **MCQ** – Select one incorrect statement regarding forensic psychiatry:
(a) Munchausen's syndrome was originally described by Dr Richard Asher in the *Lancet* in 1951.
(b) Psychopathy is associated with excess EEG posterior slow-wave theta activity.
(c) Psychopathy is associated with XYY syndrome.
(d) The prevalence of epilepsy in prisons in England and Wales is higher than that in the community.
(e) The term Munchausen's syndrome by proxy was coined by Meadow.

34. **EMI** – Nomenclature of psychopathic personality disorder
(a) DSM-IV-TR antisocial personality disorder
(b) ICD-10 dissocial personality disorder
(c) Moral imbecile
(d) Moral insanity
(e) Sociopathy
(f) Psychopathic inferiority
(g) Psychopathic personalities
(h) Psychopathic traits
(i) Psychopathy

From the above list, select the term with which each of the following is best associated with:
(i) A personality disorder usually coming to attention because of a gross disparity between behaviour and the prevailing social norms, and characterized by features such as a callous unconcern for the feelings of others and a gross and persistent attitude of irresponsibility and disregard for social norms, rules and obligations
(ii) Royal Commission for Care and Control of Feeble-Minded, 1904
(iii) Schneider, 1927
(iv) Henderson, 1930.

35. **MCQ** – Select one incorrect statement regarding the PCL-R:
(a) A short version, the PCL-SV, can be used in non-forensic populations.
(b) Around three-quarters of people with antisocial personality disorder reach the checklist criteria for psychopathy on this scale.
(c) It has been found to be a good predictor of risk.

(d) It was devised by Hare.

(e) One of its two factors is that of personality traits.

36. **MCQ** – Select one incorrect statement regarding the Mental Health Act 1983 in England and Wales:

(a) A patient has the right, under the amended Act, to make an application to displace his nearest relative.

(b) It applies in prison in England and Wales.

(c) It replaced the Mental Health Act 1959 and was substantially amended by the Mental Health Act 2007.

(d) Under the amended Act, the RMO is replaced by the responsible clinician, who may be a psychologist.

(e) Under the amended Act, the role of the approved mental health professional is open to social workers, nurses, occupational therapists and psychologists.

37. **EMI** – Consent to treatment under the Mental Health Act 1983

(a) Consent

(b) Consent and second opinion

(c) Consent or second opinion

(d) No consent

This question concerns consent to treatment in England and Wales under the Mental Health Act 1983. From the above list, select the most appropriate level of consent required for each of the following types of treatment for an informal patient:

(i) ECT

(ii) Urgent treatment

(iii) Psychosurgery

(iv) Psychiatric drugs.

38. **EMI** – Consent to treatment under the Mental Health Act 1983

(a) Consent

(b) Consent and second opinion

(c) Consent or second opinion

(d) No consent

From the above list, select the most appropriate level of consent required for each of the following types of treatment for a patient compulsorily detained under the Act:

(i) ECT

(ii) Urgent treatment

(iii) Castration

(iv) Psychiatric drugs.

39. **EMI** – Civil treatment orders under the Mental Health Act 1983

(a) Section 2

(b) Section 3

(c) Section 4

(d) Section 5(2)

(e) Section 5(4)

(f) Section 135

(g) Section 136

This question concerns civil treatment orders in England and Wales under the Mental Health Act 1983. From the above list, select the most appropriate Section of the Act associated with each of the following applicants:

(i) Police officer

(ii) Magistrate

(iii) Registered mental nurse

(iv) Registered nurse for mental handicap.

40. **EMI** – Civil treatment orders under the Mental Health Act 1983

(a) Section 2

(b) Section 3

(c) Section 4

(d) Section 5(2)

(e) Section 5(4)

(f) Section 135

(g) Section 136

From the above list, select the most appropriate section of the Act associated with medical recommendations by the following:

(i) Doctor in charge of the patient's care

(ii) None

(iii) Any doctor.

41. **EMI** – Civil treatment orders under the Mental Health Act 1983

(a) Section 2

(b) Section 3

(c) Section 4

(d) Section 5(2)

(e) Section 5(4)

(f) Section 135

(g) Section 136

From the above list, select the most appropriate section of the Act associated with each of the following periods of maximum duration:

(i) 6 months

(ii) 6 hours

(iii) 28 days.

42. **MCQ** – Which of the following civil treatment orders in England and Wales under the Mental Health Act 1983 allows eligibility for appeal to a MHRT?

(a) Section 2

(b) Section 4

(c) Section 5(2)

(d) Section 135

(e) Section 136.

ANSWERS

1.

(i)   c – Women are admitted at least five times less frequently than men.

(ii) a

(iii) a

(iv) a

Reference: *Psychiatry: An evidence-based text*, **p. 1153.**

2. a

There is a small peak for women aged 40–50 years.

Reference: *Psychiatry: An evidence-based text*, **pp. 1153–1155.**

3. a

The ratio of five to one was correct for 2010 in the UK, but this preponderance is only half of what it was during the 1980s.

Reference: *Psychiatry: An evidence-based text*, **pp. 1155–1156.**

4. d

Around 28 per cent grow up to be psychopathic adults.

Reference: *Psychiatry: An evidence-based text*, **pp. 1156–1157.**

5.

(i)   b

(ii) b – Although the numbers are small, this group is responsible for about half the crime rate.

(iii) a

Reference: *Psychiatry: An evidence-based text*, **p. 1157.**

6. a

In the UK, female prisoners have more mental and physical disorders.

Reference: *Psychiatry: An evidence-based text*, **p. 1157.**

7. c

Overall, chronically mentally ill people are more likely to commit offences than those who are acutely ill.

Reference: *Psychiatry: An evidence-based text*, **p. 1159.**

8. c

Overall, people with mood disorders are under-represented in forensic psychiatry populations.

Reference: *Psychiatry: An evidence-based text*, **p. 1160.**

9.

(i)   e – Criminal responsibility is a legal concept.

(ii) c

(iii) b

(iv) e

(v)   e

Reference: *Psychiatry: An evidence-based text*, **p. 1161.**

10.

(i)   b

(ii) d

(iii) a

(iv) c – Indictable crimes are the more serious offences eligible for trial by jury.

Reference: *Psychiatry: An evidence-based text*, **pp. 1156, 1161.**

11. d

Homicide is the killing of another human being. It is not necessarily unlawful.

Reference: *Psychiatry: An evidence-based text*, **pp. 1162–1163.**

12.

(i)   f

(ii) g

(iii) b

(iv) d

Reference: *Psychiatry: An evidence-based text*, **p. 1163.**

13.

(i)   c

(ii) b

(iii) c

Reference: *Psychiatry: An evidence-based text*, **pp. 1163–1165.**

14. e

In England and Wales, successful defences have been based on: being so drunk as to be incapable of forming intent in offences requiring specific intent; developing a mental illness, e.g. psychosis, as a result of the ingestion of a drug or alcohol (as in delirium tremens); where the use of a drug, which might be legitimate, produces a mental state abnormality that could not have been anticipated by the subject, e.g. hypoglycaemia after the use of insulin.

Reference: *Psychiatry: An evidence-based text*, **pp. 1165–1167.**

15.

(i)   b – This may be used only by the Crown Court and is an alternative to remand to custody.

(ii) a – This order can be made under Subsection (3).

(iii) n – This section gives the Justice Secretary powers to direct the transfer to hospital of a person waiting for trial or sentence and who has been remanded in custody.

Reference: *Psychiatry: An evidence-based text*, **p. 1167.**

16.

(i)   c – The grounds are as for a Section 37 hospital order. It is rarely used.

(ii) d – If it is uncertain that a full Section 37 hospital order is appropriate, then this can be tested out by making an interim order.

(iii) g

Reference: *Psychiatry: An evidence-based text*, p. 1168.

17.

(i)   m – This allows the Justice Secretary to order the transfer of a sentenced prisoner following conviction if he or she has a mental disorder.

(ii) l – It has the same effect as a hospital order with restrictions without limit of time.

Reference: *Psychiatry: An evidence-based text*, p. 1169.

18.

(i)   b

(ii) c

(iii) a – These instinctive monomanias included homicide, fire-setting and alcoholism.

Reference: *Psychiatry: An evidence-based text*, p. 1179–1180.

19. a

In obsessive-compulsive disorder, the thought of carrying out the act must not in itself be pleasurable, i.e. the thought must be egodystonic. In contrast, in impulse-control disorders, the impulses are usually perceived as pleasurable (egosyntonic).

Reference: *Psychiatry: An evidence-based text*, pp. 1178, 1180.

20. e

The lifetime rate is 1.6 per cent, a figure not dissimilar to that for schizophrenia.

Reference: *Psychiatry: An evidence-based text*, pp. 1180–1181.

21. b

Being over 45 years of age is a risk factor.

Reference: *Psychiatry: An evidence-based text*, p. 1181.

22. e

The principal motivation is the sense of thrill and pleasure at the risk-taking, as reflected in changes in heart rate demonstrated during gambling.

Reference: *Psychiatry: An evidence-based text*, p. 1181.

23. a

The BGA (Brown–Goodwin Assessment) is a commonly used assessment tool of aggression. The PG-YBOCS (Pathological Gambling Modification of the Yale–Brown Obsessive Compulsive Scale) is widely used in the USA by clinicians to assess pathological gambling.

Reference: *Psychiatry: An evidence-based text*, p. 1182.

24. d

There is an increased incidence of arson in this group.

Reference: *Psychiatry: An evidence-based text*, pp. 1183.

25. d

It is certainly more prevalent in females than in males, unlike other impulse-control disorders such as intermittent explosive disorder and pyromania, where males predominate.

Reference: *Psychiatry: An evidence-based text*, pp. 1184–1186.

26.

(i)   e

(ii) b – Thereby having a sexual basis.

(iii) a

(iv) d

(v)   e

Reference: *Psychiatry: An evidence-based text*, p. 1185–1186.

27. a

In about half of cases, the mother's partner is not the biological father.

Reference: *Psychiatry: An evidence-based text*, pp. 1188–1189.

28. a

The true incidence of such abuse is obscured by the hidden nature of the behaviour and problems in definition, e.g. over the degree of violence. This category accounts in England and Wales for 16 per cent of all violent crimes and results in two homicides of females a week; 40 per cent of them are killed in the bedroom or kitchen.

Reference: *Psychiatry: An evidence-based text*, p. 1189.

29.

(i)   b

(ii) e – Other typologies include: the rejected stalker who acts through a mixture of revenge and desire for reconciliation; intimacy-seeking; and predatory stalkers.

(iii) d – Also known as morbid jealousy.

Reference: *Psychiatry: An evidence-based text*, pp. 1190–1191.

30. a

Afro-Caribbean people are also more likely to be the victims of murder in England and Wales.

Reference: *Psychiatry: An evidence-based text*, p. 1192.

31.

(i)   f
(ii) b
(iii) h
(iv) a

Reference: *Psychiatry: An evidence-based text*, **p. 1194.**

32.

(i)   b
(ii) b
(iii) a
(iv) a – e.g. a guiltless prisoner.

Reference: *Psychiatry: An evidence-based text*, **p. 1195.**

33. d

The prevalence of epilepsy in prisons in England and Wales was noted in the 1970s to be two to four times that in the general population (7.2 per 1000 compared with 4.2 per 1000, respectively). However, a more recent study in 2002 found a prevalence of about 1 per cent in prison, which is equivalent to that in the community. This is illustrated in Figure 76.7 on page 1193 of the accompanying textbook.

Reference: *Psychiatry: An evidence-based text*, **Ch. 76.**

34.

(i)   b – This is ICD-10 F60.2.
(ii) c
(iii) g
(iv) i – Henderson distinguished between three kinds of psychopathic personality: predominantly aggressive; predominantly inadequate; and predominately creative.

Reference: *Psychiatry: An evidence-based text*, **p. 1194.**

35. b

Only around one-third of people with antisocial personality disorder reach the checklist criteria for psychopathy on this scale. Also, scores on the deviancy of social behaviour factor may vary between cultures, e.g. low in Scotland compared with the USA.

Reference: *Psychiatry: An evidence-based text*, **p. 1196.**

36. b

It does not apply in prison, but treatment can be given in urgent circumstances in 'good faith' under common law.

Reference: *Psychiatry: An evidence-based text*, **pp. 1199–1200.**

37.

(i)   a
(ii) d
(iii) b
(iv) a

Reference: *Psychiatry: An evidence-based text*, **p. 1201.**

38.

(i)   b
(ii) d
(iii) b
(iv) b

Reference: *Psychiatry: An evidence-based text*, **p. 1201.**

39.

(i)   g – Admission by police.
(ii) f
(iii) e – Nurse's holding power of voluntary in-patient.
(iv) e

Reference: *Psychiatry: An evidence-based text*, **p. 1201.**

40.

(i)   d – Urgent detention of voluntary in-patient.
(ii) e
(iii) c – Emergency admission for assessment.

Reference: *Psychiatry: An evidence-based text*, **p. 1201.**

41.

(i)   b – Admission for treatment.
(ii) e
(iii) a – Admission for assessment.

Reference: *Psychiatry: An evidence-based text*, **p. 1201.**

42. a

Within 14 days.

Reference: *Psychiatry: An evidence-based text*, **p. 1201.**

Chapter 77

Legal aspects of psychiatric care, with particular reference to England and Wales

QUESTIONS

Note that for answers to extended matching items (EMIs), each option (denoted a, b, c, etc.) might be used once, more than once or not at all. For multiple-choice questions (MCQs), please select the best answer.

1. **EMI** – Legal sources and legal fields
   (a) Civil law
   (b) Common law
   (c) Criminal law
   (d) Equity
   (e) Statute law

   From the above list, select the option with which each of the following is best associated:
   (i) A legal source that arises from Acts of Parliament
   (ii) The principles of justice in cases not covered by statute or common law
   (iii) A legal field in which the state initiates proceedings on behalf of society against an individual
   (iv) A legal field that includes the Mental Health Act 1983.

2. **EMI** – Criminal courts in England and Wales
   (a) Appeal Courts (criminal division)
   (b) Crown Courts
   (c) Magistrates' courts
   (d) The Supreme Court of the UK

   From the above list, select the option with which each of the following is best associated:
   (i) Includes the Old Bailey
   (ii) Includes the Courts of Justice in the Strand
   (iii) Deal with the vast majority of all criminal prosecutions in England and Wales
   (iv) Replaced the House of Lords (Judicial Committee) in 2009.

3. **MCQ** – Select one incorrect statement regarding legal aspects of psychiatric care in England and Wales:
   (a) A magistrate should be addressed as 'your worship'.
   (b) Contracts require free full consent.
   (c) Informal psychiatric patients do not have the right to vote in a general election.
   (d) 'Mentally incapable' people are bound by contracts unless the other party or parties to the contract knew, or should have known, of the individual's incapacity.
   (e) The Chancery Division of the High Court deals with financial matters, company law, tax, trusts and wills.

4. **MCQ** – Select one incorrect statement regarding testamentary capacity in the UK:
   (a) If a doctor agrees to witness the will, he or she is said to have attested the will.
   (b) If an individual dies having left a will, he or she dies testate.
   (c) Individuals must be over the age of 18 years.
   (d) Individuals must not be of unsound mind.
   (e) The presence of mild dementia affects testamentary capacity.

5. **MCQ** – Select one incorrect statement. A marriage in England and Wales may be annulled if:
   (a) One of the partners was forced to agree to the marriage under duress
   (b) One partner did not disclose that he/she had a communicable venereal disease at the time of marriage
   (c) One partner did not disclose that he/she had a mental disorder at the time of marriage
   (d) One partner did not disclose that he/she had epilepsy at the time of marriage
   (e) There was non-consummation.

6. **MCQ** – Select one incorrect statement regarding legal aspects of psychiatric care in England and Wales:
   (a) An appointee is someone authorized by the Department of Social Security to receive and administer benefits on behalf of someone else.

(b) An enduring power of attorney cannot continue in force after the donor has lost the mental capacity to manage and administer his or her financial affairs.

(c) Mentally disordered individuals are considered incapable of committing a tort unless the disorder does not preclude them understanding the nature or probable consequences of their acts.

(d) Mentally disordered individuals may give evidence in court or make a written statement, but it is for the magistrates or the judge to determine whether they are fit to do so and can understand the nature and obligation of the oath.

(e) The UN Declaration of Rights of Mentally Retarded Persons (1971) gives the right of mentally disabled people to live with their own family.

7. MCQ – Select one incorrect statement. Under the Mental Capacity Act 2005 of England and Wales:
(a) A decision can be made on behalf of a person in respect to consent to marriage.
(b) A lasting power of attorney is like an enduring power of attorney but can make health and welfare decisions.
(c) A person is not to be treated as lacking in capacity only because he or she makes an 'unwise' decision.
(d) Everyone is assumed to have capacity, unless shown otherwise.
(e) No one is to be treated as unable to make a decision unless all practicable steps to assist have failed.

8. MCQ – Select one incorrect statement. The Mental Capacity Act 2005 (England and Wales) Deprivation of Liberty Safeguards apply to people:
(a) Aged 16 years or over

(b) In hospitals and care homes
(c) Who have a mental disorder such as dementia or a learning disability
(d) Who lack capacity to consent to arrangements made for their treatment or care
(e) Who need to have their liberty taken away in their own best interests in order to protect them from harm.

9. MCQ – In England and Wales, which of the following is/are not eligible for compensation as psychiatric damage (nervous shock)?
(a) Accident and compensation neurosis
(b) Normal grief
(c) Post-concussional syndrome
(d) Post-traumatic stress disorder
(e) Victims of torture.

10. MCQ – Which of the following is the commonest cause of psychiatric negligence in the UK?
(a) Failure to check the patient's renal function
(b) Failure to check the patient's thyroid function
(c) Failure to monitor blood levels of psychotropic medication
(d) Misdiagnosis
(e) Suicide or attempted suicide.

11. MCQ – Which of the following is not considered to be one of the four cardinal principles of ethical medical practice?
(a) Autonomy
(b) Beneficence
(c) Confidentiality
(d) Justice
(e) Non-maleficence.

ANSWERS

1.

(i)   e – Statute law trumps and sits upon common law.

(ii) d

(iii) c – Where Parliament and other courts have defined an activity as a crime.

(iv) a

> **Reference:** *Psychiatry: An evidence-based text*, **p. 1214.**

2.

(i)   b – This is the Central Criminal Court.

(ii) a

(iii) c – They deal with over 98 per cent of all criminal prosecutions in England and Wales. They try cases summarily, i.e. without a jury.

(iv) d

> **Reference:** *Psychiatry: An evidence-based text*, **p. 1214.**

3. c

Informal patients have voting rights.

> **Reference:** *Psychiatry: An evidence-based text*, **pp. 1202, 1215.**

4. e

The presence of mental disorder, such as mild dementia, does not necessarily affect testamentary capacity, although if the will is complex it may do so.

> **Reference:** *Psychiatry: An evidence-based text*, **pp. 1215–1216.**

5. c

However, the marriage may be annulled if one partner has a mental disorder at the time of marriage so as not to appreciate the nature of the contract.

> **Reference:** *Psychiatry: An evidence-based text*, **pp. 1216.**

6. b

Unlike an ordinary power of attorney, an enduring power of attorney (EPA; introduced in 1986 after the Enduring Powers of Attorney Act 1985) may continue in force after donors have lost their mental capacity to manage and administer their financial affairs, provided it has been registered with the Public Trust Office.

> **Reference:** *Psychiatry: An evidence-based text*, **pp. 1216–1217.**

7. a

Under Section 27 of the Act, no decision on consent to marriage is to be made on behalf of a person.

> **Reference:** *Psychiatry: An evidence-based text*, **pp. 1217–1219.**

8. a

The person must be aged 18 years or over.

> **Reference:** *Psychiatry: An evidence-based text*, **pp. 1219–1221.**

9. b

Normal ordinary emotional reactions such as grief are not eligible for compensation, but psychiatric damage (legal term 'nervous shock') is. Note that issues regarding psychiatric damage have arisen in respect of pathological grief.

> **Reference:** *Psychiatry: An evidence-based text*, **pp. 1221.**

10. e

This accounts for around half of all cases, according to UK medical defence societies.

> **Reference:** *Psychiatry: An evidence-based text*, **p. 1221.**

11. c

There are several reasons why patient confidentiality may have to be breached. Disclosure is allowed in the public interest. In England and Wales, exceptions to confidentiality include the following reasons:

- Court order
- Misuse of Drugs Law – notification of addicts
- Road Traffic Act 1988 – identification of drivers in road traffic accidents
- Police and Criminal Evidence Act 1984
- Prevention of terrorism
- Warrant
- Data Protection Act 1984
- Venereal Diseases Regulations 1974 – applies to health authority employees
- Human and Embryology Act 1990 and amendment of 1992

> **Reference:** *Psychiatry: An evidence-based text*, **pp. 1223, 1227–1228.**

Chapter 78

Ethics and law

QUESTION

Note that for answers to extended matching items (EMIs), each option (denoted a, b, c, etc.) might be used once, more than once or not at all.

1. **EMI** – Distinction between civil law and criminal law
   (a) Civil law
   (b) Criminal law
   (c) Neither of the above

From the above list, select the option with which each of the following is best associated:
   (i) Medical negligence
   (ii) Manslaughter
   (iii) Family law
   (iv) Mental health law
   (v) The imposition of military rule during a national emergency, such as war, with a suspension of habeas corpus and the imposition of curfews.

ANSWER

1.

(i)   a
(ii) b
(iii) a
(iv) a
(v)   c – This is martial law. Civil law is usually suspended.

Reference: *Psychiatry: An evidence-based text*, **p. 1237.**

Chapter 79

Risk assessment

QUESTIONS

Note that for answers to extended matching items (EMIs), each option (denoted a, b, c, etc.) might be used once, more than once or not at all. For multiple-choice questions (MCQs), please select the best answer.

1. **MCQ** – Select one correct statement regarding the association between mental disorder and violence:
   (a) A diagnosis of antisocial personality disorder is not statistically associated with an increased risk of violence.
   (b) A diagnosis of schizophrenia is not statistically associated with an increased risk of violence.
   (c) A diagnosis of substance misuse is not statistically associated with an increased risk of violence.
   (d) The probability of schizophrenia in men remanded on a charge of homicide is not significantly greater than that in the general population.
   (e) None of the above.

2. **MCQ** – Which of the following has a negative correlation with the risk of violence in the VRAG?
   (a) Age
   (b) Alcohol abuse
   (c) Never married
   (d) PCL-R score
   (e) Personality disorder.

3. **EMI** – HCR-20
   (a) C
   (b) H
   (c) R
   (d) None of the above

From the above list select the category, if any, of the HCR-20 with which each of the following is best associated:
   (i) Lack of insight
   (ii) Substance use problems
   (iii) Psychopathy.

4. **EMI** – HCR-20
   (a) C
   (b) H
   (c) R

From the above list select the category of the HCR-20 with which each of the following is best associated:
   (i) Major mental illness
   (ii) Stress
   (iii) Impulsivity
   (iv) Lack of personal support.

5. **MCQ** – Which of the following has a negative correlation with the risk of violence in the VRAG?
   (a) History of non-violent offending
   (b) Failure on prior conditional release
   (c) Problems at junior school
   (d) Schizophrenia
   (e) Separated from parents before age 16 years.

ANSWERS

1. e

It has been shown consistently that a diagnosis of schizophrenia is statistically associated with an increased risk of violence. The association with violence is even stronger for diagnoses such as substance misuse and antisocial personality disorder. Apparent contrary findings, which show no statistical association between schizophrenia and violence, usually arise because the control group includes diagnoses such as personality disorder that carry an even higher risk. The probability of schizophrenia in men remanded on a charge of homicide may be around 5 per cent, compared with about 1 per cent in the general population.

Reference: *Psychiatry: An evidence-based text*, **pp. 1240–1241.**

2. a

Box 79.1 on page 1244 of the accompanying textbook gives the 12 items of the VRAG (Violence Risk Appraisal Guide).

Reference: *Psychiatry: An evidence-based text*, **pp. 1243–1244.**

3.

(i)   a – This is clinical item C1.
(ii) b – This is historical item H5.
(iii) b – This is item H7.

Reference: *Psychiatry: An evidence-based text*, **pp. 1244–1245.**

4.

(i)   b – This is item H6.
(ii) c – This is risk-management item R5.
(iii) a – This is item C4.
(iv) c – This is item R3.

Reference: *Psychiatry: An evidence-based text*, **pp. 1244–1245.**

5. d

Box 79.1 on page 1244 of the accompanying textbook gives the 12 items of the VRAG (Violence Risk Appraisal Guide) and shows those four of these 12 items that are negatively correlated with risk of violence. The present correct option, schizophrenia, appears inconsistent with the answer to Question 1. This anomaly arises because the personality-disordered patients in the original study group presented even higher risks. The research literature would not support the downgrading of risk because the diagnosis is schizophrenia.

Reference: *Psychiatry: An evidence-based text*, **pp. 1243–1244.**

Mock Examination Papers

MRCPsych Paper 1

Mock examination
Time limit: 180 minutes
Number of questions: 200

MULTIPLE CHOICE QUESTIONS (MCQS)

1. Of the following theorists, who suggested the 'split mind' of schizophrenia and influenced Bleuler to develop a theory of fragmentation of mental activities in schizophrenia?
   A. Kahlbaum
   B. Kraepelin
   C. Hecker
   D. Freud
   E. Griesinger.

2. Which of the following statements regarding the gender differences in people with schizophrenia is false?
   A. Males have a bimodal peak of incidence.
   B. Males have an earlier onset.
   C. Males have a higher incidence.
   D. Males have a higher mortality.
   E. Males have more structural abnormalities.

3. A 30-year-old motorcyclist suffers from head injuries after a road traffic accident. His partner comments that his memory has become very poor. Which of the following is not a standardized test to assess his memory?
   A. Auditory – Verbal Learning Test (AVLT)
   B. California Verbal Learning Test (CVLT)
   C. Recognition Memory Test (RMT)
   D. Wechsler Memory Test (WMT)
   E. Weigl Colour–Form Sorting Test (WCFST).

4. Which of the following symptoms of schizophrenia is not a first-rank symptom?
   A. Audible thoughts
   B. Delusional perception
   C. Formal thought disorder
   D. Thought insertion
   E. Voices discussing or arguing.

5. A 50-year-old woman was admitted to the ward and the nurses are having difficulty with her. She appears to be arrogant and refuses to follow ward rules and insists on drinking alcohol in the ward. She believes she is a 'special' patient and requests first-class treatment. Her husband mentions that she tends to exploit others and that most people try to avoid her. Which defence mechanism is most often used by people with such a disorder?
   A. Acting out
   B. Denial
   C. Projection
   D. Rationalization
   E. Splitting.

6. You are a consultant on an in-patient psychiatric ward. A patient with schizophrenia is admitted to the ward and complains of suffering from tremor and rigidity after taking haloperidol. A specialist trainee has consulted you on the most appropriate scale to use to assess the potential side effects of antipsychotics. Which of the following scales would you recommend:
   A. Abnormal Involuntary Movement Scale
   B. Acute Dystonia Rating Scale
   C. Barnes Akathisia Scale
   D. Extrapyramidal Side-effect Scale
   E. Simpson Angus Scale.

7. Which of the following movement disorders is not typically associated with schizophrenia?
   A. Ambitendency
   B. Mannerism
   C. Mitgehen and mitmachen
   D. Negativism
   E. Stupor.

8. A 30-year-old man reports that he can smell a Christmas carol. The Christmas carol is associated with the smell of carnations. This phenomenon is known as:
   A. Autoscopy
   B. Functional hallucination
   C. Reflex hallucination
   D. Synaesthesia
   E. Trailing phenomenon.

9. A 40-year-old man suffers from choreic movements of the limbs and head which gradually affect his gait and speech. Recently,

he also has had periods of depression and memory impairment although he has no past history of psychiatric problems. Two of his brothers developed similar symptoms and passed them on to some of their children and grandchildren. The onset of symptoms was approximately 10 years before each one died. This 'unknown' disorder caused considerable worry and concern for the relatives and they want to find out the genetic cause. The gene associated with this disorder is most likely to be found on which chromosome?

A. Chromosome 2
B. Chromosome 4
C. Chromosome 6
D. Chromosome 8
E. Chromosome 10.

10. The chief executive officer of a banking corporation has recently recovered from a stroke and says 'a murder between two banks' instead of 'a merger between two banks' during the annual meeting of shareholders. This phenomenon is known as:

A. Dyslexia
B. Dysnomia
C. Dysphasia
D. Vorbeigehen
E. Vorbeireden.

11. An examiner asks a person to move her arm in different directions and the person is unable to resist even if it is against her will. This phenomenon is known as:

A. Automatic obedience
B. Gegenhalten
C. Mitmachen
D. Mitgehen
E. Waxy flexibility.

12. When attempting passively to move the arm of an 80-year-old man with dementia, the examiner feels that the patient is applying the same amount of force in resisting the passive movement. This phenomenon is known as:

A. Ambitendency
B. Gegenhalten
C. Mitmachen
D. Mitgehen
E. Waxy flexibility.

13. Which of the following statements about psychological imprinting is correct?

A. An example of it is when a young animal learns the characteristics of its parents.
B. Expression of inheritance is determined by the 'parent of origin' effect.
C. It involves learning that is slow.
D. It involves learning that is dependent on the consequences of behaviour.
E. This concept is studied extensively by Tolman.

14. Eugene Bleuler proposed the term 'schizophrenia' for what Emil Kraepelin had been calling 'dementia praecox'. The reason was:

A. The term 'schizophrenia' refers to a disorder with onset in young adulthood that is different from dementia, which usually occurs in old age.
B. The term 'schizophrenia' refers to chronic disorder comprising hallucinations and delusions with a downhill course.
C. The term 'schizophrenia' refers to the integration of functional psychiatric disorder and organic disorder (e.g. catatonia).
D. The term 'schizophrenia' refers to significant deterioration of social functioning and poor long-term outcome that occurred in the era of asylums.
E. The term 'schizophrenia' refers to the 'splitting' of affect from other psychological functions, leading to a dissociation between the social situation and the emotion expressed.

15. A man sees a blue car driving past him and he realises that the terrorists are going to kill him. This is most likely to be which of the following?

A. Delusion of hypochondriasis
B. Delusion of passivity
C. Delusional perception
D. Delusion of persecution
E. Visual hallucination.

16. A 25-year-old male patient with schizophrenia presents with a condition in which he keeps his limbs in the same position for long periods. The core trainee has presented a list of symptoms. Which of the following symptoms is not associated with his condition?

A. Ambitendency
B. Blepharospasm
C. Echopraxia
D. Mannerisms
E. Waxy flexibility.

17. A 40-year-old lady develops hyperventilation in a department store. All of the following symptoms are associated with hyperventilation syndrome, except:

A. Epigastric pressure
B. Paraesthesia in the upper limbs
C. Increase in salivary secretions
D. Wheezing
E. Visual hallucinations.

18. A 40-year-old man has been prescribed lithium, haloperidol and fluoxetine. His GP consults you on the potential complications with his medications. Which of the following conditions is the most likely to occur owing to drug interaction in this man?

A. Catatonia
B. Malignant hyperthermia
C. Neuroleptic malignant syndrome
D. Serotonin syndrome
E. Rhabdomyolysis.

19. A 25-year-old man with schizophrenia hears his thoughts being spoken aloud whenever he hears the sound of a train whistle. This psychopathological phenomenon is known as:
    A. Echo de la pensée
    B. An extracampine hallucination
    C. A functional hallucination
    D. Gedankenlautwerden
    E. A reflex hallucination.

20. A mother is concerned about the sensory development of her newborn child. She worries about a delay in his development and consults you. Which of the following is not expected to be developed fully at birth?
    A. Hearing
    B. Smell
    C. Taste
    D. Touch
    E. Vision.

21. Which of the following is not part of depersonalization?
    A. Numbness in emotions
    B. Loss of feelings
    C. Distortions in experience of time
    D. Has a quantity of unfamiliarity
    E. A duration of only 30 seconds.

22. A 40-year-old woman suffers from bipolar disorder and has been treated with carbamazepine. The core trainee reports that there is an electrolyte abnormality. Which of the following electrolyte abnormalities is most likely to be associated with carbamazepine?
    A. Hypocalcaemia
    B. Hypercalcaemia
    C. Hyponatraemia
    D. Hypernatraemia
    E. Hypokalaemia.

23. Which of the following statements regarding stigma is false?
    A. Poor social support and avoidance coping account for more than half of the cases where caregivers of people with mental illness feel stigmatized and depressed.
    B. Perceived stigma among caregivers of people with mental illnesses is positively associated with the caregivers' depressive symptoms.
    C. There are significant gender differences among relatives coping with a family member suffering from severe mental illness.
    D. In a group of primary school children, most of the stigma towards people with mental illness occurs among the oldest children.
    E. Young people are socialized into stigmatizing conceptions of mental illness through children's TV programmes.

24. A 40-year-old in-patient has been prescribed lithium, haloperidol and a thiazide. The air conditioning in the hospital suddenly stops working on a hot summer's day. He first develops diarrhoea and nausea, and then becomes lethargic and drowsy. After 2 days, he develops marked neurological impairment and becomes confused. The staff nurse informs you. The patient is most likely to be suffering from:
    A. Catatonia
    B. Lithium toxicity
    C. Gastroenteritis
    D. Neuroleptic malignant syndrome
    E. Rhabdomyolysis.

25. Which of the following personality disorders is included in DSM-IV-TR but is classified as 'other specific personality disorders' in ICD-10?
    A. Anankastic personality disorder
    B. Anxious personality disorder
    C. Histrionic personality disorder
    D. Narcissistic personality disorder
    E. Paranoid personality disorder.

26. Which of the following is least likely to be found in patients taking lithium when the lithium level is within therapeutic range?
    A. Changes in ECG
    B. Endocrine abnormalities
    C. Nystagmus
    D. Peripheral oedema
    E. Weight gain.

27. A British psychiatrist says to an Iraqi refugee: 'I can image how difficult it is to escape from Iraq.' The refugee replies: 'I can image how difficult it is to escape from Iraq.' The tone and accent of the British psychiatrist are repeated as well. This phenomenon is known as:
    A. Cryptolalia
    B. Echolalia
    C. Logoclonia
    D. Logorrhoea
    E. Vorbeireden.

28. You are on call and the foundation-year doctor has informed you that a patient with bipolar disorder choked during dinner. The nursing staff performed the Heimlich manoeuvre and the patient recovered from the episode. Which of the following medications is most likely to be associated with this swallowing problem?
    A. Carbamazepine
    B. Lamotrigine
    C. Lithium
    D. Sodium valproate
    E. Quetiapine.

29. A man offers a handshake, then withdraws his hand and offers it again 10 times. The examiner cannot make a handshake with him. This phenomenon is known as:
    A. Ambitendency
    B. Gegenhalten
    C. Mitmachen
    D. Mitgehen
    E. Waxy flexibility.

30. A 19-year-old librarian with an intense interest in British colonial history is suspected of suffering from Asperger's syndrome. Which of the following is not consistent with the diagnosis?
    A. Childhood photographs showing a strange posture
    B. Delayed speech development until the age of 5 years
    C. Good performance in English class
    D. Lack of friends owing to impaired social relationship
    E. Poor performance in sport owing to motor clumsiness.

31. Which of the following psychologists named six different emotions (i.e. anger, disgust, fear, happiness, sadness and surprise)?
    A. Cannon, Walter
    B. Ekman, Paul
    C. Lange, Carl
    D. Plutchik, Robert
    E. Schachter, Stanley.

32. Which of the following is the most lethal combination of medications in causing serotonin syndrome?
    A. Phenelzine and fluoxetine
    B. Phenelzine and amitriptyline
    C. Phenelzine and meperidine
    D. Methylphendiate and MDMA
    E. Moclobemide and paroxetine.

33. Which of the following personality disorders is the most prevalent at the community level in the UK?
    A. Anankastic
    B. Anxious (avoidant)
    C. Borderline
    D. Dependent
    E. Narcissistic.

34. A core trainee is envied by the other trainees as she passed the MRCPscyh Paper 1 on her first attempt. She simply practised a lot of MCQs and EMIs and did not study hard. The other trainees failed even though they studied a lot of textbooks and read a lot of journal articles. What is the best explanation for this phenomenon?
    A. Barnum effect
    B. Halo effect
    C. Primacy effect
    D. Practice effect
    E. Recency effect.

35. Which of the following statement refers to virtue ethics?
    A. Acting in the best interests of patients
    B. The character of the doctor behind his or her actions
    C. The duty of a doctor to care for patients under the code of practice
    D. The principle of causing no harm to patients
    E. The principle of maintaining justice in society.

36. The four ethical principles (autonomy, beneficence, non-maleficence, justice) were recommended for use in medical ethics by:
    A. Beauchamp and Childress
    B. Benjamin Rush
    C. R. D. Laing
    D. Thomas Percival
    E. Thomas Szasz.

37. A 33-year-old woman describes the frequent experience of seeing a child sitting behind her in the train without the need to look back. The psychopathology being described is?
    A. Extracampine hallucination
    B. Doppelganger
    C. Hypnogogic hallucination
    D. Negative autoscopy
    E. Pseudohallucination.

38. A 40-year-old woman was treated with lithium and fluoxetine. She was brought to the Accident & Emergency (A&E) department after ingesting 100 tablets of one of these two drugs. The consultant from the A&E department would like to consult you. Which of the following is more suggestive of serotonin syndrome than lithium toxicity?
    A. Ataxia
    B. Drowsiness
    C. Gastroenteritis
    D. Hyperthermia
    E. Muscle twitching.

39. A 50-year-old man with chronic schizophrenia says: 'The community psychiatric nurse syringerisperidone me fortnightly.' This psychopathology is known as:
    A. Asyndesis
    B. Cryptolalia
    C. Metonym
    D. Neologism
    E. Vorbeigehen.

40. A medical student has interviewed a patient with obsessive–compulsive disorder (OCD) who was remanded after he was arrested for an assault of a pharmacy manager. The patient tried to steal an antiseptic from the local pharmacy. He attacked the pharmacy manager who tried to apprehend him. He has history of repeated theft of antiseptics. The medical student wants to ask you some questions about OCD. Which of the following is incorrect?
    A. Shoplifting is more common in OCD patients than in the general population.
    B. The patient needs to check. This is the most common compulsion among people with OCD.
    C. The patient mentions that he has a fear of contamination. This is the most common obsession among people with OCD.
    D. The patient does not mention any obsessional image as this is a relatively uncommon obsession.
    E. If the patient undergoes brain PET scanning, this is likely to show hypermetabolism in the left orbital gyrus and both caudate nuclei.

41. A 35-year-old man is suing his company for compensation for his cognitive impairment as a result of a head injury he sustained at his workplace 6 months ago. You have referred him for formal neuropsychological assessment. The neuropsychologist has prepared the report. Which of following findings does not suggest feigned amnesia?
    A. Impairment of attention or immediate memory that is much worse than impairment of overall learning and memory
    B. Standardized scores on tests of recognition memory are higher than standardized scores on tests of free recall
    C. Reports of severe retrograde amnesia together with intact new learning and absence of neurological abnormality
    D. Gross inconsistency across tests or testing occasions
    E. Evasive or unusual test-taking behaviour.

42. Which of the following statements regarding chronic fatigue syndrome (CFS) is false?
    A. Approximately one-third of patients with CFS have hypocortisolism.
    B. Postviral symptoms cannot be discriminated from affective symptoms.
    C. Physical and mental fatigue symptoms are dissociable.
    D. Viral infection is detectable in 90 per cent of cases.
    E. At least 30 per cent of patients with CFS have a concurrent psychiatric illness.

43. A 60-year-old woman presents with bitemporal hemianopia and the CT scan shows a tumour. Which of the following sites is a possible site for the CNS tumour?
    A. Tumour compressing the optic nerve
    B. Pituitary tumour
    C. Tumour in the temporal lobe
    D. Tumour in the anterior parietal lobe
    E. Tumour in the occipital cortex.

44. A Greenland Inuit female suddenly strips off her clothes and rolls in the snow followed by echolalia and echopraxia. She has no recollection of the episode afterwards. Which of the following culture-bound syndromes does she suffer from?
    A. Amok
    B. Latah
    C. Pibloktoq
    D. Uqamairineq
    E. Windigo.

45. A 40-year-old man has been prescribed with lithium, haloperidol and fluoxetine. The core trainee consults you as the patient has developed a tremor. Which of the following features suggest that the tremor is caused by the haloperidol?
    A. Coarse tremor
    B. Dysdiadokinesis
    C. Fine tremor

D. Parkinsonism
E. Wide-based gait.

46. An elderly Chinese man complains that: 'My guts are rotten and blood has stopped flowing to my heart. I am dead.' The psychopathology being described is:
    A. Acute intestinal obstruction
    B. Delirium
    C. Delusion of control
    D. Nihilistic delusion
    E. Hypochondriasis.

47. A 20-year-old woman reports that she hears her thoughts being spoken out loud. The psychopathology being described is:
    A. Gedankenlautwerden
    B. Pseudohallucination
    C. Running commentary
    D. Second-person auditory hallucinations
    E. Third-person auditory hallucinations.

48. A core trainee finds the medical ward unfamiliar although she has worked in the ward for 6 months. This phenomenon is known as:
    A. Amnesia
    B. Déjà vu
    C. Déjà entendu
    D. Déjà pensé
    E. Jamais vu.

49. You are interviewing the husband of a woman with personality disorder and invite him to talk about his feeling towards his wife. He replies, 'Frustrated' and does not want to say more. Which of the following interview techniques is most likely to help the interview to continue?
    A. Closed-ended questions
    B. Long pause
    C. Prolonged eye contact
    D. Summation
    E. Transition.

50. A core trainee presents a list of symptoms for neuroleptic malignant syndrome (NMS). All of the following are symptoms of NMS except:
    A. NMS presents within 48 hours after the initiation of a new antipsychotic
    B. Dysphagia
    C. Labile blood pressure
    D. Leucocytosis
    E. Mutism.

51. A medical student asks you the specific type of epilepsy that is most commonly associated with olfactory hallucination. Your answer should be:
    A. Medial frontal lobe lesions and complex partial seizure
    B. Medial parietal lobe lesions and complex partial seizure
    C. Medial parietal lobe lesions and simple partial seizure

D. Medial temporal lobe lesions and complex partial seizure

E. Medial temporal lobe lesions and simple partial seizure

52. Which of the combinations of antidepressant therapy is the safest?
    A. Trimipramine and phenelzine
    B. Clomipramine and moclobemide
    C. Fluoxetine and phenelzine
    D. Venlafaxine and moclobemide
    E. Trazodone and phenelzine.

53. Which of the following statements regarding the Rey–Osterrieth Complex Figure Test is true?
    A. Patients with dyslexia show significant impairment in recalling the structures from memory compared with controls without dyslexia.
    B. Patients with frontal lobe lesions mainly have difficulty with spatial organization.
    C. Patients with left hemisphere damage tend to make more omissions compared with controls without head injury.
    D. Patients with parietal lobe lesions mainly demonstrate perseveration in copies.
    E. Patients with right hemispheric damage tend to break the drawing into smaller units and simplify drawings compared with controls without head injury.

54. An individual with bipolar affective disorder and long-term alcohol dependence develops haematemesis. He is advised by the gastroenterologist to go for an oesophago-gastroduodenoscopy (OGD) to identify the bleeding site. On assessment, he appears to have the capacity to make that decision and he is not manic. The psychiatrist advises acceding to his wish not to have the OGD. This case illustrates which of the following?
    A. The principle of respect for a person's autonomy
    B. The principle of beneficence
    C. The principle of non-maleficence
    D. Paternalism approach
    E. Utilitarian approach.

55. During an initial psychiatric interview, a 30-year-old woman presenting with anxiety and hypervigilance reveals that her parents were involved with the mafia and she witnessed a lot of violence as a child. She proceeds to reveal more related details. This piece of history:
    A. should not be mentioned until the psychiatrist is presenting the social and developmental history
    B. should be briefly alluded to in the history of the present illness and the details can be further elaborated in the social history
    C. is not relevant to the patient's current chief complaint and should not be included in the case presentation
    D. should not be included in the case presentation in order to respect the patient's privacy

E. should be mentioned in the family history section only.

56. A psychiatrist is evaluating a patient who has taken an overdose. Patient: 'I just want everything to end. What else can I do? My life has fallen apart and nothing is going to fix it.' Psychiatrist: 'It sounds like you are feeling really sad and hopeless.' In this exchange, the psychiatrist's response is:
    A. an open-ended question
    B. a close-ended question
    C. an interpretation
    D. a basic empathic statement
    E. a transition.

57. All the following are ICD-10 diagnostic criteria for delusional disorder except:
    A. There is a set of related delusions (e.g. persecutory, grandiose, hypochondriacal, jealous or erotic delusions).
    B. The duration of delusions must be present for at least 6 months.
    C. There must be no persistent hallucination.
    D. The general criteria for schizophrenia and depressive disorder should not be fulfilled.
    E. There must be no evidence of primary or secondary organic mental disorders.

58. Which of the following refers to balancing the risks and benefits of a new antipsychotic for people with schizophrenia?
    A. The principle of respect for a person's autonomy
    B. The principle of beneficence
    C. The principle of non-maleficence
    D. Paternalism approach
    E. Utilitarian approach.

59. You have decided to start a patient on lithium. The GP has ordered renal and thyroid function tests for the patient. Which of the following investigations needs to be done before starting lithium?
    A. Computed tomography
    B. Echocardiogram
    C. Electrocardiogram
    D. Electroencephalogram
    E. Electromyography.

60. Which of the following statements about cognitive dissonance theory is incorrect?
    A. Adding new explanations to support one set of cognitions can reduce cognitive dissonance.
    B. Cognitive dissonance can lead to anxiety.
    C. Cognitive dissonance can result in a change in attitudes.
    D. Selective attention can increase cognitive dissonance.
    E. This theory was proposed by Festinger in 1957.

61. A 50-year-old man presents with ptosis. The following are all possible differential diagnoses, except:
    A. Lambert–Eaton syndrome

B. Myasthenia gravis

C. Horner's syndrome

D. III nerve palsy

E. VI nerve palsy.

62. What is the percentage of psychiatric in-patients suffering from personality disorder?

A. 10 per cent

B. 20 per cent

C. 30 per cent

D. 40 per cent

E. 50 per cent.

63. An 18-year-old A-level student comes to your clinic complaining of excessive daytime sleepiness in class with hypnogogic hallucinations. What is the most likely condition he suffers from?

A. Catalepsy

B. Narcolepsy

C. Night terror

D. Sleep apnoea

E. Sleep walking.

64. A 35-year-old man presents with fever, hypertonia and autonomic lability. The following are all likely diagnoses, except:

A. Catatonia

B. Encephalitis

C. 'Locked in' syndrome

D. Meningitis

E. Neuroleptic malignant syndrome.

65. At the beginning of an interview before the psychiatrist is able to enquire about the chief complaint, the patient wants to talk about the 'diagnosis' that her family has already assigned to her illness. The psychiatrist should:

A. gently interrupt and redirect the patient to talk about the chief complaint.

B. apologize to the patient, explain that time is limited and proceed to ask close-ended questions.

C. point out that what her family believes her problem to be is not as important as how she perceives it.

D. allow the patient to talk freely for a few minutes and complete her thoughts.

E. interrupt and ask the patient where her family came from.

66. You are the specialist trainee working in adolescent liaison psychiatry and discover that a doctor from the paediatric team has forgotten to administer N-acetylcysteine, causing further suffering to a 15-year-old girl who was admitted to the ward after a paracetamol overdose. You have ensured the safety of the patient but the paediatric consultant asks you not to tell anyone about the error. No one has spoken to the parents and they are not aware of the error. What should you do first?

A. Inform the consultant psychiatrist

B. Inform the General Medical Council

C. Complete a critical incident form

D. Inform the parents

E. Inform the police.

67. You have diagnosed a 35-year-old bus driver as suffering from schizophrenia. You recommend him to notify the Driver and Vehicle Licensing Authority (DVLA) because he has a psychiatric condition that might preclude safe driving. He insists that he wants to continue his work as his bus route is simple and he has a clean driving record. Which of the following statements is correct?

A. More than half of the psychiatric disorders identified on police reports as the cause of road traffic accidents are the result of schizophrenia.

B. This patient insisted on working in spite of your advice. Under UK legislation, it is mandatory for you to inform the police.

C. This patient does not agree with your recommendation and the law. His appeal will be heard before the Crown Court.

D. He may drive the bus after being symptom-free for three consecutive years after any psychotic episode.

E. He can hold a vocational driving licence as he takes antipsychotic medication on a regular basis.

68. Which is the following is considered to be a normal development milestone in a child?

A. Tertiary circular reactions at 6 months

B. Constant babbling at the age of 7 months

C. Development of colour vision at 8 months

D. Preoperational stage at 1 year

E. Fear of darkness at 3 years.

69. A 30-year-old man suffering from bipolar disorder has been receiving an anticonvulsant for 2 months. He attends an Accident & Emergency department and complains of sudden and sharp mid-epigastric pain. His serum amylase is raised. Which of the following anticonvulsants is the most likely to cause this presentation?

A. Carbamazepine

B. Lamotrigine

C. Gabapentin

D. Sodium valproate

E. Topiramate.

70. The following are all findings from the Clinical Antipsychotic Trials of Intervention Effectiveness (CATIE) study, except:

A. More patients taking second-generation antipsychotics continue the antipsychotic treatment compared with patients taking conventional antipsychotics.

B. Olanzapine was the most effective in terms of the rates of discontinuation.

C. The efficacy of the conventional antipsychotic agent perphenazine appeared similar to that of quetiapine, risperidone and ziprasidone.

D. Olanzapine was associated with greater weight gain and increases in measures of glucose and lipid metabolism.

E. Perphenazine was associated with more discontinuation for extrapyramidal effects.

71. Which of the following anticonvulsants is the least likely to cause visual side effects?
    A. Carbamazepine
    B. Gabapentin
    C. Sodium valproate
    D. Topiramate
    E. Vigabatrin.

72. Which of the following theorist(s) demanded that: research subjects be treated with respect and dignity; a philosophical account was written about why persons should always be treated as ends in themselves, and never only as means; and a researcher must respect research subjects as having their own autonomously established goals and individual freedom to make decisions?
    A. Aristotle and Plato
    B. Beauchamp and Childress
    C. Casuists
    D. Kant
    E. Tarasoff.

73. The examiner wants to move a man's arm upwards and asks him to resist movement. Even with a slight touch of the examiner's fingertips, the person continues to move his arm upwards and then returns to the original position. This phenomenon is known as:
    A. Automatic obedience
    B. Gegenhalten
    C. Mitmachen
    D. Mitgehen
    E. Waxy flexibility.

74. Concomitant use with an irreversible monoamine oxidase inhibitor (MAOI) must be avoided for all of the following drugs except:
    A. Carbamazepine
    B. Stimulants
    C. Selective serotonin reuptake inhibitors
    D. Insulin
    E. L-tryptophan.

75. The following statement is true about primary (autochthonous) delusion:
    A. It can be preceded by delusional mood (wahnstimmung).
    B. It is considered to be a core criterion of Schneider's first-rank symptoms of schizophrenia.
    C. It has prognostic value for people with schizophrenia.
    D. It is secondary to depression or mania.
    E. It is often understood by people from the same culture.

76. A new psychiatric consultant has been appointed by the trust to head a community psychiatric team. He is known to be a 'hands off' person and is not available most of the time. He seldom gives feedback to his team members. Which of the following teams will be effective under his leadership?
    A. Assertive team members who request major decisions to be made by voting and thorough discussion among the whole team
    B. Team members who are eager to learn and request constant supervision from the consultant psychiatrist
    C. Honest team members who are good at performing routine home visits repeatedly
    D. Humble team members who prefer the consultant psychiatrist to make major decisions
    E. Trustworthy team members who are experienced in community psychiatry and skilful in dealing with complicated issues. They require minimal supervision.

77. Which of the following statements is false with regard to the consequentialist approach?
    A. An action is moral if it makes the greatest number of people happy.
    B. Different treatment options can be measured by foreseeable consequences such as quality of life years (QALYs).
    C. In managed mental healthcare, the consequentialist approach may lead to discrimination of individual patients and moral dilemmas owing to factual uncertainties.
    D. It is based on an obligation of fidelity (including a pledge for confidentiality), deontological theory and virtue ethics.
    E. Under the consequentialist approach, confidentiality is an absolute condition in psychiatric practice.

78. A 40-year-old lady develops panic disorder. She wants to know which of the following is the commonest symptom found in patients with panic disorder. Your answer is:
    A. Numbness
    B. Palpitation
    C. Trembling
    D. Shortness of breath
    E. Globus hystericus.

79. Massive budget cuts in a country have provoked long-term unemployment and sparked a wave of suicides. Of the following sociologists, who is best associated with providing an explanation for this phenomenon?
    A. Durkheim Emile
    B. Foucault Michel
    C. Goffman Erving
    D. Talcott Parsons
    E. Weber Max.

80. A 40-year-old female teacher suffering from depression has been on sick leave for the past 6 months. She has asked the core trainee to continue giving her sick leave. The core trainee is concerned and consults you. Which of the following is an indicator for not issuing a medical certificate to this patient?
    A. She is willing to continue the antidepressant as suggested by the core trainee.
    B. She is keen to see a psychologist for psychotherapy as suggested by the core trainee.
    C. She wants to be in a depressive state as her husband gives her more support when she is sick.
    D. She is very depressed and cannot focus on teaching. She needs to be exempted from her normal social role.
    E. She is very depressed and worries that the school will blame her for being responsible for causing her own depression.

81. Based on the Holmes and Rahe Social Readjustment Rating Scale, which of the following events is considered to be the most stressful event contributing to illness?
    A. Death of a close family member
    B. Death of a spouse
    C. Divorce
    D. Marital separation
    E. Imprisonment.

82. The rate of attempted suicide within contemporary Goth youth subculture in the UK is around:
    A. 17 per cent
    B. 27 per cent
    C. 37 per cent
    D. 47 per cent
    E. 57 per cent.

83. Which of the following statements is correct about Assertive Community Treatment (ACT)?
    A. Treatment is provided in vitro (in day hospitals first). Skills learned in the day hospital or protected environment can be better applied in the community at a later stage.
    B. ACT also involves the patient's partner or caregiver in an assertive manner, as evidence has suggested this will improve outcome.
    C. ACT is based on the 'brokerage' model.
    D. In the randomized controlled study of Training in Community Living (TCL) programme, improvements in clinical state and functioning of people with chronic mental illnesses were achieved without additional burden on families or other informal carers.
    E. ACT has traditionally been separated from the local mental health services and voluntary organizations.

84. A 28-year-old school teacher was referred by her GP for assessment of depression. She appears to be very thin but does not know her BMI. She insists that she was too fat in the past which resulted in interpersonal problems. She eats three meals a day but is not able to describe her diet in detail. She denies excessive exercise but induces vomiting if she eats too much. She complains of amenorrhoea and alopecia. She has been irritable throughout the interview and emphasizes that she suffers from depression but nothing else. She is only keen to continue fluoxetine given by her GP but no other treatment. She emphasizes that she is in a good physical condition and is able to teach. After the interview, the nurse measures her BMI and the result is 13 kg/m². What is the most likely diagnosis?
    A. Anorexia nervosa
    B. Borderline personality disorder
    C. Bulimia nervosa
    D. Depressive disorder
    E. Hypomania.

85. You are the adolescent psychiatrist in a community where there has recently been a significant increase in substance abuse among secondary-school students. You have conducted a focus group with the students on substance abuse and the analysis shows that they are under pressure of conformity to use drugs. The school principal wants to develop a prevention strategy and has prepared a list of factors that she thinks might have an impact on their conformity. Which of the following factors is known to influence conformity among students?
    A. Fear of ridicule
    B. Personality of the students
    C. Previous history of substance abuse
    D. The number of students with conduct disorder
    E. Public education on substance abuse provided by the local health authority.

86. A single, female consultant physician is notorious for her bad temper as she likes openly to scold junior doctors and nurses in the ward for minor mistakes. A male medical colleague has a hard time with her; she labels him as having 'absolutely no knowledge'. Your colleague wants you to comment on her personality. You suggest that she may have an authoritarian personality. Which of the following is incorrect?
    A. The authoritarian personality theory was developed by Adorno.
    B. The authoritarian personality theory is a psychodynamic theory regarding authoritarian upbringing.
    C. The authoritarian personality theory is a psychodynamic theory which explains prejudice.
    D. She is contemptuous towards the hospital chief executive.
    E. She is contemptuous towards medical students.

87. Which of the following schizophrenia symptoms is not classified as a passivity phenomenon?
    A. Made will
    B. Thought blocking
    C. Thought broadcasting
    D. Thought insertion
    E. Thought withdrawal.

88. A 55-year-old woman suffered from a heart attack and was resuscitated by the doctors in the Accident & Emergency department. She has recovered from the episode. She later consults her GP and complains of recurrent nightmares and hypervigilance. She worries that she may suffer from nervous shock and her GP has referred her for a psychiatric assessment. During the interview, she mentions that she did not have a heart attack. She thinks she developed an anaphylactic shock after an injection and wants to sue the hospital for compensation as she is incapable of working owing to the nervous shock. Which of the following statements is most likely to be correct?
    A. There is a high chance that she will be able to return to work after settlement of this case.
    B. She meets the criteria for nervous shock but not post-traumatic stress disorder.
    C. You should refer her to see a forensic psychiatrist for a formal and proper medicolegal assessment.
    D. After you write the medical report, she is likely to be unhappy with the fact that you did not support her claim of having nervous shock and will lodge a formal complaint to the chief executive through her lawyer.
    E. She should be referred to see an expert in post-traumatic stress disorder for trauma-focused CBT.

89. A pregnant woman suffering from bipolar disorder consults you on the teratogenic effect of sodium valproate. This drug affects all the following organs or structures in the fetus, except:
    A. Heart
    B. Kidney
    C. Lip
    D. Neural tube
    E. Palate.

90. A GP is interested in conducting a study to identify people with mental health problems who are at increased risk of developing metabolic syndrome. Which of the following questionnaires can be used to identify psychiatric 'caseness'?
    A. The COOP charts for Adult Primary Care Practice
    B. Global Assessment Scale (GAS)
    C. General Health Questionnaire (GHQ)
    D. Health Outcome Study Short Form–36 (SF-36)
    E. The Nottingham Health Profile (NHP).

91. Which of the following statements about fundamental attribution error is incorrect?
    A. The fundamental attribution error is the general tendency people have to make internal attributions for others' behaviour.
    B. Witnesses attribute a criminal's behaviour to a defective personality rather than social circumstances.
    C. Witnesses of a homicide have less fundamental attribution error to the murderer compared with witnesses of an episode of shoplifting to the shoplifter.

    D. Witnesses to car crashes are more likely to attribute the cause to reckless driving than to errors in road design.
    E. White Caucasian witnesses of a fight between a white man and a black man are more likely to make negative internal attributions when the black man hits the white man.

92. Which of the following is not a recognized type of validity?
    A. Constructional validity
    B. Divergent validity
    C. Dynamic validity
    D. Ecological validity
    E. Face validity.

93. Your medical colleague is preparing for the MRCP examination and complains that he keeps on forgetting the information he has learnt. He wants to seek your advice on the underlying reason for forgetting. The following are established factors which could lead to his forgetfulness except:
    A. He forgets the information owing to disuse of information after a 1-year period of unpaid leave.
    B. He forgets the information as he spent 6 months learning surgery which has displaced his knowledge of internal medicine.
    C. When his consultant asks him questions, the answer is almost at the tip of his tongue but he cannot recall it.
    D. He can recite his knowledge perfectly in his bedroom with classical music playing but cannot recall it in the examination hall.
    E. When he studies, he usually feels sad. In the examination he often puts down the answer 'don't know' when answering MCQs as he also feels sad during the examination.

94. A 32-year-old lady seen in the emergency department says: 'They think I am in the department store, drinking in the basement, masturbating in the toilet. I go to the train station. I fall down from the platform. I want to jump to be as high as the top of the world.' The psychopathology being described is?
    A. Circumstantial speech
    B. Crowding of thought
    C. Loosening of associations
    D. Flight of ideas
    E. Tangentiality.

95. A 30-year-old lady who suffers from depression attempts suicide after ingesting 25 50 mg tablets of amitriptyline prescribed by her GP. The patient looks alert and the Accident & Emergency department consultant asks you to admit this patient to the psychiatric ward as he thinks that the psychiatric risk is higher than the medical risk. You are concerned about her medical condition. Which part of the ECG would be most significant in assessing her cardiac risk?
    A. Length of P wave
    B. Length of QRS interval

C. Length of RR interval

D. T-wave inversion

E. Pathological U wave.

96. The sister of a man with schizophrenia has read about 'simple schizophrenia'. Which of the following symptoms found in her brother do not support a diagnosis of simple schizophrenia?

A. Failure to continue university studies

B. Florid third-person auditory hallucinations

C. Inability to maintain personal hygiene

D. Odd behaviour such as locking himself in the toilet and colouring the water in a bath tub

E. Progressive withdrawal and isolation.

97. A male teenager is admitted to the ward owing to florid psychotic features. He has been smoking cannabis for 9 months. His father wants to know the increased likelihood that he will develop schizophrenia as a result of the cannabis use. Your answer should be:

A. two to three times

B. four to five times

C. six to seven times

D. eight to nine times

E. 10 times.

98. A 20-year-old man is referred to the Early Psychosis Team for a first-episode of psychosis. His mother is very concerned about the prognosis. You have reviewed his medical records. Which of the following factors in this case is most likely to be associated with a poor prognosis?

A. He has history of using cannabis.

B. The diagnosis is not clear and he may suffer from severe mania with psychotic features.

C. This patient came from Nigeria 1 year ago.

D. The patient receives haloperidol and cognitive behavioural therapy.

E. The diagnosis is confirmed to be schizophrenia and he is being treated with haloperidol alone.

99. A 21-year-old female medical student is brought in by the university counsellor as she is in shock and anger after being informed that she has failed all the subjects in her examinations and that she will need to repeat the first year. When you examine her, she is in a daze with purposeless overactivity. The counsellor wants to know when her symptoms will start to disappear. Based on the ICD-10 criteria, the answer is:

A. 1 hour

B. 12 hours

C. 24 hours

D. 48 hours

E. 60 hours.

100. A 35-year-old woman suffers from a severe depressive episode. She has three young children studying in primary school. She is unemployed with no confiding relationship. Which of the following works provides an explanation in her case?

A. Brown and Harris: *Social Origins of Depression*

B. Durkheim E: *Anomie*

C. Habermas J: *The Theory of Communicative Action*

D. Parsons T: *The Social System*

E. Sullivan HS: *The Interpersonal Theory of Psychiatry*

101. A 69-year-old woman is brought in to see you by her husband owing to recent changes in her behaviour. While testing her recent memory, you ask her what she had for lunch. She replies, 'Sandwich'. Then you ask, 'What is your name?' and she says, 'Sandwich'. When you ask, 'Where do you live?', she continues to say, 'Sandwich'. This phenomenon is known as:

A. Circumstantiality

B. Dysphasia

C. Perseveration

D. Poverty of speech

E. Tangentiality.

102. A 35-year-old patient with schizophrenia previously on olanzapine was diagnosed by his GP to suffer from diabetes mellitus. Her GP has written a letter to consult you on the most suitable antipsychotics to prescribe. Which of the following antipsychotics would you recommend in this case?

A. Amisulpride

B. Chlorpromazine

C. Clozapine

D. Risperidone

E. Quetiapine.

103. The Royal College of Psychiatrists conducts a study on the test–retest reliability of the Angoff method of setting standards for MRCPsych Paper 1 MCQs. At baseline, a panel of consultants examines each multiple-choice item and estimates the probability that the 'minimally competent' candidates would answer the items correctly. Six months later, the same group of consultants are asked to examine the same set of MCQs used at baseline. The standard set by consultants using the Angoff method at baseline and after 6 months gives a reliability of 0.7. Based on this result, which of the following conclusions is most likely to be correct?

A. Different consultants give consistent estimates of the standard of the MCQs based on the Angoff method.

B. There is a moderate consistency across items within the MRCPsych Paper 1.

C. There is a moderate consistency between the first and second halves of the MRCPsych Paper 1.

D. There is a moderate consistency of using the Angoff method to set the standard of MCQs from one time to another.

E. There is a moderate consistency of using the Angoff method to set the standard of two sets of Paper 1 constructed in the same way to the same panel of consultants.

104. A 24-year-old man covers his head with a helmet because he believes that other people can receive his thoughts. The psychopathology being described is?

A. Delusional memory

B. Running commentary

C. Thought broadcasting
D. Thought echo
E. Thought insertion.

105. Which of the following personality disorders is the most disabling in terms of occupational success?
A. Borderline
B. Dependent
C. Dissocial
D. Paranoid
E. Schizoid.

106. The local government wants to build a psychiatric rehabilitation centre but the local residents strongly oppose this idea as they claim that psychiatric patients pose a risk to the community. The local MP has come up with the following techniques to change their attitude. Which of them is the most effective in changing the residents' attitude towards psychiatric patients?
A. Demonstrate the success of psychiatric rehabilitation centres in other counties.
B. Political propaganda and legislation to limit the residents' options.
C. Provide additional privileges to the residents if they accept the proposal.
D. Indoctrinate the residents with the theory of community psychiatry and psychiatric rehabilitation.
E. The MP conveys a two-sided meeting and delivers genuine messages to the residents on the proposal.

107. Which of the following personality disorders has the highest admission rate?
A. Anxious
B. Borderline
C. Dissocial
D. Dependent
E. Histrionic.

108. Which of the following statements about attention is incorrect?
A. An inexperienced driver needs to pay more attention during driving. This is an example of controlled attention.
B. An experienced driver requires less attention during driving. This is an example of automatic attention.
C. A student requires sustained attention in class. This phenomenon is known as concentration.
D. Divided attention is the ability to pay attention to two objects at the same time.
E. In focused attention, one type of information is selected for attention while the alternative information is totally ignored.

109. A 24-year-old female patient comes for review to your out-patient clinic. The in-patient consultant prescribed olanzapine and she has been taking this medication for 3 months since discharge. She complains of weight gain of 10 kg and increased appetite. She has a family history of diabetes. She requests a change in antipsychotic. Which of the following medications would you recommend?
A. Aripiprazole
B. Paliperidone
C. Quetiapine
D. Risperidone
E. Ziprasidone.

110. Which of the following is not a feature of pseudobulbar palsy?
A. Donald Duck speech
B. Emotional incontinence
C. Normal jaw jerk
D. Spastic tongue
E. Upper motor neuron lesions due to bilateral lesion above the mid-pons.

111. Which of the following statements regarding the Nuremberg Code is false?
A. It was drafted after the Second World War in Nuremberg.
B. It was a trial by American judges of Japanese doctors who conducted the '7–31' project killing civilians in northern China.
C. It is based on the Hippocratic Oath.
D. The American judges defined 10 research principles.
E. It emphasizes the importance of consent.

112. A 24-year-old man hears a voice coming from an office building across the road, describing everything he is doing in his flat. What is the psychopathology being described?
A. Delusional perception
B. Pseudohallucination
C. Running commentary
D. Second-person auditory hallucination
E. Third-person auditory hallucinations.

113. A 60-year-old lady is admitted to the geriatric ward with the complaints of visual hallucination, symmetrical Parkinsonism and neuroleptic sensitivity. Her husband consults you about whether there is a test to differentiate Lewy body dementia from Alzheimer's disease. Your answer is:
A. Computed tomography
B. Diffusion tensor imaging
C. DaTSCAN (ioflupane 123-I injection)
D. Functional magnetic resonance imaging
E. 18-F Fluorodeoxyglucose positron emission tomography.

EXTENDED MATCHING ITEMS (EMIs)

Questions 114–120 – options
- A. Aversive conditioning
- B. Chaining
- C. Flooding
- D. Habituation
- E. Insight learning
- F. Latent learning
- G. Penalty
- H. Premack's principle
- I. Reciprocal inhibition
- J. Shaping
- K. Systematic desensitization
- L. Token economy

Lead-in: From the above list of behavioural techniques select the option that best matches each of the following examples. Each option might be used once, more than once or not at all.

114. The staff of a hostel for learning disability patients want to train their clients to clean up the tables after meals. They develop a successive reinforcing schedule to reward their clients. The clients will be rewarded successively over time for removing their utensils from the dining table into the kitchen. Then they need to wash and dry the utensils and put them back into the right drawers. (Choose one option.)

115. A 2-year-old son of a woman is scared of dogs. His mother tries to reduce his fear by bringing him to see the dogs in the park. The fear-provoking situation is coupled and opposed by putting him on her lap and allowing him to drink his favourite juice. (Choose one option.)

116. A 40-year-old woman staying in London develops fear of the Tube (underground metro) and she sees a psychologist for psychotherapy. The psychologist has drafted a behavioural programme in which the patient is advised to start by travelling between two tube stations with her husband and gradually increase this to more stations without her husband. At the end of the hierarchy, she will travel alone on the long journey from a Heathrow terminal station to Cockfosters station along almost the entire length of the Piccadilly line. (Choose one option.)

117. A 40-year-old woman staying in London who develops fear of the Tube is instructed to start with the most fearful situation by taking a train on her own from a Heathrow terminal station to Cockfosters station along the Piccadilly line. (Choose one option.)

118. An 11-year-old girl is referred to the Child and Adolescent Mental Health Service (CAMHS) as she refuses to do her homework. She prefers to stay in her room and play the piano for the whole day. The team has advised the parents to adopt the following plan: the girl is allowed to play her piano for 30 minutes only after spending 1 hour on her homework. (Choose one option.)

119. A 9-year-old girl is referred to the CAMHS as she refuses to do her homework. The case manager advises the mother to reward her child with a sticker every time she has completed her homework. Once she gets 20 stickers, she can exchange them for a present. (Choose one option.)

120. In a prison, psychologists have developed an in vivo exposure programme for the prisoners to expose themselves to the images of being arrested and other social sanctions on their criminal behaviour. Some prisoners find that their urge to commit crime reduce after repeated exposures. (Choose one option.)

Questions 121–126 – options
- A. Aversive conditioning
- B. Chaining
- C. Flooding
- D. Habituation
- E. Insight learning
- F. Latent learning
- G. Penalty
- H. Premack's principle
- I. Reciprocal inhibition
- J. Shaping
- K. Systematic desensitization
- L. Token economy

Lead-in: From the above list of behavioural techniques select the option that best matches each of the following examples. Each option might be used once, more than once or not at all.

121. A 6-year-old boy is put in a maze to look for the toy box. After a few trials, he learns the cognitive map of the maze and needs a shorter time to find the toy box. (Choose one option.)

122. A 2-year-old child is undergoing toilet training. The complex behaviour is broken down into simpler steps. She is rewarded with a sticker if she informs her mother when she has the urge to urinate. The positive reinforcement continues until she can inform her mother reliably without failures. The contingencies are then altered and she needs to go to the toilet on her own before the sticker is given. (Choose one option.)

123. A patient with moderate learning disability has an aggressive tendency and tends to assault other residents in the hostel. The staff have devised a plan in response to his aggressive behaviour. His main pleasurable activity is watching TV. He will be removed from the TV room and put in a single room for a 2-hour time-out period if he assaults any resident. (Choose one option.)

124. A 14-year-old anorexia nervosa patient with a BMI of 11 kg/m² is admitted to an eating disorder unit for in-patient treatment. Initially, she is hostile to the staff and resistant to feeding. She does not like the ward environment. She later decides to comply with the treatment programme. She also wants to reach the

target weight as soon as possible, as she wants to get out of the ward. (Choose one option.)

125. A 10-year-old boy is taught by his parents not to respond to the TV sound when he is doing homework as the stimulus is not significant. (Choose one option.)

126. A 20-year-old man is sacked by his company. His partner criticizes him. He suddenly realizes that he has been lazy and irresponsible. He decides to change and wants to demonstrate his competence to his partner. The next day, he goes to the career centre to look for a job. (Choose one option.)

Questions 127–134 – options

A. Argyll Robertson pupils
B. Blepharospasm
C. Cranial third nerve palsy
D. Cranial fourth nerve palsy
E. Horner's syndrome
F. Hutchison's pupil
G. Myasthenia gravis
H. Pellagra

Lead-in: Match the above conditions to the following clinical presentations. Each option might be used once, more than once or not at all.

127. A 35-year-old man presents with dilated pupils, extraocular muscle palsies and ptosis. (Choose one option.)

128. A 40-year-old man presents with anhidrosis, miosis and ptosis. (Choose one option.)

129. A 43-year-old woman presents with great difficulty in moving her eye downwards and laterally. She also has diplopia. (Choose one option.)

130. A 45-year-old man presents with small irregular pupils. (Choose one option.)

131. A 47-year-old woman presents with ptosis, extraocular muscle palsies and progressive external ophthalmoplegia. (Choose one option.)

132. A 50-year-old woman presents with dilated pupils and miosis. (Choose one option.)

133. A 53-year-old woman presents with diarrhoea, dermatitis and dementia. (Choose one option.)

134. A 55-year-old woman presents with painful eyes and forced eye closure when the doctor examines her. She also has visual impairments. (Choose one option.)

Questions 135 –140 – options

A. Bleuler
B. Kahlbaum
C. Kasanin
D. Kraepelin
E. Langfeldt
F. Leonard
G. Hecker
H. Griesinger
I. Kane
J. Andreason
K. Crow
L. Liddle
M. Mayer-Gross
N. Kendler

Lead-in: Select one person who is best associated with introducing each of the following terms. Each option might be used once, more than once or not at all.

135. Catatonia (choose one option).

136. Cycloid psychosis (choose one option).

137. Dementia praecox (choose one option).

138. Hebephrenia (choose one option).

139. Schizophrenia (choose one option).

140. Schizoaffective disorder (choose one option).

Questions 141–145 – options

A. 0–4 per cent
B. 5–9 per cent
C. 10–14 per cent
D. 15–19 per cent
E. 20–24 per cent
F. 25–29 per cent
G. 30–34 per cent
H. 35–50 per cent
I. 60–65 per cent
J. 70–75 per cent
K. 80–85 per cent

Lead-in: A 28-year-old man has suffered from schizophrenia for 5 years. He is currently stable and recently got married. He and his wife are planning to have children. He consults you on the genetic risk of schizophrenia. Each option might be used once, more than once, or not at all.

141. The risk of schizophrenia for his child if his wife also suffers from schizophrenia. (Choose one option.)

142. The risk of schizophrenia for his child if his wife does not suffer from schizophrenia. (Choose one option.)

143. The risk of schizophrenia if he adopted a child with velocardiofacial syndrome. (Choose one option.)

144. The risk of schizophrenia in his half-siblings. (Choose one option.)

145. The risk of schizophrenia in his younger cousin. (Choose one option.)

Questions 146–148 – options

A. 1
B. 2
C. 5
D. 15
E. 25

F. 35
G. 45
H. 55
I. 65
J. 75

Lead-in: A 17-year-old man is referred to the Early Psychosis Team for the first episode of schizophrenia. You prescribe risperidone 1 mg nocte. His mother requests an answer from you on the following questions. Each option might be used once, more than once, or not at all.

146. His psychotic symptoms are not controlled. His mother wants to know the minimum effective dose (in mg) of risperidone in his case. (Choose one option.)

147. His psychotic symptoms are under control. His mother wants to know duration of antipsychotic treatment (in months) in his case. (Choose one option.)

148. After 18 months of treatment, the patient decides to stop the medication. His mother wants to know the risk of relapse as a percentage. (Choose one option.)

Questions 149–153 – options
A. Carbamazepine
B. Diazepam
C. Electroconvulsive therapy
D. Haloperidol
E. Lamotrigine
F. Lithium
G. Olanzapine
H. Quetiapine
I. Sodium valproate
J. Sertraline
K. St John's wort
L. Topiramate

Lead-in: Choose the appropriate physical treatments for the following clinical scenarios. Each option might be used once, more than once or not at all.

149. A 45-year-old man suffers from bipolar disorder. He has had five episodes of depression and one episode of hypomania over the past 5 years. He had hypothyroidism 20 years ago. He prefers to take medication. (Choose one option.)

150. A Foundation Year 2 doctor consults you about which anticonvulsant is not recommended to be used routinely in the prophylaxis of bipolar disorder. (Choose one option.)

151. A 40-year-old man suffers from bipolar disorder. He has had two episodes of depression and three episodes of mania over the past year. He has not responded well to monotherapy with lithium. You suggest augmentation therapy with another medication. (Choose one option.)

152. A 35-year-old man suffering from bipolar disorder was treated by a psychiatrist in a tropical country. He is referred by the urologist to review his psychotropic medication as he has developed renal calculi after coming back to the UK. Which medication is associated with the development of renal calculi? (Choose one option.)

153. A 45-year-old man suffers from bipolar disorder and hypertension. His GP prescribes an ACE inhibitor to treat his hypertension. The ACE inhibitor increases the serum level of a medication. (Choose one option.)

Questions 154–156 – options
A. Carbamazepine
B. Diazepam
C. Electroconvulsive therapy
D. Haloperidol
E. Lamotrigine
F. Lithium
G. Olanzapine
H. Quetiapine
I. Sodium valproate
J. Fluoxetine
K. St John's wort
L. Topiramate

Lead-in: Choose the appropriate physical treatments for the following clinical scenarios based on the NICE guidelines. Each option might be used once, more than once or not at all.

154. A 35-year-old woman with bipolar disorder is admitted to hospital owing to severe depressive symptoms. She takes lithium CR 800 mg nocte and has been compliant with this medication. She does not tolerate lamotrigine because of Stevens–Johnson syndrome. Which medication would you consider adding to the lithium? (Choose one option.)

155. A 35-year-old woman with rapid cycling bipolar disorder is admitted to hospital owing to severe depressive symptoms. She takes lithium CR 800 mg nocte and has been compliant with this medication. She does not tolerate sodium valproate because of hair loss. Which medication would you consider adding to the lithium? (Choose one option.)

156. A 35-year-old woman with rapid cycling bipolar disorder is being managed in the community. She does not respond to monotherapy. Her GP consults you on the long-term management. A combination of which two medications is recommended? (Choose two options.)

Questions 157–161 – options
A. Hippocrates
B. Ishaq bin Ali Rahawi
C. Philippe Pinel
D. W. D. Ross
E. Soranus

Lead-in: Choose the correct individuals with the following accomplishments. Each option might be used once, more than once or not at all.

157. Advocated a mild treatment policy to the mentally ill in contrast to beatings and cold baths. (Choose one option.)

158. Doctors should come for the benefit of the sick, remaining free of all intentional injustice and harm to their patients. (Choose one option.)

159. Removed the chains from psychiatric patients. (Choose one option.)

160. Wrote the first book on medical ethics. (Choose one option.)

161. Developed the concept of prima facie duties. (Choose one option.)

Questions 162–165 – options
  A. Amok
  B. Brain fag
  C. Dhat
  D. Koro
  E. Latah
  F. Pibloktoq
  G. Susto
  H. Taijin kyofusho
  I. Windigo

Lead-in: Identify which of the above resembles the following clinical scenarios. Each option might be used once, more than once or not at all.

162. A 20-year-old African university student has been preparing for a pharmacology examination and presents with a burning headache, blurred vision, difficulty in understanding the meaning of the textbook and an inability to remember the drugs he studied. (Choose one option.)

163. A 20-year-old Chinese national serviceman in Singapore is referred by the army doctor. He complains that his penis is getting shorter and that it will continue to retract into his abdomen. He measures his penis every day and he cannot concentrate on his work. (Choose one option.)

164. A 25-year-old Malaysian woman becomes dissociative after a road traffic accident, followed by echopraxia, echolalia, command obedience and the utterance of obscene words. (Choose one option.)

165. A 30-year-old indigenous Indian staying near Yellowknife, Canada, complains that he is possessed by a spirit to eat the human flesh of the tribe leader after long-term conflict with him. (Choose one option.)

Questions 166–171 – options
  A. Complex visual hallucination
  B. Dysmegalopsia
  C. Illusion
  D. Macropsia
  E. Micropsia
  F. Pareidolia
  G. Peduncular hallucination
  H. Pseudohallucination
  I. Simple visual hallucination
  J. Visual hyperaesthesia

Lead-in: A 65-year-old woman is found to be disorientated in time and place. During your assessment, she gives a history of the following experiences. Identify which of the above psychopathological terms best describes the following clinical scenarios. Each option might be used once, more than once or not at all.

166. She is terrified and shouts, 'White lady, white lady, go away.' She perceives the curtain as a female ghost. (Choose one option.)

167. The colour in the ward appears to her to be brighter and more vivid than usual. (Choose one option.)

168. She mentions that the bed and other furniture look smaller or larger than they should be. (Choose one option.)

169. She reports episodes in which everything in her environment looks huge and she feels tiny. (Choose one option.)

170. She sees the face of Jesus Christ in the callus of a tree outside the ward. (Choose one option.)

171. She reports that she saw a colourfully dressed clown and children dancing in the ward last night. (Choose one option.)

Questions 172–177 – options
  A. Déjà vu
  B. Displacement
  C. Jamais vu
  D. Proactive interference
  E. Primacy effect
  F. Recall
  G. Recency effect
  H. Recognition
  I. Recollection
  J. Relearning
  K. Retroactive interference

Lead-in: Identify which of the above resembles the following scenarios. Each option might be used once, more than once or not at all.

172. An Afghan refugee mentions that there is no point visiting a clinic in London because he has been there before, although he has never visited the UK. (Choose one option.)

173. A candidate failed the MRCPsych Paper 1 and needs to retake the examination. It is easier for him to remember and retrieve information for his second attempt. (Choose one option.)

174. A candidate sitting for the MRCPsych Paper 3 finds new learning affects his ability to recall earlier learning. (Choose one option.)

175. The process involved in answering an essay question. (Choose one option.)

176. The process involved in answering a fill-in-the-blank question. (Choose one option.)

177. The process involved in selecting the best answer out of five options in a MCQ examination. (Choose one option.)

Questions 178 –183 – options
   A. Autonomy versus shame or doubt
   B. Ego integrity versus despair
   C. Generativity versus stagnation
   D. Identity versus role confusion
   E. Industry versus inferiority
   F. Initiative versus guilt
   G. Intimacy versus isolation
   H. Trust versus mistrust

Lead-in: Identify which of the above stages from Erikson's psychosocial development theory best resembles the following scenarios. Each option might be used once, more than once or not at all.

178. A child from the nursery avoids being fed by the staff and only allows his mother to feed him as she provides a sense of reliability and affection. (Choose one option.)

179. A child from the nursery is frustrated by repeated failure in his toilet training. (Choose one option.)

180. A child studying in kindergarten wants to explore the woods near her house but worries about being scolded by her mother. (Choose one option.)

181. A primary school student is pleased that he can cope with academic demands but unhappy that he is not good at sport. (Choose one option.)

182. A middle-aged couple are determined to have children in spite of multiple miscarriages. On the weekend, they are involved in volunteer work to help poor people. (Choose one option.)

183. A 69-year-old professor enjoys his life after retirement although he has just recovered from a major heart attack. He develops a sense of fulfilment as he works 3 days a week to mentor young researchers. (Choose one option.)

Questions 184–189 – options
   A. Eymard P.
   B. Gardocki J. F.
   C. Geigy A. G.
   D. Hanaoka
   E. Maryanoff B. E.
   F. Osterloh I.
   G. Schindler W.
   H. Sternbach L.
   I. Takezaki

Lead-in: Match the name of the above people to the discovery of the following psychotropic medications. Each option might be used once, more than once or not at all.

184. These people first used carbamazepine to control mania in patients who were refractory to antipsychotics. (Choose two options.)

185. The people who first discovered carbamazepine. (Choose two options.)

186. The person who discovered the first benzodiazepine, chlordiazepoxide (Librium) in 1955. (Choose one option.)

187. The person who suggested that sildenafil had little effect on angina but that it could improve penile erection. (Choose one option.)

188. These people discovered topiramate in 1979. (Choose two options.)

189. The person who discovered the anticonvulsant properties of sodium valproate. (Choose one option.)

Questions 190–195 – options
   A. Apolipoprotein E4 gene (homozygous for ε4)
   B. Cardiovascular disease
   C. Cancer
   D. Childhood sexual abuse
   E. Death of mother before the age of 11 years
   F. Down syndrome
   G. *Dysbindin* gene
   H. Migration
   I. *Neuregulin* gene
   J. Old age
   K. Streptococcal infection
   L. Three children at home under the age of 14 years
   M. Unemployment

Lead-in: Match the above aetiological factors to the following clinical scenarios. Each option might be used once, more than once or not at all.

190. A 10-year-old boy develops obsessions and compulsive behaviour after a sore throat and fever. (Choose one option.)

191. A 19-year-old lady presents with recurrent self-harm following the end of a transient and intense romantic relationship. She has a chronic feeling of emptiness and exhibits binge-eating behaviour. (Choose one option.)

192. A 24-year-old man complains that MI5 is monitoring him and has tried to control his feelings and intentions. He heard the voices of two secret agents talking about him and they issued him with a command. (Choose three options.)

193. A 35-year-old working-class British woman living in London presents with low mood, poor sleep, poor appetite, low energy level, hopelessness and suicidal thoughts. (Choose three options.)

194. A 60-year-old man develops Alzheimer's disease. (Choose three options.)

195. A 70-year-old woman develops low mood, poor sleep, poor appetite, psychomotor retardation and suicidal thoughts. She has no past psychiatric history. (Choose two options.)

Questions 196–200 – options
   A. Addison's disease
   B. Catatonia
   C. Cushing's syndrome

D. Hyperthyroidism
E. Hypothyroidism
F. Huntington's disease
G. Neuroleptic malignant syndrome
H. Parkinson's disease
I. Phaeochromocytoma

Lead-in: Match the above disorders to the following triads of symptoms. Each option might be used once, more than once or not at all.

196. Hypertension, diaphoresis, palpitation. (Choose one option.)

197. Labile blood pressure, hyperthermia, muscle stiffness. (Choose one option.)

198. Hypothermia, fatigue, constipation. (Choose one option.)

199. Hypertension, weight gain, hirsutism. (Choose one option.)

200. Orthostatic hypotension, rigidity, tremor. (Choose one option.)

ANSWERS – MULTIPLE CHOICE QUESTIONS

1. D

Both Freud and Bleuler believed in the 'split mind' or 'fragmentation of mental activities'.

> Further reading: Puri BK, Treasaden I, eds (2010). *Psychiatry: An evidence-based text*, pp. 12–13, 106, 215, 613, 615.

2. A

Women have a bimodal peak of incidence (late 20s and 50s).

3. E

WCFST is a test mainly for executive function. AVLT is a 15-item five-trial test, from which recall (immediate and delayed) and recognition memory can be assessed. CVLT involves a list of 16 words. The list is repeated five times. Then a second list is given, serving to interfere with the first list, after which recall of the first list is requested. RMT involves recognition of non-verbal material with interference from distracters after the first initial image is presented. The WMT assesses several memory components, including concentration and summary indices that can be derived with a mean of 100. Tasks under WMT include assessment of logical memory (subjects are asked to recall the content of two stories read to them with a 30-minute delay) and a verbal paired associates test (learning word pairs, e.g. baby–cries and to recall the second word when the first word is given).

> Reference: **Trimble M (2004)**. *Somatoform Disorders – A Medico-legal Guide*. Cambridge: Cambridge University Press.

4. C

5. D

This person suffers from narcissistic personality disorder. Rationalization is the defence mechanism most commonly used by people with narcissistic personality disorder.

> Reference: **Gabbard GO, Beck JS, Holmes J (2005)**. *Oxford Textbook of Psychotherapy*. Oxford: Oxford University Press.

6. E

The questionnaires listed under options B and D do not exist.

7. B

8. D

Synaesthesia is also known as secondary sensation. Sensations in one modality give rise to sensations in a different modality (in addition to their own modality).

9. B

This man suffers from Huntington's disease. The *huntingtin* gene is located on the short arm of chromosome 4.

> Further reading: Puri BK, Treasaden I, eds (2010). *Psychiatry: An evidence-based text*, pp. 546–7, 1101.

10. C

Dysphasia or paraphasia refers to any disturbance in the expression of speech due to brain lesions.

> Further reading: Puri BK, Treasaden I, eds (2010). *Psychiatry: An evidence-based text*, pp. 91, 96, 508, 531.

11. A

Automatic obedience refers to a condition in which the person follows the examiner's instructions blindly without judgement and resistance.

> Further reading: Puri BK, Treasaden I, eds (2010). *Psychiatry: An evidence-based text*, pp. 294–5.

12. B

Gegenhalten is a form of paratonia consisting of uneven resistance of the limbs to passive movement.

> Reference: **Campbell RJ (1996)**. *Psychiatric Dictionary*. Oxford: Oxford University Press.

13. A

Psychological imprinting refers to learning occurring at a particular stage of life. The learning process is rapid and independent of the consequences of behaviour. Genetic imprinting is a different concept. When the expression of inheritance is altered, depending upon whether it was passed to the fetus through the egg or the sperm, this phenomenon is known as genetic imprinting. The term 'imprinting' refers to the fact that some genes are stamped with a 'memory' of the parent from whom they came. In the cells of an infant, it is possible to tell which chromosome copy came from the maternal chromosome and which was inherited from the paternal chromosome. This expression of the gene is called a 'parent of origin effect' and was first described by Helen Crouse in 1960.

> References: **Barlow-Stewart K (2007)**. Genetic imprinting. *Genetic Fact Sheets*, 6th edn. Sydney: Centre for Genetics Education; **Crouse HV (1960)**. The controlling element in sex chromosome behavior in *Sciara. Genetics* **45**: 1429–43.

14. E

> References: **Charlton B (2000)**. *Psychiatry and the Human Condition*. Oxford: Radcliffe Publishing; **Shorter E (1997)**. *A History of Psychiatry*. New York: John Wiley & Sons.
>
> Further reading: Puri BK, Treasaden I, eds (2010). *Psychiatry: An evidence-based text*, pp. 11, 593, 614, 624.

15. C

Further reading: Puri BK, Treasaden I, eds (2010). *Psychiatry: An evidence-based text*, p. 23.

16. B

This man probably suffers from catatonic schizophrenia and blepharospasm is not the clinical feature.

17. C

Hyperventilation is associated with a dry mouth.

Further reading: Puri BK, Treasaden I, eds (2010). *Psychiatry: An evidence-based text*, pp. 546, 650, 681.

18. D

Lithium increases the serotonin level and this may lead to serotonin syndrome.

Further reading: Puri BK, Treasaden I, eds (2010). *Psychiatry: An evidence-based text*, pp. 874–5.

19. C

A functional hallucination is defined as the hallucination that occurs when a patient simultaneously receives a real stimulus in the same perceptual field as the hallucination.

Reference: Hunter MD, Woodruff PWR (2004). Characteristics of functional auditory hallucinations. *American Journal of Psychiatry* 161: 923.

20. E

Further reading: Puri BK, Treasaden I, eds (2010). *Psychiatry: An evidence-based text*, pp. 125, 528.

21. E

The answer is E as it may last for minutes or days.

Further reading: Puri BK, Treasaden I, eds (2010). *Psychiatry: An evidence-based text*, pp. 300, 973, 979.

22. C

Further reading: Puri BK, Treasaden I, eds (2010). *Psychiatry: An evidence-based text*, pp. 532, 538, 910.

23. C

In a Swedish study, it was shown that there were minimal gender differences in coping with the burdensome situation of having a relative with a severe mental illness, although women tend to express more inner thoughts of death. Options A and B are true. Option D is also true as the youngest children viewed the terms 'mad' and 'crazy' as positive. It was also concluded that increasing awareness of mental health and illness in children is unlikely to cause harm and should be an important component of primary education. Option E is correct.

References: Östman M, Kjellin L (2002). Stigma by association: Psychological factors in relatives of people with mental illness. *British Journal of Psychiatry*; **181**: 494–8; Perlick DA, Miklowitz DJ, Link BG *et al.* (2007). Perceived stigma and depression among caregivers of patients with bipolar disorder. *British Journal of Psychiatry*; **190**: 535–536; Shah N (2004). Changing minds at the earliest opportunity. *Psychiatric Bulletin* **28**: 213–215; Wilson C, Nairn R, Coverdale J *et al.* (2000). How mental illness is portrayed in children's television: a prospective study. *British Journal of Psychiatry* **176**: 440–3.
Further reading: Puri BK, Treasaden I, eds (2010). *Psychiatry: An evidence-based text*, pp. 303, 1120–1.

24. B

The lithium toxicity is precipitated by hot weather and the use of diuretics.

Further reading: Puri BK, Treasaden I, eds (2010). *Psychiatry: An evidence-based text*, pp. 910, 915.

25. C

Further reading: Puri BK, Treasaden I, eds (2010). *Psychiatry: An evidence-based text*, p. 704.

26. C

Nystagmus occurs in lithium toxicity.

Further reading: Puri BK, Treasaden I, eds (2010). *Psychiatry: An evidence-based text*, pp. 910, 915.

27. B

This is the automatic imitation by the refugee of the psychiatrist's speech.

28. D

Sodium valproate can cause pancreatitis which results in dysphagia.

Further reading: Puri BK, Treasaden I, eds (2010). *Psychiatry: An evidence-based text*, pp. 532, 538.

29. A

Ambitendency refers to repetitive behaviour of co-operation and opposition. The person starts to make a movement but, before completing it, he starts the opposite movement.

30. B

There is usually no delay in speech development in people with Asperger's syndrome (in contrast with autistic disorder).

Further reading: Puri BK, Treasaden I, eds (2010). *Psychiatry: An evidence-based text*, pp. 1066–7, 1088–90.

31. B

Plutchik named eight primary emotions.

Further reading: Puri BK, Treasaden I, eds (2010). *Psychiatry: An evidence-based text*, pp. 166–78.

32. C

All combinations will lead to serotonin syndrome but there are reports that the combination of phenelzine and meperidine has led to death on several occasions. Meperidine is a narcotic painkiller.

Reference: Sharav VH (2007). Serotonin syndrome: a mix of medicines that can be lethal. *The New York Times.* New York: The New York Times Company.

Further reading: Puri BK, Treasaden I, eds (2010). *Psychiatry: An evidence-based text,* pp. 874–5.

33. A

The top three personality disorders in the UK are anankastic (1.7–2.2 per cent), anxious (0.5–5 per cent) and borderline (0.7–2 per cent) personality disorder.

Further reading: Puri BK, Treasaden I, eds (2010). *Psychiatry: An evidence-based text,* p. 657.

34. D

35. B

Further reading: Puri BK, Treasaden I, eds (2010). *Psychiatry: An evidence-based text,* pp. 1231, 1235.

36. A

Rush – less confining treatment in the US. Laing – a psychiatrist who came to hold anti-psychiatry views. He is the author of The Divided Self. He saw schizophrenia as a sane response to an insane society. Percival – established a code of ethics for Manchester Infirmary. Szasz – both professor of psychiatry and leading proponent of anti-psychiatry. He identifies psychiatrists as agents of social control. He also believes it is unethical to restrict a patient's actions without his consent.

Reference: Musto DF (1998). A historical perspective. In: Bloch S, Chodoff P, Green SA, eds. *Psychiatric Ethics,* 3rd edn. Oxford: Oxford University Press; Johnstone EC, Cunningham ODG, Lawrie SM, Sharpe M, Freeman CPL (2004) *Companion to Psychiatric Studies,* 7th edn. London: Churchill Livingstone.

37. A

38. D

Options A, B, C and E occur in lithium toxicity.

Further reading: Puri BK, Treasaden I, eds (2010). *Psychiatry: An evidence-based text,* pp. 874–5, 910, 915

39. D

The person exhibits neologism as the person is condensing words such as 'syringe' and 'risperidone'.

40. A

Shoplifting is not common among OCD patients. The other statements are correct.

Reference: Bluglass R, Bowden P (1990). *Principles and Practice of Forensic Psychiatry.* Edinburgh: Churchill Livingstone.

Further reading: Puri BK, Treasaden I, eds (2010). *Psychiatry: An evidence-based text,* pp. 656–9.

41. B

Standardized scores on tests of recognition are lower than standardized scores on tests of free recall in people with feigned amnesia. Furthermore, people with feigned amnesia have a forced-choice recognition test performance that is worse than chance.

Reference: Cercy SP, Schretlen DJ, Brandt J (1997). Simulated amnesia and the pseudo-memory phenomena. In: Rogers R, ed. *Clinical Assessment of Malingering and Deception.* New York: Guilford Press; **Trimble M (2004).** *Somatoform Disorders – A Medico-legal Guide.* Cambridge: Cambridge University Press.

Further reading: Puri BK, Treasaden I, eds (2010). *Psychiatry: An evidence-based text,* pp. 93–5, 149, 252–4, 260, 557–9, 581, 667, 1160, 1165.

42. D

It is not common for viral illnesses to be detected. E is correct as depression alone may occur in more than 50 per cent.

Reference: Johnstone EC, Cunningham ODG, Lawrie SM, Sharpe M, Freeman CPL (2004) *Companion to Psychiatric Studies,* (7th edn). London: Churchill Livingstone.

Further reading: Puri BK, Treasaden I, eds (2010). *Psychiatry: An evidence-based text,* p. 831.

43. B

Further reading: Puri BK, Treasaden I, eds (2010). *Psychiatry: An evidence-based text,* pp. 385, 389.

44. C

Further reading: Puri BK, Treasaden I, eds (2010). *Psychiatry: An evidence-based text,* pp. 309–18.

45. D

Option C is a side-effect of lithium and option A occurs in lithium toxicity. Options B and E are cerebellar signs.

Further reading: Puri BK, Treasaden I, eds (2010). *Psychiatry: An evidence-based text,* pp. 541–3.

46. D

47. A – Gedankenlautwerden

On the other hand, if the woman reports that the thoughts are spoken out loud just after being produced, this phenomenon is known as écho de la pensée.

Further reading: Puri BK, Treasaden I, eds (2010). *Psychiatry: An evidence-based text,* pp. 593–609.

48. E

Jamais vu refers to the illusion of failure to recognize a familiar situation.

49. B

The husband has gone through a long difficult period by living with his wife and it is difficult to express his difficult feelings all at once. A long pause would be very helpful to give him a chance to organize his thoughts and facilitate the interview. Summation refers to a brief summary of what the person has said and this technique is irrelevant, as he has not said much. Transition is a technique used gently to inform the person that the interview is going on to another topic and it is irrelevant as the interview has not been progressing. Close-ended questions and prolonged eye contact would not facilitate a response from the husband.

Further reading: Puri BK, Treasaden I, eds (2010). *Psychiatry: An evidence-based text*, pp. 43, 75, 318–9, 1047–8.

50. A

NMS can occur at any time during the course of antipsychotic treatment.

Further reading: Puri BK, Treasaden I, eds (2010). *Psychiatry: An evidence-based text*, pp. 874, 925.

51. D

Seizures are associated with medial temporal lobe lesions and complex partial seizures are known as uncinate seizures which can give rise to olfactory hallucinations.

Reference: Cummings JL, Mega MS, eds (2003). *Neuropsychiatry and Behavioural Neuroscience*. New York: Oxford University Press.

Further reading: Puri BK, Treasaden I, eds (2010). *Psychiatry: An evidence-based text*, p. 532.

52. A

Of these options, the combination of an MAOI with a tricyclic antidepressant (TCA) is the safest, with the safest TCA being trimipramine.

53. A

Patients with frontal lobe lesions may demonstrate perseveration in copying drawings. Patients with left hemisphere damage tend to break drawings into smaller units and simplify them (e.g. by rounding angles; turning the cross into a T) compared with controls without head injury. Patients with parietal lobe lesions have difficulty with spatial organization. Patients with right hemispheric damage tend to make more omissions compared with controls without head injury.

References: Winner E, von Karolyi C, Malinsky D (2000). *Dyslexia and Visual-Spatial Talents: No Clear Link*. Boston: Boston College Perspectives; **Walsh K, Darby D (2002)**. *Neuropsychology: A Clinical Approach*. Edinburgh: Churchill Livingstone.

54. A

Further reading: Puri BK, Treasaden I, eds (2010). *Psychiatry: An evidence-based text*, p. 1231.

55. B

56. D

Further reading: Puri BK, Treasaden I, eds (2010). *Psychiatry: An evidence-based text*, p. 21.

57. B

It should be 3 months. Bizarre delusions are not associated with delusional disorders but correspond to the first-rank symptoms of schizophrenia.

Reference: World Health Organization (1992). *ICD-10: The ICD-10 Classification of Mental and Behavioural Disorders: Clinical Descriptions and Diagnostic Guidelines*. Geneva: World Health Organization.

58. E

Further reading: Puri BK, Treasaden I, eds (2010). *Psychiatry: An evidence-based text*, pp. 677, 837–8, 1159–60.

59. C

60. D

Humans are good at rationalizing and use the following techniques: selective exposure, selective perception, selective attention and selective interpretation to focus on the things they want to see and hear. By doing so, cognitive dissonance can be reduced.

Further reading: Puri BK, Treasaden I, eds (2010). *Psychiatry: An evidence-based text*, pp. 287–8.

61. E

Cranial VIth nerve palsy causes horizontal diplopia on looking out, but not ptosis.

Further reading: Puri BK, Treasaden I, eds (2010). *Psychiatry: An evidence-based text*, pp. 336–8, 351, 525–7.

62. D

The rates are as follows: community, 10 per cent; patients seeing GP, 20 per cent; psychiatric out-patients, 30 per cent; psychiatric in-patients, 40 per cent.

63. B

The classical symptoms of narcolepsy are excessive daytime sleepiness, sleep paralysis or cataplexy, hypnogogic hallucinations (hypnopompic hallucinations are possible but less common) and automatic behaviour.

Further reading: Puri BK, Treasaden I, eds (2010). *Psychiatry: An evidence-based text*, pp. 845, 847–8, 851.

64. A

Catatonia is not associated with fever and autonomic lability.

Further reading: Puri BK, Treasaden I, eds (2010). *Psychiatry: An evidence-based text*, pp. 579, 925.

65. D

66. A

The consultant psychiatrist should consider how best to address this issue in such a way that the parents become aware (as they are entitled to) of the mistake. This would need to be done in accordance with local procedures and under the principle of justice acting in the best interests of the patient.

67. D

Option A is incorrect and it should be dementia (dementia, 68 per cent; hypomania, 12 per cent; schizophrenia = suicide = substance abuse, 8 per cent).

Option B is incorrect and should be the DVLA. Option C is incorrect. It will be heard before the Magistrates' Court. Option D is correct. The 1-year symptom-free period is for non-vocational drivers. The symptom-free period should be 3 years (the same period is required for alcohol abstinence) for a vocational driver.

Option E is incorrect as the DVLA may only allow vocational drivers taking SSRIs to hold a vocational driving licence, but not so for antipsychotics. In general, it is acknowledged that drivers with psychiatric illnesses are usually safer when they are on regular psychotropic medication.

Reference: Harris M (2000). Psychiatric conditions with relevance to fitness to drive. *Advances in Psychiatric Treatment* 6: 261–9.

68. B

Tertiary circular reaction (part of sensorimotor stage, Piaget's cognitive model) occurs at 12–18 months. Development of colour vision occurs at 4–5 months. Development of fear of darkness occurs at 8–11 months. Preoperational stage (Piaget's cognitive model) occurs at 2 years.

Further reading: Puri BK, Treasaden I, eds (2010). *Psychiatry: An evidence-based text*, pp. 119–20, 280–1.

69. D

The patient develops pancreatitis after taking sodium valproate.

Further reading: Puri BK, Treasaden I, eds (2010). *Psychiatry: An evidence-based text*, pp. 532, 538.

70. A

The majority of patients in both groups discontinued their assigned treatment owing to inefficacy or intolerable side effects or for other reasons. Quetiapine had the highest rate of discontinuation for any cause (82 per cent) versus 79 per cent for ziprasidone, 75 per cent for perphenazine, 74 per cent for risperidone and 64 per cent for olanzapine. Discontinuation of the drug because of lack of efficacy was highest among patients on quetiapine (28 per cent) and lowest for those on olanzapine (15 per cent). Nineteen per cent of patients on olanzapine cited intolerability as the reason for stopping the drug, while intolerability caused 10 per cent of patients on risperidone to stop the drug. It was reported that 30 per cent of olanzapine-treated patients gained more than 7 per cent of their body weight during the study, which was significantly greater than weight gain with other study drugs. Predictors of an earlier time to drug discontinuation included higher PANSS score, younger age and long duration of antipsychotic use. CATIE involved 1493 patients with schizophrenia. They were randomly assigned to receive olanzapine (7.5–30 mg/day), perphenazine (8–32 mg/day), quetiapine (200–800 mg/day) or risperidone (1.5–6.0 mg/ day) for up to 18 months.

Reference: Lieberman JA, Stroup TS, McEvoy JP (2005). Effectiveness of antipsychotic drugs in patients with chronic schizophrenia. *New England Journal of Medicine* 353: 1209–23.

71. C

In general, new anticonvulsants are more likely to cause visual side effects than the older anticonvulsants. For example, carbamazepine causes visual hallucination, but relatively rarely. Gabapentin causes visual-field defects, photophobia, bilateral or unilateral ptosis and ocular haemorrhage. Topiramate causes acute onset of decreased visual acuity and/or ocular pain. Vigabatrin causes concentric visual-field defects.

Further reading: Puri BK, Treasaden I, eds (2010). *Psychiatry: An evidence-based text*, pp. 532, 538.

72. D

Aristotle and Plato: virtue ethics; Beauchamp and Childress: four ethical principles; Casuists are supporters of casuistry which focuses on decision-making based on previous cases; Tarasoff: an influential case on duty to protect and example of casuistry where the murderer (Poddar) told the therapist (Dr Moore) of killing Tarasoff but Dr Moore did not disclose this to Tarasoff or the police. The court held that mental health professionals have a duty to protect someone who may be harmed by patients.

73. D

Mitgehen refers to excessive cooperation and limb movement in response to slight pressure of an applied force even if the person is asked to resist movement.

74. A

Further reading: Puri BK, Treasaden I, eds (2010). *Psychiatry: An evidence-based text*, **pp. 425, 907.**

75. A

Further reading: Puri BK, Treasaden I, eds (2010). *Psychiatry: An evidence-based text*, **pp. 23–4.**

76. E

This case refers to laissez-faire leadership. Option A is for democratic leadership. Option B applies to both autocratic and democratic leadership. Options C and D are suitable for autocratic leadership.

Further reading: Puri BK, Treasaden I, eds (2010). *Psychiatry: An evidence-based text*, **pp. 292, 118.**

77. E

Confidentiality is recognized as a prima facie obligation.

Reference: Green SA (1998). The ethics of managed mental health care. In Bloch S, Chodoff P, Green SA *Psychiatric Ethics*, 3rd edn. Oxford: Oxford University Press.

78. B

Globus hystericus refers to the feeling of choking and difficulties in swallowing which can occur in panic disorder but it is not the commonest symptom.

Further reading: Puri BK, Treasaden I, eds (2010). *Psychiatry: An evidence-based text*, **pp. 649–51.**

79. A

The phenomenon described refers to anomic suicide when suicide resulted from chronic anomie (long-term unemployment). This concept was proposed by Emile Durkheim, who believed that a major cause of suicide could be seen in terms of social forces.

80. C

The patient has an obligation to get well. The others are criteria that a person has to fulfil for Parsons' sick role.

Further reading: Puri BK, Treasaden I, eds (2010). *Psychiatry: An evidence-based text*, **pp. 299, 682.**

81. B

Death of a spouse is considered to be the most stressful event with 100 life change units (LCU), followed by divorce (73 LCU), marital separation (65 LCU), imprisonment (63 LCU) and death of a close family member (63 LCU).

Reference: Holmes TH, Rahe RH (1967). The Social Readjustment Rating Scale. *Journal of Psychosomatic Research* 11: 213–8.

Further reading: Puri BK, Treasaden I, eds (2010). *Psychiatry: An evidence-based text*, **pp. 155–6.**

82. D

Reference: Young R, Sweeting H, West P (2006). Prevalence of deliberate self-harm and attempted suicide within contemporary Goth youth subculture: longitudinal cohort study. *British Medical Journal* **332**, pp. **1058–61**.

Further reading: Puri BK, Treasaden I, eds (2010). *Psychiatry: An evidence-based text*, **pp. 309–18.**

83. D

The Training in Community Living (TCL) study was conducted in the US in the 1970s. It was found that community living was significantly less expensive than standard care, which relied more on psychiatric hospitals. Option A is false. Treatment is provided in vivo in community settings, as skills learned in the community can be better applied in the community. Option B is false. Only the patients are engaged in an assertive manner in ACT, but not the caregivers. Option C is false as ACT is a pure form of clinical case management and 'brokerage' is based on an earlier model. Option E is false as ACT depends on the local mental health service if the service user needs admission. Voluntary organizations also play a key role in delivering some of the services in the community.

Reference: Stein LI, Test MA (1980). Alternative to mental hospital treatment. I. Conceptual model, treatment program and clinical evaluation. *Archives of General Psychiatry* 37: 392–7.

Further reading: Puri BK, Treasaden I, eds (2010). *Psychiatry: An evidence-based text*, **pp. 605, 1125–6.**

84. A

In clinical practice, it is not uncommon to encounter patients with anorexia nervosa minimizing symptoms of eating disorder and attributing their low body weight to something else. It is often more useful to pay attention to objective signs such as low BMI and amenorrhoea to establish the diagnosis of anorexia nervosa.

Further reading: Puri BK, Treasaden I, eds (2010). *Psychiatry: An evidence-based text*, **pp. 687–703, 1063.**

85. A

Peer pressure is the most significant factor to influence conformity among students. The vulnerability to group pressure is low in students with high intelligence, social effectiveness, expressiveness and thoughtfulness. A history of substance abuse is not important as a lot of drug-naive students will use drugs in a group setting owing to de-individuation or loss of individual identity.

Reference: Hill P (1997). *Human development and Basic Psychology.* Guildford Revision Course.

Further reading: Puri BK, Treasaden I, eds (2010). *Psychiatry: An evidence-based text*, **p. 975.**

86. D

She is probably obedient to the hospital chief executive as she sees this person as superior.

Reference: Atkinson RL, Atkinson RC, Smith EE, Bern DJ (1993). *Introduction to Psychology*, 11th edn. Orlando, FL: Harcourt Brace.

Further reading: Puri BK, Treasaden I, eds (2010). *Psychiatry: An evidence-based text*, **p. 294.**

87. B

Thought interference including insertion, withdrawal and broadcasting belong to the passivity phenomenon.

88. D

This is a case of compensation neurosis and her unreasonable request may stop after being informed by her own lawyer that the chance of success is low and that there is a high cost to pay if she pursues the case. Option A is incorrect as more than 50 per cent of cases are not able to work after a settlement. Option B is incorrect. She does not meet the criteria for both nervous shock and PTSD. Nervous shock is a legal concept where the patient must be suffering from a positive psychiatric illness and there is a clear and reasonable chain of causation between the negligent act and psychiatric illness. In this case, the chain of causation is not clear. Options C and E are not necessary.

Reference: Gunn J, Taylor PJ (1993). *Forensic Psychiatry. Clinical, Legal and Ethical Issues.* Oxford: Butterworth-Heinemann.

Further reading: Puri BK, Treasaden I, eds (2010). *Psychiatry: An evidence-based text*, p. 660.

89. B

The greatest teratogenic effect is neural tube defect (1–1.5 per cent).

90. C

Reference: Whittaker W, Sutton M, Maxwell M *et al.* (2010). Predicting which people with psychosocial distress are at risk of becoming dependent on state benefits: analysis of routinely available data. *British Medical Journal* 341: 3838

91. C

The fundamental attribution error increases with the seriousness of the consequences of one's behaviour.

Further reading: Puri BK, Treasaden I, eds (2010). *Psychiatry: An evidence-based text*, p. 278.

92. C

Further reading: Puri BK, Treasaden I, eds (2010). *Psychiatry: An evidence-based text*, pp. 76, 490–1.

93. E

The state-dependent effect should theoretically facilitate recall. His low mood during the examination may lead to pseudodementia where the patient has poor motivation to attempt the questions rather than memory deficit or forgetfulness. Option A refers to the decay or trace decay theory. Option B refers to displacement theory. Option C refers to cue-dependent forgetting and option D refers to context-dependent forgetting.

94. D

95. B

96. B

Further reading: Puri BK, Treasaden I, eds (2010). *Psychiatry: An evidence-based text*, pp. 593–609.

97. A

At an individual level, cannabis use confers an overall twofold increase in the relative risk for later schizophrenia.

Reference: Arseneault L, Cannon M, Witton J, Murray RM (2004). Causal association between cannabis and psychosis: examination of the evidence. *British Journal of Psychiatry* 184: 110–7.

Further reading: Puri BK, Treasaden I, eds (2010). *Psychiatry: An evidence-based text*, pp. 412, 596–7.

98. E

The diagnosis of schizophrenia and treatment with first-generation antipsychotics alone indicate the worst prognosis for schizophrenia.

Further reading: Puri BK, Treasaden I, eds (2010). *Psychiatry: An evidence-based text*, pp. 311, 1063.

99. D

Based on the ICD-10 criteria for acute stress disorder. For transient stress which can be relieved, the symptoms begin to diminish after 48 hours.

Further reading: Puri BK, Treasaden I, eds (2010). *Psychiatry: An evidence-based text*, p. 660.

100. A

Reference: Brown G, Harris T (1978). *Social Origins of Depression. A Study of Psychiatric Disorder in Women.* London: Tavistock.

101. C

The answer is perseveration, as the same answer is being repeated for different questions. The presence of perseveration may indicate frontal lobe dementia.

Further reading: Puri BK, Treasaden I, eds (2010). *Psychiatry: An evidence-based text*, pp. 92, 95, 510, 525.

102. A

Amisulpride appears not to elevate plasma glucose and seems not to be associated with diabetes. Chlorpromazine, clozapine, risperidone and quetiapine have been associated with impaired glucose tolerance and diabetes.

Reference: Taylor D, Paton C, Kapur S (2009). *The Maudsley Prescribing Guidelines.* London: Informa Healthcare.

Further reading: Puri BK, Treasaden I, eds (2010). *Psychiatry: An evidence-based text*, pp. 425–7, 603.

103. D

This study only reported the test–retest reliability but not the other types of reliability. Option A refers to inter-rater reliability. Option B refers to internal consistency reliability. Option C refers to split-half reliability and option E refers to parallel-forms reliability.

Further reading: Puri BK, Treasaden I, eds (2010). *Psychiatry: An evidence-based text*, **pp. 35–6, 75, 491.**

104. C

105. C

People with dissocial personality disorder may break the law, resulting in a criminal record. This will reduce the chance of getting a job. Furthermore, some of them may have to serve sentences in prison and cannot work in society.

Further reading: Puri BK, Treasaden I, eds (2010). *Psychiatry: An evidence-based text*, **p. 668.**

106. E

The most effective method is persuasive communication.

Further reading: Puri BK, Treasaden I, eds (2010). *Psychiatry: An evidence-based text*, **p. 114.**

107. B

The rates are as follows: A, 5 per cent; B, 52 per cent; C, 13 per cent; D, 2 per cent; E, 2 per cent

Reference: Dasgupta P, Barber J (2004). Admission patterns of patients with personality disorder. *Psychiatric Bulletin* **28:** 321–3.

Further reading: Puri BK, Treasaden I, eds (2010). *Psychiatry: An evidence-based text*, **pp. 707, 709.**

108. E

In focused attention, the alternative information is processed simultaneously by dichotic listening.

Further reading: Puri BK, Treasaden I, eds (2010). *Psychiatry: An evidence-based text*, **pp. 179–94, 502–3.**

109. A

The other antipsychotics may produce weight gain.

Further reading: Puri BK, Treasaden I, eds (2010). *Psychiatry: An evidence-based text*, **pp. 425–6, 604, 904.**

110. C

Candidates are advised to be familiar with the differences between bulbar and pseudobulbar palsies. The differences are summarized as follows:

	Bulbar palsy	Pseudobulbar palsy
Lesions	Lower motor neuron	Upper motor neuron
Causes	Motor neuron diseases, Guillain–Barré syndrome, polio, syringobulbia, brainstem tumours, central pontine myelinolysis in people with alcohol misuse	Bilateral lesions above the mid-pons. For example, in the corticobulbar tracts in multiple sclerosis, motor neuron disease and stroke. It is commoner than bulbar palsy
Tongue	Flaccid and fasciculating	Spastic
Jaw jerk	Normal	Increased
Speech	Quiet, hoarse and nasal	Donald Duck speech, inappropriate laughter or emotional incontinence

Reference: Longmore M, Wilkinson I, Turmezei T, Cheung CK (2007). *Oxford Handbook of Clinical Medicine*, 7th edn. Oxford: Oxford University Press.

Further reading: Puri BK, Treasaden I, eds (2010). *Psychiatry: An evidence-based text*, **pp. 544, 554.**

111. B

The Nuremberg Code is based on a trial of the Nazi doctor Karl Brandt, who conducted a Nazi euthanasia programme.

112. C

Further reading: Puri BK, Treasaden I, eds (2010). *Psychiatry: An evidence-based text*, **pp. 593–609.**

113. C

Further reading: Puri BK, Treasaden I, eds (2010). *Psychiatry: An evidence-based text*, **pp. 1106–7.**

ANSWERS – EXTENDED MATCHING ITEMS

114. J – shaping

Further reading: Puri BK, Treasaden I, eds (2010). *Psychiatry: An evidence-based text*, p. 204.

115. I

Reciprocal inhibition is a concept developed by Joseph Wolpe. Opposing emotions cannot exist simultaneously.

Further reading: Puri BK, Treasaden I, eds (2010). *Psychiatry: An evidence-based text*, pp. 655, 990.

116. K

Systemic desensitization was developed by Wolpe.

Further reading: Puri BK, Treasaden I, eds (2010). *Psychiatry: An evidence-based text*, p. 990.

117. C

Flooding involves exposure to the top stimulus in the hierarchy in vivo, while implosion involves exposure to the top stimulus in imagination.

Further reading: Puri BK, Treasaden I, eds (2010). *Psychiatry: An evidence-based text*, pp. 665, 991.

118. H

Premack's principle uses high-frequency behaviour in this case (e.g. playing piano) to reinforce the low-frequency behaviour (e.g. doing homework). Premack's principle is useful when it is difficult to identify reinforcers. The high-frequency behaviour does not need to be pleasurable.

119. L – token economy

120. A – aversive conditioning

This type of aversive conditioning is known as covert sensitization, in which the prisoners imagine the adverse outcomes.

121. F

Latent learning shows that learning can take place in the absence of reinforcement.

Further reading: Puri BK, Treasaden I, eds (2010). *Psychiatry: An evidence-based text*, pp. 207, 222.

122. B – chaining

123. G

Penalty refers to the removal of a pleasant stimulus following undesirable behaviour. It is different from punishment that gives an unpleasant outcome, e.g. caning.

124. A

This example demonstrates escape conditioning, an example of aversive conditioning.

125. D

Sensitization is the opposite of habituation. In sensitization, the strength of response is increased as the subject is told that the stimuli are significant.

Further reading: Puri BK, Treasaden I, eds (2010). *Psychiatry: An evidence-based text*, p. 990.

126. E

Insight learning involves a spontaneous and sudden gaining of insight and solution to the problems.

Further reading: Puri BK, Treasaden I, eds (2010). *Psychiatry: An evidence-based text*, p. 949.

127. C – cranial third nerve palsy

128. E – Horner's syndrome

Further reading: Puri BK, Treasaden I, eds (2010). *Psychiatry: An evidence-based text*, pp. 526, 531

129. D – cranial fourth nerve palsy

130. A – Argyll Robertson pupils

131. G – myasthenia gravis

Further reading: Puri BK, Treasaden I, eds (2010). *Psychiatry: An evidence-based text*, pp. 533–4.

132. F

133. H – pellagra

Further reading: Puri BK, Treasaden I, eds (2010). *Psychiatry: An evidence-based text*, pp. 561–2.

134. B – blepharospasm

135. B – Kahlbaum

136. F – Leonard

137. D – Kraepelin

Further reading: Puri BK, Treasaden I, eds (2010). *Psychiatry: An evidence-based text*, **pp. 11, 593, 614, 624.**

138. G – Hecker

139. A – Bleuler

Further reading: Puri BK, Treasaden I, eds (2010). *Psychiatry: An evidence-based text*, **p. 593.**

140. C

An oneiroid state consists of a strange, dream-like, psychotic experience with narrowing of consciousness. It can occur in catatonia.

141. H (36–50 per cent)

142. C (13 per cent)

143. E (23 per cent)

144. A (4 per cent)

145. A (2.4 per cent)

Further reading: Puri BK, Treasaden I, eds (2010). *Psychiatry: An evidence-based text*, **pp. 474–5, 597, 599.**

146. B

147. D (12–24 months)

Reference: Taylor D, Paton C, Kapur S (2009) *The Maudsley Prescribing Guidelines*. London: Informa Healthcare.

148. J

149. E – lamotrigine

If the patient does not have hypothyroidism, lithium monotherapy is also an option.

Further reading: Puri BK, Treasaden I, eds (2010). *Psychiatry: An evidence-based text*, **pp. 532, 536, 906, 910.**

150. L – topiramate

Further reading: Puri BK, Treasaden I, eds (2010). *Psychiatry: An evidence-based text*, **pp. 538, 699, 905, 910.**

151. I – sodium valproate

Further reading: Puri BK, Treasaden I, eds (2010). *Psychiatry: An evidence-based text*, **pp. 532, 538.**

152. L – topiramate

This may cause renal calculi if there is poor hydration during hot weather.

Further reading: Puri BK, Treasaden I, eds (2010). *Psychiatry: An evidence-based text*, **pp. 538, 699, 905, 910.**

153. F

Lithium is increased through sodium depletion.

Further reading: Puri BK, Treasaden I, eds (2010). *Psychiatry: An evidence-based text*, **pp. 613, 623, 630, 632, 633, 909–10.**

154. H – quetiapine

Reference: Bioplar Disorder Guideline Development Group (2006). *Clinical Guidance 38 Bipolar Disorder*. London: National Institute for Health and Clinical Excellence.

Further reading: Puri BK, Treasaden I, eds (2010). *Psychiatry: An evidence-based text*, **pp. 426, 601, 904.**

155. E

For rapid cycling bipolar disorder, the NICE guidelines recommend increasing the dose of an antimanic drug or adding lamotrigine.

Reference: Bioplar Disorder Guideline Development Group (2006). *Clinical Guidance 38 Bipolar Disorder*. London: National Institute for Health and Clinical Excellence.

Further reading: Puri BK, Treasaden I, eds (2010). *Psychiatry: An evidence-based text*, **pp. 532, 536, 906, 910.**

156. F and I

For long-term management of rapid cycling bipolar disorder, the NICE guidelines recommend a combination of lithium and valproate as first-line treatment. Lithium monotherapy is a second-line treatment. Antidepressants should be avoided and thyroid function tests should be checked every 6 months.

Further reading: Puri BK, Treasaden I, eds (2010). *Psychiatry: An evidence-based text*, **pp. 532, 613, 623, 630, 632, 633, 905, 909–10.**

157. E – Soranus

158. A – Hippocrates

159. C – Philippe Pinel

Further reading: Puri BK, Treasaden I, eds (2010). Psychiatry: An evidence-based text, p. 7.

160. B – Ishaq bin Ali Rahawi

161. D – W. D. Ross

162. B – Brain fag

163. D – Koro

164. E – Latah

165. I – Windigo

Further reading: Puri BK, Treasaden I, eds (2010). Psychiatry: An evidence-based text, pp. 309–18.

166. C – illusion

It is an involuntary false perception in which a transformation of a real object (i.e. curtain) takes place.

Further reading: Puri BK, Treasaden I, eds (2010). Psychiatry: An evidence-based text, pp. 234–7.

167. J – visual hyperaesthesia

168. B – dysmegalopsia

This is also known as the Alice in Wonderland effect. There is an illusory change in the size and shape (both reduction and increase in size).

169. D – macropsia

The visual sensation of objects being larger than their actual size.

170. F – pareidolia

This refers to the type of intense imagery (i.e. Jesus' face) that persists even when the person looks at a real object (callus of a tree) in the external environment.

171. G – peduncular hallucination

This is a form of vivid and colourful visual hallucination.

172. A – déjà vu

173. J – relearning

The candidate relearns information that has been learned in a previous attempt.

174. K – retroactive interference

Further reading: Puri BK, Treasaden I, eds (2010). Psychiatry: An evidence-based text, pp. 259–60.

175. I – recollection

The candidate needs to rely on the information remembered and reconstructs the information and transforms it into logical arguments.

176. F – recall

This refers to the process of accessing the information without being cued and a fill-in-the-blank test provides minimal cues.

Further reading: Puri BK, Treasaden I, eds (2010). Psychiatry: An evidence-based text, pp. 94, 250.

177. H – recognition

This involves identifying information that was encountered before.

Further reading: Puri BK, Treasaden I, eds (2010). Psychiatry: An evidence-based text, pp. 94, 250.

178. H – trust versus mistrust in infancy

179. A – autonomy versus shame or doubt in early childhood

180. F – initiative versus guilt in preschool children

181. E – industry versus inferiority in school-aged children

182. C – generativity versus stagnation in middle adulthood

183. B – ego integrity versus despair in elderly

Further reading: Puri BK, Treasaden I, eds (2010). Psychiatry: An evidence-based text, pp. 124–5.

184. D and I – Hanaoka and Takezaki

185. C and G – Schindler W. and Geigy A. G.

186. H – Sternbach L.

187. F – Osterloh I.

188. B and E – Maryanoff B. E. and Gardocki J. F.

189. A – Eymard P.

190. K

This patient suffers from paediatric autoimmune neuropsychiatric disorder associated with streptococcal infection (PANDAS).

Further reading: Puri BK, Treasaden I, eds (2010). *Psychiatry: An evidence-based text*, p. 551.

191. D

This patient suffers from borderline personality disorder and childhood sexual abuse is an important aetiological factor.

Further reading: Puri BK, Treasaden I, eds (2010). *Psychiatry: An evidence-based text*, pp. 707, 709.

192. G, H, I

This patient suffers from schizophrenia and dysbindin, neuregulin and migration may be aetiological factors.

Further reading: Puri BK, Treasaden I, eds (2010). *Psychiatry: An evidence-based text*, pp. 593–609.

193. E, L, M

This working-class woman is suffering from a moderate depressive episode. Loss of mother before the age of 11 years, having three or more children at home under the age of 14 years and not working outside the home were previously considered to be three important aetiological factors according to Brown and Harris' research.

194. A, F, J

Further reading: Puri BK, Treasaden I, eds (2010). *Psychiatry: An evidence-based text*, pp. 1103–4.

195. B, C

This woman suffers from late-onset depression. Medical diseases such as cancer and cardiovascular disease are important aetiological factors.

Reference: Brown GW, Harris TO (1978). *Social Origins of Depression: A Study of Psychiatric Disorder in Women*. London: Tavistock Publications.

Further reading: Puri BK, Treasaden I, eds (2010). *Psychiatry: An evidence-based text*, p. 616.

196. I – phaeochromocytoma

197. G – neuroleptic malignant syndrome

Further reading: Puri BK, Treasaden I, eds (2010). *Psychiatry: An evidence-based text*, pp. 874, 925.

198. E – hypothyroidism

Further reading: Puri BK, Treasaden I, eds (2010). *Psychiatry: An evidence-based text*, pp. 576–6, 1081.

199. C – Cushing's syndrome

Further reading: Puri BK, Treasaden I, eds (2010). *Psychiatry: An evidence-based text*, pp. 388, 573–4, 612.

200. H – Parkinson's disease

Further reading: Puri BK, Treasaden I, eds (2010). *Psychiatry: An evidence-based text*, pp. 541–3.

MRCPsych Paper 2

Mock examination
Time limit: 180 minutes
Number of questions: 200

MULTIPLE CHOICE QUESTIONS (MCQS)

1. The copying of a genetic message from mRNA to protein via tRNA is known as:
   A. Coding
   B. Degradation
   C. Polyadenylation
   D. Translation
   E. Transcription.

2. Which of the following statements regarding molecular genetics is false?
   A. PCR can detect small changes caused by mutations.
   B. PCR requires large amounts of DNA.
   C. Southern blotting can detect large triplet repeat expansions better than can PCR.
   D. Northern blotting involves analysis of RNA.
   E. In expression microarray, mRNA from the tissue is converted to cDNA using reverse transcriptase and the cDNA is then labelled using different coloured fluorochromes.

3. What is the increased risk for developing Alzheimer's disease in an individual with $\varepsilon 2/\varepsilon 4$ alleles for the *ApoE4* gene compared with the general population?
   A. Four times higher
   B. 10 times higher
   C. 15 times higher
   D. 20 times higher
   E. 25 times higher.

4. Which of the following diseases has an autosomal dominant form in a proportion of cases?
   A. Hunter syndrome
   B. Niemann–Pick disease
   C. Hurler's syndrome
   D. Parkinson's disease
   E. Rett syndrome.

5. Mutations in which of the following gene(s) are associated with the development of schizophrenia?
   A. Dopamine D_3 receptor gene
   B. 5-HT$_{2A}$ receptor gene
   C. *Dysbindin* gene
   D. *Neuregulin* gene
   E. All of the above.

6. Genetic knockout mice lacking the gene for which of the following neuropeptides have been reported to exhibit narcolepsy?
   A. Cholecystokinin
   B. Orexin
   C. Neuropeptide Y
   D. Substance P
   E. Vasoactive intestinal peptide.

7. Which of the following statements regarding trisomy and non-disjunction of chromosome 21 is false?
   A. Non-disjunction involves failure of a pair of chromosomes to separate normally during one of the meiotic divisions.
   B. In 50 per cent of Down syndrome cases, the non-disjunction event occurs during anaphase in maternal meiosis.
   C. If non-disjunction occurs during anaphase in maternal meiosis, this results in two maternal copies of chromosome 21 plus one paternal copy.
   D. If non-disjunction occurs during maternal meiosis, then the fetus inherits two copies of one of its mother's number 21 chromosomes.
   E. Non-disjunction occurs more frequently in maternal than in paternal meiosis owing to its longer duration in the former.

8. Which of the following statements regarding Klinefelter's syndrome is false?
   A. The incidence is approximately 1 in 1000 newborn boys.

B. 80 per cent of males with Klinefelter's syndrome have a 47,XXY karyotype with the additional X chromosome being derived equally from meiotic errors in each parent.
C. Newborn boys with Klinefelter's syndrome are clinically normal.
D. Fertility in Klinefelter's syndrome is severely impaired and risks to offspring are usually irrelevant.
E. Patients with Klinefelter's syndrome usually have affected siblings.

9. Which of the following syndromes does not involve chromosomal deletion?
A. Angelman syndrome
B. Cri-du-chat syndrome
C. DiGeorge syndrome (velocardiofacial syndrome)
D. Fragile X syndrome
E. William syndrome.

10. A 25-year-old woman comes to consult you for management of her insomnia. Since adolescence, she has never managed to get to sleep before 3 a.m. As a result, she used to skip most of the morning lectures when she was in the university. She has recently taken a job which requires her to wake up at 6 a.m. Which of the following is the most likely diagnosis?
A. Circadian rhythm sleep disorder
B. Delayed sleep phase syndrome
C. Poor sleep hygiene
D. Restless legs syndrome
E. Sleep disorder related to chaotic lifestyle at university.

11. Which of the following is false with regard to the triphasic wave in the EEG?
A. Triphasic waves occur in around 25 per cent of patients with hepatic encephalopathy.
B. Triphasic waves are rarely seen in patients younger than 30 years.
C. Triphasic waves are more common in men.
D. Regardless of the underlying aetiology, patients with predominant triphasic waves usually have cognitive impairment.
E. The three most common causes of triphasic waves are hepatic encephalopathy, renal failure and anoxic injury.

12. Which of the following psychiatric conditions is the least likely to be associated with triphasic waves in the EEG?
A. Alzheimer's disease
B. Creutzfeldt–Jakob disease
C. Lithium toxicity
D. Neuroleptic malignant syndrome
E. Serotonin syndrome.

13. A foundation year trainee has read some books on hypnotherapy and intends to refer a person with anxiety disorder to a hypnotherapist. Which of the following is correct?

A. Hypnosis is recommended by the NICE guidelines for treatment of anxiety disorders or PTSD.
B. Hypnosis is found to be superior to relaxation exercise.
C. Suggestion with hypnosis is found to be superior to suggestion without hypnosis.
D. Sudden removal of symptoms by suggestion under hypnosis can lead to rebound depression and anxiety.
E. Evidence has shown that hypnosis can aid recall in psychotherapy, which leads to a better outcome.

14. Which of the following is false?
A. Carbamazepine, phenothiazine and chloral hydrate induce their own metabolism.
B. Phenothiazine and haloperidol inhibit the metabolism of tricyclic antidepressants.
C. Slow acetylators predominate in both Europe and Japan.
D. For cytochrome P450 2D6, poor acetylator status is inherited as an autosomal recessive trait.
E. Cytochrome P450 3A4 has a profound effect on pre-systemic drug metabolism.

15. Which of the following is the most likely drug to increase bleeding with warfarin?
A. Carbamazepine
B. Lamotrigine
C. Lithium
D. Phenobarbitone
E. Valproate.

16. Which of the following is false?
A. The *DRD3* Ser9Gly polymorphism has been significantly correlated with the development of tardive dyskinesia.
B. The *HLA* gene has been implicated in the development of agranulocytosis in people taking clozapine.
C. The serotonin transporter-linked polymorphic region has been associated with clinical response to tricyclic antidepressants and SSRIs.
D. The serotonin transporter gene is implicated in the response to methylphenidate among young people with ADHD.
E. The $5HT_{2A}$ gene has been implicated in the response to ECT.

17. Which of the following is false?
A. Phenytoin, valproate and clomipramine are 90–95 per cent protein bound.
B. Amitriptyline, imipramine, chlorpromazine and diazepam are 95–99 per cent protein bound
C. If a drug is highly protein bound, the volume of distribution is reduced and close to the plasma volume.
D. Ionized drugs cross the blood–brain barrier rapidly.

E. The therapeutic window is the range of plasma concentrations that yields therapeutic success.

18. Which of the following statements regarding the pharmacokinetics of psychotropic drugs is false?
   A. Psychotropic drugs are absorbed from the gastrointestinal tract as they are lipophilic.
   B. Psychotropic drugs must reach the central nervous system in adequate amounts to produce therapeutic effects.
   C. Psychotropic drugs are mainly metabolized by the liver.
   D. Psychotropic drugs are mainly excreted by the liver.
   E. Psychotropic drugs are not highly ionized at physiological pH levels.

19. The pharmacodynamic action of agomelatine involves:
   A. Alpha agonist
   B. Cholinergic agonist
   C. Histaminergic agonist
   D. Melatonergic antagonist
   E. $5-HT_{2C}$ antagonist.

20. All of the following neuroanatomical areas demonstrate significant changes before and after antipsychotic treatment in the first episode of schizophrenia, except:
   A. Amygdala
   B. Cerebellum
   C. Frontal eye fields
   D. Postcentral gyrus
   E. Prefrontal cortex.

21. An 18-year-old woman suffers from borderline personality disorder. She complains of frequent mood swings and poor impulse control. She finds antidepressant treatment is not helpful and is keen to try a mood stabilizer. Her current BMI is 30 kg/m². Which of the following drugs cause weight loss?
   A. Carbamazepine
   B. Gabapentin
   C. Lamotrigine
   D. Topiramate
   E. Valproate.

22. Which of the following changes is implicated in the neuropathology of obsessive–compulsive disorder?
   A. Mesolimbic activation
   B. Mesolimbic deactivation
   C. Orbitofrontal activation
   D. Orbitofrontal deactivation
   E. Prefrontal activation.

23. Which of the following statements is correct?
   A. Adenine always pairs with guanine.
   B. Introns are not expressed in the final protein product.
   C. Telomeres play a key role in chromosome assortment during cell division.

D. The lagging strand is formed continuously, moving in the 5′ to 3′ direction during DNA replication.
E. The leading strand is formed in blocks during DNA replication.

24. A 30-year-old woman with a history of bipolar disorder presents with confusion, slurred speech and ataxia. Her partner finds the lithium bottle empty. Her serum level of lithium is 4 mmol/L. What is the best management?
   A. Administer an antidote to reduce the toxic effects of lithium.
   B. Control hyperthermia by rapid cooling.
   C. Consult a renal physician and seek their advice for dialysis.
   D. Fluid replacement to dilute the lithium concentration.
   E. Ventilatory support or intubation.

25. A 55-year-old black African man suffers from hypertension and bipolar disorder. His GP wants to consult you about the safest diuretic to prescribe, as he takes lithium. Your recommendation is:
   A. Amiloride
   B. Bendroflumethiazide
   C. Chloralidone
   D. Furosemide
   E. Indapamide.

26. A 35-year-old woman with agoraphobia is gradually exposed to crowded areas while relaxed. The periods of exposure gradually become longer and longer until she can confidently go to the market without an anxious response. This phenomenon is known as:
   A. Desensitization
   B. Extinction
   C. Flooding
   D. Habituation
   E. Sensitization.

27. The big five factors of personality do not include which of the following?
   A. Agreeableness
   B. Carelessness
   C. Conscientiousness
   D. Extraversion
   E. Neuroticism.

28. Based on the experiments conducted by H. Wimmer and J. Perner, the theory of mind develops after the age of:
   A. 6 months
   B. 1 year
   C. 2 years
   D. 4 years
   E. 6 years.

29. Which of the following statements regarding the Hayling and Brixton test is false?
   A. People with frontal lobe impairment perform poorly in the Hayling and Brixton test.

B. The Hayling and Brixton test was developed by Paul Burgess and Tim Shallice.

C. The Brixton test is a spatial awareness test.

D. The Brixton test is a response initiation and response suppression test.

E. The Hayling test is a sentence completion test.

30. A 14-year-old female adolescent develops non-epileptic fits when she is stressed. Her response was initially reinforced by attention from her teachers and peers. The non-epileptic fit is subsequently ignored until the non-epileptic fits no longer occur. This phenomenon is known as:
A. Desensitization
B. Extinction
C. Flooding
D. Habituation
E. Sensitization.

31. The neuroanatomical area involved in face recognition is:
A. Angular gyrus
B. Fusiform gyrus
C. Heschl gyrus
D. Postcentral gyrus
E. Precentral gyrus.

32. Which of the following statements regarding the Camberwell Family Interview is false?
A. Both verbal responses and non-verbal uses are used to assess expressed emotion.
B. It has five components: critical comments, hostility, emotional over-involvement, warmth and positive comments.
C. It is used to assess expressed emotion.
D. The interview is audio-taped.
E. The Camberwell Family Interview does not measure the perception of the patient.

33. Tardive dyskinesia is associated with supersensitivity of which of the following receptors?
A. D_1
B. D_2
C. D_3
D. D_4
E. D_5.

34. A 30-year-old man with a dual diagnosis of schizophrenia and alcohol dependence is admitted to hospital. He presents with tender hepatomegaly and jaundice. The level of aspartate transaminase (AST) is 250 IU/L (normal value 3–35 IU/L) and the level of alanine transaminase (ALT) is 150 IU/L (normal value 3–35 IU/L). He is disturbed by third-person auditory hallucinations and a delusion of persecution. The medical consultant consults you about which antipsychotic to prescibe. Your recommendation is:
A. Amisulpiride
B. Chlorpromazine
C. Haloperidol
D. Risperidone
E. Quetiapine.

35. A 22-year-old nurse suffers from depression and needs to work night shifts. She does not like to take medication on a daily basis. Which of the following antidepressants is the most suitable for her?
A. Amitriptyline
B. Citalopram
C. Fluoxetine
D. Mirtazapine
E. Paroxetine.

36. Which of the following statements regarding duloxetine is true?
A. Duloxetine induces cytochrome P450 enzymes.
B. Duloxetine is safe to be co-administered with a monoamine oxidase inhibitor (MAOI).
C. Duloxetine is beneficial to people with urinary stress incontinence.
D. Its half-life is 4 hours.
E. There is clear evidence that duloxetine offers efficacy benefits over tricyclic antidepressants in the treatment of depression.

37. A 30-year-old American woman suffering from depression asks to take reboxetine, as her British friend has recommended this medication. Which of the following statements regarding reboxetine is true?
A. Based on previous study findings, there is clear evidence that reboxetine offers efficacy benefits over other antidepressants in treatment of depression.
B. Reboxetine does not have anticholinergic effects.
C. Reboxetine exerts more influence on serotonin reuptake than noradrenaline reuptake.
D. Reboxetine is metabolized by cytochrome P450 3A4.
E. Reboxetine is available in the United States.

38. The heritability of bipolar disorder is:
A. 55 per cent
B. 65 per cent
C. 75 per cent
D. 85 per cent
E. 95 per cent.

39. A 40-year-old man with bipolar disorder has severe red plaques on his palms and soles that interfere with his work and leisure activities. Which of the following mood stabilizers is contraindicated?
A. Carbamazepine
B. Lamotrigine
C. Lithium
D. Sodium valproate
E. Topiramate.

40. A 32-year-old woman suffering from depression is currently 35 weeks pregnant and she needs to take antidepressant treatment. Which of the following antidepressants is the most likely to cause withdrawal in the neonate after birth?
A. Duloxetine

B. Mirtazapine
C. Paroxetine
D. Sertraline
E. Trazodone.

41. A medical student is interested in mirtazapine and wants to find out more about its pharmacodynamics. Which of the following is the mechanism of action of mirtazapine?
   A. α_2 receptor antagonism
   B. $5HT_{1A}$ receptor antagonism
   C. $5HT_{2A}$ receptor agonism
   D. $5HT_{2C}$ receptor agonism
   E. $5HT_3$ receptor agonism.

42. Which of the following neuroanatomical areas is associated with obsessive–compulsive disorder?
   A. Dorsolateral prefrontal cortex
   B. Inferior frontal gyrus
   C. Orbitofrontal cortex
   D. Prefrontal cortex
   E. Primary motor cortex.

43. A 20-year-lady suffers from borderline personality disorder and is admitted to the ward. Her parents want to know which of the following symptoms is the easiest to treat with medication or psychotherapy. Your answer is:
   A. Demandingness and manipulativeness
   B. Impulsive acts and self-mutilation
   C. Identity disturbance and hostility
   D. Irritability and moodiness
   E. Mercuriality and substance misuse.

44. Which of the following statements regarding the MacArthur Competence Assessment (MacCAT-CA) is false?
   A. The assessment begins with a vignette of a hypothetical offence.
   B. The MacCAT-CA comprises 30 items that are organized into five sections.
   C. The MacCAT-CA differs notably from earlier competence assessment instruments [e.g. Competence to Stand Trial Assessment Instrument, Interdisciplinary Fitness Interview (IFI) and Fitness Interview Test (FIT)].
   D. The MacCAT-CA is used to assess a defendant's competence to stand trial.
   E. The respondents are asked to make judgements about their own cases and to explain their reasoning.

45. A foundation-year trainee is interested in buspirone and he wants to find out more about its pharmacodynamics. Which of the following is the mechanism of action of buspirone?
   A. $5HT_{1A}$ receptor partial agonism
   B. $5HT_{1A}$ receptor partial antagonism
   C. $5HT_{2A}$ receptor partial agonism
   D. $5HT_{2A}$ receptor partial antagonism
   E. $5HT_{2C}$ receptor partial agonism.

46. When people with Down syndrome reach the age of 40 years, they have a high risk of developing Alzheimer's disease. The gene that accounts for this association is:
   A. *Amyloid precursor protein*
   B. *Apolipoprotein E*
   C. *Neuregulin*
   D. *Presenilin 1*
   E. *Presenilin 2.*

47. Functions of astrocytes include all of the following, except:
   A. Formation of the myelin sheath
   B. Maintenance of the blood–brain barrier
   C. Providing metabolic support to the brain
   D. Providing structural support to the brain
   E. Phagocytosis of injured nerve cells.

48. The ventral tegmental area is located in the:
   A. Locus coeruleus
   B. Medulla
   C. Midbrain
   D. Pons
   E. Reticular formation.

49. Which of the following is characteristic of tau protein found in Alzheimer's disease?
   A. Achromatic
   B. Eosinophilic
   C. Granulovacuolar
   D. Hyperphosphorylated
   E. Spongiform.

50. Which of the following enzymes are involved in the metabolism of serotonin?
   A. Catechol-*O*-methyl transferase (COMT) and tyrosine hydroxylase
   B. Dopa decarboxylase and sulfotransferase
   C. GABA transaminase and glutamatic acid decarboxylase
   D. Monoamine oxidase A (MAO-A) and aldehyde dehydrogenase
   E. Phenylalanine hydroxylase and tyrosine hydroxylase.

51. Which of the following is a type of glutamate receptor?
   A. Amino methylisoxazole propionic acid (AMPA) receptor
   B. Cannabinoid (CB) receptor
   C. γ-Aminobutyric acid (GABA) receptor
   D. 3,4-Methylenedioxymethamphetamine (MDMA) receptor
   E. Sigma-1 (σ_1) receptor.

52. A 24-year-old man with schizophrenia complains of third-person auditory hallucinations. Which of the following gyri is involved?
   A. Angular gyrus
   B. Heschl gyrus
   C. Inferior frontal gyrus
   D. Postcentral gyrus
   E. Supramarginal gyrus.

53. A 30-year-old woman with borderline personality disorder wants to find out more about dialectical behaviour therapy (DBT). Which of the following statements regarding DBT is true?
    A. DBT uses thinking and techniques drawn from Shinto philosophy emphasizing harmony with the environment.
    B. DBT does not promote the use of metaphor as DBT is strongly influenced by cognitive behaviour therapy.
    C. DBT does not promote the judicious use of humour or irreverence to reinforce the boundary between therapist and patient.
    D. Dialectical thinking refers to the way of thinking that emphasizes the limitations of linear ideas about causation.
    E. Out-of-therapy telephone contact by a case manager is usually available on a 24-hour basis to prevent self-harm.

54. A 50-year-old woman suffers from schizophrenia and she has taken quetiapine for 2 years. Her GP notices that she has developed postural hypotension. The GP wants to find out the pharmacodynamic pathway involved in causing the postural hypotension. Your answer is:
    A. Blocking alpha-1 adrenergic receptor
    B. Stimulating alpha-1 adrenergic receptor
    C. Blocking alpha-2 adrenergic receptor
    D. Stimulating alpha-2 adrenergic receptor
    E. Blocking beta receptor.

55. All the following symptoms found in patients with bulimia nervosa are the focus of interpersonal therapy (IPT), except:
    A. Binge eating, guilt and self-induced vomiting
    B. Conflict avoidance and difficulty with role expectations
    C. Confusion regarding the needs for closeness and distance
    D. Difficulty in managing negative emotions
    E. Social anxiety, sensitivity to conflict and rejection.

56. Which of the following neurotransmitters is involved in long-term potentiation for learning and memory formation?
    A. Acetylcholine
    B. Dopamine
    C. γ-Aminobutyric acid (GABA)
    D. Glutamate
    E. Glycine.

57. A 65-year-old man complains of poor memory because he worries about the significant increase in the risk of acquiring Alzheimer's disease after the age of 65 years. He wants to find out more about the risk. Your answer is:
    A. The risk doubles for every 3 years of increase in age.
    B. The risk doubles for every 5 years of increase in age.
    C. The risk doubles for every 8 years of increase in age.

D. The risk triples for every 5 years of increase in age.
E. The risk triples for every 8 years of increase in age.

58. What is the female-to-male ratio for developing paraphrenia?
    A. 2:1
    B. 8:1
    C. 30:1
    D. 40:1
    E. 50:1.

59. A medical consultant wants to find out from you the best sedative to prescribe to a 50-year-old man with a history of chronic alcohol misuse and severe hepatic impairment. Your answer is:
    A. Diazepam
    B. Flurazepam
    C. Midazolam
    D. Nitrazepam
    E. Oxazepam.

60. The autopsy report of a man who died of Creutzfeldt–Jakob disease shows spongiform change in his brain. Which of the following pathological findings is associated with the spongiform change?
    A. Amyloid beta deposition in the entorhinal cortex
    B. Hirano bodies in hippocampal pyramidal cells
    C. Hyaline eosinophilic bodies in the neocortex
    D. Neurofibrillary tangles in raphe nuclei
    E. Vacuolation of the glial cells.

61. Which of the following genes is associated with Pick's disease?
    A. *Amyloid precursor protein* gene on chromosome 21
    B. *Apolipoprotein E* gene on chromosome 19
    C. *Presenilin 1* gene on chromosome 14
    D. *Presenilin 2* gene on chromosome 1
    E. *Tau* gene on chromosome 17.

62. A 60-year-old man suffers from mild cognitive impairment and his son wants to find out the rate of conversion into dementia every year. Your answer is:
    A. 2–5 per cent
    B. 10–15 per cent
    C. 20–25 per cent
    D. 30–35 per cent
    E. 40–45 per cent.

63. A medical student wants to find out the principal component of the mesolimbic reward system which plays a key role in addiction. Your answer is:
    A. Basal nucleus of Meynert
    B. Mammillary body
    C. Nucleus accumbens
    D. Purkinje cell
    E. Raphe nuclei.

64. Buprenorphine acts as a partial agonist at which of the following receptors?
    A. Beta opioid receptor
    B. Delta opioid receptor

C. Mu opioid receptor
D. Kappa opioid receptor
E. Sigma opioid receptor.

65. Deletion in which of the following genes is associated with ubiquitin-positive and tau-negative frontotemporal dementia (FTD)?
A. *Epidermal growth factor* gene
B. *Latent-transforming growth factor beta-binding protein* gene
C. *Nerve growth factor* gene
D. *Neurotrophin* gene
E. *Progranulin* gene.

66. The following are all common auras associated with complex partial seizures, except:
A. Auditory hallucination
B. Déjà vu
C. Epigastric sensation
D. Myoclonus
E. Olfactory hallucination.

67. Which of the following statements correctly describes confounding bias?
A. This bias occurs in clinical trials when treatment is chosen by personnel involved without randomization.
B. This bias occurs when comparisons are made between groups of participants that differ with respect to determinants of outcome other than those under study.
C. This bias occurs when the methods of measurements are consistently dissimilar among groups of participants.
D. This bias occurs when participants in one group are more likely to remember past events than participants in another study group.
E. This bias occurs when studies based on the prevalence produce very different results compared with studies based on incidence of a disease.

68. Zopiclone acts as a full agonist predominantly at which of the following sites?
A. $GABA_A$ receptor (α subunit)
B. $GABA_A$ receptor (β subunit)
C. $GABA_A$ receptor (γ subunit)
D. $GABA_B$ receptor
E. $GABA_C$ receptor.

69. A 40-year-old woman suffers from depression and has taken tranylcypromine for 2 years. She presents to the Accident & Emergency (A&E) department with blood pressure of 220/120 mmHg. A few hours ago, she went for a buffet dinner and consumed a large amount of mature cheese, red wine and smoked salmon. The A&E department consultant wants to find out from you the best medication to reduce her blood pressure. Your answer is:
A. Lisinopril

B. Phentolamine
C. Propranolol
D. Nifedipine
E. Thiazide.

70. A 4-year-old child is referred to you with delayed speech and language. He was initially suspected to suffer from autism. He has gaze aversion and social avoidance. His IQ is 60. He also has attention deficit. Physical examination shows enlarged testes, large ears, a long face and flat feet. Mental state examination reveals limited eye contact, perseveration of words, echolalia and hand flapping. The genetic mutation responsible for this disorder is:
A. CAA repeats
B. CCC repeats
C. CAG repeats
D. CCG repeats
E. CGG repeats.

71. A 75-year-old man seems to develop Alzheimer's disease. His daughter has read an article stating that an MRI scan can establish the diagnosis of early Alzheimer's disease. Which of the following MRI findings is associated with the diagnosis of early Alzheimer's disease?
A. Atrophy of frontal lobe
B. Atrophy of lateral parietal lobe
C. Atrophy of medial parietal lobe
D. Atrophy of lateral temporal lobe
E. Atrophy of medial temporal lobe.

72. Rivastigmine is a:
A. Reversible acetylcholinesterase inhibitor
B. Pseudo-irreversible acetylcholinesterase inhibitor
C. Reversible butyrylcholinesterase inhibitor
D. Reversible acetylcholinesterase and butyrylcholinesterase inhibitor
E. Pseudo-irreversible acetylcholinesterase and butyrylcholinesterase inhibitor.

73. Based on the statistics provided by the Office for National Statistics, *Mental Health in Children and Young People in Great Britain*, the prevalence in young people between the ages of 1 and 15 years of suffering from a mental health disorder is:
A. 1 in 5
B. 1 in 10
C. 1 in 15
D. 1 in 20
E. 1 in 25.

74. Which of the following risk factors causes the late onset (ages 12–14 years) of delinquent behaviour in males?
A. Difficulty concentrating
B. Dishonesty
C. Hyperactivity
D. Neglect
E. Physical problems.

75. A 25-year-old woman suffers from depression and has taken fluoxetine for 2 weeks. She complains of insomnia at night. Her GP wants to find out the receptor involved in causing the insomnia. Your answer is:
    A. Agonism of $5HT_1$ receptors
    B. Agonism of $5HT_2$ receptors
    C. Agonism of $5HT_3$ receptors
    D. Agonism of $5HT_4$ receptors
    E. Agonism of $5HT_6$ receptors.

76. A 35-year-old middle-class man has been dependent on heroin and is highly motivated to remain abstinent. He wants to take an opioid antagonist with a relatively long half-life. Your recommendation is:
    A. Buprenorphine
    B. Dihydrocodeine
    C. Methadone
    D. Naloxone
    E. Naltrexone.

77. A 13-year-old obese white Caucasian boy with a learning disability is referred. He presents with an irresistible hunger drive and incessant skin picking with compulsion and anxiety. His mother reports that he tends to talk to himself. On physical examination, he has almond-shaped eyes, a fish-shaped mouth, micro-orchidism and truncal obesity. Which of the following is the most likely finding by molecular genetic testing?
    A. Microdeletion of chromosome 15q 11–13 of maternal origin
    B. Microdeletion of chromosome 15q 11–13 of paternal origin
    C. Microdeletion of chromosome 16p 13.3
    D. Microdeletion of chromosome 17q 21–31 of maternal origin
    E. Microdeletion of chromosome 17q 21–31 of paternal origin.

78. The Royal College of Psychiatrists wants to assess the quality of the MRCPsych Paper 2. The Royal College selects the Paper 2 used in spring 2008. The items in the exam paper are split into two tests equivalent in content and difficulty. The two tests are administered to a group of 100 volunteer candidates. The correlation of two separate tests is assessed with an adjustment for the test length by the Kuder–Richardson formula. What is the Royal College trying to measure?
    A. The degree of agreement among the same candidates at different times
    B. The degree of agreement among different candidates within the same time-frame
    C. The internal consistency of the MRCPsych Paper 2 used in spring 2008
    D. The stability of the MRCPsych Paper 2 used in spring 2008 under identical conditions at different times
    E. The validity of the MRCPsych Paper 2 in measuring the competency of trainees.

79. A 13-year-old adolescent suffering from depressive disorder was referred to a psychologist for psychotherapy. She missed three psychotherapy sessions and her father finds her missing. Today, her father informs the psychologist that the patient has committed suicide. Which of the following parental factors is not associated with suicide in this young person?
    A. Her parents' divorce when she was 6 years old
    B. Early death of her mother owing to kidney disease
    C. Poor education level of both parents
    D. Her father also suffers from depressive disorder
    E. Upper social class and high expectation of children.

80. A 40-year-old man presents with depression, anxiety, aggression and sensory pain. He shows cerebellar ataxia on physical examination and severe deficits on cognitive assessment. He passes away shortly after admission. He worked as a food factory worker and processed meat products made from cows infected with bovine spongiform encephalopathy (BSE). Following the death of the patient, a postmortem examination is performed. In which of the following neuroanatomical areas are florid plaques and spongiform changes most likely to be found?
    A. Brainstem
    B. Occipital cortex
    C. Parietal cortex
    D. Prefrontal cortex
    E. Temporal cortex.

81. An economic study compares the outcome of 300 patients randomly assigned to haloperidol, risperidone and olanzapine. The results are summarized as follows:

	Haloperidol ($n = 100$)	Risperidone ($n = 100$)	Olanzapine ($n = 100$)
Monthly drug and health service costs (per patient)	£30	£50	£100
Monthly benefits in terms of employment income (per patient)	£1500	£3000	£2500

The above analysis is known as a:
    A. Cost–benefit analysis
    B. Cost–effectiveness analysis
    C. Cost–efficacy analysis
    D. Cost–minimization analysis
    E. Cost–utility analysis.

82. What is the lifetime prevalence of non-suicidal self-injury among adolescents?
    A. 2–12 per cent
    B. 13–23 per cent
    C. 24–34 per cent
    D. 35–45 per cent
    E. 56–66 per cent.

83. A 60-year-old woman suffering from bipolar disorder has developed acute renal failure. You are given a list of psychotropic medication the patient has taken (see options below). The renal

consultant wants to find out which medication has the highest percentage of excretion unchanged in urine. Your response is:

A. Amisulpiride
B. Lithium
C. Lamotrigine
D. Mirtazapine
E. Olanzapine.

84. The son of a 75-year-old man with Alzheimer's disease consults you on the predicted risk of developing Alzheimer's disease among the first-degree relatives like himself. Your response is:

A. 5–9 per cent
B. 10–14 per cent
C. 15–19 per cent
D. 20–24 per cent
E. 25–29 per cent.

85. The Department of Health announces that women are becoming pregnant while using oral contraceptives and St John's wort. Which of the following constituents of the herbal extract is most likely to be responsible for this observation?

A. Hyperfourin
B. Hypericin
C. Hyperoside
D. Pseudohypericin
E. Rutin.

86. A researcher has conducted the following experiments on 10 people with schizophrenia and 10 people without schizophrenia. Each participant is presented with a sequence of letters, and the task consists of indicating when the current letter matches the one from five steps earlier in the sequence while undergoing functional magnetic resonance imaging. Which of the following neuroanatomical areas shows less activation in people with schizophrenia compared with controls?

A. Dorsolateral prefrontal cortex
B. Frontal eye fields
C. Orbitofrontal cortex
D. Primary motor cortex
E. Ventromedial prefrontal cortex.

87. A 20-year-old motorcyclist complains that he has forgotten the way to ride a motorcycle. Damage in which of the following neuroanatomical areas accounts for his symptom?

A. Amygdala
B. Dentate gyrus
C. Entorhinal cortex
D. Dorsal striatum
E. Hippocampus.

88. A 25-year-old man with bipolar disorder has tried different types of mood stabilizers and antipsychotics without much success in controlling his manic symptoms. The consultant psychiatrist has read an article stating that the calcium channel blocker verapamil has been extensively studied for the treatment of mania. This article also suggests that psychiatrists faced with patients with mania who do not respond to other anti-mania agents may consider using verapamil as adjunctive therapy. The

consultant is very keen to add verapamil to the following list of medications. Which of the following drugs has the highest risk of causing toxicity when combined with verapamil?

A. Amitriptyline
B. Lamotrigine
C. Lithium
D. Valproate
E. Risperidone.

89. A medical consultant wants to find out which subset of the verbal scale of the Wechsler Adult Intelligence Scale (WAIS) is the most sensitive to detecting organic brain disease. Your answer is:

A. Arithmetic
B. Comprehension
C. Digit span
D. Similarities
E. Vocabulary.

90. The Department of Health announces that there are 8.4 stillbirths for every 1000 live births and stillbirths from 2009 to 2010. This figure refers to the:

A. Age-specific mortality rate
B. Infant mortality rate
C. Neonatal mortality rate
D. Perinatal mortality rate
E. Stillbirth rate.

91. A 60-year-old man is brought in by his partner as he has been aggressive and disinhibited. He has suffered a severe contracoup head injury from a fall in the bathtub. The MRI scan reveals a brighter area that represents contusions resulting from the contracoup injury. Which of the following neuroanatomical areas is the most likely to be involved?

A. Contracoup in occipital lobe
B. Contracoup in orbitofrontal lobe
C. Contracoup in parietal lobe
D. Contracoup in primary motor cortex
E. Contracoup in temporal lobe.

92. 'The heritability of autism is 0.6.' What does this statement mean?

A. 60 per cent of people with autism have specific alleles in coupling at linked loci more or less often than would be expected by chance.
B. 60 per cent of people with autism have two or more loci at which alleles show linkage.
C. 60 per cent of total phenotypic variance of autism in a population results from genetic factors.
D. The constant proportion of different genotypes of autism in a population is 60 per cent.
E. The proportion of autism resulting from mutation in an allele is 60 per cent.

93. Which of the following is the mechanism of action of acamprosate?

A. GABA antagonist
B. Glutamate antagonist
C. Inhibition of alcohol dehydrogenase
D. Inhibition of alcohol aldehyde dehydrogenase
E. Opioid antagonist.

94. The origin of neural crest is found between the neural plate and:
    A. Ectoderm
    B. Endoderm
    C. Mesenchyme
    D. Mesoderm
    E. Somitomere.

95. Lofexidine is used in the treatment of opioid withdrawal. Its mechanism of action involves:
    A. α_1-adrenergic receptor agonist
    B. α_1-adrenergic receptor antagonist
    C. α_2-adrenergic receptor agonist
    D. α_2-adrenergic receptor antagonist
    E. β_1-receptor agonist.

96. A developing country is financially very poor and the government can only purchase one type of antipsychotic. The government administers a survey to 800 patients with schizophrenia and they are given two drugs from which to choose. The government informs the patients that drug A can cure 300 people and make them free of psychotic symptoms, while drug B has a 60 per cent chance of failure. Both drugs have the same expected benefits of curing around 300 patients. Ninety per cent of respondents chose drug A while only 10 per cent chose drug B. This phenomenon is known as:
    A. Cognitive bias
    B. Cognitive dissonance
    C. Cognitive distortion
    D. Cognitive framing
    E. Cognitive representation.

97. A 35-year-old man suffering from treatment-resistant schizophrenia has taken clozapine for 6 months. He is disturbed by excessive saliva drooling from his mouth. His GP wants to know the pharmacodynamics related to this side effect. Your response is:
    A. α_1-adrenergic receptor agonism and M_3 muscarinic receptor antagonism

B. α_1-adrenergic receptor antagonism and M_3 muscarinic receptor agonism
C. α_1-adrenergic receptor agonism and M_5 muscarinic receptor antagonism
D. α_2-adrenergic receptor agonism and M_4 muscarinic receptor antagonism
E. α_2-adrenergic receptor antagonism and M_4 muscarinic receptor agonism.

98. A 50-year-old man has taken warfarin and fluoxetine for 6 months. What is the increase in risk of non-gastrointestinal tract bleeding compared with patients taking warfarin without a selective serotonin reuptake inhibitor (SSRI)?
    A. Twofold
    B. Threefold
    C. Fourfold
    D. Fivefold
    E. Sixfold.

99. Which of the following has the least impact on the cognitive representation of disease among people with chronic schizophrenia?
    A. Aetiology of schizophrenia
    B. Impact of schizophrenia on patients' lives
    C. Measures and strategies available to control schizophrenia
    D. Positive symptoms
    E. Prevalence of schizophrenia.

100. A 40-year-old woman suffering from treatment-resistant schizophrenia has taken clozapine 450 mg/day for 2 months. Which of the following side effects would not improve even the dose is reduced?
    A. Hypotension
    B. Neutropenia
    C. Sedation
    D. Seizure
    E. Weight gain.

EXTENDED MATCHING ITEMS (EMIs)

Questions 101–106 – options
- A. Deletion
- B. Insertion
- C. Frame shift
- D. Missense mutation
- E. Nonsense mutation
- F. Regulatory (transcription) mutations
- G. RNA processing mutation
- H. Silent mutation
- I. Substitution
- J. Transition
- K. Transversion

Lead-in: Select the above mutations to match the following descriptions. Each option might be used once, more than once or not at all.

101. This mutation involves a change to a single nucleotide. (Choose one option.)

102. Substitution of a purine for a purine. (Choose one option.)

103. Owing to the degeneracy of the genetic code, this mutation does not alter the amino acid being encoded. (Choose one option.)

104. This mutation results in the substitution of one amino acid for another. (Choose one option.)

105. This mutation creates a new stop codon (UAA, UPG or UGA) and results in premature termination of translation. (Choose one option.)

106. The mutation usually results in a shortened (truncated) protein product. (Choose one option.)

Questions 107–111 – options
- A. Adoption studies
- B. Association studies
- C. Family studies
- D. Segregation analysis
- E. Twin studies

Lead-in: Select the above options to the match the following descriptions. Each option might be used once, more than once or not at all.

107. The morbid risk of the illness is determined within families, and rates of occurrence in the different degrees of relatives are compared with those the general population. (Choose one option.)

108. It compares the concordance rates of diagnosis in twins, both monozygotic and dizygotic, thus allowing researchers the possibility of dissecting the role of genes from that of the environment. (Choose one option.)

109. Genetic study to delineate inherited and environmental factors. (Choose one option.)

110. It compares the likelihood for the observed frequency of illness in a pedigree with multiple cases of affective disorder with those that can be predicted by different modes of transmission. (Choose one option.)

111. It allows researchers to follow up regions of interest identified in linkage analyses or to examine the candidate genes of *a priori* interest. (Choose one option.)

Questions 112–114 – options
- A. Chromosome 1
- B. Chromosome 4
- C. Chromosome 5
- D. Chromosome 6
- E. Chromosome 7
- F. Chromosome 8
- G. Chromosome 9
- H. Chromosome 10
- I. Chromosome 15
- J. Chromosome 17
- K. Chromosome 22

Lead-in: Select the chromosome that is affected in each of the presentations below. Each option might be used once, more than once or not at all.

112. A 10-year-old girl presents with a small head, happy face, jerk movement and ataxia. She is known to have a history of epilepsy and learning disability. (Choose one option.)

113. A 14-year-boy is referred to the Early Psychosis Service. He has features of a round face, cleft palate, low-set ears, learning disability and congenital heart disease with frequent infections. (Choose one option.)

114. A 7-year-old girl is admitted to the paediatric ward for self-injury. She also presents with hyperactivity, severe learning disability, attention-seeking and sleep disturbance. The mother reports that she cried like a cat at birth. (Choose one option.)

Questions 115–121 – options
- A. Slowing of the occipital rhythm with the increasing amounts of theta and delta frequencies.
- B. Alpha frequencies are replaced with increasing theta and delta waves.
- C. High-amplitude, slow, triphasic, and sharp waves.
- D. Predominantly frontal triphasic slow waves and generalized slow activity.
- E. EEG trace may be normal until clouding of consciousness.
- F. Diffuse irregularity and excess fast activity.
- G. Generalized fast activity in the early stages, followed by loss of alpha activity, a subsequent increase in the amplitude and amount of theta and delta activities. At the end, there is a burst suppression effect.

Lead-in: Match the EEG patterns to the following conditions. Each option might be used once, more than once or not at all.

115. Alcohol intoxication (choose one option).

116. Anaesthesia (choose one option).

117. Chronic haemodialysis with dementia as complication (choose one option).

118. Hyperglycaemia (choose one option).

119. Hypoxia (choose one option).

120. Liver failure (choose one option).

121. Renal failure (choose one option).

Questions 122–125 – options
  A. Diffuse slow activity with episodic, bilaterally synchronous and symmetrical bursts of rhythmic waves.
  B. Unusual appearance of episodic discharges, recurring every 1–3 seconds and variable focal slow waves over the temporal areas.
  C. Periodic stereotyped repetitive discharges at a rate of 1 per second.
  D. High-amplitude, repetitive, bilaterally synchronous and symmetrical, polyphasic sharp-wave and slow-wave complexes, occurring every 4–15 seconds.

Lead-in: Match the EEG patterns to the following conditions. Each option might be used once, more than once or not at all.

122. Acute encephalitis (choose one option).

123. Creutzfeldt–Jakob disease (choose one option).

124. Herpes simplex encephalitis (choose one option).

125. Subacute sclerosing panencephalitis (choose one option).

Questions 126–130 – options
  A. 1
  B. 2
  C. 3
  D. 4
  E. 5
  F. 6
  G. 7
  H. 8
  I. 9
  J. 10

Lead-in: Match the above number to fill in the blank of the following statements regarding the epidemiology of psychiatric disorders in the UK. Each option might be used once, more than once or not at all.

126. 1 in __ British adults experience at least one diagnosable mental health problem in 1 year. (Choose one option.)

127. __ in 10 British meet the diagnostic criteria for mixed anxiety and depression. (Choose one option.)

128. 1 in __ British women and 1 in __ British men with depression receive treatment. (Choose two options.)

129. Depression affects ___ in 5 older people living in the community and ___ in 5 living in care homes. (Choose two options.)

130. 1 in ___ prisoners has no mental disorder. (Choose one option.)

Questions 131–134 – options
  A. Mildly abnormal EEG with brief bursts of moderately slow-wave and complex activity between attacks.
  B. Decrease or loss of spindles, with diminished or absent reactivity in the EEG.
  C. Non-specific EEG abnormalities.
  D. Diminished alpha frequencies and fast activities over the affected hemisphere.

Lead-in: Match the EEG patterns to the following conditions. Each option might be used once, more than once or not at all.

131. Dementia pugilistica (choose one option).

132. Head trauma with prolonged coma (choose one option).

133. Migraine (choose one option).

134. Space-occupying lesion (choose one option).

Questions 135–139 – options
  A. Generalized very fast activity, followed by rhythmic activity at approximately 10 Hz with rapidly increasing amplitude.
  B. Spike and wave complexes at 3 Hz with faster and slower complexes at the beginning and end of the attacks.
  C. Slow (2 Hz) complexes in prolonged runs with gradual cessation. These discharges are enhanced in non-REM sleep.
  D. High-amplitude mixed delta slow waves and multifocal spikes which tend to cluster to give an apparent burst-suppression appearance during sleep and constitute a chaotic appearance.
  E. The EEG findings may vary from no EEG correlates to polyspikes.

Lead-in: Match the EEG patterns to the following disorders. Each option might be used once, more than once or not at all.

135. Absence (petit mal) seizure (choose one option).

136. Hypsarrhythmia (choose one option).

137. Lennox–Gastaut syndrome (choose one option).

138. Myoclonus (choose one option).

139. Tonic–clonic attacks (grand mal) (choose one option).

Questions 140–144 – options

A. A significant increase in fast activity, persisting for up to 2 weeks after the drug has been stopped.

B. Minor increases in alpha frequencies at therapeutic levels, but slow waves, paroxysmal complex activity and possible convulsions at higher doses.

C. EEG abnormalities correlate to the levels of medication.

D. Slow waves appear initially. Generalized, irregular, slow waves with bilaterally synchronous bursts may persist for at least a month after a course of treatment.

E. Both excess fast and slow activities.

Lead-in: Match the EEG patterns to the following disorders. Each option might be used once, more than once or not at all.

140. Benzodiazepines (choose one option).

141. ECT (choose one option).

142. First-generation antipsychotics (choose one option).

143. Lithium (choose one option).

144. Barbiturate (choose one option).

Questions 145–148 – options

A. Aggressive obsession
B. Contamination obsession
C. Symmetry obsession
D. Religious obsession
E. Somatic obsession
F. Sexual obsession
G. Checking compulsion
H. Cleaning compulsion
I. Counting compulsion
J. Hoarding obsession
K. Ordering compulsion
L. Repeating compulsion
M. Saving compulsion

Lead-in: A 35-year-old man suffers from treatment refractory obsessive–compulsive disorder (OCD). The core trainee wants to find out more about OCD symptoms and the relationship with treatment outcome. Each option might be used once, more than once or not at all.

145. Name two symptoms associated with poor response to selective serotonin reuptake inhibitors (SSRIs). (Choose two options.)

146. Name two symptoms associated with poor response to cognitive behaviour therapy (CBT). (Choose two options.)

147. Name the most common obsession. (Choose one option.)

148. Name the most common compulsion. (Choose one option.)

Questions 149–155 – options

A. Altruism
B. Acting out
C. Anticipation
D. Denial
E. Displacement
F. Humour
G. Idealization
H. Identification
I. Intellectualization
J. Introjection
K. Isolation of affect
L. Projection
M. Projective identification
N. Rationalization
O. Reaction formation
P. Repression
Q. Regression
R. Splitting
S. Sublimation
T. Suppression
U. Undoing
V. Ascetism

Lead-in: A 25-year-old woman is admitted to the psychiatric ward with a history of emotionally unstable personality disorder, borderline type, and alcohol dependence. She was physically abused by her parents as a child and she mentions that she feels, as with her parents, the hospital staff have become abusive towards her. Select the most appropriate defence mechanisms for each of the following situations. Each option might be used once, more than once or not at all.

149. The nurse asks the client if she can go through her things to ensure there aren't any sharp objects that she could use to self-harm. The client becomes upset and feels like punching the nurse. Later when the client sees a psychotherapist she realizes that her desire to hit the nurse was related to her mother hitting her as a child. (Choose one option.)

150. The client tells the core trainee that she has thoughts of harming her partner and she has to tap on a table five times in order to dispel these thoughts. (Choose one option.)

151. The core trainee enquires about her alcohol dependence and the client informs her that she is not dependent on alcohol and that drinking is a way to ease the stress in her life. She feels that her drinking was within reason and gives an explanation for this. (Choose one option.)

152. After speaking to the core trainee, she believes that the trainee is the best doctor she has ever seen. From now on, the patient only wants to see this core trainee as her doctor. (Choose two options.)

153. The core trainee asks you to give some examples of primitive defences. (Choose seven options.)

154. On the second day, the client worries that the consultant may give her a warning for hitting the nurse and behaving like a child on the ward. (Choose one option.)

155. Her behaviour becomes uncontrollable and she almost sets fire to part of the ward. The consultant decides to send her to a secure hospital. She complains that no one cares about her. She was chased away by her parents and is now being chased away by the consultant. This verifies her belief that hospital staff are as abusive as her parents. (Choose one option.)

Questions 156–163 – options
- A. Altruism
- B. Acting out
- C. Anticipation
- D. Denial
- E. Displacement
- F. Humour
- G. Idealization
- H. Identification
- I. Intellectualization
- J. Introjection
- K. Isolation of affect
- L. Projection
- M. Projective identification
- N. Rationalization
- O. Reaction formation
- P. Repression
- Q. Regression
- R. Splitting
- S. Sublimation
- T. Suppression
- U. Undoing
- V. Ascetism

Lead-in: A 20-year-old man is referred by his GP for assessment for abnormal grief. His father, a businessman, died suddenly during an elective operation 4 weeks ago and his family intends to take legal action against the hospital seeking compensation as they believe his death was preventable. Select the most appropriate defence mechanism for each of the following situations. Each option might be used once, more than once or not at all.

156. The GP mentioned in his referral letter that the client has tried to separate himself from his emotions since his father died. (Choose one option.)

157. During the interview, the client tells you that he has tried to block and expel grief from entering his mind. (Choose one option.)

158. During the interviewing, the client refers to abstract philosophy to explain his current state. (Choose one option.)

159. The core trainee asks you to give examples of neurotic defences devised by Anna Freud. (Choose nine options.)

160. The client appears to be coping well and informs you that he has an active plan to take over his father's business. (Choose one option.)

161. One month later, the client appears to take on the quality of his father by behaving like him. (Choose one option.)

162. Two months later, the client informs you that he has internalized the hostility of his father to scold other staff in the business as he feels sad about his father's sudden death. (Choose one option.)

163. You speak to his mother who expresses sympathy to doctors as they are always busy and medical errors seem to be inevitable. She wants to apologize to the doctor who looked after her husband as she was rude to him. Two weeks later, the client informs you that his mother is proceeding with the legal case and hopes to get a huge amount of compensation from the hospital. What is the defence mechanism being used by his mother? (Choose one option.)

Questions 164–169 – options
- A. Ask to reflect
- B. Breach confidentiality
- C. Clarification
- D. Containment
- E. Show empathy
- F. Transference interpretation

Lead-in: A 30-year-old man presents with mixed anxiety after he contracts a sexually transmitted disease (STD) from his female partner. He feels that he has been symbolically castrated by her, as all women are trying to avoid him. This also reminds him of the remarks made by his mother who threatened to castrate him when he was a child. She probably ridiculed him and tried to undermine his sense of masculinity but the client took her remarks very seriously. Furthermore, his father abandoned the family when he was a child. The client sees his father as passive and irresponsible. A male psychotherapist offers brief psychodynamic psychotherapy to this client. Select the most appropriate psychodynamic technique for each of the following situations. Each option might be used once, more than once or not at all.

164. The issues of STD and castration are anxiety-provoking. The therapist tries to modify and return to the difficult issues in a way that the client can tolerate (Choose one option.)

165. During the second session, the client is very frustrated with the STD and wants to end his life. (Choose two options.)

166. During the fourth session, the client is 30 minutes late. (Choose one option.)

167. During the sixth session, the client mentions that he had a dream in which he saw himself arguing with his girlfriend in his childhood house. (Choose one option.)

168. During the eighth session, the client mentions that he has been abusing the son of his partner. (Choose two options.)

169. During the last session, the client feels frustrated as the psychotherapy is coming to an end and he will be left alone. The client is angry and feels as if the therapist is going to abandon him. (Choose two options.)

Questions 170–174 – options
- A. Eclectic family therapy
- B. Strategic family therapy

C. Structural family therapy

D. Systemic family therapy

Lead-in: You are seeing a 30-year-old woman, Cindy, who suffers from emotionally unstable personality disorder, borderline type, and from benzodiazepine dependence. Cindy is the eldest and one of her sisters, Mary, is close to her but suffers from alcohol dependence. Cindy and Mary often have arguments with the youngest sister, Lynette, who is a lesbian. They live together with their parents. Her father is very frustrated with the whole family situation and hits Mary one night when she is drunk. You have decided to refer this family for family therapy. Select the most appropriate type of therapy for each of the following situations. Each option might be used once, more than once or not at all.

170. You discover that her parents are often not at home and ask the youngest daughter, Lynette, to supervise Cindy for her medication intake. Lynette always uses the medication to threaten Cindy unless she offers something in return. Cindy feels that there is no hierarchy in the family. (Choose one option.)

171. Cindy informs you that her family members hold opposite views on the incident when her father hit Mary. She sympathizes with Mary but the other members feel that her father was right to have hit Mary. You want to ask each family member to comment on the incident. (Choose one option.)

172. During the therapy, you also clarify the gains and losses experienced by each family member from the incident. (Choose one option.)

173. After talking to other family members, you discover that the main problem lies in a lack of communication and a tendency to keep secrets among a few family members, leading to misunderstandings. You come up with some practical advice to help deal with this dysfunctional pattern of communication. (Choose one option.)

174. You discover that Lynette has a tendency to cut her wrists. Owing to her age, you decide to refer her to a child and adolescent psychiatrist. The child and adolescent psychiatrist recommends that Lynette undergo family therapy with her parents. Her parents are busy with work and they request family therapy focusing on the present situation and communication in the family. (Choose one option.)

Questions 175–180 – options
  A. < 1 per cent
  B. 2 per cent
  C. 5 per cent
  D. 10 per cent

Lead-in: A couple has adopted a child with Down syndrome. They want to find out the chances of their child developing a psychiatric disorder when he or she becomes an adult. Match the correct number to each of the following psychiatric co-morbidities. Each option might be used once, more than once or not at all.

175. Anxiety disorders (choose one option).

176. Depressive disorder (choose one option).

177. Dementia (choose one option).

178. Obsessive–compulsive disorder (choose one option).

179. Schizophrenia (choose one option).

180. Self-injury (choose one option).

Questions 181–183 – options
  A. 5 per cent
  B. 9 per cent
  C. 13 per cent
  D. 45 per cent

Lead-in: A 28-year-old man suffers from a first episode of schizophrenia. His family members want to find out their risk of developing schizophrenia. Match the correct number to the following psychiatric co-morbidity. Each option might be used once, more than once or not at all.

181. The risk of his brother developing schizophrenia. (Choose one option.)

182. The risk of his son developing schizophrenia. (Choose one option.)

183. The risk of his father developing late-onset schizophrenia. (Choose one option.)

Questions 184–187 – options
  A. Gene map
  B. Genomic library
  C. Linkage map
  D. Physical map

Lead-in: Match the above genetic terminology to the following descriptions. Each option might be used once, more than once or not at all.

184. It is constructed from total cellular DNA and the desired target sequence is screened by a complementary DNA (cDNA) by hybridization. (Choose one option.)

185. It shows the positions of two genes in terms of recombination frequency. (Choose one option.)

186. It shows the DNA sequence (e.g. location of introns, exons, promoters, etc.) of a gene. (Choose one option.)

187. It shows the position of two genes in terms of base pairs. (Choose one option.)

Questions 188–192 – options
  A. Absent P waves
  B. Biphasic P waves
  C. PR interval = 100 ms
  D. PR interval = 300 ms
  E. QRS complex = 200 ms
  F. QTc = 500 ms
  G. RR interval 450 ms

H. RR interval = 1500 ms
I. R wave in V6 = 30 mm
J. ST segment depression
K. ST segment elevation
L. Diffuse ST segment elevation
M. ST segment elevation with saddle
N. Absent T wave
O. Diffuse T wave inversion
P. Tall T waves
Q. Q wave
R. Heart rate: 120/minute
S. Heart rate: 30/minute

Lead-in: Match the above electrocardiogram (ECG) findings to the most typical ECG features found in the following scenarios. Each option might be used once, more than once or not at all.

188. A 40-year-old married woman with major depression checks into a hotel and takes 100 amitriptyline tablets (100 mg each). She remains in a drugged state at the Accident & Emergency (A&E) department and is about to be transferred to an intensive care unit. (Choose three options.)

189. A 40-year-old man suffering from treatment-resistant schizophrenia has been taking clozapine for the past 5 years. He experiences tiredness, shallow and difficult breathing and chest pain. The temperature is 39°C. (Choose three options.)

190. A 55-year-old man suffering from depression does not respond to various types of antidepressants. His antidepressant treatment is augmented with thyroxine. He presents to the A&E department presenting with a 2-hour history of chest pain, nausea and sweatiness. (Choose four options.)

191. A 35-year-old woman complains of a 3-month history of ankle swelling, together with increased abdominal distension and breathlessness over the past week. She admits to having taken amphetamines on a daily basis for the last 5 years. (Choose four options.)

192. A 70-year-old man with Alzheimer's disease is admitted because of a blackout. He has taken donepezil on a daily basis for the past year. (Choose two options.)

Questions 193–198 – options
A. Alzheimer's disease
B. Bipolar disorder
C. Chronic depression
D. Huntington's disease
E. Lewy body dementia
F. Obsessive–compulsive disorder
G. Progressive supranuclear palsy
H. Schizophrenia
I. Variant Creutzfeldt–Jakob disease
J. Wernicke's encephalopathy
K. Wilson's disease

Lead-in: Match the above neuropsychiatric conditions to the following magnetic resonance imaging (MRI) changes. Each option might be used once, more than once or not at all.

193. Atrophy of the head of caudate nucleus. (Choose one option.)

194. Atrophy of the midbrain. (Choose one option.)

195. Hockey-stick sign. (Choose one option.)

196. Hyperintensities in bilateral mammillary bodies. (Choose one option.)

197. Periventricular white matter hyperintensities. (Choose one option.)

198. Pulvinar sign. (Choose one option.)

Questions 199–200 – options
A. Adiponectin
B. Cholecystokinin
C. Leptin
D. Orexins
E. Neuropeptide Y
F. Neurotensin
G. Somatostatin
H. Substance P
I. Vasoactive intestinal peptide

Lead-in: Match the above neuropeptides to the following sources of secretion. Each option might be used once, more than once or not at all.

199. Secreted by adipose tissue and correlates with body fat percentage in adults.

200. Secreted by the gut and hypothalamus to stimulate feeding.

ANSWERS – MULTIPLE CHOICE QUESTIONS

1. D

Further reading: Puri BK, Treasaden I, eds (2010). *Psychiatry: An evidence-based text*, p. 467.

2. B

A small amount of DNA is required.

Further reading: Puri BK, Treasaden I, eds (2010). *Psychiatry: An evidence-based text*, pp. 466–7.

3. A

It is three to four times higher. If the individual is homozygous for ε4/ε4 alleles for the *ApoE4* gene, the risk of developing Alzheimer's disease is 10 times higher.

Further reading: Puri BK, Treasaden I, eds (2010). *Psychiatry: An evidence-based text*, pp. 1103–4.

4. D

Parkinson's disease with mutation in the *alpha synuclein* gene, which is involved in neuronal plasticity, follows an autosomal dominant pattern of inheritance.

Further reading: Puri BK, Treasaden I, eds (2010). *Psychiatry: An evidence-based text*, pp. 541–3.

5. E

6. B

Orexin promotes wakefulness.

Reference: Chemelli RM, Willie JT, *et al.* (1999). Narcolepsy in orexin knockout mice: molecular genetics of sleep regulation. *Cell* **98**: 437–451.

7. B

In 95 per cent of Down syndrome cases, the non-disjunction event occurs in anaphase of maternal meiosis.

Further reading: Puri BK, Treasaden I, eds (2010). *Psychiatry: An evidence-based text*, pp. 467, 1082, 1087–8.

8. E

Option E is false as Klinefelter's syndrome usually occurs as sporadic familial cases. Option C is correct as the diagnosis is usually first suspected in childhood because of mild learning disabilities, or in adulthood because of infertility.

Further reading: Puri BK, Treasaden I, eds (2010). *Psychiatry: An evidence-based text*, pp. 467, 754, 763.

9. D

Further reading: Puri BK, Treasaden I, eds (2010). *Psychiatry: An evidence-based text*, pp. 1082, 1088, 1091.

10. B

The prevalence of delayed sleep phase syndrome is 3 in 2000 with no clear aetiology. Both sleep architecture and total time of sleep are normal. Patients usually feel sleepy in the morning. Depression is a common co-morbidity. Treatment strategies involve adaptation to late-night sleep, regular sleep schedule, good sleep hygiene, light therapy and melatonin.

11. C

There is no difference in the occurrence of triphasic waves in the EEG between men and women.

12. D

13. D

Hypnosis is not commonly used in psychiatry and not recommended by the NICE guidelines to treat psychiatric disorders. Hypnosis is not found to be superior to other psychological treatments.

Further reading: Puri BK, Treasaden I, eds (2010). *Psychiatry: An evidence-based text*, p. 141.

14. C

Slow acetylators predominate in Europe (fast:slow = 40:60) but not Japan (fast:slow = 85:15).

15. E

Valproate increases the bleeding effects of warfarin by inhibiting platelet aggregation and inhibits the P450 system.

16. D

Option D is false as the dopamine transporter gene is implicated.

17. D

Ionized drugs (highly basic or acidic) cross the blood–brain barrier slowly. For option E, therapeutic window refers to 'toxic dose' divided by 'therapeutic dose'.

18. D

Psychotropic drugs are mainly excreted by the kidneys.

19. E

Agomelatine is an antidepressant which resynchronizes the circadian rhythm. It is a melatonergic agonist at MT_1 and

MT$_2$ receptors and a 5-HT$_{2C}$ antagonist. It has no affinity for alpha, beta, adrenergic, histaminergic, cholinergic, dopaminergic and benzodiazepine receptors.

20. D

The postcentral gyrus is the somatosensory cortex and shows the least change in activity after antipsychotic treatment. Changes in prefrontal and amygdala activity during olanzapine treatment have been reported in people with schizophrenia and these areas are involved in emotional processing. Increased activations in both frontal eye fields and the cerebellum can signify improvement in attentional and sensorimotor systems after antipsychotic treatment.

References: Blasi G, Popolizio T, Taurisano P (2009). Changes in prefrontal and amygdala activity during olanzapine treatment in schizophrenia. *Psychiatry Research* **173**: 31–8; Keedy SK, Rosen C, Khine T (2009). An fMRI study of visual attention and sensorimotor function before and after antipsychotic treatment in first-episode schizophrenia. *Psychiatry Research* **172**: 16–23.

21. D

Further reading: Puri BK, Treasaden I, eds (2010). *Psychiatry: An evidence-based text*, pp. 538, 699, 905, 910.

22. C

Reference: Drummond LM, Finberg NA (2007). Phobias and obsessive compulsive disorder. In: Stein G, Wilkinson G, eds. *Seminars in General Adult Psychiatry*. London: Gaskell.

23. B

Adenine pairs with thymine while guanine pairs with cytosine. The centromere plays a key role in chromosome assortment during cell division. The leading strand is formed continuously, moving in the 5′ to 3′ direction during DNA replication. The lagging strand (Okazaki fragments) is formed in blocks during DNA replication.

Further reading: Puri BK, Treasaden I, eds (2010). *Psychiatry: An evidence-based text*, p. 467.

24. C

25. A

Potassium-sparing diuretics (e.g. amiloride) are recommended as potassium depletion may induce lithium toxicity. There is an unpredictable rise in the lithium concentration when it is combined with thiazide diuretics (e.g. bendroflumethiazide, chloralidone and indapamide). Loop diuretics (e.g. furosemide) are not very useful in treating hypertension and may lead to lithium toxicity.

Reference: Taylor D, Paton C, Kapur S (2009). *The Maudsley Prescribing Guidelines*, 10th edn. London: Informa Healthcare.

26. A

27. B

Further reading: Puri BK, Treasaden I, eds (2010). *Psychiatry: An evidence-based text*, pp. 79, 282.

28. D

Further reading: Puri BK, Treasaden I, eds (2010). *Psychiatry: An evidence-based text*, pp. 22, 290–1, 974, 1089.

29. D

The Hayling test is a response initiation and response suppression test.

Further reading: Puri BK, Treasaden I, eds (2010). *Psychiatry: An evidence-based text*, p. 516.

30. B

Extinction also occurs in operant conditioning when positive reinforcement (i.e. attention from others) is removed.

Further reading: Puri BK, Treasaden I, eds (2010). *Psychiatry: An evidence-based text*, pp. 208, 503.

31. B

Further reading: Puri BK, Treasaden I, eds (2010). *Psychiatry: An evidence-based text*, pp. 332–5.

32. E

The Camberwell Family Interview rates the patient's perception of how his family feels about him and the disorder, although the patient is absent when the family is interviewed.

Reference: Vaughn C, Leff J (1976). The measurement of expressed emotion in the families of psychiatric patients. *British Journal of Social and Clinical Psychology* **15**: 157–65.

33. B

Further reading: Puri BK, Treasaden I, eds (2010). *Psychiatry: An evidence-based text*, pp. 604, 903.

34. A

This man suffers from moderate alcohol hepatitis. Amisulpride is predominantly excreted by the kidneys and dosage reduction is not necessary as this man is floridly psychotic.

Reference: Taylor D, Paton C, Kapur S (2009). *The Maudsley Prescribing Guidelines*, 10th edn. London: Informa Healthcare.

Further reading: Puri BK, Treasaden I, eds (2010). *Psychiatry: An evidence-based text*, p. 425.

35. C

Fluoxetine is less sedative than other antidepressants and has a long half-life. Hence, fluoxetine is suitable for this patient as it can be taken every other day.

Further reading: Puri BK, Treasaden I, eds (2010). *Psychiatry: An evidence-based text*, **pp. 698, 708, 724, 762.**

36. C

Duloxetine does not induce cytochrome P450 enzymes. Co-administration with an MAOI may lead to potentially serious drug interactions. Its half-life is 12 hours and there is no clear evidence that it offers benefits over tricyclic antidepressants in efficacy.

Further reading: Puri BK, Treasaden I, eds (2010). *Psychiatry: An evidence-based text*, **p. 907.**

37. D

Reboxetine is an ineffective and potentially harmful antidepressant. It has anticholinergic properties and does not inhibit serotonin reuptake. At the time of writing, reboxetine is not licensed in the US.

Reference: Eyding D, Lelgemann M, Grouven U (2010). Reboxetine for acute treatment of major depression: systematic review and meta-analysis of published and unpublished placebo and selective serotonin reuptake inhibitor controlled trials. *British Medical Journal* **341: c4737**

Further reading: Puri BK, Treasaden I, eds (2010). *Psychiatry: An evidence-based text*, **pp. 425, 907.**

38. D

Further reading: Puri BK, Treasaden I, eds (2010). *Psychiatry: An evidence-based text*, **p. 468.**

39. C

This man suffers from psoriasis and lithium may exacerbate the psoriasis.

40. C

Paroxetine has a shorter half-life compared with other antidepressants and is associated with discontinuation syndrome.

Further reading: Puri BK, Treasaden I, eds (2010). *Psychiatry: An evidence-based text*, **p. 717.**

41. A

The mechanism of action of mirtazapine includes $5HT_{1A}$ agonism, $5HT_{2A}$ antagonism, $5HT_{2C}$ antagonism and $5HT_3$ antagonism.

Further reading: Puri BK, Treasaden I, eds (2010). *Psychiatry: An evidence-based text*, **pp. 426, 661, 907, 1110–11.**

42. C

Further reading: Puri BK, Treasaden I, eds (2010). *Psychiatry: An evidence-based text*, **pp. 333, 1181.**

43. B

Reference: Stone MH (2010). Recovery from borderline personality disorder. *American Journal of Psychiatry* **167: 618–19.**

Further reading: Puri BK, Treasaden I, eds (2010). *Psychiatry: An evidence-based text*, **pp. 707, 709.**

44. B

The MacCAT-CA comprises 22 items that are organized into three sections. The first section is 'Understanding, assesses defendants' ability to understand general information about the legal system and the process of adjudication'; the second section is 'Reasoning, evaluates defendants' ability to discern the legal relevance of information and their capacity to reason about specific choices that confront defendants during the course of a typical criminal proceeding' and the third section is 'Appreciation, assesses defendants' ability to appreciate the meaning and consequences of their own legal circumstances'.

Reference: Pinals DA, Tillbrook CE, Mumley DL (2006). Practical application of the MacArthur Competence Assessment Tool-Criminal Adjudication (MacCAT-CA) in a public sector forensic setting. *Journal of the American Academy of Psychiatry and the Law* **34: 179–88.**

45. B

Further reading: Puri BK, Treasaden I, eds (2010). *Psychiatry: An evidence-based text*, **pp. 426, 648, 912.**

46. A

The *amyloid precursor protein* gene is located on chromosome 21.

Further reading: Puri BK, Treasaden I, eds (2010). *Psychiatry: An evidence-based text*, **pp. 473, 1104.**

47. A

Oligodendrocytes form the myelin sheath.

Further reading: Puri BK, Treasaden I, eds (2010). *Psychiatry: An evidence-based text*, **p. 436.**

48. C

The ventral tegmental area is part of the mesolimbic dopamine pathway.

Further reading: Puri BK, Treasaden I, eds (2010). *Psychiatry: An evidence-based text*, **p. 997.**

49. D

Further reading: Puri BK, Treasaden I, eds (2010). *Psychiatry: An evidence-based text*, **p. 436.**

50. D

Further reading: Puri BK, Treasaden I, eds (2010). *Psychiatry: An evidence-based text*, **pp. 413–4.**

51. A

There are three main types of glutamate receptors: AMPA receptors, kainite receptors and *N*-methyl-D-aspartic acid (NMDA) receptors.

Further reading: Puri BK, Treasaden I, eds (2010). *Psychiatry: An evidence-based text*, **pp. 351, 358, 410, 416–7.**

52. B

Heschl's gyrus (superior temporal gyrus) contains frequency strips which correspond to the tonal frequencies of sound. An fMRI study has demonstrated an increase in the blood oxygen level-dependent (BOLD) signal in Heschl's gyrus when patients experience auditory hallucinations.

Reference: Dierks T, Linden DEJ, Jandl M (1999). Activation of Heschl's gyrus during auditory hallucinations. *Neuron* **22:** 615–21.

Further reading: Puri BK, Treasaden I, eds (2010). *Psychiatry: An evidence-based text*, **pp. 332–5.**

53. D

DBT is based on Zen Buddhism. DBT promotes the use of metaphor and irreverence. Out-of-therapy telephone contact is determined by the treatment contract between the patient and the therapist but is not generally available on a 24-hour basis.

Palmer RL (2002). Dialectical behaviour therapy for borderline personality disorder. *Advances in Psychiatric Treatment* **8:** 10–16.

54. A

Further reading: Puri BK, Treasaden I, eds (2010). *Psychiatry: An evidence-based text*, **pp. 421, 695.**

55. A

IPT does not focus on the direct symptoms associated with bulimia nervosa but allows for identification of problem areas that have contributed to the emergence of bulimia nervosa over time.

Reference: Robin AF (1999). Interpersonal therapy for bulimia nervosa. *Psychotherapy in Practice* **55:** 715–25.

Further reading: Puri BK, Treasaden I, eds (2010). *Psychiatry: An evidence-based text*, **p. 693.**

56. D

Further reading: Puri BK, Treasaden I, eds (2010). *Psychiatry: An evidence-based text*, **p. 419.**

57. B

Further reading: Puri BK, Treasaden I, eds (2010). *Psychiatry: An evidence-based text*, **pp. 1103–4.**

58. B

Reference: Almeida OP, Howard RJ, Levy R, David AS (1995). Psychotic states arising in late life (late paraphrenia). *British Journal of Psychiatry.* **166:** 215–28.

59. E

Reference: Taylor D, Paton C, Kapur S (2009). *The Maudsley Prescribing Guidelines*, 10th edn. London: Informa Healthcare.

60. E

Further reading: Puri BK, Treasaden I, eds (2010). *Psychiatry: An evidence-based text*, **pp. 571–3, 1101.**

61. E

Further reading: Puri BK, Treasaden I, eds (2010). *Psychiatry: An evidence-based text*, **pp. 95, 438, 463, 1107.**

62. B

Reference: Petersen RC, Doody R, Kurz A *et al.* (2001). Current concepts in mild cognitive impairment. *Achieves of Neurology* **58:** 1985–92.

Further reading: Puri BK, Treasaden I, eds (2010). *Psychiatry: An evidence-based text*, **pp. 524, 1103**

63. C

Further reading: Puri BK, Treasaden I, eds (2010). *Psychiatry: An evidence-based text*, **p. 997.**

64. C

Reference: Ho RCM, Chen KY, Broekman B, Mak A (2009). Buprenorphine prescription, misuse and service provision: a global perspective. *Advances in Psychiatric Treatment* **15:** 354–63.

Further reading: Puri BK, Treasaden I, eds (2010). *Psychiatry: An evidence-based text*, **pp. 717, 1037, 1039–40.**

65. E

Progranulin is a growth factor protein and its genetic locus deletion is associated with frontotemporal dementia.

Reference: Gijselinck I, van der Zee J, Engelborghs S (2008). Progranulin locus deletion in frontotemporal dementia. *Human Mutation* **29:** 53–8.

Further reading: Puri BK, Treasaden I, eds (2010). *Psychiatry: An evidence-based text*, **pp. 507, 1107.**

66. D

Myoclonus is not part of the aura associated with complex partial seizure.

67. B

Option A refers to selection bias, option C refers to measurement bias, option D refers to recall bias, and option E refers to Neyman bias.

Further reading: Puri BK, Treasaden I, eds (2010). *Psychiatry: An evidence-based text*, **pp. 43, 72, 74, 75, 86.**

68. A

Further reading: Puri BK, Treasaden I, eds (2010). *Psychiatry: An evidence-based text*, p. 912.

69. B

This lady suffers from hypertensive crisis owing to consumption of food containing high levels of tyramine.

Further reading: Puri BK, Treasaden I, eds (2010). *Psychiatry: An evidence-based text*, pp. 425, 426, 708, 907.

70. E

This child suffers from fragile X syndrome.

Further reading: Puri BK, Treasaden I, eds (2010). *Psychiatry: An evidence-based text*, pp. 1082, 1088, 1091.

71. E

Reference: Duara R, Loewenstein DA, Potter E *et al.* (2008). Medial temporal lobe atrophy on MRI scans and the diagnosis of Alzheimer disease. *Neurology* **71**: 1986–92.

Further reading: Puri BK, Treasaden I, eds (2010). *Psychiatry: An evidence-based text*, pp. 1103–4.

72. E

Option D refers to tacrine and option A refers to donepezil and galantamine.

Further reading: Puri BK, Treasaden I, eds (2010). *Psychiatry: An evidence-based text*, pp. 906, 1104, 1106.

73. B

Reference: http://www.mentalhealth.org.uk/information/mental-health-overview/statistics/#children

74. A

Options B to E are risk factors for early-onset (ages 6–11 years) delinquent behaviour.

Reference: Office of the Surgeon General (2001). *Youth Violence: A Report of the Surgeon General*. Washington, DC: US Department of Health and Human Services, Office of the Secretary, Office of Public Health and Science, Office of the Surgeon General. Retrieved from: www.surgeongeneral.gov/library/youthviolence

Further reading: Puri BK, Treasaden I, eds (2010). *Psychiatry: An evidence-based text*, pp. 1156–7.

75. B

Further reading: Puri BK, Treasaden I, eds (2010). *Psychiatry: An evidence-based text*, pp. 698, 708, 724, 762.

76. E

Both naloxone and naltrexone are opioid antagonists. Naltrexone has a longer half-life (4 hours) than naloxone (< 1 hour).

Further reading: Puri BK, Treasaden I, eds (2010). *Psychiatry: An evidence-based text*, p. 913.

77. B

This person suffers from Präder–Willi syndrome. Option A refers to Angelman syndrome.

Further reading: Puri BK, Treasaden I, eds (2010). *Psychiatry: An evidence-based text*, pp. 471, 1086, 1091.

78. C

Here, the Royal College of Psychiatrists is trying to measure the split-half reliability of the MRCPsych Paper 2 used in spring 2008. Option A refers to intra-rater reliability, option B refers to inter-rater reliability and option D refers to test–retest reliability.

79. E

The parental risk factors should be low social class but not high social class. Parental factors associated with an increased risk of suicide in young people include suicide or early death, admission to hospital for a mental illness, unemployment, low income, poor schooling, divorce, as well as mental illness in siblings and mental illness and short duration of schooling in the young people themselves. The strongest risk factor is mental illness in the young people.

Reference: Agerbo E, Nordentoft M, Mortensen PB (2002). Familial, psychiatric, and socioeconomic risk factors for suicide in young people: nested case-control study. *British Medical Journal* **325**: 74.

Further reading: Puri BK, Treasaden I, eds (2010). *Psychiatry: An evidence-based text*, pp. 855–6.

80. B

This man suffers from variant Creutzfeldt–Jakob disease (vCJD) where immunohistochemistry for prion protein often shows strong staining of plaques in the occipital cortex. In contrast, conventional CJD and kuru-type plaques are commonly found in the cerebellar cortex.

Reference: Sánchez-Juan P, Houben J, Hoff I, Jansen C *et al.* (2007). The first case of variant Creutzfeldt-Jakob disease in the Netherlands. *Journal of Neurology* **254**: 958–60.

Further reading: Puri BK, Treasaden I, eds (2010). *Psychiatry: An evidence-based text*, pp. 572–3.

81. A

Cost–benefit analysis measures costs and benefits in monetary terms.

Further reading: Puri BK, Treasaden I, eds (2010). *Psychiatry: An evidence-based text*, p. 41.

82. B

Reference: Jacobson CM, Gould M (2007). The epidemiology and phenomenology of non-suicidal self-injurious behaviour among adolescents: a critical review of the literature. *Archive of Suicide Research* **11**: 129–47.

83. B

Only lithium and sulpiride are 95 per cent excreted unchanged in urine. The percentages for the other options are as follows: mirtazapine (75 per cent), olanzapine (57 per cent), amisulpride (50 per cent) and lamotrigine (<10 per cent).

Reference: Taylor D, Paton C, Kapur S (2009). *The Maudsley Prescribing Guidelines*, 10th edn. London: Informa Healthcare.

84. B

The risk for the general population is 5 per cent.

Reference: Liddel MB (2001). Genetic risk of Alzheimer's disease: advising relatives. *British Journal of Psychiatry* **178**: 7–11.

Further reading: Puri BK, Treasaden I, eds (2010). *Psychiatry: An evidence-based text*, pp. 1103–4.

85. A

86. A

The task described here is known as the 'n-back' task which is a continuous performance task that assesses working memory. Lesions in dorsolateral prefrontal cortex cause negative symptoms and working memory impairment in people with schizophrenia.

Reference: Tan HY, Choo WC, Fones CS, Chee MW (2005). fMRI study of maintenance and manipulation processes within working memory in first-episode schizophrenia. *American Journal of Psychiatry* **162**: 1849–58.

Further reading: Puri BK, Treasaden I, eds (2010). *Psychiatry: An evidence-based text*, pp. 332–3, 340.

87. D

This motorcyclist has lost his procedural memory. Procedural memory is formed by the cerebellum, basal ganglia and motor cortex. The dorsal striatum is part of the basal ganglia and damage in this area would affect procedural memory. Procedural memory is not affected by damage to the amygdala, dentate gyrus, entorhinal cortex or hippocampus.

Further reading: Puri BK, Treasaden I, eds (2010). *Psychiatry: An evidence-based text*, pp. 335, 339–41, 352, 509, 803.

88. C

Multiple cases of toxicity when combining lithium and verapamil, particularly neurotoxicity, have been reported.

References: Singh GP, Sidana A, Sharma RP (2004). Renewed interest in calcium channel blockers as antimania agents in the third millennium. *Hong Kong Journal of Psychiatry* **14**: 12–15; Freeman MP, Stoll AL (1998). Mood stabilizer combinations: A review of safety and efficacy. *American Journal of Psychiatry* **155**: 12–21.

89. C

Further reading: Puri BK, Treasaden I, eds (2010). *Psychiatry: An evidence-based text*, p. 516.

90. D

91. B

Further reading: Puri BK, Treasaden I, eds (2010). *Psychiatry: An evidence-based text*, pp. 557–9.

92. C

Further reading: Puri BK, Treasaden I, eds (2010). *Psychiatry: An evidence-based text*, p. 468.

93. B

Acamprosate is a GABA agonist and glutamate antagonist.

Further reading: Puri BK, Treasaden I, eds (2010). *Psychiatry: An evidence-based text*, p. 913.

94. A

Reference: Huang X, Saint-Jeannet JP (2004). Induction of the neural crest and the opportunities of life on the edge. *Developmental Biology* **275**: 1–11.

95. C

Further reading: Puri BK, Treasaden I, eds (2010). *Psychiatry: An evidence-based text*, p. 1040.

96. D

Cognitive framing is a concept used in psychology and social science. Cognitive frames are formed based on our life experiences. Drug A is associated with the word 'cure' and evokes a positive frame in which it offers hope of cure although it benefits only around 40 per cent of patients. Drug B is associated with the word 'failure' and evokes a negative frame. The choices made by patients in this survey were influenced by the positive and negative frames.

97. E

Further reading: Puri BK, Treasaden I, eds (2010). *Psychiatry: An evidence-based text*, pp. 425–7, 603.

98. A

Reference: Schalekamp T (2008). Increased bleeding risk with concurrent use of selective serotonin reuptake inhibitors and coumarins. *Archives of Internal Medicine* **168**: 180–5.

Further reading: Puri BK, Treasaden I, eds (2010). *Psychiatry: An evidence-based text*, p. 540.

99. E

The cognitive representation of a disease is the belief that patients have in relation to their illness at a given time. Cognitive representation is determined by five factors: aetiology, symptoms, impact of the disease on patients' lives, measures for controlling the disease and progress of the disease.

100. B

Neutropenia is not dose-related.

Further reading: Puri BK, Treasaden I, eds (2010). *Psychiatry: An evidence-based text*, pp. 425–427, 603.

ANSWERS – EXTENDED MATCHING ITEMS

101. I

102. J

103. H

104. D

105. E

106. C

Further reading (for Q. 101–106): Puri BK, Treasaden I, eds (2010). *Psychiatry: An evidence-based text*, **pp. 466, 467.**

107. C

Further reading: Puri BK, Treasaden I, eds (2010). *Psychiatry: An evidence-based text*, **p. 469.**

108. E

Further reading: Puri BK, Treasaden I, eds (2010). *Psychiatry: An evidence-based text*, **p. 469.**

109. A

Further reading: Puri BK, Treasaden I, eds (2010). *Psychiatry: An evidence-based text*, **p. 469.**

110. D

Further reading: Puri BK, Treasaden I, eds (2010). *Psychiatry: An evidence-based text*, **p. 474.**

111. B

Further reading: Puri BK, Treasaden I, eds (2010). *Psychiatry: An evidence-based text*, **pp. 41, 77, 78, 470.**

112. I

This is a case of Angleman's syndrome with deletion of maternal chromosome 15.

Further reading: Puri BK, Treasaden I, eds (2010). *Psychiatry: An evidence-based text*, **p. 471.**

113. K

This is a case of DiGeorge syndrome or velocardiofacial syndrome.

114. C

This is a case of cri-du-chat syndrome.

115. F

116. G

117. C

118. E

119. A

120. D

121. B

Reference (for Q. 115–121): Morgan H (1993). Clinical neurophysiology. In: Morgan G, Butler S, eds. *Seminar in Basic Sciences*. London: Gaskell.
Further reading: Puri BK, Treasaden I, eds (2010). *Psychiatry: An evidence-based text*, **pp. 400–9, 563.**

122. A

123. C

Further reading: Puri BK, Treasaden I, eds (2010). *Psychiatry: An evidence-based text*, **pp. 571–3, 1101.**

124. B

Further reading: Puri BK, Treasaden I, eds (2010). *Psychiatry: An evidence-based text*, **pp. 95, 404, 568.**

125. D

Reference (for Q. 122–125): Morgan H (1993). Clinical neurophysiology. In: Morgan G, Butler S, eds. *Seminar in Basic Sciences*. London: Gaskell.
Further reading: Puri BK, Treasaden I, eds (2010). *Psychiatry: An evidence-based text*, **pp. 404, 569–70.**

126. D

127. I

128. D, J

129. A, B

130. J

Reference: The Office for National Statistics (2001). *Psychiatric Morbidity Report*. London: ONS.

131. C

Further reading: Puri BK, Treasaden I, eds (2010). *Psychiatry: An evidence-based text*, pp. 439–40, 558.

132. B

133. A

Further reading: Puri BK, Treasaden I, eds (2010). *Psychiatry: An evidence-based text*, p. 520.

134. D

Reference (for Q. 131–134): Morgan H (1993). Clinical neurophysiology. In: Morgan G, Butler S, eds. *Seminar in Basic Sciences*. London: Gaskell.
Further reading: Puri BK, Treasaden I, eds (2010). *Psychiatry: An evidence-based text*, p. 519; Morgan H (1993). Clinical neurophysiology. In: Morgan G, Butler S, eds. *Seminar in Basic Sciences*. London: Gaskell.

135. B

Further reading: Puri BK, Treasaden I, eds (2010). *Psychiatry: An evidence-based text*, p. 403; Morgan H (1993). Clinical neurophysiology. In: Morgan G, Butler S, eds. *Seminar in Basic Sciences*. London: Gaskell.

136. D

137. C

Further reading: Puri BK, Treasaden I, eds (2010). *Psychiatry: An evidence-based text*, p. 403; Morgan H (1993). Clinical neurophysiology. In: Morgan G, Butler S, eds. *Seminar in Basic Sciences*. London: Gaskell.

138. E

Further reading: Puri BK, Treasaden I, eds (2010). *Psychiatry: An evidence-based text*, p. 523; Morgan H (1993). Clinical neurophysiology. In: Morgan G, Butler S, eds. *Seminar in Basic Sciences*. London: Gaskell.

139. A

Reference (for Q. 135–139): Morgan H (1993). Clinical neurophysiology. In: Morgan G, Butler S, eds. *Seminar in Basic Sciences*. London: Gaskell.

140. A

141. D

142. B

143. C

144. E

Reference (for Q. 140–144): Morgan H (1993). Clinical neurophysiology. In: Morgan G, Butler S, eds. *Seminar in Basic Sciences*. London: Gaskell.

145. J, M – hoarding and saving compulsions

146. G, J – checking and hoarding compulsions

147. B – contamination obsession (45 per cent)

148. G – checking compulsion (63 per cent)

References (for Q. 145–148): Rufer M, Fricke S, Moritz S, Kloss M, Hand I (2006). Symptom dimensions in obsessive-compulsive disorder: prediction of cognitive-behavior therapy outcome. *Acta Psychiatrica Scandinavia* **113**: 440–6; Mataix-Cols D, Wooderson S, Lawerence N, Brammer MJ, Speckens A, Phillips ML (2004). Distinct neural correlates of washing, checking and hoarding symptom dimensions in obsessive compulsive disorder. *Archives of General Psychiatry* **61**: 564–76; Saxena S, Maidment KM, Vapnik T *et al.* (2002). Obsessive-compulsive hoarding: symptom severity and response to multimodal treatment. *Journal of Clinical Psychiatry* **63**: 21 – 27.

149. B

Acting out is enacting an unconscious wish or fantasy impulsively as a way of avoiding painful affect.

Further reading: Puri BK, Treasaden I, eds (2010). *Psychiatry: An evidence-based text*, pp. 940, 948–9.

150. U

Undoing is an attempt to negate sexual, aggressive or shameful implications from a previous comment or behaviour by elaborating, clarifying, or doing the opposite.

151. N

Rationalization refers to the justification of unacceptable attitudes, beliefs, or behaviours and making them tolerable to oneself.

152. G, R

Idealization refers to the attribution of perfect or near-perfect qualities to others as a way of avoiding anxiety or negative feelings. Splitting is compartmentalizing experiences of self and others such that integration is not possible.

153. B, D, G, L, M, Q, R

Melanie Klein described projection and splitting but not denial.

154. Q

Regression refers to an earlier phase of functioning to avoid the conflicts and tensions associated with current situation.

155. M

Projective identification has two phases: (i) the client first projected an internal object (i.e. uncaring parents in this case) to the consultant; (ii) then pressure is placed on the consultant to take on characteristics of the uncaring parents.

Further reading: Puri BK, Treasaden I, eds (2010). *Psychiatry: An evidence-based text,* pp. 949–50, 979.

156. K

Isolation of affect refers to the separation of an idea from its associated affect to avoid emotional turmoil.

157. T

Suppression refers to conscious effort not to attend to the certain state, feeling or impulse. On the other hand, repression refers to blockage or expulsion of unacceptable ideas or impulses in the inner states from entering the consciousness.

158. I

Intellectualization refers to the excessive use of abstract ideation to avoid difficult feelings.

159. E, H, I, J, K, N, O, P, U

160. S

161. H

Identification refers to internalization of the qualities of another person by behaving like that person.

162. J

Introjection means internalizing aspects of a significant person as a way of dealing with the loss of that person.

163. O

Reaction formation refers to the transformation of an unacceptable wish or impulse into its opposite.

164. D

165. C, E

166. A

167. A

168. C, B

169. E, F

Further reading (for Q. 164–169) : Puri BK, Treasaden I, eds (2010). *Psychiatry: An evidence-based text,* pp. 947–54.

170. C

171. D

172. D

173. B

174. A

Further reading (for Q. 170–174): Puri BK, Treasaden I, eds (2010). *Psychiatry: An evidence-based text,* pp. 955–66, 978.

175. A

Anxiety disorders are uncommon among people with Down syndrome. The prevalence is around 0.3 per cent.

176. D

177. D

Dementia is the one of most common psychiatric co-morbidities with a prevalence of 6–10 per cent.

178. C

179. B

180. C

References (for Q.175–180): Collacott RA (1992). The effect of age and residential placement on adaptive behaviour of adults with Down's syndrome. *Br J Psychiatry* **161**: 675–9; Myers BA, Pueschel SM (1991). Psychiatric disorders in a population with Down syndrome. *Journal of Nervous and Mental Disease* **179**: 609–13.

Further reading: Puri BK, Treasaden I, eds (2010). *Psychiatry: An evidence-based text*, pp. 467, 1082, 1087–8.

181. B

182. C

183. A

Further reading (for Q. 181–183): Puri BK, Treasaden I, eds (2010). *Psychiatry: An evidence-based text*, pp. 593–609.

184. B

Further reading: Puri BK, Treasaden I, eds (2010). *Psychiatry: An evidence-based text*, pp. 468–9.

185. C

Further reading: Puri BK, Treasaden I, eds (2010). *Psychiatry: An evidence-based text*, p. 470.

186. A

187. D

Reference (for Q. 184–187): Young ID (2005). *Medical Genetics*. Oxford: Oxford University Press.

188. E, F, R

QRS complex = 200 ms, QTc = 500 ms, heart rate = 120/minute. This patient suffers from tricyclic antidepressant overdose.

Reference: Olgun H, Yildirim ZK, Karacan M, Ceviz N (2009). Clinical, electrocardiographic, and laboratory findings in children with amitriptyline intoxication. *Pediatric Emergency Care* **25**: 170–3.

189. M, O, R

ST segment elevation with saddle, heart rate = 120/minute, diffuse T wave inversion. This man suffers from clozapine-induced myocarditis.

Reference: Feldman AM, McNamara D (2000). Myocarditis. *New England Journal of Medicine* **343**: 1388–98.

190. K, P, Q, R

ST segment elevation, tall T waves, Q wave, heart rate = 120/minute. This man suffers from acute myocardial infarction caused by thyroxine treatment.

191. B, I, R

Biphasic P waves, heart rate = 120/minute, R wave in V6 = 30 mm, Q wave. This patient suffers from amphetamine-induced left ventricular hypertrophy.

Reference: Crean AM, Pohl JEF (2004). Ally McBeal heart? – Drug induced cardiomyopathy in a young woman. *British Journal of Clinical Pharmacology* **58**: 558–9.

192. D and S

PR interval = 300 ms, heart rate = 30/minute. This patient suffers from acetylcholinesterase inhibitor-induced sinus bradycardia and first-degree AV block

Reference: Rowland JP, Rigby J, Harper AC, Rowlan R (2007). Cardiovascular monitoring with acetylcholinesterase inhibitors: a clinical protocol. *Advances in Psychiatric Treatment* **13**: 178–84.

193. D – Huntington's disease

194. G – progressive supranuclear palsy

195. I – variant Creutzfeldt–Jakob disease

The hockey-stick sign refers to bilateral symmetrical regions of hyperintensity in the pulvinar and the dorsomedial nuclei of the thalami.

Reference: Sánchez-Juan P, Houben J, Hoff I, Jansen C *et al.* (2007). The first case of variant Creutzfeldt–Jakob disease in the Netherlands. *Journal of Neurology* **254**: 958–60.

196. J – Wernicke's encephalopathy

197. C – chronic depression

198. I – variant Creutzfeldt–Jakob disease

199. A

200. E

MRCPsych Paper 3

Mock examination
Time limit: 180 minutes
Number of questions: 200

MULTIPLE CHOICE QUESTIONS (MCQS)

1. A 10-year-old child presents with bedwetting at night. Which of the following features is <u>not</u> associated with nocturnal enuresis?
   A. Tall stature
   B. Family history of enuresis
   C. Minor neurological abnormalities
   D. Tends to recur if there is an abrupt withdrawal of imipramine
   E. Male gender.

2. Which of the following is the least common feature of Cushing's syndrome of endogenous origin?
   A. Cognitive impairment
   B. Delusion of guilt
   C. Depression
   D. Mania
   E. Second-person auditory hallucination.

3. A person dependent on opiates does not respond to oral methadone treatment. He has heard from his friends that a recent trial was conducted in the UK and showed some promising data on injectable opioid maintenance therapy. He wants to know which of the following injectable opioids shows the highest retention rate:
   A. Injectable buprenorphine
   B. Injectable methadone
   C. Injectable heroin
   D. Injectable lofexidine
   E. Injectable naltrexone.

4. Which of the following randomization methods is the least likely to produce bias in a randomized controlled trial?
   A. Allocation by order of arrival time in the clinic (before 11.00 am to antipsychotic A and after 11.00 am to antipsychotic B).
   B. Allocation of patients by month of birth. (Patients born in odd-numbered months receive antipsychotic A and those born in even-numbered months receive antipsychotic B.)
   C. Allocation by gender. (Patients are subdivided into strata and individuals within each stratum undergo further randomization to antipsychotic A and antipsychotic B.)
   D. Allocation by status of patients. (In-patients to antipsychotic A and out-patients to antipsychotic B.)
   E. Allocation by laboratory results. (Patients with metabolic syndrome to antipsychotic A and patients without metabolic syndrome to antipsychotic B.)

5. Which of the following conditions is most frequently seen with autism?
   A. Enuresis
   B. Gilles de la Tourette's syndrome
   C. Hyperkinetic disorder
   D. Pica
   E. MMR vaccination.

6. An 18-year-old lady complains of low mood, irritability and insomnia prior to her menses. Which of the following medication would you recommend?
   A. Sertraline
   B. Sex hormone such as progesterone
   C. St John's wort
   D. Low-dose sulpiride
   E. Sleeping pills.

7. The mother of a 14-year-old boy with ADHD wants to ask you about the side effects of methylphenidate medication. Which of the following statements is incorrect?
   A. Methylphenidate almost always delays physical growth.
   B. A drug holiday is required to facilitate growth.
   C. Methylphenidate suppresses appetite.
   D. Methylphenidate combined with clonidine is better than placebo in controlling tics and ADHD symptoms.

E. Dependence is common in patients who continue methylphenidate long term.

8. A 12-year-old girl was sexually assaulted by a gang of classmates 2 months ago. She developed flashbacks, nightmares, hypervigilance and school avoidance. Which of the following antidepressants has the best evidence to support its use as treatment in her case?
   A. Citalopram
   B. Clomipramine
   C. Mirtazapine
   D. Paroxetine
   E. Sertraline.

9. Which of the following statements regarding the standard error of the mean (SEM) is false?
   A. It measures the variability of the sample statistic (mean or proportion) in relation to the true but unknown population characteristic.
   B. It is a measure of the variability of the observations.
   C. It is used in constructing confidence intervals for a mean or proportion.
   D. As the sample size (n) increases, the SEM decreases.
   E. As the standard deviation increases, the SEM increases.

10. A 50-year-old man with a history of alcohol misuse presents with tremors and anxiety. He admits to drinking a lot of alcohol 1 day ago. Which is the most likely metabolic abnormality?
    A. Hypoglycaemia
    B. Hyperglycaemia
    C. Hypokalaemia
    D. Hyperkalaemia
    E. Hyponatraemia.

11. Which of the following is false?
    A. Routine investigations for hypoparathyroidism include U&Es, liver function tests, serum calcium and phosphate.
    B. In patients with suspected hypoparathyroidism, $25(OH)D_3$ is a reliable indicator of total body stores of vitamin D.
    C. Chronic hypocalcaemia causes alopecia, cataracts and papilloedema.
    D. Treatment of hypoparathyroidism involves a combination of alfacalcidol and calcitriol.
    E. The MEN 1 syndrome involves parathyroid tumour, pituitary adenoma and phaeochromocytoma.

12. A 13-year-old boy has dropped out of secondary school. He is odd and is not accepted by his classmates. Your consultant recommends ruling out Asperger's syndrome. Which of the following features would not support such a diagnosis?
    A. Restricted and repetitive behaviours
    B. Marked clumsiness
    C. Socially withdrawn
    D. Worries about the welfare of his classmates
    E. Language delay.

13. A 55-year-old woman is concerned about developing dementia and consults you on supplementation that she can use to prevent dementia. Which of the following medications or supplements would you recommend?
    A. NSAIDs
    B. Vitamin E
    C. Statin
    D. Hormone replacement therapy
    E. Do not recommend any of the above.

14. When assessing a patient with features of dementia, which of the following would suggest subcortical dementia rather than cortical dementia?
    A. Preservation of calculation
    B. Absence of neurological signs
    C. Reduced awareness of oneself
    D. Euthymic mood
    E. Absence of dysarthria.

15. A 55-year-old shopkeeper presented to the Accident & Emergency department with memory loss. You are the psychiatric specialist trainee on call tonight. Which of the following features do not suggest transient global amnesia?
    A. He cannot remember the events which occurred in the afternoon.
    B. He cannot recall the name of his shop.
    C. He is disorientated in time and place.
    D. He demonstrates anterograde amnesia after admission to the ward.
    E. He demonstrates retrograde amnesia for variable durations.

16. Which of the following statements regarding reading disorder is incorrect?
    A. The prevalence of dyslexia in the UK is 5 per cent.
    B. The prevalence of genuine dyslexia and mild dyslexia is 10 per cent.
    C. In the US, 17–20 per cent of elementary school children are estimated to suffer from reading disabilities.
    D. In the US, 17–20 per cent of the population display a reading disability.
    E. A survey conducted across Japan, Taiwan and the US concluded that using more than one criterion, the percentage of children who were reading-disabled was 8 per cent in Japan, 8 per cent in Taiwan and 7 per cent in the USA.

17. Antidepressant A was found to be more likely to reduce the Hamilton Depression Scale score by 50 per cent from baseline in 6 months when compared with a placebo [n = 3000 depressed patients, 10 centres, relative risk (RR) for remaining depressed = 0.30, CI = 0.2–0.6; absolute risk difference (ARR) = 0.42, CI = 0.2–0.6]. What is the 95 per cent confidence interval for the number needed to treat (NNT) with antidepressant A to prevent one additional patient from remaining depressed?
    A. 1.37–4.7
    B. 1.47–4.8

C. 1.5–4.9
D. 1.67–5
E. 1.7–5.1

18. A core trainee consults you about a 50-year-old man with chronic liver disease who has developed alcohol withdrawal. Which of the following sedative medications is the most appropriate?
   A. Chlordiazepoxide
   B. Diazepam
   C. Flurazepam
   D. Lorazepam
   E. Oxazepam.

19. Which of the following offences is the most common first presentation of conduct disorder?
   A. Fire-setting
   B. Shoplifting
   C. Robbery
   D. Assaulting someone
   E. Molesting someone.

20. A 20-year-old man suffering from schizophrenia was admitted beacause of worsening of psychotic symptoms. The urine cannabis screen is negative (level of cannabinoids < 20 ng/mL) despite the fact that his partner confirms that he is a heavy user of cannabis. The core trainee wants to consult you on the underlying reason. All the following are possible reasons, except:
   A. The urine screen was done on the fourth day after admission and the active ingredient of cannabis was not detectable.
   B. The person adulterated his urine sample with vinegar.
   C. The person drank a lot of water and alcohol prior to the urine test.
   D. The person took 10 tablets of aspirin 12 hours before the urine test.
   E. The person took a lot of vitamin B prior to the test and then diluted his urine with water.

21. Henry is a 40-year-old office worker who has been dependent on alcohol for 20 years. He wants to find out from you the risk of his 14-year-old son developing alcohol dependence when he becomes an adult compared with adolescents whose fathers do not drink. What would you tell Henry?
   A. Two times
   B. Three times
   C. Four times
   D. Five times
   E. Six times.

22. In HIV clinics, what percentage of patients have neurocognitive impairment?
   A. < 5 per cent
   B. 5–15 per cent
   C. 15–30 per cent
   D. 30–50 per cent
   E. > 50 per cent.

23. A 25-year-old patient was diagnosed with schizophrenia and Gilles de la Tourette's syndrome. The consultant would like to clarify the diagnosis further. He asks which of the following features is the most suggestive of the diagnosis of Gilles de la Tourette's syndrome:
   A. Frequent hand-washing
   B. Age of onset is 19 years
   C. Repeated purposeless movements
   D. Not responding to clozapine
   E. Shouting at the voices.

24. With regards to enuresis and encopresis, which of the following statements is incorrect?
   A. 70 per cent of enuresis is caused by organic causes.
   B. Regressive encopresis is associated with a good prognosis.
   C. Encopresis is associated with aggression and a short attention span.
   D. Diurnal enuresis is more common in females.
   E. If a child presents with both enuresis and encopresis, enuresis should be treated first.

25. All of the following may increase the power of a study, except:
   A. High potency of a medication
   B. High compliance rate with treatment
   C. Comparison of active treatment with placebo
   D. Use of observer-rated questionnaires rather than self-reported questionnaires
   E. Focus more on the number of collaborating centres rather then the number of subjects.

26. A medical student is revising a syndrome related to learning disability. She would like to find out from you which of the following is inherited in an autosomal dominant fashion:
   A. DiGeorge syndrome
   B. Hunter's syndrome
   C. Hurler's syndrome
   D. Phenylketonuria
   E. Mucopolysaccharidosis III.

27. Henry is a 40-year-old unemployed man who has been dependent on alcohol for 20 years. He wants to find out from you the risk to his 14-year-old son of developing alcohol dependence compared with those adolescents whose biological fathers do not drink. His son has been adopted away to a family who do not drink. What would you tell Henry?
   A. Two times
   B. Three times
   C. Four times
   D. Five times
   E. Six times.

28. A 22-year-old woman develops her first episode of anorexia nervosa. Her mother is very concerned and gathers some information on the outcome of her illness. Which of the following statements is correct?
   A. This patient has good prognosis as she has a relatively late onset.

B. The most common switch in pattern is from anorexia nervosa to bulimia nervosa.

C. The most common switch in pattern is from bulimia nervosa to anorexia nervosa.

D. The outpatient treatment should be of 3 months' duration for those patients without hospitalization.

E. 30 per cent will have a duration of illness longer than 12 years.

29. Which of the following regarding the water deprivation test is false?

A. In normal subjects, urine osmolality rises as urine volume falls.

B. In patients with cranial diabetes insipidus, urine osmolality fails to rise and a relative diuresis continues despite the increasing plasma osmolality.

C. In patients with nephrogenic diabetes insipidus, the urine concentrates normally in response to desmopressin.

D. With primary polydipsia, excessive fluid intake prior to the test may result in an apparent continued diuresis despite fluid restriction.

E. With primary polydipsia, plasma osmolality remains below 295 mosmol/kg after fluid restriction.

30. An elderly woman suffers from somatoform pain disorder and her son wants to find out from you whether this condition is common in the community. What is the one-year prevalence of this condition?

A. 8 per cent

B. 18 per cent

C. 28 per cent

D. 38 per cent

E. 48 per cent.

31. A 5-year-old boy presents with autism. Which of the following is false?

A. Attachments tend to be rigid.

B. There is a tendency to echolalia and pronoun reversal.

C. Stimulants can relieve the stereotyped behaviours.

D. IQ is the most important prognostic factor.

E. He may suffer from fragile X syndrome or tuberous sclerosis.

32. A 20-year-old female university student suffers from bulimia nervosa. She finds medication ineffective and requests psychotherapy. Choose the most appropriate psychotherapy for her:

A. Psychodynamic psychotherapy

B. Interpersonal psychotherapy

C. Cognitive analytical therapy

D. Mentalization-based therapy

E. Dialectical behavioural therapy.

33. A 58-year-old woman presents with dementia and peripheral neuropathy. Which of the following cancers is most likely?

A. Brain tumour

B. Colon cancer

C. Hepatic tumour

D. Renal cell carcinoma

E. Pancoast's tumour.

34. Which of the following statements regarding melatonin is incorrect?

A. If an adolescent takes melatonin and the oral contraceptive pill concurrently, melatonin has less propensity to cause drug interactions.

B. A prolonged-release formulation of melatonin is licensed for the short-term treatment of insomnia in children in the UK.

C. Meta-analyses of small RCTs comparing melatonin with placebo in children with insomnia show consistent improvement in sleep, with earlier sleep onset and increased total sleep duration.

D. Melatonin can worsen asthma and seizure in the short term.

E. The optimal dose of melatonin in the treatment of insomnia in children and adolescents is unknown.

35. A newborn child with Down syndrome is found on genetic testing to have an unbalanced Robertsonian translocation and you are asked to counsel the parents. Which of the following statements is incorrect?

A. Both parents should be offered chromosomal analysis as one may carry the translocation in a balanced form.

B. If the mother is found to be a carrier then the recurrence risk is 50 per cent.

C. Ultrasound monitoring of nasal bone formation will be useful in future antenatal screening for Down syndrome.

D. If the parents are carriers of translocation, they have 46 chromosomes.

E. In translocation, patients with Down syndrome have 46 chromosomes.

36. Which of the following statements is false in respect of the findings of the Multimodal Treatment Study (MTA) on ADHD?

A. There is a small but detectible reduction in overall growth in height for children who remain on stimulants.

B. Loss of growth is maximal in the first year of treatment.

C. 35 per cent showed a moderate and gradual improvement and 50 per cent showed significant improvement over the 3-year study period.

D. 15 per cent initially responded well but deteriorated over 3 years.

E. Drug treatment was associated with a reduction in the rate of delinquency and substance abuse in children with ADHD compared with the rate found in normal controls.

37. Which of the following statements is true about measures of central tendency?
    A. The mean is a good measure of central tendency in a sample of skewed distribution.
    B. The mode is greater than the median in a positively skewed distribution.
    C. The median is greater than the mean in a positively skewed distribution.
    D. The mean is less than the median in a negatively skewed distribution.
    E. The median is greater than the mode in a negatively skewed distribution.

38. The male to female ratio in hypothyroidism is:
    A. 1:2
    B. 1:8
    C. 1:16
    D. 1:32
    E. 1:64.

39. Which of the following statements is false about meta-analysis?
    A. Meta-analysis offers greater precision as a result of larger sample size.
    B. 'Publication bias' may skew results of meta-analyses because of the tendency to publish studies with positive results.
    C. Combining results of RCTs and open-label trials in one forest plot is appropriate.
    D. The Cochrane Collaboration produces and disseminates systematic reviews of healthcare interventions, and promotes the search for evidence in the form of clinical trials and other studies of the effects of interventions.
    E. Systemic review of RCTs is level 1A evidence.

40. Which of the following complications is most likely in a man who recovered from herpes encephalitis and subsequently developed a very good appetite, weight gain and high sexual drive?
    A. Churg–Strauss syndrome
    B. Devic's syndrome
    C. Klüver–Bucy syndrome
    D. Hallervorden–Spatz disease
    E. Tolosa–Hunt syndrome.

41. Which of the following statements is false?
    A. Hypomagnesaemia is associated with hyperparathyroidism.
    B. After treatment of hyperthyroidism, psychiatric symptoms usually resolve.
    C. Hypothyroidism causes hirsutism.
    D. One-third of patients with hyperthyroidism meet the criteria for major depressive disorder.
    E. Delusions and hallucinations are equally common in hypothyroidism.

42. Which of the following is true about exhibitionism?
    A. Exhibitionism is commonly associated with homosexual behaviour.
    B. Exhibitionism is commonly associated with exposure of the genitalia to an unsuspecting stranger of the opposite gender.
    C. Exhibitionism is commonly associated with sexual assault.
    D. Exhibitionism is commonly associated with voyeurism.
    E. Exhibitionism is commonly associated with young men.

43. You are a specialist trainee in forensic psychiatry and are asked to write a court report for a man convicted of a sexual offence. Which of the following is the strongest predictor of sexual recidivism?
    A. Alcohol and opioid misuse
    B. Diagnosis of bipolar disorder
    C. Low remorse and victim blaming
    D. Being a victim of sexual abuse
    E. Young age of first sexual offence conviction.

44. Select the statement that is most likely to be true. Progressive supranuclear palsy is associated with:
    A. Autoimmune disorder
    B. Abnormal vestibulo-ocular reflexes
    C. Bedridden patients in the later stages, owing to rigidity
    D. Fluent speech
    E. Difficulty moving the eyes, particularly horizontally.

45. Which of the following regarding hyperparathyroidism is false?
    A. It leads to an increase in serum magnesium.
    B. Affective disturbance and personality change occur when the serum calcium is 3–4 mmol/L.
    C. Delirium, impaired cognition and psychosis occur when the serum calcium is 4–4.75 mmol/L.
    D. Somnolence and coma occur when the serum calcium is higher than 4–4.75 mmol/L.
    E. One-third of patients with hyperparathyroidism have severe psychiatric problems.

46. Parents of a child with Down syndrome request chromosomal analysis as they are worried about the increased chance of having another affected child. Which of the following chromosome abnormalities will lead to an increased chance of having a second child with Down syndrome?
    A. Disomy 21
    B. Mosaicism
    C. Meiotic non-disjunction or trisomy 21
    D. Translocation of chromosome 21
    E. Trisomy 22.

47. A 20-year-old woman suffers from anorexia nervosa and she is 30 weeks pregnant. The obstetrician consults you on the potential problems that might occur during the delivery. The use of which of the following obstetric procedures is known to be increased in pregnant women with anorexia nervosa?
   A. Caesarean section
   B. Episiotomy
   C. Forcep delivery
   D. Induction of labour
   E. Vacuum delivery.

48. A 50-year-old woman with a strong family history of depression has been taking venlafaxine 225 mg daily and mirtazapine 45 mg daily for 6 months. She is admitted because of a severe depressive episode but she refuses electroconvulsive therapy and psychotherapy. She does not have any other medical illness. Which of the following treatment strategies is best recommended?
   A. Augment with mianserin, continue with venlafaxine and mirtazapine.
   B. Augment with mianserin, continue with venlafaxine but stop mirtazapine.
   C. Augment with lithium and continue with venlafaxine and mirtazapine.
   D. Augment with lithium, continue with venlafaxine but stop mirtazapine.
   E. Augment with lamotrigine, continue with venlafaxine and mirtazapine.

49. Which of the following features is associated with Rett syndrome?
   A. Midline hand-wringing or hand-washing stereotypes are seen.
   B. Purposeful hand movements are maintained.
   C. The child develops normally until 36 months.
   D. Microcephaly at birth.
   E. Developmental delays are seen later in the course of the illness.

50. The risk of future antisocial personality disorder in a 14-year-old child with conduct disorder is:
   A 10 per cent
   B. 20 per cent
   C. 30 per cent
   D. 40 per cent
   E. 50 per cent.

51. A 55-year-old man presents with coronary artery disease (CAD). His wife asks you what is the percentage of patients with CAD who develop depression. Your answer is:
   A. 3 per cent
   B. 10 per cent
   C. 20 per cent
   D. 40 per cent
   E. 60 per cent.

52. Which of the following statements regarding the treatment of ADHD is true?
   A. Very low birth weight and perinatal insult are risk factors for ADHD.
   B. The half-life of atomoxetine is 15 hours.
   C. Atomoxetine can be given only as second-line agent under all circumstances.
   D. There is evidence to support the use of second-generation antipsychotics to treat hyperactivity in ADHD.
   E. Hyperactivity and epilepsy are mutually exclusive.

53. A 20-year-old woman suffers from anorexia nervosa and she is 30 weeks pregnant. The neonatologist consults you on the potential complications for her fetus. Which of the following is not known to be found in fetuses born to mothers suffering from anorexia nervosa?
   A. APGAR (Appearance, Pulse, Grimace, Activity, Respiration) score of 2 at 1 minute and 3 at 5 minutes
   B. Small head circumference
   C. Low birth weight
   D. Small for gestational age
   E. Microcephaly at 3 years.

54. A core trainee has informed you that a patient taking quetiapine has developed amenorrhoea with raised prolactin. What of the following actions is correct?
   A. Reassure the patient that it is caused by quetiapine
   B. No further intervention and check the prolactin level in 3 months
   C. Order a CT brain scan
   D. Order an MRI brain scan
   E. Prescribe bromocriptine.

55. A new screening test for dementia has been developed to help GPs. It is found to have a sensitivity of 80 per cent and a likelihood ratio for negative results of 0.5. The prevalence of depression in a community is around 5 per cent. The likelihood ratio for a positive result would be:
   A. 0.3
   B. 1.3
   C. 2.3
   D. 3.3
   E. 4.3.

56. A 65-year-old bus driver suffers from post-CVA cognitive impairment and he is referred for assessment of pre-morbid intelligence. A junior psychologist consults you about which test to use. Which of the following would you recommend?
   A. Hayling and Briston tests
   B. National Adult Reading Test
   C. Luria–Nebraska neuropsychological battery
   D. Mini-mental state examination
   E. Verbal fluency test.

57. The mortality from suicide in Hungtington's disease is increased by:
    A. 5 times
    B. 10 times
    C. 15 times
    D. 25 times
    E. 30 times.

58. A male adolescent suffers from depression as he has difficulty in coping with changes associated with puberty. He wants to know the average duration of puberty in boys. Your answer is:
    A. 1–2 years
    B. 3–4 years
    C. 5–6 years
    D. 7–8 years
    E. 9–10 years.

59. A 40-year-old man presents with memory loss and ataxia. The radiologist gives you a call as he has discovered the pulvinar sign in his MRI scan. This MRI finding is associated with which of the following conditions?
    A. CJD
    B. Kuru
    C. Gerstmann–Straussler–Scheinker syndrome
    D. Familial fatal insomnia
    E. New variant CJD.

60. A 55-year-old lady was admitted to a psychiatric ward after the accidental death of her son which occurred 3 months ago. She complains of low mood, poor sleep, poor appetite and hearing her son's voice. What is the diagnosis?
    A. Bereavement – phase I: shock and protest
    B. Bereavement – phase II: preoccupation
    C. Bereavement – phase III: disorganization
    D. Major depressive disorder
    E. Pathological grief.

61. A 70-year-old man is admitted to a general hospital because of pain when passing urine. Three days later he begins complaining to his relatives that the ward staff are not treating him well and are poisoning his food. He also sees insects crawling on the wall. The likely diagnosis is:
    A. Delirium
    B. Delusional disorder
    C. Late-onset schizophrenia
    D. Lewy body dementia
    E. Psychotic depression.

62. A new screening test for dementia has been developed to help GPs. It is found to have a sensitivity of 80 per cent and a likelihood ratio for negative results of 0.5. The prevalence of depression in a community is around 5 per cent. From the Fagan's nomogram below, calculate the probability of a person having dementia when they test negative on the new screening test by the GP. Choose one answer:
    A. 0.5 per cent
    B. 1 per cent
    C. 2 per cent
    D. 3 per cent
    E. 10 per cent.

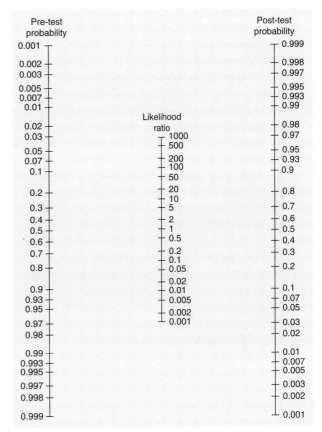

Reproduced from Fagan (1975) with permission from the *New England Journal of Medicine*

63. Which of the following is not usually found in Addison's disease?
    A. Low sodium
    B. Low potassium
    C. High urea
    D. Low glucose
    E. Hypercalcaemia.

64. A 40-year-old woman is arrested multiple times for stealing a baby from a nursery. She admits to the police that she is emotionally deprived owing to her unfulfilled wish to have children. Which of the following psychiatric conditions is most likely to be associated with her offending?
    A. Anxious personality
    B. Borderline personality
    C. Dependent personality
    D. Hysterical personality
    E. Obsessive–compulsive personality.

65. A 5-year-old girl presents with compulsive acts, without any prior or concomitant obsessions. Which of the following conditions is most likely?
    A. Learning disability
    B. Basal ganglia lesion
    C. Autism
    D. ADHD
    E. Rett syndrome.

66. A 15-year-old boy presents with an annular rash (ring-shaped lesion) on the palm. He also presents with low mood. Which of the following is the most likely diagnosis?
    A. Atopic dermatitis
    B. Contact dermatitis
    C. Infectious mononucleosis
    D. Erythema migrans
    E. Secondary syphilis.

67. A 15-year-old boy is referred for assessment of Gilles de la Tourette's syndrome. The following are all common symptoms of Tourette's syndrome, except:
    A. Tremor
    B. Echolalia
    C. Echopraxia
    D. Coprolalia
    E. Coprophagia.

68. A 13-year-old boy presents with bilateral involuntary movements after pharyngeal infection 2 weeks ago. His emotion is labile. What is the most likely diagnosis?
    A. Meningitis
    B. Huntington's chorea
    C. Sydenham's chorea
    D. Myoclonic epilepsy
    E. Tourette's syndrome.

69. Ten depressed patients are given venlafaxine and matched with another 10 patients given amitriptyline. The Hamilton Depression Scale scores of the 20 patients are measured. Which of the following tests is used to compare treatment effect?
    A. Mann–Whitney U-test
    B. Confidence intervals for the mean difference
    C. Paired t-test
    D. Independent sample t-test
    E. McNemar test.

70. Which of the following is a measure of external validity of a randomized controlled trial?
    A. Research design
    B. Research setting
    C. Instruments used
    D. Reliability of study results
    E. Generalizability of study results.

71. A 35-year-old drug dealer is stopped by the police who find a lot of bottles containing urine in his car. He seems to be incoherent and violent. Which of the following illicit substances is he most likely to have consumed?
    A. Amphetamine
    B. Cocaine
    C. Methylenedioxymethamphetamine (MDMA)
    D. Heroin
    E. Ketamine.

72. A 17-year-old male is referred for somnambulism. Which of the following statements is correct?
    A. Somnambulism is more common in young adults than in children.
    B. Somnambulism is a rapid eye movement (REM) sleep phenomenon.
    C. This child will have a higher prevalence of psychiatric abnormality than children who do not sleepwalk.
    D. If the patient commits an offence while sleepwalking, it is classed as a disease of mind in the UK.
    E. It is usually helpful to wake the child up while they are sleepwalking.

73. Which of the following statements about correlation coefficients is false?
    A. Correlation describes the strength of the linear relationship between variables which is denoted by the correlation coefficient (r).
    B. The value of a correlation coefficient can range from -1 to $+1$.
    C. A correlation coefficient can be strong but statistically non-significant because of the sample size.
    D. The range of values 0.2–0.5 signifies moderate correlation.
    E. Spearman's and Kendall's rank correlation coefficients are the non-parametric alternatives to Pearson's correlation coefficient.

74. Which of the following statements regarding Student's *t*-test is false?
    A. The calculated *t*-value = (observed difference in means)/(standard error of the difference in means).
    B. The calculated *t*-value is compared with a critical *t*-value from tables at a predetermined significance level and appropriate degrees of freedom. The larger the value of *t* (positive or negative), the smaller the value of *p* and the stronger the evidence that the null hypothesis is untrue.
    C. The paired *t*-test compares the means of two small paired observations, either on the same individual or on matched individuals.
    D. The independent sample *t*-test is used to compare the effects of two drugs on a particular patient, at different points in time.
    E. The standard deviations must be approximately the same in the two groups.

75. You see a 14-year-old boy with Tourette's syndrome, who also has hyperkinetic disorder. The most effective treatment for this boy would be:
    A. Tricyclic antidepressant medication
    B. Risperidone
    C. Pemoline
    D. Methylphenidate
    E. Atomoxetine.

76. Which of the following percentages with regard to ADHD is incorrect?
    A. The heritability is 90 per cent
    B. 80 per cent concordance rate for monozygotic twins
    C. 40 per cent concordance rate for dizygotic twins
    D. 30 per cent show residual symptoms in adulthood
    E. If a parent has ADHD, there is 50 per cent chance that the child will develop ADHD.

77. A 35-year-old man is charged for molesting a woman in her house. The defendant is known to the woman and her husband. He was invited to stay in their house as a guest after a drink in the pub. The defendant suffers from somnambulism and he walked into the couple's room at night. He removed her underwear and was discovered by her husband. Concerning the defence of 'not guilty by reason of insanity' in this case, which of the following statements is true?
    A. Somnambulism is classified as sane automatism.
    B. Somnambulism is classified as insane automatism.
    C. There is a fixed maximum punishment for legal automatisms.
    D. Voluntary intoxication with alcohol is classified as sane automatism.
    E. Voluntary intoxication with alcohol is classified as insane automatism.

78. A woman is arrested after killing her 10-month-old daughter. The infant is described as having been very noisy and having cried excessively. Which of the following conditions is the most common predisposing factor?
    A. Battering father
    B. Battering mother
    C. Elder brother with conduct disorder
    D. Mother suffering from depression
    E. Father suffering from depression.

79. An infarct in which of the following regions of the brain is most likely to result in depression?
    A. Occipital lobe
    B. Basal ganglia
    C. Medulla
    D. Cerebellum
    E. Parietal lobe.

80. Which one of the following disorders is recognized as causing schizophrenia-like psychosis in a 40-year-old man?
    A. CADASIL
    B. MELAS syndrome
    C. Huntington's disease
    D. Kennedy's disease
    E. POEMS syndrome.

81. A core trainee wants to find out more about the medical causes of dementia. Which of the following is not associated with dementia?
    A. Carcinoma of the lung
    B. Cardiac arrest
    C. Carbon monoxide poisoning
    D. Cardiopulmonary bypass surgery
    E. Crohn's disease.

82. A 25-year-old married woman with a history of anorexia nervosa of 8 years' duration presents to an obstetrician asking for help with infertility. She wants medication to induce ovulation as she does not have menses. She keeps her BMI strictly at 12 kg/m^2, eats mainly vegetables and jogs 2 km every day. She is determined that she will not gain weight. The obstetrician is worried by her request. He seeks a consultation from you. Which of the following recommendations is inappropriate?
    A. To highlight to the obstetrician the ambivalence inherent in her request.
    B. To explore the symbolic significance of bypassing normal conception to achieve motherhood.
    C. To take a full developmental history, paying particular attention to her psychosexual development and conflicts with her own parents.
    D. To explore the psychodynamic issues relating to the patient and her partner.
    E. To respect her request to become pregnant and offer the best intervention to induce ovulation.

83. Which of the following antidepressants may cause arrhythmia?
    A. Bupropion
    B. Citalopram
    C. Moclobemide
    D. Venlafaxine
    E. All of the above.

84. Which of the following is uncommonly associated with pica?
    A. Learning disability
    B. Psychosis
    C. Eating non-nutritive substances
    D. Iron deficiency anaemia
    E. Lead poisoning.

85. Which of the following is true for a case–control study?
    A. Bias can be adjusted for at the analysis stage.
    B. It is often difficult to find age-matched controls in a case–control study.
    C. Confounding factors are defined as any factors which affect the outcome.
    D. In the design of a case–control study, confounding factors must be completely excluded.
    E. Linear regression or logistic regression can only adjust for one factor at a time.

86. The presence of eosinophilic inclusion bodies is most likely to be found in which of the following types of the dementia?
    A. Alzheimer's disease
    B. Frontotemporal lobe dementia
    C. Lewy body dementia
    D. Huntington's disease
    E. Vascular dementia.

87. A 20-year-old man is brought in by his parents as he insists on waiting for a man to take revenge on him at the bus station. He appears to be odd in his speech and behaviour. Which of the following support the diagnosis of schizotypal disorder?
    A. Abnormal ideas but consistent with cultural norms
    B. Compulsive checking behaviour
    C. First-rank symptoms
    D. Good rapport with the interviewer
    E. The onset of symptoms occured at the age of 14 years.

88. Which of the following statements is false?
    A. Hypothalamic harmatoma is associated with epilepsy, precocious puberty and hypothalamic rage.
    B. Type I diabetes mellitus patients have more cognitive impairment than Type II diabetes mellitus patients
    C. Hyperparathyroidism can cause cognitive impairment.
    D. Diabetes insipidus is associated with generalized anxiety.
    E. Addison's disease is associated with hypercalcaemia, hyponatraemia and lethargy.

89. Which of the following statements regarding various types of offenders is correct?
    A. A hepatologist refers a patient with hepatitis B to you. She is a 55-year-old woman with no previous offences and is an active member of her church. She has just been convicted of shoplifting. In this case, the most likely cause is depression.
    B. In the UK, homicide of the father is more common than that of the mother.
    C. Castration of violent offenders and reduction of testosterone have been found to be associated with significant reductions in violent offending.
    D. Cautioning is not a common disposal method for female offenders.
    E. Studies have suggested that raised levels of serotonin turnover and alterations in dopamine metabolism occur in violent offenders.

90. Which of the following is contraindicated in prednisolone-related depression?
    A. Amitriptyline
    B. Fluoxetine
    C. Mirtazapine
    D. Sertraline
    E. Venlafaxine.

91. The syndrome of inappropriate antidiuretic hormone (SIADH) is more likely to be associated with which of the following psychotropic medications?
    A. Carbamazepine
    B. Lithium
    C. Lamotrigine
    D. Phenytoin
    E. Valproate.

92. Which of the following offences or types of misconduct is not more likely to be committed by male offenders?
    A. Murder and manslaughter
    B. Robbery with violence
    C. Sexual aggression
    D. Homosexual offences
    E. Threat and fraud.

93. Which of the following statements regarding exhibitionism is false?
    A. Exhibitionism is included in both DSM and ICD.
    B. One of the best predictors of recidivism is lack of empathy.
    C. 50 per cent of sexual offences seen by courts are related to exhibitionism.
    D. Exhibitionists are more likely to be married than other sexual offenders.
    E. The reconviction rate is low after a first conviction but high after second conviction.

94. A 22-year-old university student suffers from her first episode of schizophrenia. She has great difficulty with her studying. Which of the following neurocognitive functions is most likely to be impaired?
    A. Language functions
    B. Immediate verbal memory
    C. Visuospatial skills
    D. Working memory
    E. Vigilance.

95. Which of the following findings from the National Confidential Inquiry into Suicide and Homicide (UK) is incorrect?
    A. Approximately 25 per cent of people who committed suicide had been in recent contact with the mental health services.
    B. The period of highest risk of suicide after discharge from in-patient care is the first 14 days.
    C. Over one-fifth of individuals who commit suicide have not adhered to their medication in the month preceding their death.
    D. In the UK, around 50 homicides per year are committed by those in recent contact with the mental health services.
    E. The rate of 'stranger homicides' committed by those with mental illness has increased sharply.

96. Which of the following is a plot of sensitivity versus $(1 - \text{specificity})$?
    A. Blobbogram
    B. Forest plot
    C. Funnel plot
    D. Galbraith plot
    E. Receiver operating characteristic curve.

97. A randomized controlled trial (RCT) comparing two antipsychotics is published showing that the power of the trial is designed to detect a 25 per cent difference ($\alpha = 0.5$, $\beta = 0.8$). Comparing the relapse rate in 1 year for patients on antipsychotics A and B, those on antipsychotic B have a relative risk of 1.5 and a 95 per cent confidence interval of 0.7–1.9. Which of the following statements is false?
    A. A difference in relapse rate in 1 year of 20 per cent between the drugs would not be statistically significant in the trial.
    B. If the authors claim there is a significant difference this would be a type 1 error.
    C. If the authors claim they demonstrated there is no difference between the two drugs, this would be a type 2 error.
    D. The P will be less than 0.05.
    E. The RCT result is compatible with antipsychotic B being associated with lower relapse rate than antipsychotic A.

98. A 10-year-old child presents with bedwetting at night and his father asks about prognostic factors. Which of the following is not a poor prognosis factor?
    A. Psychiatric disorder in the child
    B. Chronic family stress
    C. Lack of parental concern
    D. Diurnal enuresis
    E. Immature child.

99. You are the specialist trainee based at a local substance misuse service. An advanced practice nurse wants to incorporate a structured interview to assess both substance misuse and psychiatric disorders among the service users. Which of the following would you recommend?
    A. Assessment of Lifestyle Instrument (DALI)
    B. Chemical Use, Abuse and Dependence (CUAD) survey
    C. Inventory of Substance Abuse Treatment Services (SATS)
    D. Psychiatric Research Interview for Substance and Mental Disorders (PRISM)
    E. Stages of Change Readiness and Treatment Eagerness Scale (SOCRATES).

100. A 25-year-old with schizophrenia on risperidone complains of sexual dysfunction. Which of the following tests would you order?
    A. Calcium and parathyroid hormone
    B. Cortisol level
    C. Fasting serum glucose
    D. Prolactin level
    E. Thyroid function test.

101. In a randomized controlled trial, which of the following types of bias can be minimized by blinding?
    A. Berkson's bias
    B. Measurement bias
    C. Misclassification bias
    D. Neyman bias
    E. Volunteer bias.

102. Which of the following theories explains the gender-typed behaviour in a 4-year-old?
    A. Freud's psychosexual development theory
    B. Cognitive-developmental theory
    C. Kohlberg's stages of gender development
    D. Erikson's psychosocial development
    E. Social cognitive theory.

103. A core trainee consults you on how to avoid causing amenorrhoea, in a 25-year-old female patient with schizophrenia, resulting from prescribing her with antipsychotics. The core trainee shows you the following list of antipsychotics. Which is the most likely to cause amenorrhoea?
    A. Amisulpride
    B. Aripiprazole
    C. Clozapine
    D. Olanzapine
    E. Quetiapine.

104. A 14-year-old adolescent is admitted to the paediatric ward for the management of anorexia nervosa. The paediatrician wants to find out from you the most common cardiac complication in anorexia nervosa. Your answer is:
    A. First-degree heart block and hypotension
    B. Cardiomyopathy
    C. Right bundle branch block
    D. Left bundle branch block
    E. Pulmonary embolism.

105. Which of the following is recommended to treat pathological crying?
    A. Fluoxetine
    B. Haloperidol
    C. Moclobemide
    D. Mirtazapine
    E. Venlafaxine.

106. Which of the following statements regarding the chi-squared test is false?
    A. A chi-squared test can only be used on count data and the categories of data used must be mutually exclusive and discrete.
    B. In a chi-squared test for a 5 × 3 contingency table, there are 15 degrees of freedom.
    C. At least 80 per cent of cells must have expected values greater than 5.
    D. It requires a Yates correction if the total of the cells is less than 100 or any cell has a value of less 10.
    E. 'Goodness of fit' tests whether the data depart significantly from a theoretical distribution.

107. Which of the following antipsychotics should be avoided in patients with renal impairment?
    A. Amisulpride
    B. Clozapine
    C. Haloperidol
    D. Olanzapine
    E. Quetiapine.

108. The conclusion that can be reached from the forest plot below is:
    A. New antidepressants are more efficacious than placebos.
    B. Placebo is more efficacious than new antidepressants.
    C. Placebo and new antidepressants are equally efficacious.
    D. New antidepressants have higher drop-out rates than placebos.
    E. It is difficult to reach any conclusions owing to the heterogeneity among the studies.

109. Which of the following statements regarding conduct of a randomized trial is correct?
    A. A patient can withdraw from a RCT at any time and a valid reason is required.
    B. A RCT should be guided by the certainty principle where both investigators and subjects are fully informed about the efficacy of the trial drug and the gold-standard treatment.
    C. An open-label study can be granted retrospective research ethics committee approval.
    D. Placebo treatment is not advised in chronic and severe illness.
    E. A single-centre RCT is preferred as results are more homogeneous.

110. Which of the following statements regarding the impact of divorce on children is incorrect?
    A. Children of divorced parents are sexually active at a younger age.
    B. If the mother remarries, her son has a better relationship with the stepfather compared with her daughter.
    C. The mother-to-daughter bond is more affected than the mother-to-son bond if the mother remarries.
    D. Parental divorce causes more anxiety in the children than does parental death.
    E. On average, girls are more distressed than boys by parental divorce.

111. Which of the following personality disorders is most associated with suicide in the elderly?
    A. Anxious PD
    B. Dependent PD
    C. Histrionic PD
    D. Paranoid PD
    E. Schizoid PD.

Study name	Statistics for each study							Std diff in means and 95% CI
	Std diff in means	Standard error	Variance	Lower limit	Upper limit	Z-Value	p-Value	
Koseoglu 2007	1.193	0.201	0.041	0.798	1.588	5.924	0.000	
Quadri 2004	0.277	0.264	0.069	-0.239	0.794	1.052	0.293	
Bottiglieri 2001	0.606	0.409	0.167	-0.195	1.407	1.483	0.138	
Lehmann 1999	0.472	0.186	0.035	0.108	0.837	2.538	0.011	
Quadri 2005	0.416	0.223	0.050	-0.021	0.853	1.868	0.062	
	0.628	0.103	0.011	0.426	0.830	6.089	0.000	

-4.00   -2.00   0.00   2.00   4.00

Favours placebo   Favours new antidepressant

112. Which of the following statements regarding the confidence interval (CI) is false?
  A. The CI is the interval or range about which the 'true' statistic (parameter) is believed to be found within a given population with a known probability.
  B. Ninety-nine per cent of sample means under a normal distribution curve lie within a distance of 2.56 SD from the true population mean, so that we can be 99 per cent confident that this interval contains the true population mean.
  C. A 99 per cent CI will be wider than a 95 per cent CI.
  D. The width of the CI also depends on the sample size: larger samples provide wider CIs.
  E. For a relative risk or odds ratio, if the CI contains 1, then the results are not significantly different.

113. Which of the following statements regarding regression analysis is false?
  A. A regression line is a line that minimizes the sum of the squares of the vertical distances to the line of each data point, i.e. 'least-squares regression' ($Y = a + bX$).
  B. It is used when the main purpose is to develop a predictive model, i.e. to predict Y for a given value of X, using the equation $Y = a + bX$.
  C. As with the correlation coefficient (r), a slope of 0 represents no linear relationship between the variables.
  D. Multiple linear regression is used to predict the probability of a binary outcome occurring, e.g. psychosis /no psychosis, using several predictor or explanatory variables, e.g. age, cannabis misuse and family history.
  E. In case–control studies, regression allows for the correction of multiple potential confounding factors.

114. All the following statements regarding modafinil are true, except:
  A. It increases the release of dopamine.
  B. It increases the release of histamine.
  C. It increases the release of noradrenaline.
  D. It increases the GABAergic neurotransmission.
  E. Severe side-effects such as Steven–Johnson syndrome have been reported.

115. Which of the following statements regarding the standard deviation (SD) is true?
  A. SD is more difficult to calculate than the quartile distribution.
  B. SD can have negative values.
  C. SD has the same units as the original observation.
  D. The variance is the square root of the SD.
  E. For a sample size of 20, a good estimate of the population SD can be obtained by using 20 in the denominator of the equation.

116. Which of the following antipsychotic agents when used prophylactically reduces the occurrence of postoperative delirium?
  A. Chlorpromazine
  B. Haloperidol
  C. Olanzapine
  D. Risperidone
  E. Trifluoperazine.

117. For comparing the response (graded as minimal, mild, moderate and high responses) to venlafaxine of a group of depressed patients with the responses of a control group to amitriptyline, which of the following tests would be the most appropriate?
  A. McNemar's test
  B. Sign test
  C. Mann–Whitney U test
  D. Wilcoxon test
  E. Spearman correlation test.

118. The mechanism of action of a galantamine is:
  A. A reversible inhibition of the enzymes AChE and BChE
  B. A reversible inhibition of the enzyme AChE
  C. Irreversible inhibition of the AChE
  D. Irreversible inhibition of the enzymes AChE and BChE
  E. NMDA antagonism.

119. A 50-year-old man develops a non-itchy, erythematous rash on his thigh after a mountain hike. He reports that he was bitten by a tick. He complains of fatigue and low mood. The most likely diagnosis is:
  A. Dengue fever
  B. Depression
  C. Lyme disease
  D. Malaria
  E. Rickettsia.

120. A 9-year-old boy is referred with night terrors. Which of the following statements is incorrect?
  A. Night terrors are arousals from non-rapid eye movement (NREM) sleep.
  B. The child cannot remember the terror the next morning.
  C. It is caused by a rapid shift from stage 4 to stage 1 sleep.
  D. Night terrors occur mostly in the second half of the night.
  E. Waking up the child before the anticipated night terror is helpful.

121. A 60-year-old man is diagnosed with atrial fibrillation and the cardiologist prescribes 40 mg verapamil three times a day. He also suffers from atypical depression and the psychiatrist has prescribed an MAOI. Which of the following complications is most likely with the addition of an MAOI to verapamil?
    A. Persistent cough
    B. Frequent nasal bleeding
    C. Hypotension
    D. Cerebrovascular accident
    E. Liver impairment.

122. All the following statements regarding orexin are true, except:
    A. Orexin increases craving for food.
    B. Orexin promotes wakefulness.
    C. A link between orexin and Alzheimer's disease has been suggested.
    D. A link between orexin and autism has been suggested.
    E. A link between orexin and narcolepsy has been suggested.

123. Which is the medication of choice for a 25-year-old woman with bipolar depression who wants to breastfeed her baby?
    A. Citalopram
    B. Fluoxetine
    C. Lamotrigine
    D. Lithium
    E. Valproate.

EXTENDED MATCHING ITEMS (EMIs)

Question 124–130 – options
  A. One-way ANOVA
  B. Two-way ANOVA
  C. Chi-squared test
  D. Kruskal–Wallis test
  E. Mann–Whitney U test
  F. McNemar's test
  G. Paired-t test
  H. Wilcoxon's rank-sum test
  I. Median and range

Lead-in: Match the above statistical tests to the following scenarios. Each option might be used once, more than once or not at all.

124. A study is conducted to analyse the effects of antidepressants on immunological functions. Thirty female depressed patients are treated with SSRIs and placebo for 6 weeks using a crossover design and a washout period in between. Cytokine levels are measured during treatment with SSRIs and placebo according to the protocol. (Choose one option.)

125. Five years ago, a group of 60-year-old patients who were diagnosed as suffering from mild cognitive impairment (MCI) were recruited into a longitudinal study. Their homocysteine levels were measured at baseline and were found to be skewed. Now, this sample is assessed for the presence or absence of dementia. The homocysteine levels are measured again and compared with levels 5 years ago. You wish to test the hypothesis that changes in homocysteine levels depend on the presence or absence of dementia. (Choose one option.)

126. Five years ago, a group of 60-year-old patients who were diagnosed as suffering from mild cognitive impairment (MCI) and a group of age-matched controls without MCI were recruited into a longitudinal study. Their homocysteine levels were measured at baseline and were classified as low, medium and high. Now, this sample is assessed for the presence or absence of dementia. Which tests will be useful: (1) to compare the baseline homocysteine status between MCI patients and normal controls; and (2) to assess the association of baseline homocysteine levels with the subsequent development, or not, of dementia? (Choose two options.)

127. A researcher wants to find out which types of antidepressants, TCAs, SSRIs or SNRIs, lead to a better quality of life in depressed patients. The health-related quality of life is measured by the SF-36 and the scores of the three groups are compared. It is assumed that SF-36 follows the normal distribution. (Choose one option.)

128. A researcher wants to find out which types of antidepressants TCAs, SSRIs or SNRIs, lead to a better quality of life in depressed patients. The patients are self-rated using the SF-36, which assesses their health-related quality of life, and the doctors independently assess the Global Assessment of Functioning (GAF) scores. Both SF-36 and GAF scores are normally distributed. The researcher will compare the SF-36 and GAF scores of patients receiving the three different types of antidepressants. (Choose one option.)

129. In a postgraduate psychiatric clinical examination which follows a close marking system (i.e. candidates usually score marks between 4 and 7: 4 = fail, 5 = pass, 7 = distinction), the chief examiner wants to compare the median examination score among local, immigrant and refugee doctors. (Choose one option.)

130. A study was conducted to test for a difference in income between schizophrenia patients and age-matched normal controls. The researchers also need to decide the best way to summarize income in the two groups. (Choose two options.)

Questions 131–133 – options
  A. Block randomization
  B. Minimization method
  C. Stratified randomization

Lead-in: Match the above randomization methods to the following scenarios. Each option might be used once, more than once or not at all.

131. In a controlled trial to study the effect of olanzapine versus placebo in the management of delirium, age and metabolic syndrome (MS) status are taken as prognostic factors and the subjects are divided into four groups – group 1: MS with age ≤ 50 years; group 2, MS with age > 50 years; group 3, non-MS with age ≤ 50 years; group 4, non-MS with age > 50 years. Thus, if a patient registered is non-MS with age < 50 years, then she will be put into group 3 and will be allocated to the control group or trial group as per a list generated for group 3. (Choose one option.)

132. In a controlled trial to study the effect of olanzapine (O) versus placebo (P) in the management of delirium, the researcher intends to create groups equal in size. He prepared six chits and wrote PPOO on chit 1, OOPP on chit 2 and so on until he reached POOP on chit 6. After folding the chits properly and mixing well in a box, the chits are drawn at the end. (Choose one option.)

133. In a controlled trial to study the effect of olanzapine versus placebo in the management of delirium, the first participant is allocated randomly to olanzapine or placebo. Each subsequent participant is allocated after determining which group would lead to a better balance between the groups with respect to age and metabolic syndrome status. (Choose one option.)

Questions 134–138 – options

    A. Cluster sampling
    B. Convenience sampling
    C. Event sampling methodology
    D. Matched random sampling
    E. Panel sampling
    F. Progressive sampling
    G. Quota sampling
    H. Snowball sampling
    I. Systematic sampling
    J. Simple random sampling

Lead-in: Match the above sampling methods to the following scenarios. Each option might be used once, more than once or not at all.

134. In this sampling, participants are first matched based on some demographic characteristics and then randomly assigned into groups. (Choose one option.)

135. In this sampling, participants are assorted with respect to areas such as inner city, suburban and rural areas and then participants from these areas are selected. (Choose one option.)

136. This sampling method involves monitoring of ongoing experiences at various times over a number of days in the ward environment. (Choose one option.)

137. This sampling refers to clinical trial where the period of study is fixed and patients enter the study at different times during the period. (Choose one option.)

138. In this sampling, participants are first identified based on their characteristics and then they are required to provide the names of other potential sample members. (Choose one option.)

Questions 139–143 – options

    A. Cost-minimization analysis
    B. Cost-effectiveness analysis
    C. Cost–utility analysis
    D. Cost–benefit analysis
    E. Sensitivity analysis

Lead-in: Match the above analyses to the following scenarios. Each option might be used once, more than once or not at all.

139. In a study comparing a new type of psychological intervention for alcohol dependence with treatment as usual, the analysis concludes that the new intervention yields an average extra cost of £5 per abstinent day compared with treatment as usual. (Choose one option.)

140. In this study, the effect of the alternative interventions on the individuals' health-related quantity and quality of life are assumed to be equal. All other resource consequences are measured in monetary terms. (Choose one option.)

141. In a study of management of schizophrenia in three sites, the analysis is as follows:

	Centre A	Centre B	Centre C
Capital cost	£10 500	£8310	£1700
Rent and maintenance	£6508	£10 230	£4490
Staff costs	£41 480	£84 320	£66 320
Utilities	£22 220	£19 920	£11 130
Contracted services (laboratory tests, pharmacists, securities)	£39 340	£237 200	£131 600
Total costs	£120 048	£359 980	£215 240
Number of clients	210	300	250
Cost per client	£518	£1200	£860

142. In a study of the management of opioid dependence, 150 patients are randomly assigned to three groups of 50 patients each. The analysis is as follows:

	Residential care and dihydrocodeine	Out-patient buprenorphine	Out-patient methadone
Savings per day during treatment by not purchasing illicit drugs	£2500	£1800	£2000
Money earned per day from workshop	£3000	£3300	£2900
Total benefits	£5500	£5100	£4900
Cost per day of treatment	£5000	£3500	£2000
Benefit to cost	1.1	1.46	2.45

143. This analysis checks the effect on the outcome if the assumptions are changed in some way, such as worst-case scenario measures. (Choose one option.)

Questions 144–148 – options

    A. Case–control study
    B. Cohort study
    C. Cross-sectional study
    D. Ecological study
    E. Randomized controlled trial

Lead-in: Match the above studies to the following scenarios. Each option might be used once, more than once or not at all.

144. A group of researchers want to find out if alcohol dependence is a risk factor for morbid jealousy in a community. (Choose one option.)

145. A group of researchers want to find out if long-term aspirin usage in patients with ischaemic heart disease protects against dementia. (Choose one option.)

146. A group of researchers want to find out the effects of cannabis misuse on the incidence of schizophrenia in a community. (Choose one option.)

147. A group of researchers want to find out the prevalence of schizophrenia in Manchester. (Choose one option.)

148. A study looked at data from the member states of the European Union and investigated whether television exposure is related to fear of terrorism. This controlled for population size, level of education, age distribution and income and wealth. (Choose one option.)

Questions 149–154 – options

A. < 1
B. 3
C. 5
D. 10
E. 15
F. 20
G. 25
H. 30
I. 35
J. 40
K. 50
L. 70
M. 80
N. 85
O. 90

Lead-in: Match the correct number to the following statements. Each option might be used once, more than once or not at all.

149. Based on ICD-10 criteria, what is the lower limit of mild learning disability? (Choose one option.)

150. Based on ICD-10 criteria, what is the lower limit of moderate learning disability? (Choose one option.)

151. Based on ICD-10 criteria, what is the lower limit of severe learning disability? (Choose one option.)

152. What is the prevalence (as a percentage) of learning disability in the South Asian community in the UK? (Choose one option.)

153. What is the prevalence (as a percentage) of learning disability in the general population at any one time? (Choose one option.)

154. What is the prevalence (as a percentage) of learning disability in prison? (Choose one option.)

Question 155–158 – options

A. 2
B. 3
C. 4
D. 10
E. 15
F. 20
G. 25
H. 30
I. 35
J. 40
K. 50
L. 70
M. 80
N. 85
O. 90

Lead-in: Match the correct number to the following statements. Each option might be used once, more than once or not at all.

155. What is the percentage of patients with mild learning disability who suffer from epilepsy? (Choose one option.)

156. What is the percentage of patients with moderate learning disability who suffer from epilepsy? (Choose one option.)

157. What is the percentage of patients with severe learning disability who suffer from epilepsy? (Choose one option.)

158. What is the percentage of patients with profound learning disability who suffer from epilepsy? (Choose one option.)

Question 159–163 – options

A. 2 per cent
B. 3 per cent
C. 4 per cent
D. 10 per cent
E. 15 per cent
F. 20 per cent
G. 25 per cent
H. 30 per cent
I. 35 per cent
J. 40 per cent
K. 50 per cent
L. 70 per cent
M. 80 per cent
N. 85 per cent
O. 90 per cent

Lead-in: Match the correct percentage to the following statements. Each option might be used once, more than once or not at all.

159. What is the prevalence of epilepsy in fragile X syndrome? (Choose one option.)

160. What is the prevalence of epilepsy in Down syndrome? (Choose one option.)

161. What is the prevalence of schizophrenia in people with learning disability? (Choose one option.)

162. What is the rate of successful control of epilepsy among those patients with learning disability who have epilepsy? (Choose one option.)

163. What is the frequency of challenging behaviour in people with learning disability? (Choose one option.)

Questions 164–167 – options

- A. < 1 per cent
- B. 3 per cent
- C. 5 per cent
- D. 10 per cent
- E. 15 per cent
- F. 20 per cent
- G. 25 per cent
- H. 30 per cent
- I. 35 per cent
- J. 40 per cent
- K. 50 per cent
- L. 70 per cent
- M. 80 per cent
- N. 85 per cent
- O. 90 per cent

Lead-in: Match the correct percentage to the following statements. Each option might be used once, more than once or not at all.

164. What is the percentage of patients with Turner syndrome who suffer from coarctation of the aorta? (Choose one option.)

165. What is the percentage of patients with Turner syndrome who suffer from renal malformations? (Choose one option.)

166. What is the percentage of patients with Turner syndrome who suffer from hypothyroidism? (Choose one option.)

167. What is the percentage of patients with Turner syndrome who suffer from meiotic error that occurred in a paternal meiotic division? (Choose one option.)

Questions 168–169 – options

- A. 1 per cent
- B. 3 per cent
- C. 5 per cent
- D. 7 per cent
- E. 10 per cent

Lead-in: Match the correct percentage to the following statements. Each option might be used once, more than once or not at all.

168. You are counselling a mother who has one child with autism and is expecting her second child. She wishes to know the risk of autism in this second child. (Choose one option.)

169. A 14-year old boy presents with Tourette's syndrome and shows an encyclopaedic interest in British colonial history. His father asks: what is the probability that he will develop Asperger's syndrome? (Choose one option.)

Questions 170–174 – options

- A. Multi-systemic therapy
- B. Duty to inform the police if not reported yet

C. Obtain informed consent from the child and his or her parents
D. Parent management training
E. Family therapy
F. Methylphenidate
G. Risperidone

Lead-in: Match the above actions/interventions to the following situations. Each option might be used once, more than once or not at all.

170. A 14-year-old boy has recently assaulted his classmates and is defiant with his father. His parents are finding it difficult to discipline him. He does not have ADHD. (Choose one option.)

171. A 15-year-old boy is aggressive in many situations, to the point that his parents have a court injunction against him. No other symptoms have been found. The aggression is directed particularly at vulnerable people and pets at home. He does not have ADHD. He refuses psychotherapy, which his parents have also not found helpful for him. (Choose one option.)

172. Your core trainee consults you as she has been requested by the GP to perform a psychiatric assessment on a 15-year-old boy who has been involved in shoplifting over a 3-month period. (Choose two options.)

173. A 15-year-old boy is referred for treatment by the children's court. He recently lit a fire which resulted in significant damage to a shop. He was previously arrested for shoplifting and fighting. Previous history shows that he does not have learning disability or attention deficit disorder. (Choose one option.)

174. An 8-year-old child has frequent loss of temper, arguments with parents and feels irritable at home but not at school. The symptoms have persisted for 8 months. The parents are asking for help. (Choose two options.)

Questions 175–178 – options

- A. Father
- B. Mother
- C. Patient
- D. Elder brother
- E. Younger brother
- F. Male stranger

Lead-in: Whilst working in a child psychiatry department, you are dealing with an 11-year-old girl who was referred by the paediatrician. She admits that she was sexually assaulted. The gynaecologist examined her vagina and it was partially torn. The social worker reports that the girl has been abused by her father but he vehemently denies this. Match the above family members to the situations below. Each option might be used once, more than once or not at all.

175. If this is a case of incest, which family members may be involved? (Choose three options.)

176. You have decided to meet the siblings of the abused child. Which family member should not be invited to the family meeting? (Choose one option.)

177. The majority of abuse is committed by which family members? (Choose two options.)

178. She was diagnosed as suffering from Munchausen syndrome-by-proxy in the past. This syndrome is associated with psychological over-dependence of which person on the child? (Choose one option.)

Questions 179–183 – options
- A. Alzheimer's disease
- B. Binswanger's disease
- C. CASDIL
- D. Frontal lobe dementia
- E. Lewy body dementia
- F. Psychogenic fugue
- G. Pseudodementia
- H. Vascular dementia
- I. Vitamin B1 deficiency

Lead-in: Match the above situations to the following diagnoses. Each diagnosis might be used more than once.

179. An 80-year-old man presents with fluctuating, progressive memory loss and emotional incontinence. He has a history of falls and is being treated for hypertension by his GP. His relatives say that his personality is preserved. (Choose one option.)

180. A 65-year-old woman presents with memory loss following the death of her husband 4 months ago. She also complains of poor sleep, lack of energy and weight loss. During the cognitive assessment, she is not keen to answer questions. (Choose one option.)

181. A 75-year-old man presents with cognitive impairment, fluctuating levels of consciousness, particularly confusion and bizarre behaviour in the evenings. His daughter claims that he has been seeing ghosts and has not been able to turn in his bed. On physical examination, he is found to have hypertonia and hypersalivation. The MMSE score is 15/30. These above symptoms worsen following the commencement of antipsychotic medication. (Choose one option.)

182. A 40-year-old woman presents with cognitive deterioration and mood changes. On physical examination, there are gait abnormalities. She has a past medical history of epilepsy and migraines with aura. She also has episodes of left-sided muscular weakness. On further inquiry, her aunt also has similar problems. (Choose one option.)

183. A 60-year-old woman is found wandering on the streets with some memory loss after the recent funeral of her husband. She is brought in by the police for psychiatric assessment. When you assess her, she is unable to recall her personal details. She is physically well and all investigations are normal. (Choose one option.)

Questions 184–186 – options
- A. 1
- B. 5
- C. 7
- D. 10
- E. 20
- F. 30
- G. 40
- H. 50

Lead-in: Match the correct number to the following scenarios. Each option might be used once, more than once or not at all.

184. The percentage of shoplifters considered to be recidivists. (Choose one option.)

185. The percentage of psychosis in prisoners. (Choose one option.)

186. The number of times suicide risk is increased in prisoners compared with the general population. (Choose one option.)

Questions 187–189 – options
- A. Adversarial system
- B. Common law
- C. Court of protection order
- D. Restriction order
- E. Hospital order
- F. Not guilty by reason of insanity (NGRI) or McNaughton rule
- G. Procedural security
- H. Relational security

Lead-in: Match the above legal terminology to the following. Each option might be used once, more than once or not at all.

187. At the time of offending, the offender does not know the act he was doing was wrong. (Choose one option.)

188. This is used by the court as an alternative to a prison sentence. (Choose one option.)

189. It takes total control over the property and affairs of a psychiatric patient without mental capacity. (Choose one option.)

Questions 190–191 – options
- A. Hyponatraemia
- B. Hypernatraemia
- C. Hypokalaemia
- D. Hyperkalaemia
- E. Hypocalcaemia
- F. Hypercalcaemia
- G. Hypomagnesaemia
- H. Hypermagnesaemia

Lead-in: Identify one metabolic disturbance for each of the following scenarios:

190. A 65-year-old man presents with malaise and low back pain. He complains of increasing nausea and constipation. On physical examination, he is dehydrated and there is tenderness over his lumbar spine. According to his wife, he has been confused. ECG shows shortening of the QT interval. (Choose one option.)

191. You are asked to see a 65-year-old man with schizophrenia who has benign prostate hypertrophy. He suddenly develops

vomiting and appears breathless. He is lethargic. On physical examination, there is an enlarged bladder. ECG shows tented T waves, diminished P waves and broadened QRS complexes. (Choose one option.)

Questions 192–195 – options

A. Anorexia nervosa
B. Coeliac disease
C. Crohn's disease
D. Hyperthyroidism
E. Iatrogenic cause
F. Whipple's disease

Lead-in: Match the above causes of weight loss to the following situations. Each option might be used once, more than once or not at all.

192. A 68-year-old woman with a history of type II diabetes mellitus was referred by the geriatrician for assessment for depression. She complains of low mood and weight loss. Physical examination reveals oedema in her lower limbs. Echocardiogram shows congestive heart failure. Her medications include fluoxetine, metformin and furosemide.

193. A 40-year-old Irish woman was referred by her GP for assessment of depression. She complains of having lethargy, frequent diarrhoea with offensive stools and weight loss. She appears to be pale, and physical examination shows clubbing, abdominal distension and oral ulceration. Barium follow-through is abnormal. Her medications include iron and vitamin D supplements.

194. A 16-year-old girl was referred by the paediatrician for assessment of depression. She was admitted because of fever, weight loss, diarrhoea and abdominal pain. She appears to be thin and pale. Physical examination shows clubbing, aphthous ulceration, abdominal tenderness and perianal skin tags. She is a smoker. Her medication includes paracetamol and she is currently nil by mouth.

195. A 40-year-old man was referred by the rheumatologist for assessment of depression. He complains of weight loss and migratory polyarthritis. He appears to be pale. Physical examination reveals clubbing and pigmentation. His medications include sulphamethoxazole and trimethoprim.

Questions 196–198 – options

A. Edinburgh Postnatal Depression Scale (EPDS)
B. Hamilton Depression Rating Scale (HDRS)
C. Hospital Anxiety and Depression Scale (HADS)
D. Montgomery–Åsberg Depression Scale (MADS)
E. Patient Health Questionnaire (PHQ-9)
F. General Health Questionnaire (GHQ)
G. Ask two questions on low mood and loss of interest during the past month

Lead-in: Match the above questionnaires to the following situations. Each option might be used once, more than once or not at all.

196. A 30-year-old lady delivered her first-born 4 weeks ago. This is her first visit to her GP. The GP has a busy clinic and wants to screen for possible depression as quickly as possible. (Choose one option.)

197. A 30-year-old lady has been diagnosed with postnatal depression. The health visitor wants the patient to answer a questionnaire to monitor the outcome. (Choose three options.)

198. A 30-year-old lady has been diagnosed with postnatal depression. The core trainee wants to rate her mood objectively during the follow-up visit. (Choose two options.)

Questions 199–200 – options

A. Alcohol
B. Benzodiazepine
C. Opiate
D. Tobacco

Lead-in: Match the above substance misuse to the following situations where the mothers took the substance throughout the pregnancy. Each option might be used once, more than once or not at all.

199. The neonate developed floppy baby syndrome after he was born. On physical examination, he was noted to have cleft palate. (Choose one option.)

200. A 4-year-old child developed attention deficit and hyperactivity. (Choose one option.)

ANSWERS – MULTIPLE CHOICE QUESTIONS

1. A

Nocturnal enuresis is associated with short stature.

Further reading: Puri BK, Treasaden I, eds (2010). *Psychiatry: An evidence-based text*, pp. 482–483, 1067.

2. D

Mania is less common than depression in Cushing's syndrome of endogenous origin, but the converse holds true in exogenous cases, in which mania is common.

Further reading: Puri BK, Treasaden I, eds (2010). *Psychiatry: An evidence-based text*, p. 574.

3. C

Treatment with supervised injectable heroin leads to significantly lower use of street heroin than does supervised injectable methadone or optimized oral methadone.

Reference: Strang J, Metrebian N, Lintzeris N, Potts L *et al.* (2010). Supervised injectable heroin or injectable methadone versus optimised oral methadone as treatment for chronic heroin addicts in England after persistent failure in orthodox treatment (RIOTT): a randomised trial. *Lancet* **29**; 375: 1885–95.

4. C

It is stratified randomization while the other options are quasi-randomization.

Further reading: Puri BK, Treasaden I, eds (2010). *Psychiatry: An evidence-based text*, pp. 16, 38, 74, 77.

5. C

Further reading: Puri BK, Treasaden I, eds (2010). *Psychiatry: An evidence-based text*, pp. 109, 1066–7, 1088–90.

6. A

SSRIs are efficacious in treating both physical and psychological symptoms of premenstrual syndrome.

Reference: Henshaw CA (2007). Premenstrual syndrome: diagnosis, aetiology, assessment and management. *Advances in Psychiatric Treatment* **13**: 139–146.

7. E

Most patients do not develop dependence on methylphenidate if the stimulant is used over the long term. Check the ECG before prescribing methylphenidate and clonidine. Methylphenidate is also indicated for narcolepsy.

Reference: Semple D, Smyth R, Burns J, Darjee R, McIntosh A (2005). *Oxford Handbook of Psychiatry*. Oxford: Oxford University Press.

8. E

The NICE guidelines do not recommend any specific antidepressants for PTSD in young people. Mirtazapine and paroxetine are recommended for adults with PTSD. The FDA approved sertraline for OCD in children > 6 years and PTSD in adults. Hence, sertraline has the best evidence compared with the other antidepressants.

References: NICE guidelines on PTSD treatment: www.nice.org.uk/nicemedia/pdf/PTSD_2ndcons_publicinfo.pdf; Cohen JA, Mannarino AP, Perel JM, Staron V (2007). A pilot randomized controlled trial of combined trauma-focused CBT and sertraline for childhood PTSD symptoms. *Journal of the American Academy of Child and Adolescent Psychiatry* 46: 811–9.

9. B

Option B refers to standard deviation.

Further reading: Puri BK, Treasaden I, eds (2010). *Psychiatry: An evidence-based text*, pp. 49, 51, 52.

10. A

Alcohol-induced hypoglycaemia occurs in people who are dependent on alcohol after a large drink.

11. E

MEN 1 syndrome involves hyperparathyroidism, pituitary adenoma and pancreatic islet cell tumour.

12. E

Young people with Asperger's syndrome usually do not have language delay.

Further reading: Puri BK, Treasaden I, eds (2010). *Psychiatry: An evidence-based text*, p. 1099.

13. E

The NICE guidelines advise not to use the above drugs as specific treatment for the primary prevention of dementia. If this question had asked which medication may reduce the risk of dementia, then the answer would be selegeline because it has an antioxidant effect.

Reference: Sano M, Ernesto C, Thomas RG, *et al.* (1997). A controlled trial of selegiline, alpha-tocopherol, or both as treatment for Alzheimer's disease. The Alzheimer's Disease Cooperative Study. *New England Journal of Medicine* **336**: 1216–22

14. A

The dominant parietal lobe is involved in calculation. Subcortical dementia is associated with altered behaviour and personality and a dysexecutive syndrome, whereas cortical dementia gives rise to a classic neuropsychological deficit syndrome of amnesia, agnosia and apraxia.

Further reading: Puri BK, Treasaden I, eds (2010). *Psychiatry: An evidence-based text*, p. 512.

15. D

Transient global amnesia usually lasts for a few hours and seldom recurs. It will not lead to anterograde amnesia.

Further reading: Puri BK, Treasaden I, eds (2010). *Psychiatry: An evidence-based text*, **pp. 95, 557.**

16. C

It should be 2–8 per cent. For E, it was supported by Stevenson's study which showed that the prevalence of reading disorders is similar in US, Taiwan and Japan.

Reference: Stevenson HW *et al.* (1982). Reading disabilities: the case of Chinese, Japanese, and English. *Child Development* **53:** 1164–81.

17. D

(1/0.6 to 1/ 0.2) while NNT = 2.

Further reading: Puri BK, Treasaden I, eds (2010). *Psychiatry: An evidence-based text*, **p. 87.**

18. E

Further reading: Puri BK, Treasaden I, eds (2010). *Psychiatry: An evidence-based text*, **pp. 872–3.**

19. B

Further reading: Puri BK, Treasaden I, eds (2010). *Psychiatry: An evidence-based text*, **p. 1059.**

20. A

This applies to the first-time user but not a heavy user. The active ingredient (Δ^9-THC) is detectable in the urine of the first-time or occasional user after 48–72 hours, but in a heavy user it is detectable up to 6 weeks as it is stored in the body fat. 'B' is possible and the other agents include toilet cleaning agent. 'D' is possible as aspirin may interfere with the enzyme immunoassays. 'E' is possible and the excessive consumption of vitamin B has darkened his urine. This made the laboratory staff less suspicious that his urine was diluted.

Further reading: Puri BK, Treasaden I, eds (2010). *Psychiatry: An evidence-based text*, **pp. 412, 1031.**

21. C

22. E

Further reading: Puri BK, Treasaden I, eds (2010). *Psychiatry: An evidence-based text*, **p. 789.**

23. C

Tics are sudden, rapid and involuntary movements of circumscribed muscle groups without serving any purpose.

Further reading: Puri BK, Treasaden I, eds (2010). *Psychiatry: An evidence-based text*, **p. 550.**

24. E

The encopresis should be treated first. Aggressive encopresis is associated with a poor prognosis. Diurnal enuresis is more common in females owing to a higher prevalence of urinary tract infections.

Further reading: Puri BK, Treasaden I, eds (2010). *Psychiatry: An evidence-based text*, **p. 1068.**

25. E

Having more collaborating centres does not necessarily mean more subjects, which would increase the power of the RCT.

Further reading: Puri BK, Treasaden I, eds (2010). *Psychiatry: An evidence-based text*, **p. 52.**

26. A

DiGeorge syndrome (velocardiofacial syndrome) is inherited in an autosomal dominant fashion. Mucopolysaccharidosis III refers to Sanfilippo syndrome.

27. C

Reference: Goodwin, DW, Hermansen L, Guze SB *et al.* (1973). Alcohol problems in adoptees raised apart from alcoholic biological parents. *Archives of General Psychiatry* **28:** 238–243.

28. B

Normal weight bulimia nervosa develops in 25 per cent of anorexia nervosa patients. 'D' is false, it should be 6 months according to NICE guidelines. 'E' is false; only 5 per cent will be longer than 12 years (30 per cent, < 3 years; 35 per cent, 3–6 years; 30 per cent, 6–12 years).

Reference: Treasure J (2007). Anorexia nervosa and bulimia nervosa. In: Stein G, Wilkinson G. *Seminars in General Adult Psychiatry*. London: Gaskell; **NICE guidelines for antenatal and postnatal mental health:** http://guidance.nice.org.uk/CG45.

29. C

This refers to cranial diabetes insipidus. There is failure to concentrate urine in response to desmopressin in nephrogenic diabetes insipidus.

30. A

The 1-year prevalence of somatoform pain disorders is 8 per cent and the lifetime prevalence is 12.7 per cent.

Reference: Nickel R, Hardt J, Kappis B *et al.* (2009). Somatoform disorders with pain as the predominant symptom: results to distinguish a common group of diseases. *Schmerz* **23:** 392–8.

Further reading: Puri BK, Treasaden I, eds (2010). *Psychiatry: An evidence-based text*, **p. 840.**

31. C

Stimulants reduce hyperactivity but not stereotyped behaviour.

Further reading: Puri BK, Treasaden I, eds (2010). *Psychiatry: An evidence-based text*, **pp. 109, 1066–7, 1088–90.**

32. B

Both CBT and IPT are useful in the management of bulimia nervosa.

Further reading: Puri BK, Treasaden I, eds (2010). *Psychiatry: An evidence-based text*, **pp. 687–703, 1063.**

33. E

Pancoast's tumour or lung cancer causes peripheral neuropathy and it may metastasize to the brain.

34. B

A prolonged-release formulation was licensed in the UK as a short-term treatment of insomnia in patients > 55 years. 'A' is correct as melatonin is a hormone from the pineal gland and is secreted in a circadian manner with a nocturnal rise in level. This natural chemical does not cause much drug interaction and it is metabolized by the liver. It has not been evaluated in children and adolescents. The dose of melatonin varies from 500 µg (physiological dose) to 5 mg.

Reference: Taylor D, Paton C, Kapur S (2009). *The Maudsley Prescribing Guidelines*, 10th edn. **London: Informa Healthcare.**

35. B

It is incorrect and the recurrence risk is 10–15 per cent.

Reference: Gelder M, Mayou R, Cowen P (2001). *Shorter Oxford Textbook of Psychiatry.* Oxford: Oxford University Press.

36. E

The MTA study shows that children with ADHD continue to show higher than normal rates of delinquency (four times) and substance use (two times). In the MTA study, 485 children took part in the 3-year follow-up study. Their mean age was 12 years. The primary outcome measures were ADHD and oppositional defiant disorder symptoms, reading scores, social skills, level of impairment and diagnosis. At the end of the first year, the research protocol was dropped, allowing for more naturalistic and personalized treatment.

Reference: Bates G (2009). Drug treatments for attention-deficit hyperactivity disorder in young people. *Advances in Psychiatric Treatment* **15:** 162–71.

37. D

Please refer to figures below for explanation.

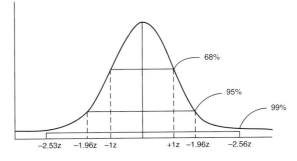

a. Normal distribution (Mean = Median = Mode)

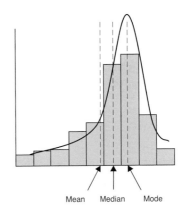

b. Left skewed/ Negatively skewed/ Ceiling Effect (Mean < Median < Mode)

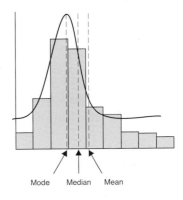

c. Right skewed/ Positively skewed / Floor effect (Mode < Median < Mean)

38. B

Further reading: Puri BK, Treasaden I, eds (2010). *Psychiatry: An evidence-based text*, **pp. 576–7, 1081.**

39. C

We cannot combine both in one forest plot.

Further reading: Puri BK, Treasaden I, eds (2010). *Psychiatry: An evidence-based text*, **pp. 67–69, 74.**

40. C

Devic's syndrome, also known as neuromyelitis optica, is a variant of multiple sclerosis. Churg–Strauss syndrome presents with asthma, pulmonary infiltrates, the vasculitic phase involving the peripheral and central nervous systems, heart, lungs, kidneys and gastrointestinal tract. Hallervorden–Spatz disease is a rare familial disorder with extrapyramidal symptoms, aggression and the gradual development of dementia. Tolosa–Hunt syndrome presents with unilateral orbital pain with third, fourth and sixth cranial nerve palsies.

Reference: Kay R (2002). *Casebook of Neurology.* Hong Kong: Lippincott Williams and Wilkins.

Further reading: Puri BK, Treasaden I, eds (2010). *Psychiatry: An evidence-based text*, p. 568.

41. C

Hypothyroidism is associated with hair loss.

Further reading: Puri BK, Treasaden I, eds (2010). *Psychiatry: An evidence-based text*, pp. 576–7, 1081.

42. B

Exhibitionism describes the continual or repetitive desire to expose one's genitals to strangers, usually of the opposite sex, without seeking or desiring any further contact.

Further reading: Puri BK, Treasaden I, eds (2010). *Psychiatry: An evidence-based text*, pp. 749, 762, 766–7.

43. E

A history of sexual offending has been found to be amongst the strongest predictors of sexual recidivism. Predictors for recidivism are classified into two categories: static and dynamic factors. Static factors refer to historical characteristics that cannot be altered (e.g. age, prior offence history, childhood abuse and age at first sex offence arrest or conviction). Dynamic factors are characteristics, circumstances and attitudes that can change throughout one's life. Examples of dynamic characteristics include drug or alcohol use, poor attitude (e.g. low remorse and victim blaming), deviant sexual preferences, negative peer influences, poor self-regulation and intimacy problems.

Reference: Recidivism amongst serious violent and sexual offenders (http://www. scotland.gov.uk/Publications/2002/11/15729/12635); Hanson RK, Harris A (1998). *Dynamic Predictors of Sexual Recidivism.* Ottawa: Solicitor General of Canada.

44. C

It is a degenerative disorder, with normal vestibulo-ocular reflexes, dysarthria and difficulty with downwards vertical gaze (supranuclear ophthalmoplegia).

Further reading: Puri BK, Treasaden I, eds (2010). *Psychiatry: An evidence-based text*, pp. 440, 544–5.

45. A

It leads to reduction in magnesium.

46. D

About 95 per cent of cases of Down syndrome result from trisomy 21 and 1 per cent are mosaic. The remaining 4 per cent are caused by translocations of part of one chromosome to another. The extra chromosome is usually of maternal origin and error occurs during first meiotic division. The risk of recurrence of translocation is 10 per cent.

Further reading: Puri BK, Treasaden I, eds (2010). *Psychiatry: An evidence-based text*, pp. 467, 1082, 1087–8.

47. A

Pregnant women with active eating disorders have a greater chance of delivery by Caesarean section and may develop postpartum depression.

Reference: Franko DL, Blais MA, Becker AE *et al.* (2001). Pregnancy complications and neonatal outcomes in women with eating disorders. *American Journal of Psychiatry* **158**: 1461–6.

48. C

Based on the NICE guidelines, a trial of lithium augmentation should be considered for patients whose depression has failed to respond to several antidepressants, such as venlafaxine and mirtazapine. Augmentation with lithium has better evidence for efficacy than augmentation with mianserin. Removing mirtazapine or venlafaxine may worsen the patient's mood.

Reference: NICE guidelines on depression (http://www.nice.org.uk/nicemedia/pdf/ CG23NICEForConsultation.pdf).

49. A

B is incorrect as there is loss of purposeful hand movements. D is incorrect as there is acquired microcephaly.

Further reading: Puri BK, Treasaden I, eds (2010). *Psychiatry: An evidence-based text*, p. 1067.

50. D

Reference: Gelhorn HL, Sakai JT, Price RK, Crowley TJ (2007). DSM-IV conduct disorder criteria as predictors of antisocial personality disorder. *Comprehensive Psychiatry* **48**: 529–38.

51. C.

Further reading: Puri BK, Treasaden I, eds (2010). *Psychiatry: An evidence-based text*, p. 613.

52. A

'B' is incorrect as its half-life is approximately 5 hours. 'C' is incorrect as atomoxetine is a first-line treatment in

ADHD patients with tics. 'D' is incorrect as there is no evidence for the use of second-generation antipsychotics to treat hyperactivity, although risperidone may be useful in the treatment of aggression in ADHD in learning disability patients. 'E' is incorrect. Hyperactivity is often a manifestation of epilepsy.

Reference: Baker P (2004). *Basic Child Psychiatry, 7th edn.* London: Blackwell; Taylor D, Paton C, Kapur S (2009). *The Maudsley Prescribing Guidelines,* 10th edn. London: Informa Healthcare.

53. A

The other features are found in fetuses born to mothers with past or active eating disorders. The majority of the women with eating disorders have a normal length of pregnancy (mean length 39 weeks). Their babies usually have a normal Apgar score (at 1 and 5 minutes after birth, the scores are 8 and 9 points, respectively).

Reference: Koubaa S, Hällström T, Lindholm C, Hirschberg AL (2005). Pregnancy and neonatal outcomes in women with eating disorders. *Obstetrics & Gynecology* **105**: 255–60.

54. D

Quetiapine is not commonly associated with hyperprolactinaemia and the core trainee needs to rule out pituitary microadenoma.

Further reading: Puri BK, Treasaden I, eds (2010). *Psychiatry: An evidence-based text,* pp. 426, 601, 904.

55. B

Prevalence = pre-test probability = 5 per cent; likelihood ratio for a negative result = 0.5. LR(–) = (1 – sensitivity)/specificity, i.e. 0.5 = (1 – 0.8)/specificity and hence specificity = 0.2 / 0.5 = 0.4. LR(+) = sensitivity / (1 – specificity), i.e. = 0.8 / (1 – 0.4) = 1.33.

Further reading: Puri BK, Treasaden I, eds (2010). *Psychiatry: An evidence-based text,* p. 37.

56. B

The National Adult Reading Test (NART) is the most widely used to estimate premorbid ability.

Further reading: Puri BK, Treasaden I, eds (2010). *Psychiatry: An evidence-based text,* pp. 93, 97, 98, 515, 535.

57. B

Further reading: Puri BK, Treasaden I, eds (2010). *Psychiatry: An evidence-based text,* p. 546.

58. C

Boys enter puberty at an average age of 11 years (1–2 years later than girls) but it may occur any time between 9 and 14 years.

Further reading: Puri BK, Treasaden I, eds (2010). *Psychiatry: An evidence-based text,* pp. 120–1.

59. E

The pulvinar sign refers to symmetrical hyperintensity in the posterior nuclei of the thalamus.

Further reading: Puri BK, Treasaden I, eds (2010). *Psychiatry: An evidence-based text,* pp. 572–3.

60. D

The differences between normal grief, grief with depressive features and major depressive disorder remain controversial and will be in debate in the upcoming DSM-5 and ICD-11. The key factor lies in the duration of symptoms. As the patient presents with depressive symptoms 3 months after the death of her son, her diagnosis is major depressive disorder, as the DSM-IV-TR criteria state that uncomplicated grief sometimes includes depressive symptoms in the first 2 months. On the other hand, if she presents with the above features 3 weeks after the death of her son, her diagnosis would become uncomplicated grief.

Further reading: Puri BK, Treasaden I, eds (2010). *Psychiatry: An evidence-based text,* p. 881.

61. A

This patient presents with agitation, aggression, confusion and hallucinations.

Further reading: Puri BK, Treasaden I, eds (2010). *Psychiatry: An evidence-based text,* p. 880.

62. D

Prevalence = pre-test probability = 5 per cent; likelihood ratio for a negative result = 0.5. Then plot a line from across the points on the nomogram.

63. B

It should be high potassium.

64. D

Those with hysterical personality are over-emotional and have over-dramatic personality traits. They may crave attention and be manipulative. Under stress, they have an increased vulnerability to developing dissociative disorders and are also prone to parasuicidal acts.

Further reading: Puri BK, Treasaden I, eds (2010). *Psychiatry: An evidence-based text,* p. 666.

65. C

This could be the stereotyped behaviour associated with autism.

Further reading: Puri BK, Treasaden I, eds (2010). *Psychiatry: An evidence-based text,* pp. 109, 1066–7, 1088–90.

66. D

Erythema migrans is the earliest sign in Lyme disease at the site of the tick bite. It occurs 7–10 days after the bite. It evolves from an erythematous macule initially to form a large, annular lesion if left untreated. Secondary syphilis is a possible diagnosis but unlikely in a 15-year-old. The other possibility is erythema marginatum associated with active carditis, dermatophytes and tinea infection.

67. E

Coprophagia refers to eating faeces. Coprolalia refers to the complex vocal tics involving inappropriate social vocalizations. Less than one-third of cases display tremor, echolalia and echopraxia. Mental coprolalia is more common than overt coprolalia.

Further reading: Puri BK, Treasaden I, eds (2010). *Psychiatry: An evidence-based text*, pp. 523, 550–1, 1068.

68. C

Sydenham's chorea occurs in 10 per cent of rheumatic fever triggered by β-haemolytic streptococci.

Further reading: Puri BK, Treasaden I, eds (2010). *Psychiatry: An evidence-based text*, pp. 523, 581.

69. D

An independent sample *t*-test is used to compare the post-treatment Hamilton Depression Scale Scores in two groups. A paired *t*-test can be used to assess the equality of the means of one group before and after intervention.

Further reading: Puri BK, Treasaden I, eds (2010). *Psychiatry: An evidence-based text*, pp. 57–58.

70. E

Candidates should be aware that the concepts of validity and reliability also apply to a randomized, double-blind, placebo-controlled trial (RCT). A to D are measures of internal validity of a RCT.

Further reading: Puri BK, Treasaden I, eds (2010). *Psychiatry: An evidence-based text*, pp. 16, 38, 74, 77.

71. E

Ketamine is associated with moderate to severe lower urinary tract symptoms, i.e. frequency, urgency, dysuria, urge incontinence and occasionally painful haematuria.

Reference: Chu PS, Ma WK, Wong SC *et al.* (2008). The destruction of the lower urinary tract by ketamine abuse: a new syndrome? *BJU International* **102**: 1616–22.

72. D

The answer is D or automatism. 'A' is incorrect as sleepwalking is more common in children (30 per cent at least one episode). 'B' is incorrect as it is a non-rapid eye movement (NREM) phenomenon. Waking the child in sleepwalking is not helpful.

Further reading: Puri BK, Treasaden I, eds (2010). *Psychiatry: An evidence-based text*, pp. 850, 1165–66.

73. D

Explanation: *r* value (degree of correlation): 0–0.2 (negligible), 0.2–0.5 (weak), 0.5–0.8 (moderate), 0.8–1.0 (strong).

Further reading: Puri BK, Treasaden I, eds (2010). *Psychiatry: An evidence-based text*, pp. 59–65.

74. D

A paired *t*-test can be used to compare the effects of two drugs on a particular patient at different points in time.

Further reading: Puri BK, Treasaden I, eds (2010). *Psychiatry: An evidence-based text*, pp. 54–55, 78.

75. E

Atomoxetine is indicated in the patients with hyperkinetic disorder and Tourette's syndrome.

Further reading: Puri BK, Treasaden I, eds (2010). *Psychiatry: An evidence-based text*, pp. 523, 550–1, 1068.

76. A

The heritability is 75 per cent.

Further reading: Puri BK, Treasaden I, eds (2010). *Psychiatry: An evidence-based text*, pp. 1059–60.

77. B

The man cannot use voluntary intoxication with alcohol as a defence, as voluntary intoxication does not constitute a defence by itself. Legal automatisms result in decreased punishment or even acquittal but there is no fixed maximum punishment.

Further reading: Puri BK, Treasaden I, eds (2010). *Psychiatry: An evidence-based text*, pp. 1165–66.

78. B

The battering mother lost her temper and killed the infant in response to her child's behaviour. In the UK, the rate of infanticide has remained relatively constant with about 20 convictions per year. If the scenario in the question were to change and instead state that the infant was calm and stable, then the most common predisposing factor would become severe postpartum mental illness.

Further reading: Puri BK, Treasaden I, eds (2010). *Psychiatry: An evidence-based text*, pp. 719, 726, 1165.

79. B

Patients with depression have been reported as having a higher number and larger volume of infarcts affecting the prefrontosubcortical circuits, particularly the caudate and pallidum in basal ganglia, and genu of internal capsule, with left-sided predominance.

Reference: Vataja R, Pohjasvaara T, Leppävuori A *et al.* (2001). Magnetic resonance imaging correlates of depression after ischemic stroke. *Archives of General Psychiatry* **58**: 925–31.

80. C

CADASIL: cerebral autosomal dominant arteriopathy with subcortical infarcts and leucoencephalopathy with older age of onset; MELAS syndrome: mitochondrial encephalomyopathy leading to stroke and seizure but mean age of death is mid-30s; Kennedy's disease: X-linked recessive spinobulbar muscular atrophy; POEMS syndrome: polyneuropathy, organomegaly, endocrinopathy, monoclonal gammopathy and skin changes (pigmentation/tethering).

Reference: Kay R (2002). *Casebook of Neurology.* Hong Kong: Lippincott Williams and Wilkins.

Further reading: Puri BK, Treasaden I, eds (2010). *Psychiatry: An evidence-based text*, pp. 546–47, 1101.

81. E

82. E

The psychiatrist should not accept the problem as presented by the patient but help the obstetrician to explore the patient's denial of chronic illness. The patient may be looking for an untenable solution to a problem which she does not fully understand. Her present condition is clearly not an ideal one with respect to considering becoming pregnant at this time.

83. E.

Reference: Taylor D, Paton C, Kapur S (2009). *The Maudsley Prescribing Guidelines*, 10th edn. London: Informa Healthcare.

84. E

Pica may lead to lead poisoning but is not common. It may persist into adulthood as geophagy (i.e. eating clay and dirt).

Further reading: Puri BK, Treasaden I, eds (2010). *Psychiatry: An evidence-based text*, p. 716.

85. B

Bias cannot be adjusted and confounding factors cannot be completely excluded. Linear regression or logistic regression can adjust for several factors simultaneously.

Further reading: Puri BK, Treasaden I, eds (2010). *Psychiatry: An evidence-based text*, pp. 40, 73.

86. C

The eosinophilic intracytoplasmic inclusion bodies refer to Lewy bodies that contain accumulated alpha synuclein.

Further reading: Puri BK, Treasaden I, eds (2010). *Psychiatry: An evidence-based text*, pp. 1106–7.

87. E

Schizotypal disorder runs a chronic course (at least 2 years). People with schizotypal disorder may have odd beliefs inconsistent with cultural norms, obsessive ruminations without inner resistance, transient quasi-psychotic episodes but not as intensified as first-rank symptoms and poor rapport.

Further reading: Puri BK, Treasaden I, eds (2010). *Psychiatry: An evidence-based text*, pp. 593–609.

88. B

Patients with type I diabetes mellitus tend to have less cognitive impairment than those with type II diabetes mellitus.

Further reading: Puri BK, Treasaden I, eds (2010). *Psychiatry: An evidence-based text*, pp. 621–22.

89. E

'A' is false as only 1 per cent have depressive disorder and the most common cause is not related to psychiatric disorder. 'B' is false as matricide (killing one's own mother) is more common than patricide (killing one's own father). Thirty per cent of mothers who committed filicide (killing one's own children) have a psychiatric illness. 'C' is false as physical castration has no impact while chemical castration shows conflicting results. Cautioning is the main disposal used for female offenders (50 per cent in females *v.* 30 per cent of males).

Reference: Chiswick D, Cope R (1995). *Seminars in Forensic Psychiatry.* Gaskell: London; D'Orban PT (1979). Women who kill their children. *British Journal of Psychiatry* **134**: 560–71.

90. A

Tricyclic antidepressant treatment co-prescribed with prednisolone can lead to deterioration in mental state and psychotic features in depressed patients.

91. A

Carbamazepine may cause SIADH. The mechanism for this is uncertain, but may involve increased release of ADH (vasopressin) and/or potentiation of the action of this hormone.

Further reading: Puri BK, Treasaden I, eds (2010). *Psychiatry: An evidence-based text*, p. 431.

92. E

The male-to-female ratio for recorded crime is approximately 10:1 and the age distribution of female offenders is similar to that of males owing to a secondary peak of middle-aged shoplifters. A–D are exclusively male offences. Predominantly male offences include breaking and entering, sex offences of any kind, non-sexual aggression to the person, grievous bodily harm, larceny and motoring offences. Women are responsible for over one-third of all homicides in which the offender has a psychiatric disorder.

Women predominate among depressive homicides and the commonest victim is their child.

Child-stealing is almost exclusively committed by females. There are three types:

- Comforting offence – usually committed by a young woman who has a need to look after a young child. She is more likely to take a child whom she has already known. She often has a history of personality disorder and delinquency.
- Manipulative offence – usually committed by a woman to maintain a relationship by claiming the baby to replace the one lost by miscarriage.
- Impulsive psychotic offence – usually committed by a woman during the acute relapse of a psychotic illness.

Reference: Chiswick, D and Cope R (1995). *Seminars in Forensic Psychiatry.* Gaskell: London.

93. C

The true answer is only 25 per cent. Less than 20 per cent of indecent exposers will reoffend.

References: Stone JH, Roberts M, O'Grady J, Taylor AV, O'Shea K (2000). *Faulk's Basic Forensic Psychiatry,* 3rd edn. Oxford: Blackwell Science; **Gelder M, Mayou R, Cowen P (2001).** *Shorter Oxford Textbook of Psychiatry.* Oxford: Oxford University Press; **Gunn J, Taylor PJ (1993).** *Forensic Psychiatry. Clinical, Legal and Ethical Issues.* Oxford: Butterworth-Heinemann.

94. B

The meta-analytical review given in the reference below has reported that neurocognitive deficits are maximal in immediate verbal memory and processing speed in people suffering from first-episode schizophrenia.

Reference: Mesholam-Gately RI, Giuliano AJ, Goff KP *et al.* (2009). Neurocognition in first-episode schizophrenia: a meta-analytic review *Neuropsychology* 23: 315–336.

95. E

There is no increase in 'stranger homicide' committed by psychiatric patients. In the UK, 35 per cent of homicide is committed by offenders with psychiatric illnesses. Among those with psychiatric illnesses, schizophrenia is the most common psychiatric disorder associated with homicide (55 per cent), followed by personality disorder (26 per cent) and affective disorder (19 per cent). Less than 50 per cent of psychotic offenders describe psychotic motivation. Around 160–200 psychiatric in-patients commit suicide annually and the most common method is hanging.

Reference: Gelder M, Mayou R, Cowen P (2001). *Shorter Oxford Textbook of Psychiatry.* Oxford: Oxford University Press; **Swinson N (2007).** National Confidential Inquiry into Suicide and Homicide by People with Mental Illness: new directions. *Psychiatric Bulletin* 31: 161–3.

96. E

Further reading: Puri BK, Treasaden I, eds (2010). *Psychiatry: An evidence-based text,* p. 38.

97. D

The confidence interval crosses 1.

Further reading: Puri BK, Treasaden I, eds (2010). *Psychiatry: An evidence-based text,* pp. 44, 46, 49. 51, 52, 57.

98. E

Immaturity is unlikely to predict the outcome of bedwetting.

Further reading: Puri BK, Treasaden I, eds (2010). *Psychiatry: An evidence-based text,* **pp. 482, 1067.**

99. D

The PRISM is used for the assessment of substance abuse and psychiatric comorbidity. It is a structured diagnostic interview and emphasizes that the assessment of alcohol and substance misuse is to be performed before the assessment of psychiatric disorders, so that the history of substance misuse can be linked to the development of psychiatric illnesses.

Reference: Goldberg D, Hilier VP (1979). A scaled version of the General Health Questionnaire (GHQ-28). *Psychological Medicine* 9: 139–45.

100. D

Risperidone leads to an increase in prolactin level and sexual dysfunction.

Further reading: Puri BK, Treasaden I, eds (2010). *Psychiatry: An evidence-based text,* p. 632.

101. B

Measurement bias includes observer or interview bias which can be minimized by blinding.

Reference: Puri BK, Treasaden I, eds (2010). *Psychiatry: An evidence-based text,* p. 86.

102. E

Social cognitive theory was developed by Bandura. There is a 'model of causation' that links three sets of variables, all of which influence each other: behaviour (e.g. activity patterns), person (e.g. expectations, intentions, goals) and environment (e.g. modelling, reinforcement). Gender-typed behaviour is heavily dependent on parental and peer responses to gender stereotypes (e.g. masculine and feminine).

Reference: The Open University and BBC on family and child development (http://open2.net/healtheducation/family_childdevelopment/2005/extractone.html)

103. A

Other antipsychotics which have a strong hyperprolactinaemia effect include risperidone and sulpiride.

Further reading: Puri BK, Treasaden I, eds (2010). *Psychiatry: An evidence-based text,* p. 425.

104. A

Besides bradycardia, option 'A' is the most common cardiac complication. Note that cardiac arrest is the most common cause of death in anorexia nervosa. Other common causes of death include fluid imbalance, suicide, renal failure and electrolyte imbalance.

Further reading: Puri BK, Treasaden I, eds (2010). *Psychiatry: An evidence-based text*, pp. 687–703, 1063.

105. A

106. B

Degrees of freedom in a 5×3 table $= (5 - 1) \times (3 - 1) = 8$.

Further reading: Puri BK, Treasaden I, eds (2010). *Psychiatry: An evidence-based text*, pp. 58–59, 77–78.

107. A

Reference: Taylor D, Paton C, Kapur S (2009). *The Maudsley Prescribing Guidelines*, 10th edn. London: Informa Healthcare.

108. A

Further reading: Puri BK, Treasaden I, eds (2010). *Psychiatry: An evidence-based text*, p. 68.

109. D

'A' is against the Declaration of Helsinki which states that research subjects can withdraw without giving any reason. 'B' is false as a RCT should be guided by the uncertainty principle and both investigators and subjects do not know the efficacy of trial and gold-standard medication. 'C' is false as ethical approval should be obtained beforehand. 'E' is false as more centres are preferred to assess the effects of a trial drug in different ethnic groups owing to variation in pharmacokinetics.

Further reading: Puri BK, Treasaden I, eds (2010). *Psychiatry: An evidence-based text*, pp. 16, 38, 74, 77.

110. E

On average, boys are more distressed than girls by parental divorce while girls are more distressed than boys if their mothers remarry. Previous studies have shown that there is a rise in conduct problems, anxiety and depression a year or two following the divorce. Eventually, most of the children become well-functioning individuals but the divorce may leave a lasting impression on their own intimate relationships, which may be associated with failure of a child's marriage.

Reference: Goodman R, Scott S (2005). *Child Psychiatry*, 2nd edn. Oxford: Blackwell.

111. A

Higher levels of neuroticism, lower scores for openness to experience, and having a restricted range of interests are personality characteristics associated with suicide in the elderly.

Reference: Duberstein PR, Conwell Y, Caine ED (1994). Age differences in the personality characteristics of suicide completers: preliminary findings from a psychological autopsy study. *Psychiatry* **57**: 213–24.

112. D

A larger sample produces a narrower CI.

Further reading: Puri BK, Treasaden I, eds (2010). *Psychiatry: An evidence-based text*, pp. 44, 46, 49, 51, 52, 57.

113. D

This should be logistic regression. Multiple linear regression predicts a single dependent or response variable using a number of independent variables, e.g. PANSS (Positive and Negative Symptom Scale) scores predicted by age, duration of untreated psychosis and duration of illness. Multiple linear regression can only be used for normally distributed responses, and not for binary outcomes, e.g. disease/no disease.

Further reading: Puri BK, Treasaden I, eds (2010). *Psychiatry: An evidence-based text*, pp. 59–65.

114. D

Modafinil is a stimulant which causes a reduction in GABAergic neurotransmission.

Further reading: Puri BK, Treasaden I, eds (2010). *Psychiatry: An evidence-based text*, pp. 848, 912.

115. C

For 'B', the standard deviation never takes negative values. For 'E', the denominator should be 19; degrees of freedom $= n - 1$.

Further reading: Puri BK, Treasaden I, eds (2010). *Psychiatry: An evidence-based text*, pp. 44, 46, 64, 78.

116. B

Further reading: Puri BK, Treasaden I, eds (2010). *Psychiatry: An evidence-based text*, p. 881.

117. C

The data are not paired, hence B and D are incorrect.

118. B

Further reading: Puri BK, Treasaden I, eds (2010). *Psychiatry: An evidence-based text*, pp. 906, 1104.

119. C

Lyme disease is transmitted by tick bites and its manifestations include diffuse muscular pain and a spreading erythematous discoloration of the skin.

120. D

Night terrors usually occur in the first half of the night.

Further reading: Puri BK, Treasaden I, eds (2010). *Psychiatry: An evidence-based text*, **pp. 850, 1166.**

121. C

Verapamil is a calcium channel blocker. MAOIs may enhance the hypotensive effect.

122. D

Orexin is not implicated in autism. Mutation in the (hypocretin) orexin receptor 2 gene is associated with narcolepsy. Orexin is implicated in Alzheimer's disease as it controls the diurnal variation of beta-amyloid levels.

Reference: Lin L, Faraco J *et al.* (1999). The sleep disorder canine narcolepsy is caused by a mutation in the hypocretin (orexin) receptor 2 gene. *Cell* **98:** 365–76; Kang JE, Lim MM, Bateman RJ *et al.* (2009). Amyloid-β dynamics are regulated by orexin and the sleep-wake cycle. *Science* **326:** 1005–7.

123. E

Valproate can be used in breastfeeding when there is adequate protection against pregnancy. Citalopram, lithium and fluoxetine are present in breast milk at relatively high levels. Lamotrigine is not recommended because it may cause life-threatening rashes in babies.

Reference: Taylor D, Paton C, Kapur S (2009). *The Maudsley Prescribing Guidelines*, 10th edn, London: Informa Healthcare.

ANSWERS – EXTENDED MATCHING ITEMS

124. G

125. H

It tests the difference between paired homocysteine levels in the same patient at baseline and five years later.

Further reading: Puri BK, Treasaden I, eds (2010). Psychiatry: An evidence-based text, pp. 55–6, 78.

126. C, E

The Mann–Witney *U* test is used because we are testing the ranked homocysteine levels between two independent patient groups: with and without dementia.

Further reading: Puri BK, Treasaden I, eds (2010). Psychiatry: An evidence-based text, pp. 55–6, 58–9, 77–8.

127. A

128. B

129. D

Further reading: Puri BK, Treasaden I, eds (2010). Psychiatry: An evidence-based text, p. 57.

130. H, I.

Income is usually skewed.

Further reading: Puri BK, Treasaden I, eds (2010). Psychiatry: An evidence-based text, pp. 55–56, 78.

131.C

Further reading: Puri BK, Treasaden I, eds (2010). Psychiatry: An evidence-based text, pp. 38, 43, 74, 86, 902.

132.A

Further reading: Puri BK, Treasaden I, eds (2010). Psychiatry: An evidence-based text, pp. 38, 43, 74, 86, 902.

133.B

Further reading: Puri BK, Treasaden I, eds (2010). Psychiatry: An evidence-based text, pp. 38, 43, 74, 86, 902.

134. D

Further reading: Puri BK, Treasaden I, eds (2010). Psychiatry: An evidence-based text, pp. 42, 52, 74–75.

135. A

Further reading: Puri BK, Treasaden I, eds (2010). Psychiatry: An evidence-based text, pp. 42, 52, 74–75.

136. C

Further reading: Puri BK, Treasaden I, eds (2010). Psychiatry: An evidence-based text, pp. 42, 52, 74–75.

137. F

Further reading: Puri BK, Treasaden I, eds (2010). Psychiatry: An evidence-based text, pp. 42, 52, 74–75.

138. H

Further reading: Puri BK, Treasaden I, eds (2010). Psychiatry: An evidence-based text, pp. 42, 52, 74–75.

139. B

Further reading: Puri BK, Treasaden I, eds (2010). Psychiatry: An evidence-based text, pp. 41–2.

140. A

Further reading: Puri BK, Treasaden I, eds (2010). Psychiatry: An evidence-based text, p. 41.

141. A

Further reading: Puri BK, Treasaden I, eds (2010). Psychiatry: An evidence-based text, p. 41.

142. D

Further reading: Puri BK, Treasaden I, eds (2010). Psychiatry: An evidence-based text, p. 41.

143. E

Further reading: Puri BK, Treasaden I, eds (2010). Psychiatry: An evidence-based text, pp. 37, 76.

144. A

Morbid jealousy is a rare disease.

Further reading: Puri BK, Treasaden I, eds (2010). Psychiatry: An evidence-based text, pp. 40, 73, 1009.

145. A

It could be considered unethical to withhold aspirin from patients with ischaemic heart disease.

Further reading: Puri BK, Treasaden I, eds (2010). Psychiatry: An evidence-based text, pp. 40, 73, 1009.

146. B

Further reading: Puri BK, Treasaden I, eds (2010). *Psychiatry: An evidence-based text*, pp. 40–1, 73, 86, 107, 1009.

147. C

Further reading: Puri BK, Treasaden I, eds (2010). *Psychiatry: An evidence-based text*, pp. 40, 73, 106–7.

148. D

Further reading: Puri BK, Treasaden I, eds (2010). *Psychiatry: An evidence-based text*, p. 41.

149. K

150. I

151. F

Less than 20 per cent of people with learning disability are classified as having profound learning disability.

152. F

153. B

2.5 per cent have mild learning disability and 0.5 per cent have moderate to severe learning disability.

154. D

Further reading: Puri BK, Treasaden I, eds (2010). *Psychiatry: An evidence-based text*, p. 1081.
Reference: O'Hara J (2003). Learning disabilities and ethnicity: achieving cultural competence. *Advances in Psychiatric Treatment* 9: 166–76.

155. C

156. F

157. H

158. K

Further reading (for Q. 155–158): Puri BK, Treasaden I, eds (2010). *Psychiatry: An evidence-based text*, pp. 538, 1080, 1086.

159. G

Further reading: Puri BK, Treasaden I, eds (2010). *Psychiatry: An evidence-based text*, pp. 1082, 1088, 1091.

160. D

Further reading: Puri BK, Treasaden I, eds (2010). *Psychiatry: An evidence-based text*, pp. 167, 1082, 1087–8.

161. B

Further reading: Puri BK, Treasaden I, eds (2010). *Psychiatry: An evidence-based text*, pp. 1079–99.

162. L

163. F

Reference (for Q. 159–163): Fraser W, Kerr M (2003). *Seminars in the Psychiatry of Learning Disabilities*, 2nd edn. Gaskell: London.

164. E

165. J

166. F

167. M

Further reading (for Q. 164–167): Puri BK, Treasaden I, eds (2010). *Psychiatry: An evidence-based text*, p. 467.

168. B

Further reading: Puri BK, Treasaden I, eds (2010). *Psychiatry: An evidence-based text*, p. 477.

169. E

170. D

The Parent Management Programme draws on operant-behavioural and cognitive-behavioural approaches involving consistent strategies that reward desired behaviours but ignore undesired behaviours.

Further reading: Puri BK, Treasaden I, eds (2010). *Psychiatry: An evidence-based text*, p. 1059.

171. G

Short-term risperidone (at a dose of 0.25–2 mg) can be used in adolescents with conduct disorder with aggressive behaviour who refuse psychological treatment.

Further reading: Puri BK, Treasaden I, eds (2010). *Psychiatry: An evidence-based text*, pp. 1058–9.

172. B, C

This may be a case of juvenile delinquency with ethical, legal and clinical problems. Aetiological factors may include living in an inner city area, lack of caring supervision and lower socioeconomic class. The male:female ratio is 3–10:1. In the UK, the African-Caribbean rates are around double the rates in Caucasians. The trainee needs to be aware that there are differences between potential forensic and therapeutic assessments. The trainee needs to obtain consent from the adolescent and his parents. She also needs to inform them that there are circumstances in which the clinical information gathered could be used in court proceedings.

From the forensic aspect, she needs to assess the mode of shoplifting and the nature of the items stolen. Risk assessment is important. She also needs to assess the adolescent's awareness of the implications of conviction and the impact on himself and his family. The past forensic history may shed light on how previous offences may affect the current situation. Clinical issues involve assessment of the developmental stage, school situation, family reaction to the shoplifting, the adolescent's reaction to and explanation for the shoplifting, evidence of psychiatric illness, substance abuse and social history. One-quarter of juvenile offenders will be repeat offenders.

Reference: Goodman R, Scott S (2005). *Child Psychiatry*, 2nd edn. Oxford: Blackwell Publishing.

173. A.

This is a case of juvenile delinquency after excluding common causes for fire-setting in young people. Multisystemic therapy is the treatment of choice in juvenile delinquency. It involves family therapy focusing on effective communication, systematic reward and punishment systems and taking a problem-solving approach to day-to-day conflicts. It also encourages the adolescent to spend more time with his or her peers without delinquency and to avoid those with delinquency. Individual therapy involves assertiveness training against negative peer influences. The therapist also needs to liaise with the education authority (to improve learning and academic performance), the correctional services (regular monitoring of antisocial behaviour) and the social worker (to help the family to cope).

Further reading: Puri BK, Treasaden I, eds (2010). *Psychiatry: An evidence-based text*, pp. 1156–7.

174. D, E.

Family therapy and parent management training are both possible treatments for oppositional defiant disorder.

175. A, D, E

Further reading: Puri BK, Treasaden I, eds (2010). *Psychiatry: An evidence-based text*, p. 773.

176. A

177. A, B

178. B

(For Q. 176–178): In childhood sexual abuse, the abuse is usually inside the family and disclosure is less likely if incest occurs. In the UK, sexual intercourse under 13 years is regarded in law as statutory rape. Father–daughter incest usually takes place when the girl is aged about 10 or 11 years. The father who has an incestuous relationship with his daughter usually does not suffer from a psychiatric abnormality. Mother–son incest is often associated with neurotic states, personality difficulties and occasionally psychosis. Victims of sexual abuse are more likely to develop inability to control sexual impulses, precocious sexual play, weakened gender identity, increased incidence of homosexuality, increased incidence of child molestation and eating disorders.

In the UK, incest is legally defined as occurring when a man has sexual intercourse with a female whom he knows to be his daughter, granddaughter, sister, half-sister or mother, or when a woman aged over 16 years permits a man whom she knows to be of such consanguinity to have sexual intercourse with her. Family relationships which do not involve consanguinity (e.g. stepfather–daughter) generally do not fall within the legal definition of incest.

Munchausen syndrome (or factitious illness) by proxy was first described by Meadow in 1977. The main psychiatric associations with the mother are personality, somatization, affective and eating disorders. The perpetrator often appears to be an exemplary mother with nursing experience and the father is either emotionally or physically absent.

Reference: Chiswick D, Cope R (1995). *Seminars in Forensic Psychiatry*. London: Gaskell.

179. H

Further reading: Puri BK, Treasaden I, eds (2010). *Psychiatry: An evidence-based text*, p. 1105.

180. G

Further reading: Puri BK, Treasaden I, eds (2010). *Psychiatry: An evidence-based text*, p. 93.

181. E

Further reading: Puri BK, Treasaden I, eds (2010). *Psychiatry: An evidence-based text*, p. 1106.

182. C

183. F

Fugue is present with loss of semantic memory (details of events or facts), but procedural memory is usually retained.

References (for Q. 179–182): Kay R (2002). *Casebook of Neurology.* Hong Kong: Lippincott Williams and Wilkins Asia; Butler R, Pit B (1998). *Seminars in Old Age Psychiatry.* London: Gaskell.

184. D

185. B

Psychotic illness is more common in male prisoners than female prisoners.

186. D

187. F

Further reading: Puri BK, Treasaden I, eds (2010). *Psychiatry: An evidence-based text,* pp. 1162–3, 1168.

188. E

Approximately 15 per cent of hospital orders are created with restriction on discharge.

Further reading: Puri BK, Treasaden I, eds (2010). *Psychiatry: An evidence-based text,* p. 1168.

189. C

Further reading: Puri BK, Treasaden I, eds (2010). *Psychiatry: An evidence-based text,* pp. 1112, 1202, 1219.

190. F

Hypercalcaemia resulting from myeloma.

191. D

Hyperkalaemia owing to renal failure and bladder outflow obstruction.

192. E

The three medications mentioned can cause unintentional weight loss in the elderly. Fluoxetine is stronger than other SSRIs in causing an anorectic effect.

193. B

This patient suffers from coeliac disease. Investigations include FBC ($\downarrow$haemoglobin) and detection of antigliaden antibody. Treatment involves a gluten-free diet, iron supplementation and immunosuppression.

194. C

This patient suffers from Crohn's disease. Investigations include FBC ($\downarrow$haemoglobin), $\uparrow$CRP, $\uparrow$ESR, $\downarrow$B12 and folate. Sigmoidoscopy and colonoscopy show patch inflammation, and biopsy may show granuloma. Small-bowel follow-through may show fistulae. Corticosteroids and azathioprine may be prescribed in the short term and long term, respectively.

195. F

This patient suffers from Whipple's disease which is caused by *Tropheryma whipplei* (formerly *whippelii*). Jejunal biopsy characteristically shows large foamy macrophages in the lamina propria which contain positive periodic acid–Schiff staining material. The treatment is to continue sulphamethoxazole and trimethoprim for 1 year. Other causes of malabsorption include chronic pancreatitis, tropical sprue (rare in the UK), giardiasis (often with a history of travelling to infected areas), small-bowel syndrome and following gastric surgery.

Reference (for Q. 192–195): Firth JD, Collier JD (2001). *Medical Masterclass: Gastroenterology and Hepatology.* London: Royal College of Physicians.

196. G

197. A, C, E

Further reading: Puri BK, Treasaden I, eds (2010). *Psychiatry: An evidence-based text,* pp. 516, 635, 786, 880.

198. B, D

199. B

Benzodiazepines are contraindicated in the first trimester. They may cause floppy baby syndrome if taken near term.

200. D

Tobacco also causes intrauterine growth retardation, low birth weight and developmental delay.

Index

NOTE

Reference to individual questions and their answers are given in the form of page numbers followed by a question number (e.g. 1 (Q3) for page 1, question 3).

Where a significant topic is *only* mentioned in the answer (and not in the question), index entries will give the page number of the answer (e.g. 6(A2)). Topics covering a whole chapter range are given a normal page range reference without any mention of the question numbers.

Abbreviations

ADHD - attention-deficit hyperactivity disorder; CBT - cognitive-behavioural therapy; OCD - obsessive-compulsive disorder; PTSD - post-traumatic stress disorder

14-3-3 protein 185(A20)

Abbreviated Mental Test Score (AMTS) 317(Q7)
abducens nerve 112(Q12), 358–9(Q61)
absence seizure, EEG pattern 394(Q135)
absolute risk reduction 33(Q4), 33–4(Q6)
absorption of drugs 257(Q1)
abstraction, auditory operational processing 122(Q4), 122(Q5)
acalculia 38(Q11)
acamprosate 260(Q33), 391(Q93)
acceptance, Kübler-Ross stage 251–2(Q6)
accessory nerve, damage 174(Q6)
accommodation (ocular) 77(Q3)
acculturation strategies 103(Q1), 103(Q2)
ACE inhibitors 367(Q153)
acetazolamide 176(Q22)
N-acetyl aspartate (NAA) 155–6(Q7)
acetylators, slow 384(Q14)
acetylcholine 141(Q2), 141(Q3), 142(Q11)
    functions and synthesis 142(Q11)
    metabolite 258(Q15)
    precursor 258(Q14)
    REM sleep 134(Q6)
    repeated ECT effect 265(Q4)
    synthesis pathway 142–3(Q12)
acetylcholine receptor antagonists 176(Q21)
acetylcholinesterase 141(Q2), 142(Q11)
    pseudo-irreversible 389(Q72)
    reversible inhibition 421(Q118)
acetylcholinesterase inhibitors 259(Q25), 389(Q72), 421(Q118)
    effect on sleep 237(Q4)
    sinus bradycardia 397–8(Q192)
acetyl-CoA 142–3(Q12)
N-acetylcysteine 359(Q66)
achievement motivation 74(Q10)
acrophobia 196(Q14)
ACTH *see* adrenocorticotrophic hormone (ACTH)
acting in 273(Q1)
acting out 395(Q149), 395(Q153)
action potential, neuronal 117(Q4)

action slips, types 65(Q12)
activity factor, attitudes 95(Q5)
actus rea 334(Q10)
acute dystonic reactions 249(Q3)
acute stress disorder 363(Q99)
adaptation, normal adjustment phase 251(Q5)
Adaptive Behaviour Assessment System (ABAS) 314(Q8)
addiction psychiatry 301–5
    mesolimbic reward system 388(Q63)
    see also substance abuse/misuse
addictive behaviour, social learning theory and 69(Q21)
Addison's disease 221(Q1), 416(Q63), 418(Q88)
adenine 159(Q6), 159–60(Q7)
adenylate cyclase 144(Q25), 144(Q26)
adiponectin 398(Q199)
adjustment (normal), to diagnosis of life-threatening illness 251(Q5)
admission rate bias 18(Q20)
adolescent mothers, postnatal depression 307(Q1)
adolescent psychiatry 307–11
    anxiety disorders 309(Q16)
    conduct disorder with aggression 426(Q171)
    depression 308(Q11), 309(Q16)
    non-suicidal self-injury 390(Q82)
    obsessive-compulsive disorder 308(Q12)
    shoplifting and 426(Q172)
    substance abuse, and fear of ridicule 361(Q85)
    suicide risk factors 390(Q79)
adoption studies 393(Q109)
adrenal cortex 123(Q10)
adrenal gland, ACTH stimulation of 56(Q7)
adrenaline
    Schachter and Singer's experiment 59–60(Q6)
    Schachter and Wheeler's experiment 60(Q7)
    synthesis pathway 142(Q8)
adrenoceptors 144(Q25), 392(Q95)

α-adrenoceptors 144(Q25)
    α_1-adrenoceptor blocker 388(Q54)
    α_2-adrenergic receptor agonist 392(Q95)
    α_2-adrenoceptor antagonism 392(Q97)
β-adrenoceptors 144(Q25)
    antagonists/blockers 176(Q22), 207(Q3)
adrenocortical insufficiency, primary 181(Q22)
adrenocorticotrophic hormone (ACTH) 56(Q7), 129(Q5), 130(Q7)
    stimulation test 130(Q9)
adverse drug reactions, type A 260(Q34)
A & E department, attendees 329(Q1)
aerial perspective 77(Q4)
affective psychoses 191(Q4), 191–3
    drug therapy 191(Q2)
    historical developments 192(Q3), 192(Q12)
    see also bipolar disorder; depression/depressive disorders
Afro-Caribbean people, criminal justice system 337(Q30)
after-image 78(Q5)
age
    arson and 336(Q24)
    as continuous variable, and ratio 15(Q1)
    crime by women 333(Q2)
    disorientation, schizophrenia 37(Q1)
    pathological gambling risk factor 336(Q21)
    suicide rates 105(Q17)
    Violence Risk Appraisal Guide (VRAG) and 349(Q2)
age of criminal responsibility 334(Q9)
aggression
    antipsychotic drugs for 313(Q5)
    in conduct disorder, therapy 426(Q171)
    orbitofrontal lobe contracoup injury 391(Q91)
    penalty, behavioural technique 365(Q123)
    theories 95(Q1)
agitation, anticipatory drug for 252(Q7)

agomelatine, pharmacodynamics 385(Q19)
agoraphobia 31(Q5), 195(Q6), 196(Q11), 385(Q26)
Agouti-related protein (AgRP) 146(Q38)
agranulocytosis 260(Q34)
agraphia 38(Q11)
agreeableness 92(Q8), 92(Q12)
air rage 260(Q32)
alanine aminotransferase 302(Q13)
alarm reaction stage 56(Q7)
albumin, serum 203(Q5), 221(Q1)
alcohol
 abuse
  hypoglycaemia 410(Q10)
  learning disability and 313(Q4)
  sedatives in 388(Q59)
 acute intoxication
  DSM-IV-TR 304(A10)
  EEG pattern 393–4(Q115)
  ICD-10 301(Q6)
 AUDIT, assessment by 221–2(Q5)
 benzodiazepine interaction 260(Q32)
 binding sites 301(Q1)
 CAGE assessment 221–2(Q5)
 dependence
  arson and 336(Q24)
  heritability 160(Q15)
  risk in offspring 411(Q21), 411(Q27)
  with schizophrenia 386(Q34)
 effect on sleep 237(Q5), 238(Q8)
 excessive intake, indicators 221(Q1)
 hazardous drinking 329(Q1)
 misuse, management 303(Q18)
 problem drinking among in-patients 329(Q1)
 voluntary intoxication, legal issues 417(Q77)
 withdrawal, DSM-IV-TR 302(Q10)
 withdrawal syndrome 302(Q11), 411(Q18)
alcoholic liver disease 302(Q13)
alcoholism, psychotherapy 269(Q1)
aldosterone 123(Q10)
Alexander basal ganglia–thalamocortical circuit 113(Q16), 113(Q17)
Alice in Wonderland effect 368(Q168)
aliphatic phenothiazine 259(Q18)
all-or-nothing thinking 287–8(Q6)
Allport, DA 51(Q2)
alpha adrenoceptors see α-adrenoceptors
alpha rhythms, EEG 51(Q3), 137(Q5), 137–8(Q6), 238(Q12)
alprostadil 211–12(Q6)
altruism 95(Q2), 283–4(Q5)
alveolar ventilation 133(Q2)
Alzheimer's disease
 aetiological factors 369(Q194)
 APOE4 alleles 369(Q194), 383(Q3)
 APP mutations 160(Q14)
 diagnosis 317–18(Q8)
 Down syndrome and 369(Q194), 387(Q46)
 early, pathology 389(Q71)
 ECG pattern 397–8(Q192)
 EEG 138(Q7)
 heritability 160(Q13), 391(Q84)
 Lewy body dementia vs 318(Q9), 364(Q113)
 MRI scan 389(Q71)
 neuropathology 151(Q2)
 orexin and 438(A122)
 prevalence 105(Q15), 317(Q7)
 risk 391(Q84)
  age relationship 388(Q57)
  familial 391(Q84)
 sleep patterns 239(Q18)
 tau protein 387(Q49)
 treatment 145(Q31), 259(Q25)
amacrine cell pathway 121(Q1)
ambiguous figure 78(Q6)
ambitendency 355(Q29)
amenorrhoea 207(Q1), 361(Q84), 414(Q54)
 antipsychotics causing 419(Q103)
amiloride 385(Q25)
amiodarone, hypothyroidism association 182(Q27)
amisulpride 258(Q11), 259(Q19)
 avoidance in renal impairment 420(Q107)
 indications 386(Q34), 419(Q103)
amitriptyline 257(Q5), 362–3(Q95)
 contraindication 418(Q90)
 mechanism of action 258(Q16)
amnesia 170(Q5)
 anterograde 84(Q5), 410(Q15)
 feigned 357(Q41)
 retrograde 170(Q5), 265(Q6), 357(Q41)
 transient global 410(Q15)
amnesic syndrome 170(Q5)
amok 105(Q12), 105(Q13)
AMPA receptors 387(Q51)
amphetamines 4(Q13), 257(Q4)
 adverse effects 397–8(Q191)
 binding sites 301(Q5)
 dependence 260(Q33)
 ECG associated 397–8(Q191)
 effect on sleep 237(Q5)
 MAOI related to 259(Q26)
amputation 329(Q4)
amputee identity disorder 329(Q4)
amyloid β peptide 151(Q6), 160(Q14)
amyloidosis, familial, Finnish type 151(Q3)
amyloid precursor protein (APP) 160(Q14), 387(Q46)
 see also APP gene
amyotrophic lateral sclerosis (ALS) 179(Q5), 179–80(Q6)
anabolic steroids 301(Q3), 301(Q4)
anaesthesia, EEG pattern 393–4(Q116)
analgesic ladder 251(Q1)
anankastic personality disorder 196(Q10), 205(Q3), 205(Q4), 356(Q33)
anaphase 159(Q5)
Andrews, J et al 3(Q4)
androgen-insensitivity syndrome 217(Q3)
Angelman syndrome 160(Q11), 393(Q112)
anger
 Ax's experiment 59(Q5)
 Kübler-Ross stages 251–2(Q6)
Angoff method 363(Q103)
angular gyrus, lesions 38(Q10)
ankle, reflex, spinal root transmitting 174(Q7)
anomalous monism 11(Q6)
anomic suicide 360(Q79)
anophthalmia 228(Q8)
anorexia nervosa 361(Q84)
 aversive conditioning 365–6(Q124)
 cardiac complications 420(Q104)
 causes of death 437(A104)
 heritability 160(Q13)
 incidence and DSM-IV-TR 203(Q2)
 infertility management 418(Q82)
 pathognomic feature 203(Q1)
 predictor of death 203(Q5)
 in pregnancy 414(Q47), 414(Q53)
 psychological defences 269–70(Q8), 270(Q11)
 risk factor 203(Q3)
 switch to bulimia nervosa 411–12(Q28)
anorgasmia 212(Q9)
ANOVA 19(Q30), 20(Q32)
 one-way 423(Q127)
 two-way 423(Q128)
anterior cerebral artery ischaemia 174–5(Q13)
anterior pituitary hormones 129(Q5)
anterograde amnesia 84(Q5), 410(Q15)
anticholinergic side-effects 260(Q28)
anticipation, genetic 185(A26)
anticipatory drugs 251–2(Q6), 252(Q7)
 in care of dying 251(Q4), 252(Q7)
anticonvulsants (antiepileptic drugs) 175(Q14), 175–6(Q20), 259(Q23), 259(Q24), 367(Q150)
 adverse effects 175–6(Q20), 359(Q69), 360(Q71)
antidepressants 191(Q2)
 arrhythmia due to 418(Q83)
 breastfeeding and 422(Q123)
 combination, safest 358(Q52)
 contraindications 418(Q90)
 ECG features and 397–8(Q188), 397–8(Q190)
 mechanism of action 145(Q31)
 persistent somatoform pain disorder 234(Q6)
 in pregnancy 207(Q5), 386–7(Q40)
 for PTSD in young people 410(Q8)
 REM sleep and 238(Q7)
 treatment effect comparison, statistics 416(Q69)
 see also tricyclic antidepressants; individual antidepressants
antidiuretic hormone (ADH) 123(Q10)
anti-emetics 252(Q7)
antiepileptic drugs see anticonvulsants
antihistaminergic effects, tricyclic antidepressants 260(Q28)
anti-manic medication 191(Q2)
antipsychotic drugs 386(Q34)
 adverse effects 260(Q34), 353(Q6)
  extrapyramidal 38(Q12), 259(Q20)
  sedative effects 259(Q22)
  weight gain 259(Q21)
 aggressive behaviour in intellectual disability 313(Q5)

amenorrhoea association 419(Q103)
atypical 259(Q17), 262(A18)
avoidance in renal impairment
    420(Q107)
CATIE study 359–60(Q70)
D$_2$R partial agonists 260(Q29)
in diabetes 363(Q102)
duration of therapy 366–7(Q147)
eating disorders and 203(Q6)
first generation 187(Q4), 187(Q5)
    EEG pattern 395(Q142)
metabolism and CYP3A4 allele
    106(Q20)
minimum effective dose 366–7(Q146)
postoperative delirium reduction
    421(Q116)
prolactin levels and 130(Q11),
    436(A103)
relapse risk 187(Q4)
REM sleep and 238(Q7)
risks/benefits 358(Q58)
second-generation 4(Q12), 187(Q5)
sleep disorders associated 237(Q3)
trials, in schizophrenia 187(Q5)
typical 262(A18)
antipyrine, metabolism 106(Q20)
antisocial personality disorder 105(Q14),
    205(Q1), 304(A2), 337–8(Q35)
risk, in conduct disorder 414(Q50)
violence and 349(Q1)
anxiety
    Cattell's second-order factors and
        92(Q7)
    depression with 195(Q1), 394(Q127)
    insomnia in 238(Q13)
    of pathological degree, Cushing's
        syndrome 181(Q21)
    performance relationship 196(Q13)
    phobic 199(Q2)
    prepartum 207(Q3), 207(Q5)
    symptoms 195(Q3)
anxiety disorders
    children/adolescents 309(Q16)
    cognitive processes associated 287(Q3)
    Down syndrome and 397(Q175)
    generalized see generalized anxiety
        disorder
    heritability 160(Q15)
    separation, in childhood 308(Q10)
    thinking, changes in 287(Q2)
anxiety hysteria 199(Q2)
anxious personality disorder 356(Q33),
    420(Q111)
APGAR score 414(Q53)
apolipoprotein E4 gene 369(Q194),
    383(Q3)
apomorphine 4(Q11)
apotemnophilia 218(Q8)
apparent movement 78(Q7)
Appeal Courts 343(Q2)
appetite, cannabis intoxication 302(Q15)
APP gene 151(Q3), 387(Q46)
    mutations 160(Q14)
appointee 343–4(Q6)
apraxia, oral 170(Q11)
arbitrary inference 191(Q3)
archetypes 5(Q14), 273(Q4)

arcuate nucleus 129(Q3)
arginine vasopressin (VVP) 129(Q4)
Argyll Robertson pupils 366(Q130)
aripiprazole 187(Q4), 259(Q21), 259(Q22),
    260(Q29)
    indications 364(Q109)
L-aromatic amino acid decarboxylase
    142(Q8)
arousal 133–5
arrhythmia, antidepressants causing
    418(Q83)
arsenic intoxication 181(Q16)
arson, epidemiology 336(Q24)
arterial spin labelling (ASL) 156(Q10)
art therapy 269(Q1), 291(Q1), 291(Q3)
    separation differentiation 291(Q2)
ascertainment bias 18(Q20)
Asia, suicide methods in 243(Q3)
'ask to reflect', psychodynamic therapy
    396(Q166), 396(Q167)
aspartate aminotransferase 141(Q2),
    302(Q13)
aspartylglycosaminuria 313(Q3)
Asperger's syndrome 356(Q30), 410(Q12)
    Tourette's syndrome and 426(Q169)
asphyxiophilia 218(Q9)
aspirin 424–5(Q145)
assaults 426(Q170)
Assertive Community Treatment (ACT)
    361(Q83)
assimilation, acculturation strategy
    103(Q1)
association studies 393(Q111)
astrocytes, function 387(Q47)
astrocytoma 151–2(Q8)
astrocytosis 151(Q1)
astroglia 141(Q1)
ataque depression nervios 105(Q13)
atomoxetine 258(Q8), 414(Q52),
    417(Q75)
atrioventricular block 397–8(Q192)
attachment behaviour 43(Q4)
    anxious-avoidant temperament
        43(Q7)
    development 43(Q2), 43(Q3)
    insecure-ambivalent 43(Q4)
    insecure-avoidant 43(Q4)
    secure 43(Q4)
attachment figure 43(Q3)
    separation from 47(A4)
attachment theory 43(Q1), 273(Q4),
    279(Q2)
attention 63–6, 364(Q108)
    anatomical loop 114(Q26)
    assessment 37(Q3), 63(Q2)
    divided (dual-task) 65(Q9)
    focused 364(Q108)
        auditory 63(Q3), 63(Q4)
        Deutsch–Norman theory 64(Q7)
        single-channel theories (Broadbent)
            63(Q5)
        Treisman's attenuation model
            64(Q6)
        visual 64–5(Q8)
    limited-capacity theory (Kahneman)
        65(Q10)
    models 63(Q1)

multi-store model of memory 83(Q3)
selective 358(Q60)
    see also attention, focused
serial 66(A8)
visual 64–5(Q8)
attention deficit hyperactivity disorder
    (ADHD) 228(Q8), 308(Q8), 384(Q16)
    heritability 417(Q76)
    methylphenidate in 409–10(Q7)
    Multimodal Treatment Study (MTS)
        412(Q36)
    risk factors 414(Q52)
    substance abuse and 428(Q200)
    treatment 414(Q52)
attenuation model (Treisman's) 64(Q6),
    66(A8)
attitudes 95(Q4), 95(Q5)
    measurement 95(Q4)
attorney, power of 343–4(Q6), 344(Q7)
attribution, types, and emotions 60(Q8),
    60(Q9)
attrition 18(Q20)
attunement 12(Q8)
AUDIT (Alcohol Use Disorders Inventory)
    221–2(Q5)
auditory attention, selective 64–5(Q8)
auditory cortex, primary 112(Q6),
    121(Q2), 122(Q3)
auditory hallucinations 363(Q96),
    364(Q112)
    Parkinson's disease therapy and
        179(Q4)
    schizophrenia 104(Q9), 387(Q52)
    third-person 363(Q96), 386(Q34),
        387(Q52), 387(Q52)
auditory operational processing 122(Q3),
    122(Q4), 122(Q5)
auditory pathway 121(Q2), 122(Q3)
Auditory Verbal Learning Test (AVLT)
    353(Q3)
auras, complex partial seizures 389(Q66)
authoritarian personality theory
    361(Q86)
autism 314(Q7)
    genetic counselling 426(Q168)
    heritability 391(Q92), 426(Q168)
    hyperkinetic disorder with 409(Q5)
    stereotyped behaviour 416(Q65)
    stimulants effect 412(Q31)
autistic speech 87–8(Q7)
autobiographical memory 84(Q6)
autochthonous delusion see delusion(s),
    primary
autoerotic, term 212(Q12)
autoerotic asphyxia 220(A9)
autogynaephilia 215(Q1)
autoimmune disorder 196(Q10)
autokinetic effect 78(Q8)
automatic obedience 354(Q11)
automatism 335(Q14)
    legal, punishment 417(Q77)
    somnambulism and 417(Q77),
        434(A72)
autonomy, patient's 358(Q54)
autonomy vs shame or doubt 369(Q179)
autosomal dominant cerebellar ataxia
    177(A8)

autosomal dominant disorders 383(Q4)
  learning disability 313(Q3), 411(Q26)
  movement disorders 180(Q9), 182(Q26)
autosomal recessive disorders 159(Q1),
    159(Q2), 159(Q3), 174(Q12), 411(Q26)
  learning disability 313(Q3)
  movement disorders 180(Q9), 182(Q26)
aversive conditioning 365(Q120),
    365-6(Q124)
avoidance learning 69(Q15), 69(Q16),
    69(Q18)
avoidant personality disorder 205(Q1)
awareness 51-4
  impairment states 169(Q2)
Ax, AF, fear and anger 59(Q5)
axonal transport 118(Q6)

babbling 88(Q8), 359(Q68)
baby battering 336(Q27)
backward selection 21(Q43)
baclofen 258-9(Q16)
bacterial meningitis 175(Q15), 175(Q16),
    175(Q17)
Baddeley's working memory model
    65(Q11)
Balint group 283(Q2)
Balint's syndrome 169(Q3)
Bandura, Albert 43(Q1), 95(Q1),
    436(A102)
barbiturates 258(Q9)
  EEG pattern associated 395(Q144)
bargaining stage (Kübler-Ross) 251(Q4),
    251-2(Q6)
baroreceptors 123(Q10)
basal forebrain 113-14(Q24)
basal ganglia 113(Q15), 144(Q26)
  connections 114(Q26)
  infarct, depression 417(Q79)
  spongiform change 179(Q2)
basal ganglia-thalamocortical circuit
    113(Q16), 113(Q17)
basal metabolic rate 74(Q7)
basic assumption mentality (Bion's)
    270(Q10), 270(Q12)
Bateman, A 205(Q5)
Bateson, G 275(Q2)
battering mother 417(Q78)
Beard, George 4(Q8)
Beck, Aaron 192(Q12), 287(Q4)
Beck Depression Inventory (BDI)
    221-2(Q5)
before-after studies 17(Q16)
behaviour
  acute disturbances 249(Q1), 249(Q2)
  analysis, Skinner and 69(Q20)
  challenging, in learning disability
    426(Q163)
  control, frontal lobe region 170(Q9)
  dysfunctional, psychotherapy
    269(Q2)
  gender-typed in child 419(Q102)
  integrated, neurophysiology 121-5
  late-onset delinquent 389(Q74)
  law of effect and 68(Q8)
  non-regulatory, sexual 123(Q8)
  problems in preschool children
    308(Q7)

  purpose, in marital therapy 279(Q2)
  sexual 123(Q8)
  stereotyped 412(Q31), 416(Q65)
behavioural development
  attachment see attachment behaviour
  gene-environment interaction 43(Q1)
behavioural techniques 365(Q114)-
    366(Q126)
behaviourism 49(Q2), 67(Q1)
Behçet's disease 180(Q10)
beliefs 78-9(Q11)
Bell's palsy 174(Q6)
belonging, motive 74(Q9)
Benlate 228(Q8)
benzamides, substituted 259(Q18),
    259(Q19)
Benzedrine (amphetamine) 4(Q13)
benzodiazepines 207(Q3)
  adverse reaction 260(Q34)
  alcohol interaction 260(Q32)
  binding sites 301(Q5)
  discovery 369(Q186)
  EEG pattern 395(Q140)
  floppy baby syndrome 428(Q199)
  opiate detoxification 302(Q16)
bereaved, care of 251-4
bereavement 252(Q8), 252(Q10),
    415(Q60)
  dual-process model of coping 252(Q9)
  four-phase model 252(Q11)
  outcomes 252(Q12)
  researchers on 252(Q9), 252-3(Q13)
  stress of 361(Q81)
  theory, psychosocial transition
    252(Q9)
  Two-Track Model 252(Q9), 252(Q10)
  see also grief
Berkson's bias 18(Q20)
bestiality 212(Q13)
beta activity, EEG 138(Q8)
beta-adrenoceptors 144(Q25)
  beta-blockers 176(Q22), 207(Q3)
beta-amyloid protein 151(Q6), 160(Q14)
Bethlem 3(Q4), 4(Q8)
bias 17-18(Q19), 18(Q20), 418(Q85)
  avoidance in randomization 409(Q4)
  confounding 389(Q67)
  measurement 419(Q101)
  minimization 419(Q101)
  publication 413(Q39)
  types 18(Q20)
biastophilia 218(Q8)
bifrontal triphasic waves 137-8(Q6),
    138(Q7)
binary data 23(A4)
binomial distribution 15(Q2)
  model 18(Q25)
bioavailability, drugs 257(Q2)
Bion, Wilfred 270(Q10), 270(Q12),
    283(Q3)
bipolar disorder
  carbamazepine side-effect 355(Q22)
  diagnosis and classification 191(Q1)
  diuretics in 385(Q25)
  dysphagia and sodium valproate
    355(Q28)
  ethnicity and 31(Q5)

  gender ratio 31(Q4)
  heritability 160(Q13), 386(Q38)
  lithium treatment see lithium
  mood stabilizers 260(Q31)
  prophylaxis (anticonvulsant)
    367(Q150)
  psoriasis in 386(Q39)
  rapid-cycling 192(Q9), 367(Q155),
    367(Q156)
  renal failure and 390-1(Q83)
  severity/diagnostic rating 192(Q10)
  sleep deprivation effect 239(Q16)
  suicide and 192(Q13), 244(Q9),
    244(Q14)
  therapy 367(Q149), 367(Q151),
    367(Q153), 367(Q154), 367(Q155),
    367(Q156)
    breastfeeding and 422(Q123)
    see also lithium
  see also depression/depressive disorder;
    mania
bipolar I disorder 191(Q1)
bipolar II disorder 191(Q1)
bisphosphonates 203(Q6)
bitemporal hemianopia 357(Q43)
blepharospasm 354(Q16), 366(Q134)
Bleuler, Paul Eugen 3(Q6), 4(Q9),
    187(Q1), 366(Q139)
  'four A's' 4(Q9), 187(Q1)
  origin of term schizophrenia 354(Q14),
    366(Q139)
  'split mind' theory of schizophrenia
    353(Q1)
block design, WAIS subtest 175(Q18)
blood-brain barrier 384(Q17)
blood oxygen level-dependent (BOLD)
  signal 402(A52)
blood pressure 123(Q10), 134(Q7)
  monitoring 249(Q2)
  in NREM sleep 52(Q10)
body dysmorphic disorder 12(Q8),
    199(Q4)
body mass 75(A7)
body mass index (BMI) 361(Q84)
body temperature
  core temperature 133(Q2)
  interval scale 15(Q2)
  monitoring, acute behavioural
    disturbance 249(Q2)
Bonferroni correction 21(Q37)
Boolean logic symbols 33(Q2)
bootstrapping 17(Q18)
borderline personality disorder 205(Q4),
    205(Q6), 356(Q33), 364(Q107),
    369(Q191)
  symptoms 387(Q43)
  therapy 385(Q20), 387(Q43)
    dialectical behaviour therapy
    269(Q3), 388(Q53)
Bowlby, Sir John 252(Q11), 252-3(Q13),
    273(Q4)
Bowlby's attachment theory 43(Q1)
box plot 19(Q26), 22(Q46)
Braddick, OJ 78(Q8)
Bradford-Hill criteria 18(Q21)
brain
  anatomical loops 114(Q26)

anatomy, neuroimaging 155(Q1), 156(Q10)
   see also neuroanatomy
chemistry, neuroimaging 155(Q1), 156(Q10)
hypoxic-ischaemic injury 127(Q4)
neurone number 117(Q1)
scans 414(Q54)
tumours 137(Q3), 357(Q43)
brain-derived neurotrophic factor (BDNF) 146(Q40)
brain fag 368(Q162)
brainstem damage/lesions 173–4(Q5)
   generalized slow waves 137(Q3)
brainstem nuclei 133(Q4)
breach confidentiality 396(Q168)
breastfeeding 422(Q123)
British Misuse of Drugs Regulations (2001) 301(Q3), 301(Q4)
Brixton test 385–6(Q29)
Broadbent's theory 63(Q5)
Broca's aphasia (dysphasia) 170(Q7), 170(Q8), 170(Q11)
Broca's area, lesion 38(Q10)
Brodmann area 4 111(Q1)
Brodmann area 17 112(Q6)
Brodmann areas 44 and 45 111(Q3)
Brown–Goodwin Assessment (BGA) 336(Q23)
Brown–Peterson technique 83(Q4)
Bucknill, J 3(Q5)
bulbar palsy 378(A110)
bulimia nervosa 203(Q2), 203(Q3)
   in anorexia nervosa patients 411–12(Q28)
   first-line treatment 203(Q4)
   fluoxetine 203(Q6)
   psychotherapy 412(Q32)
     CBT 269(Q5)
     interpersonal therapy 388(Q55)
buprenorphine 302(Q16), 388–9(Q64)
   legal classification 302–3(Q17)
bupropion 418(Q83)
buspirone 387(Q45)
butyrylcholinesterase inhibitor 389(Q72)
bystander effect 95(Q2)

CADASIL 151(Q3), 174(Q8), 180(Q11), 427(Q182), 435(A80)
Cade, J 192(Q13)
Caesarean section, in anorexia nervosa 414(Q47)
caffeine 257(Q4)
   dependence 260(Q33)
   effects on sleep 237(Q5), 238(Q8)
caffeine-induced sleep disorder 165(Q1), 237(Q5)
CAGE questionnaire 221–2(Q5)
calcium ions 117(Q2), 144(Q22)
calculation, subcortical dementia 410(Q14)
California Verbal Learning Test (CVLT) 353(Q3)
Camberwell Assessment of Need - Clinical Version 321(Q4)
Camberwell Family Interview 386(Q32)

cAMP response element binding protein(CREB) 146(Q40)
cancer, survival, stress effect 56(Q10)
cannabinoid, binding sites 301(Q1)
cannabinoid system 141(Q5)
cannabis 141(Q4), 329(Q1)
   intoxication 302(Q15)
   legal classification 301(Q4)
   schizophrenia and 187–8(Q7), 363(Q97), 411(Q20)
   screening for 411(Q20)
canonical correlation analysis 21–2(Q45)
carbamazepine 360(Q71)
   discovery 369(Q185)
   electrolyte abnormalities and 355(Q22)
   first use in mania 369(Q184)
   hypothyroidism association 182(Q24)
   MAOIs interactions 360(Q74)
   SIADH association 418(Q91)
carbon dioxide, PCO_2 134(Q7)
carbon monoxide poisoning 180(Q13)
carboxyhaemoglobin 180(Q13)
cardiac arrest 437(A104)
carotid dissection 174–5(Q13)
CART 21–2(Q45)
case–control study 17(Q14), 17(Q17), 418(Q85), 424–5(Q144), 424–5(Q145)
case vignettes 179–80(Q6)
castration, consent 338(Q38)
casuists 360(Q72)
cataplexy 238(Q10), 238(Q11)
catastrophizing 288(Q7)
catatonia 359(Q64), 366(Q135)
catatonic schizophrenia 104(Q8), 372(A16)
catatonic symptoms 354(Q16)
cat faeces, toxoplasmosis and 181(Q19)
catharsis 283–4(Q5)
CATIE trial 187(Q5)
Cattell's second-order factors 92(Q7)
cauda equina, neuroepithelial tumours 152(Q11)
caudate nucleus 113(Q15)
   atrophy 151(Q7), 398(Q193)
causal inference, Bradford-Hill criteria 18(Q21)
cautioning 418(Q89)
CB receptors 141(Q5)
cell division 134(Q7)
central nervous system cells 113(Q22)
central pontine myelinolysis 181(Q17)
central tendency, measures 413(Q37)
cerebellar dysfunction 173(Q3), 357(Q45)
cerebellum, neuroepithelial tumours 152(Q11)
cerebral blood flow 196(Q10)
   ECT effect 265(Q3)
   neuroimaging 155(Q1), 156(Q10)
   'shivers-down-the-spine' inducing music 291(Q4)
cerebral cortex
   embryology 127(Q2), 127(Q3), 127(Q4)
   see also brain
cerebral hemispheres
   dominant, praxis 170(Q11)

left
   language 170(Q8)
   lesions 374(A53)
   neuroepithelial tumours 151–2(Q8), 152(Q11)
   right, lesions 374(A53)
cerebral infarcts 417(Q79)
cerebral plasticity 127–8
cerebrospinal fluid (CSF)
   analysis 175(Q19)
   appearance 175(Q16)
   in CJD 181(Q20)
   5-HIAA and suicide 244(Q8)
   in meningitis and encephalitis 175(Q16), 175(Q17)
   protein levels 175(Q17), 181(Q20)
cervical adenocarcinoma 227–8(Q6)
cervicogenic tension headache 173(Q1)
C fibres 233–4(Q5)
CGG repeats 185(A26), 389(Q70)
chaining 365(Q122)
Chancery Division, High Court 343(Q3)
character neurosis 337(Q31)
chargrilled meat, CYP1A2 induction 258(Q12)
chemicals, multiple chemical sensitivity 227(Q3)
cherry-red discoloration 180(Q13)
child abuse 221(Q2), 336(Q27)
   defence mechanisms and 395(Q149)–396(Q155)
   persistent effects 43(Q5)
   rates of death 307–8(Q6)
   sexual *see* sexual abuse
childhood sexuality 212(Q12)
child protection 307–8(Q6)
child psychiatry 307–11
children
   anxiety disorders 309(Q16)
   CBT in 269(Q5)
   depression 308(Q11)
   difficult 43(Q6), 44(Q7), 44(Q8)
   divorce impact on 420(Q110)
   easy 43(Q6), 44(Q8)
   EEG 137(Q5)
   encopresis and enuresis 411(Q24)
   Mozart effect and 291(Q5)
   obsessive-compulsive disorder 308(Q12)
   prevalence of mental disorders 389(Q73)
   schizophrenia 308(Q13)
   sleepwalking 416(Q72)
   slow-to-warm-up 43(Q6), 44(Q8)
   stigma 355(Q23)
   suicide attempts 244(Q14)
   temperament 43(Q6), 44(Q7), 44(Q8)
child-stealing 416(Q64), 436(A92)
China
   dementia prevalence 105(Q15)
   neurasthenia 104(Q11)
   suicide rate 246(A4)
chi-squared test 20(Q32), 20(Q34), 20(Q35), 21(Q38), 21(Q41), 420(Q106), 423(Q126)
chloral hydrate 4(Q11), 8(A11)
chlordiazepoxide 369(Q186)

chloride ions 117(Q3), 143(Q17)
chlorpromazine 4(Q11), 60(Q7), 259(Q18)
cholecystokinin (CCK) 129(Q4), 145(Q35)
    receptors 145(Q35)
choline 142-3(Q12), 258(Q14), 258(Q15)
    MR spectroscopy 156(Q12)
choline acetyltransferase 141(Q3),
    142-3(Q12)
cholinergic pathway 113-14(Q24)
cholinesterase inhibitors see
    acetylcholinesterase inhibitors
chorea 173(Q4)
chorea gravidarum 207(Q2)
choreic movements 353-4(Q9)
choreoacanthocytosis 182(Q26)
choroid plexus cells 113(Q22)
chrematistophilia 218(Q9)
chromatolysis, central 151(Q1)
chromosomal abnormalities 160(Q8),
    160(Q12), 160(Q16), 384(Q9),
    393(Q112)-393(Q114)
    Down syndrome see Down syndrome
    Huntington's disease 160(Q12),
        353-4(Q9)
    Prader-Willi syndrome 390(Q77)
    Robertsonian translocation 412(Q35)
    trisomy 21 and non-disjunction
        383(Q7)
chronic fatigue syndrome see myalgic
    encephalomyelitis
chunking, memory 83(Q2)
Churg-Strauss syndrome 432(A40)
cigarette smoke 258(Q9)
ciliary ganglion 112(Q8)
cingulate gyrus 113(Q18)
circadian rhythm 51(Q4), 133-4(Q5)
circularities, interaction pattern 275(Q3),
    275-6(Q5)
circular questioning 275-6(Q5)
cirrhosis 302(Q13)
citalopram 258(Q8), 418(Q83), 422(Q123)
citrulline 122(Q6)
civil law 343(Q1), 347(Q1)
civil treatment orders 338(Q39),
    338(Q40), 338(Q41), 338(Q42)
clarification, psychodynamic therapy
    396(Q165), 396(Q168)
classification and regression tree analysis
    21-2(Q45)
classification of mental disorders 165-7
    see also DSM-IV-TR; ICD-10
Cleckley, H 337(Q31)
Clinical Antipsychotic Trials of
    Intervention Effectiveness (CATIE)
    359-60(Q70)
clinical psychology 49(Q3)
clinical psychopharmacology 257-63
clinical trials
    randomization not possible 16(Q13)
    type for SSRIs 16(Q10)
    see also randomized controlled trials
        (RCT)
clitoral engorgement, in REM sleep
    52(Q10)
clomipramine, metabolism 106(Q20)
clonazepam 239(Q20)
close-ended questions 357(Q49)

clozapine 145(Q32), 187(Q4), 187(Q5)
    anti-suicidal effect 244(Q15)
    indications 363(Q102)
    introduction (historical) 4(Q12)
    metabolism 258(Q8)
    side-effects 260(Q34), 384(Q16),
        392(Q97), 392(Q100)
        life-threatening 249(Q7)
    therapeutic drug monitoring 258(Q13)
    treatment-resistant psychosis 321(Q5)
cluster analysis 22(Q45)
cluster headache 173(Q1)
cluster randomized trial 16(Q13)
cluster sampling 424(Q135)
coarctation of aorta 426(Q164)
cocaine
    binding sites 301(Q1)
    legal classification 301(Q3), 301(Q4)
    misuse, psychotherapy 269(Q4)
cochlea 122(Q3)
cochlear hair cells 121(Q2)
cochlear nuclear complex 121(Q2)
Cochrane Collaboration 413(Q39)
'cock-walk' 181(Q15)
codeine 251(Q2), 301(Q3)
coeliac disease 428(Q193)
coenaesthesia 12(Q8)
coeruleospinal pathway 114(Q25)
cognitive analytical therapy (CAT)
    205(Q5)
cognitive approach, personality 91(Q4)
cognitive assessment 37(Q3), 37(Q5),
    169-71
cognitive-behavioural therapy (CBT)
    269(Q2), 287-9
    in bulimia nervosa 203(Q4)
    evidence-based effectiveness 269(Q5),
        297(Q1)
    five-areas assessment model 287(Q1)
    in OCD 395(Q146)
    in persistent somatoform pain disorder
        234(Q6)
    trial/research methods 16(Q10)
cognitive-behaviour marital therapy
    279(Q3), 279-80(Q4), 280(Q5)
cognitive development 87(Q1)
    theory 43(Q1)
cognitive dissonance theory 95(Q4),
    358(Q60)
cognitive distortions 191(Q3), 287(Q5),
    287-8(Q6), 288(Q7)
cognitive epistemology, Piaget's model
    44(Q9), 44(Q10)
Cognitive Estimates Test 38(Q9)
cognitive framing 392(Q96)
cognitive impairment
    cannabis association 141(Q4)
    head injury and 357(Q41)
    schizophrenia 37(Q1)
    type 1 vs type 2 diabetes 418(Q88)
cognitive labelling theory 60(Q7)
cognitive models 287(Q4)
    personality 92(Q9)
cognitive processes 287(Q3)
cognitive psychology 49(Q4)
cognitive representation 392(Q99)
cognitive screening test 319(A6)

cognitive triad 192(Q12)
cogwheel rigidity 180-1(Q14)
Cohen's kappa 15(Q3)
cohesion, group success and 273(Q5)
cohort study 424-5(Q146)
    prospective/retrospective 17(Q17)
collective unconscious 273(Q2)
colours, focal, language and 87(Q3),
    87(Q4)
colour vision, development 359(Q68)
coma, EEG pattern 394(Q132)
comfort eating 233(Q4)
commentary, running 364(Q112)
common fate, Gestalt laws of perception
    77(Q1)
common law 343(Q1)
communication
    persuasive 364(Q106)
    styles, schizophrenia risk 187-8(Q7)
community reinforcement approaches
    269(Q4)
compensation, for psychiatric damage
    344(Q9)
compensation neurosis 362(Q88)
competence, impression of stranger
    95(Q6)
competence motives 74(Q10)
complex, Jung's concept 273(Q4)
comprehension
    in dysphasias 170(Q7)
    WAIS subtest 175(Q18)
compulsions 395(Q145), 395(Q146)
    autism and 416(Q65)
    most common 395(Q148)
    see also obsessive-compulsive disorder
        (OCD)
computed tomography (CT) 155(Q1)
computed tomography (CT) angiography
    175(Q19)
Comte, Auguste 11(Q1)
COMT gene 106(Q20)
concentration, assessment 37(Q3)
concrete operations stage 44(Q9),
    44(Q10)
conditioned reflexes 37(Q6)
conditioning 67(Q1), 169(Q4)
    aversive 365(Q120), 365-6(Q124)
    backward 67(Q3), 68(Q6)
    classical 67(Q2), 67(Q3), 69(Q15)
    escape 379(A124)
    operant 68(Q7), 73(Q4)
    Pavlovian 67(Q2), 67(Q4), 67-8(Q5)
    strength 68(Q7)
conduct disorder 308(Q7), 333(Q4),
    411(Q19)
    aggression with, therapy 426(Q171)
    antisocial personality disorder risk
        414(Q50)
conduction dysphasia 170(Q7)
confidence interval 17-18(Q19), 19(Q29),
    31(Q2), 410-11(Q17), 419(Q97),
    421(Q112)
confidentiality 344(Q11), 360(Q77)
    disclosures, reasons 344(Q11)
conformity, influencing factors 361(Q85)
confounding, residual 18(Q21)
confounding bias 389(Q67)

confounding factors 418(Q85)
confusional state 137(Q3)
congenital adrenal hyperplasia 217(Q3)
Conolly, John 4(Q7)
consciousness
    impaired 221(Q3)
    primary/secondary 51(Q1)
    research 51(Q2)
consent to treatment 338(Q37), 338(Q38)
consequentialist approach 360(Q77)
consistency 95(Q3)
CONSORT diagram 16(Q12)
constipation 251(Q3), 302(Q14)
constructivist theory 78(Q9)
consultant psychiatrist 359(Q66),
    360(Q76)
consultation 359(Q65)
containment, psychodynamic therapy
    396(Q164)
content validity 15(Q5)
context and expectations, perceptual set
    78-9(Q11)
contiguity, law of 69(Q17)
contingency table 20(Q34), 21(Q37)
continuity, law of 80(A7)
contracoup head injury 391(Q91)
control event risk 33-4(Q6)
conus medullaris, neuroepithelial tumours
    151-2(Q8)
Conversational Model, art therapy
    291(Q3)
conversion disorders see dissociative
    (conversion) disorders
coping
    adaptive 55-6(A6), 56(Q9)
    dual-process model 252(Q9)
    emotion-focused 56(Q8)
    intrapsychic 56(Q8)
    maladaptive 55-6(A6), 56(Q9)
    strategies 56(Q8)
    types 55-6(A6), 56(Q9)
copper metabolism, disorder 174(Q12)
coprolalia 416(Q67)
coprophagia 416(Q67)
copy number variation 16(Q13)
core beliefs 287(Q4)
core-optional theory 54(A14)
cornea, sensory innervation 112(Q10)
Cornelia de Lange syndrome 314(Q10)
corona radiata 114(Q27)
coronary artery disease, depression and
    414(Q51)
corpus striatum 113(Q15)
correlation coefficient 21(Q39), 416(Q73)
correspondence analysis 22(Q45)
Corti, Alfonso Giacomo Gaspare 127(Q1)
cortical plate 128(A3)
cortical-striatal-thalamic-cortical loops
    114(Q26)
corticofugal fibres 114(Q25)
corticoneurogenesis 127(Q1)
corticotrophin-releasing hormone (CRH)
    129(Q4), 130(Q9)
    stimulation test 130(Q9)
cortisol 130(Q7), 130(Q9)
    receptors 129(Q6)
cosmetic surgery 329(Q2), 329(Q3)

cost-benefit analysis 390(Q81),
    424(Q142)
cost-effectiveness acceptability curve
    (CEAC) 26(A18)
cost-effectiveness analysis 17(Q15),
    17(Q18), 424(Q139)
cost-effectiveness plane 17(Q18)
cost-minimization analysis 424(Q140),
    424(Q141)
co-transcriptional processing 21(Q44)
counselling, client-centred 92(Q11)
countershock phase 56(Q7)
countertransference 273(Q1)
court, evidence by mentally disordered
    person 343-4(Q6)
court of protection order 427(Q189)
Courts of Justice 343(Q2)
cranial fossae 111(Q2), 111(Q5)
cranial nerves 112(Q7), 112(Q8), 112(Q9),
    112(Q10), 112(Q12)
    accessory nerve damage 174(Q6)
    palsy 173(Q2), 174(Q6), 358-9(Q61),
        366(Q127), 366(Q129)
Creutzfeldt-Jakob disease (CJD)
    181(Q20), 317(Q20)
    EEG 137-8(Q6), 175(Q19), 394(Q123)
    neuropathology 151(Q4), 388(Q60),
        403(A80)
cribriform plate 111(Q2)
Crick and Mitchison's reverse learning
    54(A14)
cri-du-chat syndrome 393(Q114)
crime 334(Q10), 364(Q105)
    age/gender relationship 333(Q2)
    left realism and 100(Q12)
    motivation 334(Q7)
    victims 321(Q2)
    see also offenders
criminal anthropology 4(Q8)
criminal courts (England/Wales)
    343(Q2)
Criminal Justice Act 2003 218(Q12)
Criminal Justice and Court Services Act
    2000 218(Q12)
criminal law 343(Q1), 347(Q1)
criminal responsibility, age of 334(Q9)
criminology 333(Q3)
criterion validity 15(Q5)
critical appraisal 9(Q2), 9(Q3)
    GATE frame 33(Q3)
Crohn's disease 428(Q194)
Cronbach's alpha 15(Q4)
cross-dressing 215(Q2), 217(Q5)
cross-modal analysis 122(Q4), 122(Q5)
crossover trials 16(Q13)
cross-sectional study 17(Q15), 17(Q17),
    424-5(Q147)
Crown Courts 343(Q2)
crying, pathological 420(Q105)
CST3 gene 151(Q3)
CTG repeat 160(Q16), 185(A26)
cue-dependent forgetting 84(Q11)
cues
    meaningless sensory 79(Q13)
    non-pictorial 77(Q3)
    pictorial 77(Q4)
Cullen, William 195(Q5)

culturally neutral observations 103-
    4(Q3)
cultural psychiatry 103-8, 104(Q4)
culture(s)
    dementia and 105(Q15)
    focal colours 87(Q4)
    pharmacodynamics/pharmacokinetics
        106(Q20)
    psychiatric disorders 104(Q11),
        105(Q14), 105(Q15)
    psychiatric symptoms 104(Q7)
    schizophrenia rates 104(Q5)
    suicide and 105(Q16), 105(Q17),
        105(Q18)
    see also ethnic group; ethnocultural
        groups
culture-bound disorders 105(Q12),
    105(Q13), 105(Q14)
Cushing's syndrome 409(Q2)
    neuropsychiatric feature 181(Q21),
        409(Q2)
    symptoms 369-70(Q199)
CUtLASS 1 trial 187(Q5)
CUtLASS 2 trial 187(Q5)
cyclic GMP 212(Q7)
cyclizine 252(Q7)
cycloid psychosis 366(Q136)
CYP1A2 257(Q4), 258(Q8), 258(Q9)
    inducers 258(Q9), 258(Q12)
CYP2C9, inducers 258(Q12)
CYP2C19 257(Q6), 258(Q8)
CYP2D6 257(Q4), 257(Q6), 258(Q7),
    258(Q8), 258(Q9), 259(Q25),
    384(Q14)
    allele 105-6(Q19), 106(Q20)
    inducers 258(Q9)
CYP3A4 257(Q4), 257(Q5), 258(Q8),
    258(Q9), 259(Q25), 384(Q14)
    allele 106(Q20)
    inducers 258(Q9)
    reboxetine metabolism 386(Q37)
cyproheptadine 249(Q8)
cytochrome enzymes 257(Q4), 257(Q5),
    257-8(Q6), 258(Q7), 258(Q8),
    258(Q9), 384(Q14)
    inducers 258(Q9), 258(Q12)
    see also entries beginning CYP
cytosine 159(Q6), 159-60(Q7)

D2 receptor see dopamine receptors
data, types 15(Q1), 15(Q2)
DaTSCAN 364(Q113)
daytime sleepiness 237(Q6), 238(Q10)
debriefing, in PTSD 234(Q6)
decay theory, forgetting 84(Q11)
Declaration of Helsinki 437(A109)
declarative memory 84(Q7), 169(Q4)
defence mechanisms 395(Q149)-
    395(Q155), 396(Q156)-396(Q163)
    in narcissistic personality disorder
        353(Q5)
    neurotic 396(Q159)
defensive strategy, kleptomania 336(Q26)
degrees of freedom 19(Q29), 20(Q34),
    420(Q106)
dehydration 221(Q1)
déjà vu 368(Q172)

delayed ejaculation 212(Q8)
delayed post-anoxic leucoencephalopathy 179(Q2)
delayed sleep phase syndrome 384(Q10)
deliberate self-harm *see* self-harm
delinquent behaviour 412(Q36)
  late-onset, risk factors 389(Q74)
delirium 221(Q3), 317(Q5), 415(Q61)
  postoperative, reduction 421(Q116)
  postpartum 208(Q10)
  pregnancy complication 207(Q2)
  in toxic/metabolic disorders 181(Q17)
delta waves 52(Q6)
delusion(s)
  duration 358(Q57)
  of infidelity 337(Q29)
  nihilistic 357(Q46)
  partition 318(Q11)
  primary 13(A5), 360(Q75)
  secondary 13(A5), 221(Q3)
  understandable 11(Q5)
delusional atmosphere 11(Q5)
delusional awareness 11(Q5)
delusional disorders 358(Q57)
delusional idea 11(Q5)
delusional perception 11(Q5), 354(Q15)
delusional states, chronic, pregnancy and 208(Q8)
'delusion-like ideas' 11(Q5)
'delusions proper' 11(Q5)
dementia
  causes 317(Q1), 317(Q2), 317(Q5), 417(Q81)
  co-morbid conditions, screening 317(Q4)
  cortical 429(A14)
  Down syndrome and 397(Q177)
  EEG 137-8(Q6), 138(Q7)
  eosinophilic inclusion bodies 418(Q86)
  focal, EEG 138(Q7)
  folate deficiency 317(Q3)
  frontotemporal *see* frontotemporal lobar dementia (FTLD)
  Lewy body *see* Lewy body dementia
  mild, testamentary capacity 343(Q4)
  mild cognitive impairment relationship 388(Q62)
  in Pancoast's tumour 412(Q33)
  prevalence 105(Q15), 317(Q7)
  prevention 410(Q13)
  in progressive supranuclear palsy 179-80(Q6)
  in sarcoidosis 179(Q3)
  screening, probabilities and 414(Q55), 415(Q62)
  sleep patterns 239(Q18)
  subcortical 410(Q14)
  vascular 317(Q2), 427(Q179)
  in vitamin B12 deficiency 179(Q1)
dementia paralytica 4(Q7)
dementia praecox 354(Q14), 366(Q137)
dementia pugilistica 151(Q6), 394(Q131)
demyelination, diffuse white matter 179(Q2)
denial 273(Q1), 395(Q153)
dentate nucleus, discoloration 152(Q10)

dentatorubralpallidoluysian atrophy (DRPLA) 180(Q9)
deoxyhaemoglobin 155(Q6)
dependent personality disorder 205(Q3)
depersonalization 99(Q6), 355(Q21)
depolarization 117(Q4), 118(Q6)
depression/depressive disorder 191(Q3)
  anxiety with 195(Q1), 394(Q127)
  causes 191(Q4), 192(Q7), 369(Q193)
  children/adolescents 308(Q11), 309(Q16)
  chronic, MRI 398(Q197)
  chronic pain and 233(Q3)
  clinical features 191(Q6), 196(Q8)
    core and common symptoms 191(Q5), 191(Q6), 192(Q14)
  cognitive processes associated 287(Q3)
  in coronary artery disease 414(Q51)
  Cushing's syndrome 181(Q21), 409(Q2)
  diagnosis in ICD-10 191(Q5), 192(Q14)
  differential diagnosis 196(Q8)
  Down syndrome and 397(Q176)
  drugs associated with 192(Q7)
  duration of episodes 191(Q4)
  elderly people 394(Q129)
  epidemiology 394(Q127), 394(Q128), 394(Q129)
    prevalence 104(Q11)
  gender differences 191(Q4)
  HPA axis in 130(Q7), 130(Q9)
  hypothyroidism and 191(Q2)
  infarcts causing 417(Q79)
  late-onset, aetiology 369(Q195)
  learned helplessness and 69(Q19)
  major 191(Q6)
    grief relationship 415(Q60)
  management 192(Q8)
    NICE guidelines 414(Q48)
    NICE stepped-care model 192(Q8)
    NIMH Treatment program 297(Q2)
  postnatal/postpartum *see* postnatal depression
  prednisolone-related 418(Q90)
  prepartum 207(Q5)
  psychological defences 269-70(Q8), 270(Q11)
  questionnaire 221-2(Q5)
  as reaction to loss 191(Q3)
  rebound, hypnosis and 384(Q13)
  severe, ECT for 265(Q5)
  sick role and 361(Q80)
  sleep control 238-9(Q14), 239(Q15), 239(Q16)
  social origins/factors 191(Q4), 363(Q100)
  spontaneous abortion and 208(Q8)
  suicide and 244(Q9)
  therapy 386(Q35), 386(Q36), 386(Q37)
    antidepressants and thyroxine, ECG 397-8(Q190)
    CBT in 269(Q5)
    failure to respond 414(Q48)
    prevalence 394(Q128)
  thinking, changes in 287(Q2)
  vulnerability factors 100(Q8)
  weight loss and disorders causing in 428(Q192)-428(Q195)

depressive episode, major 191(Q6), 415(Q60)
'depressive position' 192(Q12), 273(Q2)
Deprivation of Liberty Safeguards 344(Q8)
depth cues
  non-pictorial 77(Q3)
  pictorial 77(Q4)
depth perception 77(Q3), 77(Q4)
Descartes, R 233(Q1)
desensitization
  in agoraphobia 385(Q26)
  systematic 195(Q5), 365(Q116)
Deutsch–Norman theory of focused attention 64(Q7)
development 43-7
  delay 355(Q20)
  environmental exposure effects 228(Q8)
  history of concepts 43(Q1)
  language 44(Q11), 87(Q6), 88(Q8)
  'mirror phase' 273(Q3)
  moral (Kohlberg's) 44(Q12)
  Piaget's model 44(Q9), 44(Q10)
  psychosocial 44(Q13), 44(Q14), 44-5(Q15)
developmental disorders
  DSM-IV-TR axis 307(Q4)
  pervasive 308(Q14)
  specific 308(Q14), 309(Q17)
developmental psychology 49(Q4)
development milestone 359(Q68)
deviance 100(Q10)
Devic's syndrome 432(A40)
dexamethasone 258(Q9)
dexamethasone suppression test (DST) 130(Q10)
dexamphetamine 238(Q10)
diabetes insipidus 412(Q29), 418(Q88)
diabetes mellitus
  antipsychotics in 363(Q102), 364(Q109)
  cognitive impairment in type I *vs* type 2 418(Q88)
  type 2 and weight loss 428(Q192)
diacylglycerol (DAG) 144(Q22)
diagnosis of mental disorders 165-7
diagnostic tests, measures 16(Q8)
dialectical behaviour therapy (DBT) 269(Q3), 297(Q1), 388(Q53)
diamorphine 251(Q2)
  legal classification 302-3(Q17)
diarrhoea 180-1(Q14), 251(Q3), 302(Q14)
diet (healthy), theories/models association 73-4(Q6)
diethylstilboestrol 227-8(Q6)
differential behaviour 283(Q4)
diffusion tensor imaging (DTI) 156(Q10)
DiGeorge syndrome 393(Q113), 411(Q26)
digit span 37(Q3), 175(Q18), 391(Q89)
diphenylbutylpiperidine 259(Q19)
diplopia, symptoms 173(Q2)
DISC1 160(Q16)
discounting the positive 287(Q5)
discreditable deviance 100(Q10)
discredited deviance 100(Q10)
discriminant validity 15(Q5)

discrimination 100(Q10), 321(Q3)
disinfectants 227(Q1)
disinhibition 177(A13)
dissocial personality disorder 337(Q34),
    364(Q105)
dissociative (conversion) disorders
    199–201, 433(A64)
    precipitating factors, age of onset
        199(Q3)
dissociative fugue 199(Q1)
distortion, Ponzo illusion 78(Q6)
disulfiram 260(Q33)
diuretics 385(Q25)
divided attention, Allport's theory 63(Q1)
divorce
    impact on children 420(Q110)
    levels 313(Q4)
DM1 (myotonic dystrophy type 1)
    182(Q26)
D-motives 73(Q2)
DMPK gene 185(A26)
DNA 159(Q6)
    replication 385(Q23)
    structure 159(Q4)
doli incapax 334(Q10)
Dollard, John 95(Q1)
donepezil 145(Q31), 259(Q25), 260(Q34)
    ECG pattern 397–8(Q192)
door-in-the-face technique 95(Q3)
L-dopa 142(Q8)
dopamine 129(Q4), 130(Q11), 134(Q6),
    141(Q2), 142(Q8), 142(Q10)
    metabolism, in violent offenders
        418(Q89)
    pathological gambling and 336(Q22)
    precursor 258(Q14)
dopamine-β-hydroxylase 142(Q8),
    142(Q10)
dopamine receptors 144(Q24)
    D2 receptor 143(Q15), 144(Q24),
        145–6(Q36)
        occupancy level, antipsychotics
            187(Q4)
        partial agonist 260(Q29)
        supersensitivity 386(Q33)
    D3 receptor 144(Q24)
        gene 383(Q5)
    D4 receptor 144(Q24)
dopaminergic pathway 113–14(Q24),
    114(Q25), 114(Q27)
dopamine tracts 141–2(Q7)
dopamine transporter gene 384(Q16)
dorsal striatum 391(Q87)
dorsolateral prefrontal cortex (DLPFC)
    111(Q3), 111(Q4), 114(Q26), 123(Q10)
    in schizophrenia 391(Q86)
dorsomedial nucleus, hypothalamus
    129(Q3)
double-binding 275(Q2), 275(Q3)
double-bind theory 275(Q2)
double burden 99(Q3)
Down syndrome 313(Q3), 313(Q4),
    313–14(Q6), 314(Q7), 315(A3)
    Alzheimer's disease and 369(Q194),
        387(Q46)
    chromosomal translocation and risk
        413(Q46)

co-morbid psychiatric disorders
    397(Q175)–397(Q180)
    epilepsy prevalence 425(Q160)
    schizophrenia and 397(Q179)
    trisomy and non-disjunction 383(Q7)
    unbalanced Robertsonian translocation
        412(Q35)
drapetomania 165(Q1)
dream(s), types 239(Q23)
dreaming
    hallucinations and 52(Q11), 52(Q12)
    intense dream 237(Q4)
    in narcolepsy 238(Q9)
    theories 52(Q13), 52(Q14)
drive-reduction theory 74(Q8)
drive theory 336(Q26)
driving
    elderly people 318(Q11)
    epilepsy and 359(Q67)
    pre-accident behaviour 237(Q6)
    sleep-related accidents 237(Q6)
DRPLA 180(Q9)
drug(s)
    absorption, administration routes
        257(Q1)
    clearance 258(Q10)
    consent to treatment 338(Q37),
        338(Q38)
    dependency 260(Q33)
        bipolar disorder and 31(Q5)
    elimination rate 258(Q10)
    ionized 384(Q17)
    metabolism 257(Q3), 257(Q4), 257(Q6),
        258(Q8), 259(Q24)
    oculogyric crisis associated 249(Q4)
    protein binding 384(Q17)
    sleep disorders associated 237(Q3)
    steady state attainment 258(Q11)
    type A reactions 260(Q34)
    volume of distribution 257(Q2),
        257(Q3), 258(Q10), 384(Q17)
    weight loss associated 428(Q192)
    see also individual drugs/drug groups
drug interactions
    alcohol and benzodiazepines 260(Q32)
    carbamazepine and MAOIs 360(Q74)
    fluoxetine and warfarin 392(Q98)
    lithium and ACE inhibitor 367(Q153)
    oral contraceptives and St John's wort
        391(Q85)
drugs of abuse
    effects on sleep 237(Q5), 238(Q8)
    legal classification 301(Q3), 301(Q4),
        302–3(Q17)
DSM axes 165(Q6)
DSM-II 165(Q2), 165(Q6)
DSM-III 165(Q2)
DSM-III-R 165(Q6)
DSM-IV 91(Q1), 165(Q2), 165(Q6)
DSM-IV-TR 165(Q1), 165(Q3), 165(Q6)
    alcohol withdrawal, diagnosis
        302(Q10)
    axes 165(Q3), 165(Q4), 165–6(Q7)
    bipolar disorders 191(Q1)
    child and adolescent psychiatry
        307(Q4)
    eating disorders 203(Q2)

histrionic personality disorder
    355(Q25)
    major depressive episode 191(Q6)
    paedophilia 218(Q7)
    pervasive developmental disorders
        308(Q14)
    substance abuse diagnosis 302(Q8)
    substance dependence diagnosis
        302(Q9)
    uncomplicated grief vs depression
        433(A60)
D-state 52(Q9)
dual-memory model (multi-store model)
    83(Q3), 83(Q4)
dual-process model of coping 252(Q9)
dual-task performance 65(Q9)
dual-task technique 63(Q2)
duloxetine 257(Q6), 260(Q30), 386(Q36)
Dunedin Multi-Disciplinary Health and
    Development Study 333(Q5)
Durkheim, Emile 11(Q1), 360(Q79)
DVLA 359(Q67)
dying, care of 251–4
    anticipatory drugs 251(Q4), 252(Q7)
dynamic psychotherapy 273–4
    group 273(Q5)
    innovators 273(Q2), 273(Q3), 273(Q4)
dysarthria 38(Q12), 180–1(Q14)
Dysbindin 369(Q192), 383(Q5)
dyscalculia 38(Q11)
dysexecutive syndromes 170(Q10),
    170(Q11), 429(A14)
dysgraphia 170(Q8)
    dyspraxic 38(Q10)
dyslexia 358(Q53)
    deep 170(Q8)
    prevalence 410(Q16)
    surface 170(Q8)
dysmegalopsia 368(Q168)
dyspareunia 165(Q1)
dysphagia 355(Q28)
dysphasia 170(Q6), 170(Q7), 177(A13),
    354(Q10)
    expressive 38(Q10)
    receptive 38(Q10)
dysphoria 251(Q5)
dyspraxia, limb kinetic 170(Q11)
dystonic reactions, acute 249(Q3)

ear-by-ear recall 63(Q3), 63(Q4)
early-selection filter theory (Broadbent)
    63(Q5)
eating disorders 203–4
    culture-bound disorder 105(Q14)
    DSM-IV-TR diagnoses 203(Q2)
    see also anorexia nervosa; bulimia
        nervosa
ebonics 88(Q8)
Ebstein's anomaly 208(Q7)
echoic memory 83(Q1), 83(Q3)
echolalia 355(Q27)
eclampsia, postpartum delirium 208(Q10)
ecological study 17(Q17), 424–5(Q148)
ecstasy (MDMA)
    binding sites 301(Q5)
    class A drug 301(Q3)
edenics 103(Q3)

edic 103(Q3)
Edinburgh Postnatal Depression Scale (EPDS) 428(Q197)
Edward syndrome 160(Q8)
effect measures 33(Q4)
egocentric speech 87–8(Q7)
ego defence 84(Q11)
egodystonic and egosyntonic 336(Q19)
ego-focused emotions 59(Q4)
ego integrity *versus* despair 369(Q183)
eigenvalues 31(Q3)
ejaculatory problems 165(Q1), 212(Q8)
Ekbom's syndrome 239(Q21), 239(Q22)
elaborated code, linguistic 87(Q5)
elderly people
    acute behavioural disturbance 249(Q1)
    Alzheimer's disease 369(Q194)
    anxious personality disorder and suicide 420(Q111)
    depression 394(Q129)
    psychiatry 317–19
electrocardiography (ECG) 358(Q59), 362–3(Q95)
    features, in psychiatric disorders 397(Q188)–398(Q192)
    QRS complex 397–8(Q188)
    ST segment elevation 397–8(Q189), 397–8(Q190)
electroconvulsive therapy (ECT) 207(Q5), 265–6
    bilateral *vs* right 265(Q6)
    consent 338(Q37), 338(Q38)
    EEG pattern associated 395(Q141)
    effects 265(Q3)
    mechanism of action 265(Q2)
    repeated 265(Q4)
electroencephalography (EEG) 51(Q2), 137(Q1), 137–9
    alpha rhythms 51(Q3)
    analytical techniques 138(Q10)
    asymmetries 137(Q5)
    beta activity 138(Q8)
    frequency bands 138(Q10)
    maturational changes 137(Q5)
    number of electrodes 137(Q2)
    patterns and conditions with 393(Q115)–394(Q121), 394(Q122)–394(Q125), 394(Q131)–394(Q134), 394(Q135)–394(Q139), 395(Q140)–395(Q144)
        acute organic states 137–8(Q6)
        dementia 137–8(Q6), 138(Q7)
        during sleep 51–2(Q6), 52(Q7), 238(Q12)
    spike-and-wave discharges 137(Q4)
    triphasic wave 384(Q11), 384(Q12)
electrolyte abnormalities
    carbamazepine and 355(Q22)
    see also hyperkalaemia
electro-oculography (EOG) 240(A1)
Ellenberger, HF 3(Q4)
embryology
    cerebral cortex 127(Q2), 127(Q3), 127(Q4)
    neural crest 392(Q94)
emergency psychiatry 249–50

emic 103(Q3)
emotion(s) 59–61
    attribution types 60(Q8), 60(Q9)
    classification 59(Q1)
    complex 59(Q2), 59(Q3)
    expressed 100(Q8)
    James–Lange theory 59(Q4)
    perceptual defence and 78–9(Q11)
    primary 59(Q1), 59(Q2), 59(Q3), 356(Q31)
emotion accida 59(Q4)
'emotional incontinence' 179–80(Q6)
emotionally focused marital therapy 279(Q2), 279–80(Q4), 280(Q5), 280(Q6)
emotional reasoning 288(Q7)
emotion-focused coping 56(Q8)
empathic statement 358(Q56)
empathy 11(G3)
    psychodynamic therapy 396(Q165), 396(Q169)
encephalitis 359(Q64)
    acute, EEG pattern 394(Q122), 394(Q124)
    causes 175(Q16), 175(Q17)
encoding, auditory operational processing 122(Q4), 122(Q5)
encopresis 411(Q24)
endocannabinoids 141(Q5)
enduring power of attorney 343–4(Q6)
Engel, G 233(Q1)
engineering model 55(Q1)
enuresis 308–9(Q15)
    diurnal 411(Q24)
    encopresis with 411(Q24)
    nocturnal 308–9(Q15), 409(Q1), 419(Q98)
environmental factors
    development, effects on 228(Q8)
    DSM-IV-TR axis 307(Q4)
eosinophilic inclusion bodies 418(Q86)
ependymal cells 113(Q22)
ependymoma, myxopapillary 151–2(Q8)
epicentre 51(Q2), 103(Q3)
epidemiology 31–2
    knowledge and understanding 9(Q2)
    psychiatric disorders in UK 394(Q126)–394(Q130)
    see also individual conditions
epilepsy
    control success 425(Q162)
    driving and 359(Q67)
    idiopathic 307(Q2)
    learning disability and 425(Q162)
    medial temporal lobe 357–8(Q51)
    prevalence
        in Down syndrome 425(Q160)
        in fragile X syndrome 425(Q159)
        in learning disability 313(Q4), 425(Q155), 425(Q156), 425(Q157), 425(Q158)
        in prisons 337(Q33)
episodic memory 37(Q6), 84(Q6), 84(Q7), 169(Q4)
    anterograde, tests 38(Q8)
Epstein–Barr virus (EBV) 181(Q18)
Epston, David 291(Q6)

equity 343(Q1)
erectile dysfunction 211–12(Q6)
erethrism 181(Q16)
Erikson's model, psychosocial development 44(Q13), 44(Q14), 44–5(Q15), 45(Q16), 369(Q178)–369(Q183)
erotophonia 212(Q10)
erythema migrans 416(Q66), 421(Q119)
escape conditioning 379(A124)
Esquirol, E 335(Q18)
essential tremor 173(Q4)
eszopiclone 237(Q2)
ethical medical practice 344(Q11)
ethical principles 356(Q36)
ethics 347–8, 437(A109)
    virtue 356(Q35)
ethmoid bone 111(Q5)
ethnic group
    data category 15(Q1)
    depression prevalence 104(Q11)
    hallucinations in schizophrenia 104(Q9)
    psychiatric symptom rates 104(Q7)
    schizophrenia rates 100(Q11), 104(Q5), 187(Q3)
    see also culture(s)
ethnocultural groups
    acculturation strategies 103(Q1), 103(Q2)
    see also culture(s)
etic 103(Q3)
eustress 55(Q1)
evaluation factor, attitudes 95(Q5)
event-related potentials (ERPs) 138(Q9)
event sampling methodology 424(Q136)
evidence-based medicine 9–10
    competence development 9(Q1)
    critical appraisal 9(Q2), 9(Q3)
    practising 33–5
evoked potentials 137–9
exams, forgetfulness 362(Q93)
excitatory postsynaptic potentials (EPSPs) 117–18(Q5)
excitatory postsynaptic receptors 144(Q26)
excitatory receptors 144(Q26)
exclusion, acculturation strategy 103(Q2)
executive function 114(Q26)
    assessment 170(Q10)
exhibitionism 212(Q13), 219(Q13), 413(Q42), 418(Q93)
    classification 217–18(Q6)
experimental event risk 33(Q4), 33–4(Q6)
experimental neurosis 68(Q6)
explicit memory 169(Q4)
expressed emotion 100(Q8), 101(A10)
expression microarray 383(Q2)
expressive dysphasia 38(Q10)
extinction 386(Q30)
    resistance to 68(Q10)
extracampine hallucination 356(Q37)
extrapyramidal side-effects 260(Q34)
    antipsychotic drugs 38(Q12), 259(Q20)
Exvia-invia 92(Q7)
eye-head system 78(Q8)

eye movements 78(Q8)
  frontal eye field controlling 111(Q1)
  limitation 173(Q2)
Eymard, P 369(Q189)
Eysenck Personality Questionnaire (EPQ)
  91(Q4), 92(Q7)
Eysenck's model of personality 92(Q10)

face processing 138(Q9)
face recognition 386(Q31)
face validity 15(Q5)
facial expression, muscles 112(Q7)
facial nerve (Q9), 112, 112(Q7), 112(Q8),
  112(Q10), 112(Q12)
  palsy 174(Q6)
facial weakness 174(Q6)
factitious disorder 199–200(Q7), 234(Q6)
factor analysis 21(Q44), 31(Q3), 91(Q5)
facultative deviation, paraphilias vs
  217(Q3)
faecal incontinence 309(Q16)
Fagan's nomogram 414(Q55), 415(Q62)
false negatives 16(Q7)
false positives 16(Q7)
family
  homeostasis 275(Q2)
  sexual abuse and 426(Q175),
    426(Q176), 427(Q177), 427(Q178)
family law 347(Q1)
family studies 393(Q107)
family therapy 269(Q1), 275–7,
  396(Q170)–397(Q174), 426(Q174)
  eclectic 396–7(Q174)
  innovators 275(Q2), 275–6(Q5)
  problem-orientated 275(Q1)
  reframing 275(Q3)
  strategic 396–7(Q173)
  structural 397(Q170)
  systemic 275(Q1), 397(Q171),
    397(Q172)
  theory 275(Q3)
fasciectomy 329(Q3)
fatty liver, alcoholic 302(Q13)
F distribution 20(Q33)
fear
  Ax's experiment 59(Q5)
  of darkness, development 359(Q68)
  of heights 196(Q14)
  of parturition 207(Q3)
  of ridicule 361(Q85)
  of strangers 43(Q2)
  see also phobia
fear management
  flooding for 365(Q117)
  reciprocal inhibition 365(Q115)
  systematic desensitization 195(Q5),
    365(Q116)
feature analysis, auditory operational
  processing 122(Q4), 122(Q5)
feedback loops, negative, prolactin
  130(Q11)
feeding neuropeptides 146(Q38)
felt stigma 100(Q10)
female sexual arousal 211(Q4)
female to male ratio see gender
  differences/ratios
fenfluramine 244(Q13)

fentanyl 251(Q2)
fetal alcohol syndrome 207(Q4),
  313–14(Q6), 314(Q7)
fetishism 217(Q2), 217(Q4)
fetishistic transvestism 215(Q2)
fibromyalgia, EEG 137–8(Q6)
fight/flight 270(Q12)
filicide 334(Q12)
finger, reflex, spinal root transmitting
  174(Q7)
fire-setting 426(Q173)
Fisher's exact probability test 21(Q37)
Fisher's transformation 21(Q39)
fissure of Rolando 111(Q4)
five-factor model 92(Q8), 92(Q12),
  385(Q27)
FLAIR 155(Q1)
flight of ideas 362(Q94)
flooding 365(Q117)
floppy infant syndrome 207(Q3),
  428(Q199)
fluency, in dysphasia 170(Q7)
fluid-attenuated inversion recovery MRI
  155(Q1)
fluoxetine 203(Q6), 386(Q35), 390(Q75)
  in breast milk 422(Q123)
  MR spectroscopy 156(Q12)
  pathological crying 420(Q105)
  warfarin interaction 392(Q98)
  weight loss and 428(Q192)
flupentixol 259(Q19)
fluphenazine 259(Q18)
fluvoxamine 258(Q7)
folate, deficiency 317(Q3)
follicle-stimulating hormone (FSH)
  129(Q5)
Fonagy, P 205(Q5)
food, intake, hormone signals 123(Q9),
  123(Q11)
food colorants 228(Q8)
foot-in-the-door technique 95(Q3)
foramen caecum 111(Q2)
foramen magnum 111(Q5)
foramen ovale 111(Q5)
foramen spinosum 111(Q5)
forensic, origin of term 333(Q2)
forensic psychiatry 333–41
  law and 334(Q10)
  syndromes in 337(Q29)
forest plot 22(Q46), 413(Q39), 420(Q108)
forgetfulness 362(Q93)
forgetting, theories 84(Q11)
formal operational stage 44(Q9), 44(Q10)
fornix 113(Q20)
forward selection 21(Q43)
Foucault, Michel 3(Q1), 6(A2)
Foulkes, SH 273(Q5)
'four A's', schizophrenia 4(Q9), 187(Q1)
fragile X-associated tremor/ataxia
  syndrome 182(Q26)
fragile X syndrome 160(Q12), 313–
  14(Q6), 314(Q7), 314(Q9), 384(Q9)
  epilepsy in 425(Q159)
  features and CGG repeats 389(Q70)
FRAMES 303(Q18)
frame shift mutation 393(Q106)
Franklin, Rosalind 159(Q4)

Freud, Anna 396(Q159)
Freud, Sigmund 3(Q5), 196(Q13), 211(Q1),
  212(Q12)
  bereavement research/book 252(Q9)
  psychoanalytic theory 73(Q4)
  'split mind' theory of schizophrenia
    353(Q1)
  unconscious processes 270(Q9)
Friedreich's ataxia 160(Q16)
frontal eye field (FEF) 111(Q1), 111(Q4)
frontal intermittent rhythmical delta
  activity (FIRDA) 137(Q3)
frontal lobe 111(Q1), 111(Q4)
  areas of 111(Q1), 111(Q3)
  control of behaviour 170(Q9)
  disorders, perseverative utilization
    behaviour 37(Q2)
  dominant inferior, lesion 38(Q10)
  function assessment 38(Q9)
  lesions 374(A53)
frontotemporal lobar dementia (FTLD)
  151(Q4), 317(Q2), 318(Q11)
  genes associated 389(Q65)
  Lund–Manchester criteria 318(Q10)
  tangle-only 151(Q5)
frotteurism 212(Q13), 219(Q13)
frustration–aggression hypothesis
  95(Q1), 95(Q2)
fugue
  organic vs dissociative 201(A1)
  psychogenic 427(Q183)
functional hallucination 355(Q19)
functional MRI (fMRI) 51(Q2), 137(Q1),
  155(Q1)
fundamental attribution error 362(Q91)
funnel plot 22(Q46)
fusiform gyrus 386(Q31)
FXTAS 182(Q26)

GAA repeat 160(Q16)
GABA 141(Q3), 143(Q14)
  precursor 258(Q14)
  psychotropic drug action 258–9(Q16)
GABA$_A$ receptor 143(Q17), 145(Q30),
  145(Q33), 389(Q68)
  antagonism 145(Q32)
  hypnotic drug action 237(Q2)
GABA$_B$ receptor 145(Q30), 146(Q39)
GABAergic neurotransmission, modafinil
  and 421(Q114)
gabapentin 360(Q71)
gait
  'magnetic' 182(Q25)
  normal-pressure hydrocephalus
    182(Q25)
  Parkinson's disease 179–80(Q6)
galantamine 259(Q25), 421(Q118)
Gall, Franz 4(Q8)
gambling, pathological 336(Q20),
  336(Q21), 336(Q22), 336(Q23)
gamma-frequency waves 138(Q10)
gamma-glutamyltransferase (γGT)
  221(Q1)
gamma-hydroxybutyrate (GBH) 301(Q1)
Gardocki, JF 369(Q188)
GATE frame 33(Q3), 33(Q5)
gatekeeping 99(Q6)

gate theory of pain 233(Q1)
gedankenlautwerden 357(Q47)
Gegenhalten 354(Q12)
Geigy, AG 369(Q185)
gelsolin 151(Q3)
gender differences/ratios 31(Q4)
  admissions to special hospitals
    333(Q1)
  coping with mental illness 355(Q23)
  crime/offences 333(Q2), 333(Q3),
    418(Q92), 435-6(A92)
  depression 191(Q4)
  fragile X syndrome 314(Q7)
  generalized anxiety disorder 31(Q4),
    195(Q6)
  hypothyroidism 413(Q38)
  mentally ill offenders 333(Q6), 334(Q7)
  morbidity from psychiatric illness
    99(Q3)
  neurotic/stress-related disorders
    195(Q6)
  paraphrenia 388(Q58)
  parasuicide 245(Q17)
  pathological stealing 336(Q25)
  psychiatric disorders in children
    307(Q5)
  rapid-cycling bipolar disorder 192(Q9)
  schizophrenia 353(Q2)
  school refusal 308(Q9)
  somatoform disorders 199(Q5)
  suicide 243(Q4), 245(Q20)
gender identity disorders 215-16
  ICD-10 215(Q2)
gender reassignment surgery 215(Q4)
gender role 217(Q3)
gene-environment interaction 43(Q1)
gene map 397(Q186)
gene mutations 393(Q101)
  types 393(Q101)-393(Q106)
  see also specific genes
general adaptation syndrome 55(Q1),
  56(Q7)
General Health Questionnaire (GHQ)
  362(Q90)
generalized anxiety disorder
  back and neck pain 233-4(Q5)
  differential diagnosis 196(Q8)
  features 195(Q2), 195(Q4), 196(Q8)
  gender ratio 31(Q4), 195(Q6)
generativity versus stagnation 369(Q182)
genetic anticipation 185(A26)
genetic imprinting 371(A13)
geneticists 159(Q4)
genetics 159-62
  amyotrophic lateral sclerosis (ALS)
    179(Q5)
  Klinefelter's syndrome 383-4(Q8)
  personality 92(Q12)
  sensitivity to rejection 95-6(Q7)
genetic understanding 13(A4), 14(A6)
genitals, exposure 212(Q13), 217-18(Q6),
  413(Q42)
genograms 276(Q6)
genomic library 397(Q184)
geophagy 435(A84)
Gerstmann's syndrome 38(Q10), 38(Q11)
Gestalt laws of perception 77(Q1)

Gestalt therapy 291(Q6), 291-2(Q7),
  292(Q8), 292(Q9), 292(Q10)
ghrelin 123(Q11), 146(Q38)
giant cell arteritis 173(Q3)
Gibson's theory of direct perception
  79(Q12), 79(Q13)
Gilles de la Tourette's syndrome 180(Q7),
  309(Q16), 411(Q23), 416(Q67),
  417(Q75)
  Asperger's syndrome probability
    426(Q169)
  tics in 411(Q23), 434(A67)
Gillespie, Nathan 97(A7)
Glasgow Coma Scale (GCS) 169(Q1)
glial acidic fibrillary protein (GFAP)
  151(Q1)
glial cells, vacuolation 388(Q60)
glibenclamide 192(Q11)
glioblastoma 152(Q11)
global assessment of functioning, DSM-
  IV-TR 165-6(Q7)
global social functioning 309(Q17)
globus hystericus 376(A78)
globus pallidus 113(Q15)
glossopharyngeal nerve 112(Q7)
  lesions 174(Q6)
glucagon-like peptide 1 (GLP1) 123(Q11)
glucocorticoid receptors (GR) 129(Q6)
glucocorticoids 123(Q9)
glucostatic theory 73(Q5)
glutamate 141(Q2), 141(Q6), 142(Q10)
  antagonist 391(Q93)
  functions 388(Q56)
  as neurotransmitter precursor
    258(Q14)
  psychotropic drug action 258-9(Q16)
  receptors 387(Q51)
  release 122(Q6)
  synthesis and recycling pathway
    143(Q13)
glutamergic pathway 114(Q25), 114(Q27)
glutamic acid decarboxylase 141(Q3)
glutaminase 142(Q10), 143(Q13)
glutamine 143(Q13)
glutamine synthetase 143(Q13)
goal-directed behaviour 74(Q8)
Goffman, E 100(Q9)
Golgi apparatus 113(Q23)
gonadotrophin-releasing hormone
  (GnRH) 129(Q2)
go-no go 176(Q23)
'good-enough' mother 273(Q3)
'goodness of fit' tests 420(Q106)
G-proteins 143-4(Q21), 145(Q30)
grand mal, EEG pattern 394(Q139)
granulomatous disease 182(Q27)
Graphic Appraisal Tool for
  Epidemiological studies 33(Q3)
Graves' disease 181-2(Q23)
Greenfield, Baroness Susan 51(Q2)
Gregory's systems 78(Q8)
Gregory's theory of perception 79(Q13)
grief 252(Q8), 252(Q10)
  abnormal 396(Q156)-396(Q163)
  complicated, risk factors 253(Q14)
  'continuing bonds model' 252-3(Q13)
  model and tasks 252-3(Q13)

  not eligible for compensation 344(Q9)
  phases/stages 252(Q11)
  researchers on 252-3(Q13)
  uncomplicated 433(A60)
  see also bereavement
Griesinger, Wilhelm 11(Q1)
group(s)
  basic assumption 270(Q10), 270(Q12)
  leadership 270(Q9)
group analysis 269(Q1), 269(Q2), 273(Q5)
group cohesion 283(Q2)
group dynamic psychotherapy 273(Q5)
group dynamics 283(Q1)
group interactions 283(Q1)
group norm 283(Q2)
group therapy 283-5
  concepts 283(Q2)
  developments 283(Q3)
  phenomena experienced during
    283-4(Q5)
  psychoanalytically oriented 187(Q6)
  Yalom's therapeutic factors 283(Q4)
growth charts 43(Q1)
growth hormone-releasing hormone
  (GHRH) 129(Q2)
guanosine 159(Q6), 159-60(Q7)
guardianship order 335(Q16)
Gudjonsson Suggestibility Scale
  335(Q14)
guilt, feelings of 104(Q11)
Gulf War illness 225(Q1)
gustatory hallucinations 52(Q11),
  112(Q9), 179(Q4)

habit disorders 335(Q18)
habituation 366(Q125)
Hadfield, James 4(Q8)
HADS 192(Q10)
haemolysis, chronic, with dementia, EEG
  in 393-4(Q117)
haemorrhagic infarction 181(Q22)
Haley, J 275-6(Q5)
Hallervorden-Spatz disease 432(A40)
hallucinations 133(Q1)
  auditory see auditory hallucinations
  in delirium 221(Q3)
  dreams and 52(Q11), 52(Q12)
  extracampine 356(Q37)
  functional 355(Q19)
  gustatory 52(Q11), 112(Q9), 179(Q4)
  hypnagogic 238(Q11), 359(Q63)
  olfactory 357-8(Q51)
  of pain 52(Q12)
  Parkinson's disease therapy association
    179(Q4)
  peduncular 368(Q171)
  schizophrenia 104(Q9)
  tactile 104(Q9)
  visual see visual hallucinations
halogenated organic compounds
  227(Q3), 227(Q4)
haloperidol 260(Q34)
  acute behavioural disturbances and
    249(Q1)
  aggressive behaviour in intellectual
    disability 313(Q5)
  introduction (historical) 4(Q12)

postoperative delirium reduction 421(Q116)
  side effects 353(Q6)
  tremor and 357(Q45)
Hamilton Depression Rating Scale (HDRS) 428(Q198)
Hanaoka, M 369(Q184)
hand-washing 414(Q49)
hand-wringing 414(Q49)
Hanwell asylum 4(Q7)
Havelock Ellis, Henry 212(Q11), 212(Q12)
Hayling test 385–6(Q29)
HCHWA-D 151(Q3)
HCHWA-I 151(Q3)
headache 173(Q1), 176(Q22), 267(Q1)
head injury 153(A6), 180(Q12), 357(Q41)
  contracoup 391(Q91)
  EEG pattern 394(Q132)
health economic studies 17(Q18)
Health of the Nation Outcome Scale 321(Q4)
heart block 420(Q104)
heavy metals 227(Q3), 227(Q4)
Hebb, DO 196(Q13)
hebephilia 218(Q7)
hebephrenia 366(Q138)
Hecker, E 366(Q138)
hedonism, theory of 73(Q4)
heights, fear of 196(Q14)
hemianopia
  bitemporal 357(Q43)
  homonymous 173(Q3), 174–5(Q13)
hemiballismus 173(Q4)
hemicrania, paroxysmal 176(Q22)
hemiparesis 174–5(Q13)
hepatic porphyria 181(Q17)
hepatocellular disease 221(Q1)
hepatocellular toxicity, paracetamol overdose 227(Q5)
herbicides 227(Q1)
heroin 390(Q76)
  injectable 409(Q3)
herpes encephalitis
  EEG 137–8(Q6), 394(Q124)
  Klüver-Bucy syndrome after 413(Q40)
Heschl gyrus 387(Q52)
hierarchy of needs 73(Q1), 73(Q2), 73(Q3)
Hilgard's non-dissociation theory of hypnosis 51(Q2)
hippocampal formation 113(Q18), 113(Q20)
hippocampus
  connections 122–3(Q7)
  inhibitory autoreceptors 144(Q27)
Hippocrates 367–8(Q158)
histamine 134(Q6)
histaminergic receptors 145(Q28)
Historical Clinical Risk 20 (HCR-20) 349(Q3), 349(Q4)
history of present illness 358(Q55)
history of psychiatry 3–8, 367–8
  classic texts 3(Q4–6), 4(Q13)
  developmental concepts 43(Q1)
  impulse-control disorders 335(Q18)
  major developments and key dates 4(Q7–12)

mood/affective disorders 192(Q3), 192(Q12)
  neurotic and stress-related disorders 195(Q5), 196(Q13)
  pain, developments 233(Q1)
  somatization 225(Q2)
history of psychology 49–50
history of science 11–14
history-taking 358(Q55)
  in physical illness 221(Q2)
histrionic personality disorder 205(Q3), 355(Q25)
Hite, Shere 211(Q1), 211(Q2), 211(Q3)
HIV infection, neurocognitive impairment 411(Q22)
HM, patient 170(Q5)
Hobbes, Thomas 75(A4)
Hobson's levels of sleep 52(Q11), 52(Q12), 52(Q13)
hockey-stick sign 398(Q195)
Holms and Rahe Social Readjustment Rating Scale 361(Q81)
homeostatic drive theory 73(Q5)
homicides 334(Q8), 334(Q11), 419(Q95), 436(A92)
  partner abuse 336–7(Q28)
  perpetrators 334(Q12)
homocysteine 423(Q125), 423(Q126)
homonymous hemianopia 173(Q3), 174–5(Q13)
hope
  as basic emotion 59(Q4)
  instillation, as therapeutic factor 273(Q5)
hormone(s)
  anterior pituitary 129(Q5)
  hypothalamic 129(Q2), 129(Q4)
  signals 123(Q9), 123(Q11)
Horne, J 54(A14)
Horner's syndrome 173–4(Q5), 174–5(Q13), 366(Q128)
Hospital Anxiety and Depression Scale (HADS) 192(Q10), 428(Q197)
hospital order 427(Q188)
5-HT receptors see serotonin (5-HT), receptors
humanist approach, personality 91(Q4)
humanistic theory 92(Q7)
humour 396(Q159)
hunger drive 73(Q5), 78–9(Q11)
hunger pangs theory 73(Q5)
Huntington's disease
  case vignette 179–80(Q6)
  chromosomal abnormality 160(Q12), 353–4(Q9)
  EEG 138(Q7)
  neurological features 317(Q2)
  neuropathology 151(Q7), 398(Q193)
  pharmacology 145(Q31)
  schizophrenia-like psychosis 417(Q80)
  suicide mortality 415(Q57)
Hutchison's pupil 366(Q132)
hwa byung 105(Q12), 105(Q13)
hybristophilia 218(Q9)
hydrocephalus, normal-pressure 182(Q25)
hydrophobic transmembrane regions 143–4(Q21)

5-hydroxyindoleacetic acid (5-HIAA) 244(Q8), 258(Q15)
5-hydroxytryptamine see serotonin (5-HT)
hyoscine 4(Q11)
hyperactivity 414(Q52)
  see also attention deficit hyperactivity disorder (ADHD)
hyperaesthesia, visual 368(Q167)
hypercalcaemia 427(Q190)
hyperemesis gravidarum 207(Q2)
hyperfourin 391(Q85)
hyperglycaemia, EEG pattern 393–4(Q118)
hyperkalaemia 416(Q63), 427–8(Q191)
hyperkinetic disorder 409(Q5), 417(Q75)
hyperparathyroidism 260(Q31), 413(Q45), 418(Q88)
hyperphosphorylation, tau protein 387(Q49)
hyperpolarization 143(Q17)
hyperprolactinaemia 414(Q54), 436(A103)
hypersomnia 238(Q13)
  idiopathic 238(Q11)
hypertension 389(Q69)
hypertensive crisis 389(Q69)
hyperthermia 249(Q5), 356(Q38)
hyperthyroidism 181–2(Q23), 413(Q41)
hyperventilation 354(Q17)
hypnagogic hallucinations 238(Q11), 359(Q63)
hypnosis 51(Q2), 384(Q13)
hypnotic drugs 237(Q2)
hypocalcaemia 410(Q11)
hypochondriacal disorder 199(Q5), 233(Q2)
hypochondriacal psychosis, monosymptomatic 199(Q6)
hypochondriasis 199–201
hypoglossal nerve 112(Q12)
hypoglycaemia 181(Q17)
  alcohol-induced 410(Q10)
hypomagnesaemia 413(Q41), 413(Q45)
hyponatraemia 355(Q22)
hypoparathyroidism 410(Q11)
hypotension 420(Q104)
hypothalamic hamartoma 418(Q88)
hypothalamic hormones 129(Q2), 129(Q4)
hypothalamic–pituitary–adrenal (HPA) axis 130(Q7), 130(Q9)
hypothalamic–pituitary–thyroid (HPT) axis 130(Q8)
hypothalamus 123(Q10)
  anatomy 129(Q1), 129(Q3)
  infarction, hypothyroidism 182(Q24)
  tumour 181–2(Q23)
hypothermia 249(Q5)
hypothyroidism 181–2(Q23), 413(Q41)
  antidepressants, response 191(Q2)
  forms 182(Q24), 182(Q27)
  male to female ratio 413(Q38)
  primary 181–2(Q23), 182(Q24)
  symptoms 369–70(Q198)
  Turner syndrome and 426(Q166)
hypovolaemia, endocrine responses 123(Q10)

hypoxia, EEG 393–4(Q119)
hypoxic-ischaemic brain injury 127(Q4)
hypoxyphilia 220(A9)
hypsarrhythmia, EEG pattern 394(Q136)
hysteria
    anxiety 199(Q2)
    St Louis 199(Q2)
hysterical personality 416(Q64)

ICD-10
    acute stress disorder 363(Q99)
    alcohol intoxication 301(Q6), 301(Q7)
    anorexia nervosa 203(Q3)
    axes 165(Q5)
    bipolar affective disorder 191(Q1)
    child and adolescent psychiatry 307(Q3), 309(Q17)
    delusional disorders 358(Q57)
    depression 191(Q5), 192(Q14)
    disinfectants, code not included 227(Q1)
    gender identity disorders 215(Q1), 215(Q2)
    learning disability 425(Q149), 425(Q150), 425(Q151)
    pathological stealing 336(Q25)
    personality disorders 355(Q25)
        dissocial personality disorder 337(Q34)
    transsexualism 215(Q3)
iconic memory 83(Q1), 83(Q3)
idealization, as defence mechanism 395(Q152), 395(Q153)
identification, neurotic defence mechanism 396(Q159), 396(Q161)
identity, newly established, persuasion and 95(Q3)
idiographic approach, personality 91(Q3)
idiographic understanding 11(Q6)
idiopathic hypersomnia 238(Q11)
idiopathic intracranial hypertension 176(Q22)
IgA, stress and 56(Q10)
illness behaviour 99(Q3), 99(Q5), 99–100(Q7), 100(Q9)
'illness of the nerves' 196(Q13)
illusions 368(Q166)
    perceptual 78(Q6)
    Rogers-Ramachandran 78(Q8)
    twisted card 78(Q6)
image-retina system 78(Q8)
imipramine 297(Q2)
imitative behaviour 285(A4)
immigrants, schizophrenia rates 99(Q4), 101(A11)
immune-related disorders 179(Q3)
Implicit Association Test 95(Q4)
implicit memory 39(A6), 169(Q4)
impressions 95(Q6)
imprinting 160(Q11)
    genetic 371(A13)
    psychological 354(Q13)
impulse-control disorders 335(Q18), 336(Q19)
impulsive personality disorder 205(Q4), 205(Q6)

impulsivity, anatomical loop 114(Q26)
inception rate 31(Q1)
incest 426(Q175)
incidence rate 31(Q1)
incremental cost-effectiveness ratio (ICER) 17(Q18)
indecent assault 217(Q2)
indictable crime 334(Q10)
indiplon 237(Q2)
individual differences, study 49(Q4)
individuation 273(Q3)
indometacin 176(Q22)
industry versus inferiority 369(Q181)
infant(s)
    EEG 137(Q5)
    sleep 54(A14)
infanticide 417(Q78)
infections/infectious diseases 181(Q18), 181(Q19)
    myalgic encephalomyelitis trigger 231(Q2)
    postpartum delirium and 208(Q10)
infectious mononucleosis 181(Q18)
inferior colliculus 121(Q2)
infertility 417(Q82)
infidelity, delusions of 337(Q29)
inflammation, peripheral 122(Q6)
inflammatory mediators 122(Q6)
influence, theories of 95(Q3)
informal psychiatric patients 343(Q3)
information, flow between stimulus and response 63(Q5)
information-processing 63–6
informed consent 426(Q172)
inheritance 160(Q13)
    modes 160(Q9)
    movement disorders 180(Q9), 182(Q26)
    psychiatric disorders 160(Q13), 160(Q15)
    see also specific disorders
inhibitory autoreceptors 144(Q27)
initiation, testing 37(Q3)
initiative versus guilt 369(Q180)
inorganic phosphate 155–6(Q7)
inositol-1,4,5-triphosphate (IP3) 144(Q22)
insane, unchaining 4(Q7)
insanity, not guilty by reason of 427(Q187)
insight, obsessive-compulsive disorder 196(Q9)
insight learning 366(Q126)
insomnia 237(Q4)
    caffeine associated 238(Q8)
    EEG 238(Q12)
    fluoxetine and 390(Q75)
    primary, types 238(Q13)
    prolonged-release melatonin 412(Q34)
    psychophysiological 238(Q13)
institutionalization 99(Q6), 99–100(Q7)
insulin 123(Q9)
integration, acculturation strategy 103(Q1)
intellectualization 396(Q158), 396(Q159)
intellectual level, ICD-10 axis 307(Q3)
intelligence
    pre-morbid, test 414(Q56)
    see also IQ

intensification 276(Q6)
intention-to-treat 16(Q13)
interference theory, forgetting 84(Q11)
interim hospital order 335(Q16)
internal acoustic meatus 111(Q5)
internal clock 51(Q4)
internal consistency 23(A4), 403(A78)
interpersonal therapy 269(Q1)
    bulimia nervosa 388(Q55), 412(Q32)
interpreter, perception influenced 78(Q10)
interstitiospinal tract 113(Q14)
interval scale 15(Q2)
intramuscular administration 257(Q1)
intranuclear cats-eye inclusions 151(Q4)
intra-observer reliability 15(Q3), 15(Q4)
intrapsychic coping 56(Q8)
intravenous administration 257(Q1)
introjection 396(Q159), 396(Q162)
introns 385(Q23)
introspectionism 49(Q1)
inverse agonism 144(Q23)
investigations, neuropsychiatric 175(Q19)
involuntary manslaughter 334–5(Q13)
iodine deficiency 182(Q27)
ion(s), concentrations across neuronal plasma membrane 117(Q3)
ion channels 117(Q2), 143(Q17)
    voltage-gated 117(Q2), 117(Q4), 143(Q18)
ionotrophic receptors 143(Q15), 143(Q16)
IQ
    assessment 37(Q5)
    distribution 313(Q2)
    learning disability definition 38(Q13)
    pre-morbid, evaluation 37(Q5)
iron deficiency, Ekbom's syndrome and 239(Q22)
iron-deficiency anaemia 207(Q2)
Ishaq bin Ali Rahawi 367–8(Q160)
Isle of Wight neuropsychiatric study 307(Q2), 307(Q5)
isolation of effect 396(Q156), 396(Q159)

Jackson, D 275(Q2), 276(Q6)
jamais vu 357(Q48)
James–Lange theory of emotions 59(Q4)
Japan, suicide rate 105(Q16), 243(Q5)
Jaspers, Karl 11(Q1), 11(Q3–Q7)
jaw claudication 173(Q3)
JC virus 181(Q18)
jealousy, morbid 340(A29), 424–5(Q144)
jobs, shift-work and performance 55(Q2), 55(Q3)
Johnson, Virginia 211(Q1), 211(Q2), 212(Q11)
judgement, assessment 37(Q3)
judicial punishment, justifications 100(Q13)
Jung, Carl 3(Q3), 5(Q14), 273(Q2), 273(Q3), 273(Q4)
juvenile delinquency 333(Q4), 441(A172), 441(A173)
    forensic vs therapeutic assessments 441(A172)

Kahlbaum, KL 366(Q135)
Kahneman limited-capacity theory of attention 65(Q10)
kainite receptors 402(A51)
Kant, Emmanuel 360(Q72)
Kaplan–Meier analysis 21(Q38)
Kasanin, J 366(Q140)
Kelly, George 291(Q6)
Kelly's construct theory 91(Q4), 92(Q10)
Kendall's tau (rank) correlation coefficient 21(Q40), 416(Q73)
Kendler, KS 192(Q12)
Kennedy's disease 435(A80)
Kernig's sign 175(Q15)
ketamine 416(Q71)
Kinsey, Alfred 211(Q2), 212(Q11), 212(Q12), 217(Q1)
Klass, D 252–3(Q13)
Klein, Melanie 6(A3), 192(Q12), 273(Q2), 273(Q4), 407(A153)
kleptomania 335(Q18), 336(Q26)
Klinefelter's syndrome 217(Q4), 383–4(Q8)
klismaphilia 218(Q9)
Klüver–Bucy syndrome 413(Q40)
knee, reflex, spinal root transmitting 174(Q7)
Kohlberg's stage theory of moral development 44(Q12)
koro 105(Q13), 368(Q163)
Kraepelin, Emil 366(Q137)
Kruskal–Wallis test 423(Q129)
Kübler-Ross, Elizabeth 251(Q4)
  stages 251–2(Q6)
Kuder-Richardson formula 15(Q4), 390(Q78)
kurtosis 17–18(Q19)
kuru 403(A80)

labelling (cognitive distortion) 287–8(Q6)
LaBerge, D 64–5(Q8)
Lacan, Jacques 273(Q3)
lactate, MR spectroscopy 156(Q12)
lactotrophs 131(A11)
Laing, RD 356(Q36)
laissez-faire leadership 360(Q76)
lambda waves 138(Q10)
lamotrigine 175–6(Q20), 367(Q149)
  breastfeeding mothers and 422(Q123)
  mechanism of action 258–9(Q16)
  rapid-cycling bipolar disorder 367(Q155)
language 87–9
  delay 410(Q12)
  development 44(Q11), 87(Q6), 88(Q8)
  disorders 170(Q8)
  focal colours 87(Q3), 87(Q4)
  influence on memory 87(Q2)
  left hemisphere 170(Q8)
  pioneers in 87(Q6)
  structure and rules 44(Q11)
  in systemic marital therapy 279(Q2)
  thought relationship 87(Q1), 87(Q6)
  see also speech
lasting power of attorney 344(Q7)
last observation carried forward (LOCR) method 17(Q16)

latah 105(Q13), 368(Q164)
latent learning 365(Q121)
latent perversion 217(Q3)
lateral geniculate nucleus 115(A6), 121(Q1), 124(A2)
lateral lemniscus, nuclei of 121(Q2)
lateral orbitofrontal circuit 116(A16)
lateral spinothalamic tract 112(Q11), 112–13(Q13)
lateral ventricles
  enlargement 152(Q9)
  neuroepithelial tumours 151–2(Q8)
late-selection filter model 64(Q7)
law
  civil 343(Q1), 347(Q1)
  common 343(Q1)
  ethics and 347–8
  family 347(Q1)
law of contiguity 69(Q17)
law of continuity 80(A7)
law of effect 68(Q8)
law of independent assortment 159(Q4)
lead encephalopathy 181(Q17)
leadership 270(Q9), 360(Q76)
lead poisoning 418(Q84)
leaky barrel model 73–4(Q6)
learned helplessness 69(Q19), 99(Q3), 191(Q3)
learning
  avoidance 69(Q15), 69(Q16), 69(Q18)
  insight 366(Q126)
  latent 365(Q121)
  long-term potentiation, glutamate and 388(Q56)
  reverse 54(A14)
learning disability 313–15, 365(Q114)
  arson and 336(Q24)
  challenging behaviour frequency 426(Q163)
  conditions associated 313–14(Q6), 314(Q7), 314(Q9), 314(Q10)
  daily living skill assessment 314(Q8)
  definition 38(Q13)
  epilepsy and 425(Q155), 425(Q156), 425(Q157), 425(Q158), 425(Q162)
  genetic causes 313(Q3)
  ICD-10 425(Q149), 425(Q150), 425(Q151)
  moderate 313(Q1)
  prevalence 425(Q153)
  prisoners 425(Q154)
  psychotherapy 269(Q1)
  schizophrenia and 425(Q161)
  South Asian community (UK) 425(Q152)
learning disability psychiatry 313–15
learning theory 67–71, 336(Q22)
  behaviourist approach 67(Q1)
  depression explanation 69(Q19)
  'least-squares regression' 421(Q113)
Leff, Julian 321(Q1)
left realism 100(Q12)
legal aspects, psychiatric care 343–5
legal concepts, forensic psychiatry and 334(Q10)
legislation
  sexual offenders and 218(Q12)
  see also law

Lennox–Gastaut syndrome 137(Q4), 394(Q137)
lentiform nucleus 113(Q15)
Leonard, K 366(Q136)
leptin 146(Q38)
Lesch-Nyhan syndrome 314(Q10)
levator palpebrae superioris 112(Q12)
levels-of-processing approach 83(Q4)
levetiracetam 175(Q14)
Lewy bodies 151(Q1)
Lewy body dementia 249(Q1), 317(Q1), 317(Q2), 317(Q5), 318(Q9), 427(Q181)
  Alzheimer's disease vs 318(Q9), 364(Q113)
  eosinophilic inclusion bodies 418(Q86)
lie scale 92(Q7)
life events, psychotherapy after 269(Q1)
Life Events Scale 55(Q5)
life expectancy 322(Q7)
life-threatening illness, normal adjustment phases 251(Q5)
ligand-gated ion channel 117(Q2)
likelihood ratio 16(Q8), 414(Q55), 415(Q62)
Likert scales 15(Q1), 21(Q40), 95(Q4)
limbic system 133(Q3), 141–2(Q7)
limb kinetic dyspraxia 170(Q11)
limited-capacity theory of attention 65(Q10)
Lindemann, E 252–3(Q13)
linear perspective 77(Q4)
linear predictor 21(Q41)
linear regression 418(Q85), 421(Q113)
linguistic codes 87(Q5)
linguistic determinism 87(Q6)
linguistic relativity hypothesis 87(Q2), 88(Q8)
linkage map 397(Q185)
lipofuscin granule 113(Q23)
lipostatic theory 73(Q5)
lithium 258(Q11), 260(Q31)
  ACE inhibitor interactions 367(Q153)
  adverse effects 260(Q31), 355(Q24), 355(Q26), 357(Q45)
  augmentation therapy 367(Q151), 367(Q154), 367(Q155), 367(Q156), 414(Q48)
  in breast milk 422(Q123)
  contraindication 386(Q39)
  Ebstein's anomaly and 208(Q7)
  EEG pattern associated 395(Q143)
  effect on REM sleep 238(Q7)
  excretion 390–1(Q83)
  hypothyroidism 182(Q24)
  investigations before 358(Q59)
  mania treatment 192(Q13)
  overdose, dialysis 385(Q24)
  serotonin syndrome and 354(Q18)
  suicide and 244(Q14)
  toxicity 355(Q24), 356(Q38), 357(Q45), 385(Q24)
    potassium depletion and 385(Q25)
    verapamil interaction 391(Q88)
Little Albert 195(Q5)
Little Hans 196(Q13)
liver disease, alcoholic 302(Q13), 411(Q18)

liver failure, EEG pattern 393–4(Q120)
locked-in syndrome 169(Q2), 359(Q64)
LOCR method 17(Q16)
locus coeruleus 113–14(Q24)
LOD (logarithm of odds) score 11(Q4), 160(Q9)
lofexidine 302(Q16), 392(Q95)
logistic regression analysis 21(Q41), 31(Q2), 418(Q85)
Lombroso, Cesare 4(Q8)
long pause technique 357(Q49)
long-range feature-tracking system 78(Q8)
long-term memory 83(Q1), 83(Q3), 84(Q9), 169(Q4)
lorazepam 249(Q1)
loss to follow-up 17(Q16)
lower motor neurone lesions 174(Q6)
Lunacy Act (1890) 4(Q9)
Lund–Manchester criteria 318(Q10)
Luria tests 170(Q10)
luteinizing hormone (LH) 129(Q2)
Lyme disease 174(Q10), 421(Q119), 434(A66)
lysergide, legal classification 302–3(Q17)

MacArthur Competence Assessment (MacCAT-CA) 387(Q44)
macropsia 368(Q169)
magistrates' courts 343(Q2)
magnesium levels 413(Q45)
magnetic resonance imaging (MRI)
   3T 155(Q4), 155(Q5)
   contraindications 155(Q5)
   magnetic field strength 155(Q4)
   psychiatric disorders and 398(Q193)– 398(Q198)
   pulvinar sign in vCJD 415(Q59)
   Susac's syndrome 179(Q3)
   T1 and T2-weighted 155(Q3)
   Wilson's disease 180(Q8)
magnetic resonance spectroscopy 155–6(Q7), 156(Q12)
malaria 181(Q18)
male to female ratio see gender differences/ratios
malingering 199–200(Q7)
mamillary bodies, hyperintensities (MRI) 398(Q196)
mamillary nucleus 129(Q1)
management of psychiatric services 327–8
manganese poisoning 181(Q15)
mania 191(Q2), 191(Q3)
   drugs inducing symptoms 192(Q11)
   management 192(Q13), 369(Q184), 391(Q88)
   see also bipolar disorder
'mania without delirium' 335(Q18), 337(Q31)
Mann–Whitney U test 421(Q117), 423(Q126)
manslaughter 334–5(Q13), 347(Q1)
MAO-A (monoamine oxidase A), serotonin metabolism 387(Q50)
MAO-B (monoamine oxidase B) 141(Q2)

MAOIs (monoamine oxidase inhibitors) 259(Q26)
   combination with tricyclic antidepressant 358(Q52)
   drug interactions 360(Q74), 422(Q121)
   foods to be avoided 259(Q27), 389(Q69)
   mechanism of action 145(Q31), 258(Q16)
MAPPAs (multi-agency public protection arrangements) 218(Q12)
marginalization, acculturation strategy 103(Q1)
marital therapists 279(Q2)
marital therapy 279–81
   techniques 279(Q1), 279(Q2), 279(Q3), 279–80(Q4), 280(Q5), 280(Q6)
marriage
   annulment 343(Q5)
   consent, Mental Capacity Act and 344(Q7)
martial law 348(A1)
Maryanoff, BE 369(Q188)
Maslow's hierarchy of needs 73(Q1), 73(Q2), 73(Q3)
Maslow's theory of self-actualization 91(Q4)
masochism 212(Q12), 213(A10)
mass killing 334(Q12)
Masters, William 211(Q1), 211(Q2), 212(Q11)
masturbation 212(Q12), 217(Q4)
matched random sampling 424(Q134)
matricide 435(A89)
Maudsley, Henry 3(Q5), 4(Q10)
maxillary nerve 112(Q10)
maximum-likelihood estimation 21(Q41)
McCrone, J 51(Q2)
McNaughton, Daniel 4(Q10)
McNaughton Rules 4(Q10), 427(Q187)
McNemar test 21(Q43)
MCQs, setting, Angoff method and 363(Q103)
MDMA see ecstasy (MDMA)
mean (statistical) 19(Q26), 431(A37)
measles virus 181(Q18)
measurement bias 419(Q101)
Mechanic, D 100(Q9)
mechanically-gated ion channel 117(Q2)
Meddis, R 52(Q13), 54(A14)
medial geniculate body 121(Q2)
medial orbitofrontal circuit 113(Q16)
medial temporal lobe 122–3(Q7)
   atrophy 389(Q71)
   sulcus 113(Q19)
median (statistical) 423(Q130), 431(A37)
medical certificate 361(Q80)
medical ethics 356(Q36)
   see also ethics
medical negligence 347(Q1)
medullary raphe group 113–14(Q24)
medulloblastoma 152(Q11)
meiotic error, Turner syndrome and 426(Q167)
α-melanocyte stimulating hormone (α-MSH) 146(Q38)
MELAS syndrome 435(A80)

melatonin 239(Q20), 412(Q34)
   as metabolite of serotonin 258(Q15)
   prolonged-release formulation 412(Q34)
   synthesis 142(Q9)
melting pot 103(Q2)
Melzack, R 233(Q1)
memantine 259(Q25)
memory 83–5
   assessment tests 353(Q3)
   autobiographical 84(Q6)
   capacity 83(Q2)
   chunking 83(Q2)
   declarative 84(Q7), 169(Q4)
   echoic 83(Q1), 83(Q3)
   encoding 84(Q10)
   episodic see episodic memory
   explicit 169(Q4)
   flashback 84(Q6)
   forms 84(Q6)
   iconic 83(Q1), 83(Q3)
   immediate verbal, in schizophrenia 419(Q94)
   impairment/loss 170(Q5), 388(Q57)
      pseudodementia 427(Q180)
      psychogenic fugue 427(Q183)
      vascular dementia 427(Q179)
      see also Alzheimer's disease; amnesia
   implicit 39(A6), 169(Q4)
   language influencing 87(Q2)
   long-term 83(Q1), 83(Q3), 84(Q9), 169(Q4)
   long-term potentiation, glutamate and 388(Q56)
   multi-store model 83(Q3), 83(Q4)
   reconstruction 84(Q10)
   rehearsal 83(Q3)
   retrieval 83(Q3)
      failure, theory 84(Q11)
   schemas 84(Q10)
   semantic see semantic memory
   sensory 83(Q1)
   short-term 83(Q1), 83(Q3)
   spatial 169(Q4)
   storage 83(Q1), 83(Q3)
   taxonomy 169(Q4)
   working see working memory
MEN 1 syndrome 410(Q11)
Mendel, Gregor 159(Q4)
meningitis 175(Q15), 359(Q64)
   causes 175(Q16), 175(Q17)
   management 175(Q15)
mens rea 334(Q10)
menstrual cycle, and violence 333(Q3)
Mental After Care Association 321(Q1)
mental arithmetic 37(Q3)
mental capacity 221(Q4)
Mental Capacity Act 2005 344(Q7), 344(Q8)
mental disorders see psychiatric disorders
Mental Health Act 1983 335(Q15), 335(Q16), 335(Q17), 338(Q36), 343(Q1)
   civil treatment orders 338(Q39), 338(Q40), 338(Q41), 338(Q42)

consent to treatment 338(Q37), 338(Q38)
mental health law 347(Q1)
mental health nurses, stress and self-esteem relationship 56(Q10)
Mental Health Treatment Act 1930 4(Q9)
mental illness
    classification and diagnostic systems 165–7
    due to drug/alcohol ingestion 335(Q14)
    offenders 333(Q6), 334(Q7), 334(Q8), 334(Q11)
    see also psychiatric disorders
'mental illnesses are brain illnesses' 11(Q1)
mental incapacity 343(Q3), 427(Q189)
mentalization-based therapy (MBT) 205(Q5), 205(Q6)
    marital therapy 279(Q1)
mentally disabled people, rights 343–4(Q6)
mental retardation
    DSM-IV-TR axis 165(Q4), 165–6(Q7), 307(Q4)
    ICD-10 axis 165(Q5)
    rights for people with 343–4(Q6)
mental-state examination 37(Q1), 37(Q3)
Merton, R 100(Q9)
mesocortical system 141–2(Q7)
mesolimbic pathway 114(Q27), 147(A7), 387(Q48)
mesolimbic reward system 388(Q63)
mesostriatal pathway 114(Q25)
meta-analyses 297(Q1), 298(A3), 413(Q39)
metabolic disorders 181(Q17), 427(Q190), 427(Q191)
metabolic rate 74(Q7), 133(Q2)
metabolic syndrome 362(Q90)
metabolism
    CYP2D6 allele and 105–6(Q19)
    phase I and phase II 257(Q3)
metabotropic receptors 143(Q20), 143–4(Q21), 144(Q23), 147(Q15), 148(A18)
    $GABA_B$ receptors 145(Q30)
    glutamate receptors (mGluRs) 145(Q29)
    signalling mechanisms 144(Q22)
metaphase 159(Q5)
methadone 207(Q6), 251(Q2), 302(Q16)
methylphenidate 240(A10), 384(Q16)
    dependence/side-effects 409–10(Q7)
Meyer, Adolf 165(Q6)
microdeletions 160(Q11)
midazolam 252(Q7)
midbrain 387(Q48)
    atrophy 398(Q194)
middle cerebral artery ischaemia 174–5(Q13)
middle-ear disease, schizophrenia and 187–8(Q7)
migraine 173(Q1)
    in CADASIL 180(Q11)
    EEG pattern 394(Q133)

Milan group 275–6(Q5)
mild cognitive impairment 317(Q6), 388(Q62)
    homocysteine and 423(Q125), 423(Q126)
Mill, John Stuart 13(A2)
Mills, TM 283(Q1)
mind, theory of 171(A9), 385(Q28)
mind-reading 287(Q5)
mineralocorticoids, receptors 129(Q6)
miniature end-plate potentials (mEPPs) 118(Q6)
minimally conscious state 169(Q2)
Mini-Mental State Examination (MMSE) 37(Q4), 37(Q5), 170(Q10)
minimization (cognitive distortion) 287(Q5)
minimization (randomization method) 16(Q11)
'mirror phase' of development 273(Q3)
mirtazapine 387(Q41), 414(Q48)
misattribution effect 60(Q10)
mismatch negativity (MMN) 139(A10)
missense mutation 393(Q104)
mitgehen 360(Q73)
mitochondria 116(A23)
mitosis, stages 159(Q5)
mixed anxiety and depression 195(Q1), 394(Q127)
moclobemide 418(Q83)
modafinil 238(Q10), 257(Q6), 258(Q12), 421(Q114)
mode (statistics) 19(Q26)
molecular genetics 383(Q1), 383(Q2)
molindone 187(Q5)
Mongomery–Åsberg Depression Scale (MADS) 428(Q198)
monoamine neurotransmitters 141(Q6)
monomania 335(Q18)
monosymptomatic hypochondriacal psychosis 199(Q6)
Monro, John 6(A2)
mood
    acute alcohol intoxication, ICD-10 301(Q6)
    sleep deprivation effect 239(Q16)
mood disorders 191–3
    historical developments 192(Q12)
    offenders 334(Q8)
    psychological aetiological factors 191(Q3)
    see also bipolar disorder; depression/depressive disorder; mania
mood stabilizers
    in bipolar disorder 260(Q31)
    see also individual drugs
moral development 44(Q12)
moral imbecile 337(Q34)
moral insanity 4(Q10)
moral treatment 321(Q1)
morbid jealousy 340(A29), 424–5(Q144)
morphine 252(Q7)
    analgesic ladder and 251(Q1)
Morris, Karen 12(Q8)
mother
    battering 417(Q78)
    loss 369(Q193), 390(Q79)

Munchausen syndrome by proxy and 427(Q178)
    sexual abuse by 427(Q177)
mother–infant bonding 207(Q3)
motion after-effects 78(Q7)
motion parallax 77(Q4)
motivated-forgetting theory 84(Q11)
motivation 73–5
    concept 73(Q4)
    hunger 78–9(Q11)
motor cortex, primary 111(Q1), 111(Q3), 111(Q4)
motor innervation 112(Q7)
motor neurone disease, neuropathology 152(Q10)
motor skills 169(Q4)
motor tics 180(Q7), 196(Q10)
mourning 252(Q8)
    tasks 252–3(Q13)
movement
    abnormal 173(Q4)
        Tourette's syndrome 180(Q7), 411(Q23), 434(A67)
    apparent 78(Q7)
    bilateral involuntary 416(Q68)
    induced 78(Q7)
    real, perception 78(Q8)
    visual perception 78(Q8)
movement disorders 180(Q8)
    genetic causes 180(Q9), 182(Q26)
    neuropathology 151(Q7), 152(Q10)151(Q1)
    schizophrenia association 353(Q7)
    Wilson's disease and 174(Q12)
Mozart effect 291(Q5)
MRI see magnetic resonance imaging (MRI)
MR spectroscopy 155–6(Q7), 156(Q12)
Mullis, Kary 159(Q4)
multi-channel theory, attention 63(Q1)
multiculturism 103(Q2)
multi-infarct dementia 138(Q7)
multimodal cortex 122(Q3)
Multimodal Treatment Study (MTS) 412(Q36)
multinomial logistic regression 21(Q42)
multi-organ illnesses/syndromes 225–6
multiple chemical sensitivity 227–9
multiple linear regression 421(Q113)
multiple sclerosis 174(Q9), 176(Q21)
multiple sleep latency test 237(Q1)
multiple system atrophy (MSA) 151(Q1), 151(Q7)
multi-store model of memory 83(Q3), 83(Q4)
multi-systemic therapy 426(Q173)
Munchausen syndrome 337(Q29), 337(Q33)
Munchausen syndrome by proxy 337(Q33), 427(Q178)
murder 337(Q30)
mu rhythms 138(Q10)
muscarinic receptors 144(Q27)
    agonism 392(Q97)
    antagonist 176(Q21)
music, 'shivers-down-the-spine' 291(Q4)
music-making, live 291(Q3)

music therapy 291(Q3)
myalgic encephalomyelitis 137(Q3), 357(Q42)
  epidemics 231(Q1)
  insomnia 238(Q13)
  mental health problems in 231–2
  triggers 231(Q2)
myasthenia gravis 366(Q131)
myelin sheath 387(Q47)
mylohyoid muscle 112(Q12)
myoclonus 389(Q66)
  EEG pattern 394(Q138)
myotonic contractions, in orgasms 211(Q5)
myotonic dystrophy 160(Q16)
  type 1 (DM1) 182(Q26)
myth of mental illness 99–100(Q7)

naloxone 390(Q76)
naltrexone 390(Q76)
narcissistic personality disorder 353(Q5)
narcolepsy 238(Q9), 359(Q63)
  gene mutation 383(Q6)
  therapy 146(Q39)
narcotics 207(Q6)
narrative therapy 291(Q6), 292(Q8), 292(Q9), 293(A11)
narratophilia 218(Q8)
NART (National Adult Reading Test) 37(Q5)
nasal bleeding 422(Q121)
National Adult Reading Test (NART) 37(Q5), 414(Q56)
National Confidential Inquiry into Suicide and Homicide (UK) 419(Q95)
National Institute for Health and Clinical Excellence see NICE guidelines
National Service Framework (NSF) 327(Q1)
National Statistics Socio-economic Classification 99(Q1)
Navaho Indian children 88(Q8)
'n-back' task 404(A86)
Necker cube 78(Q6)
necrophilia 211(Q3)
negatively skewed data 20(Q31)
negative predictive poser 16(Q7)
negotiated order 99–100(Q7)
Neisser's analysis-by-synthesis model 79(Q14)
neocortex, connections 122–3(Q7)
neo-dissociation theory, of hypnosis 51(Q2)
neologism 356(Q39)
neostriatum 113(Q15), 141–2(Q7)
nerve agents/toxins 227(Q3)
nerve biopsy 175(Q19)
nerve cells
  structure 11(Q1)
  see also neurones
nervous shock 362(Q88)
neural crest 392(Q94)
neuralgia, trigeminal 173(Q3)
neural tube defect 362(Q89)
neurasthenia 4(Q8), 104(Q11)
Neuregulin 369(Q192), 383(Q5)
neuroacanthocytosis 185(A26)

neuroanatomy 111–16, 122–3(Q7), 127(Q1)
  antipsychotics in schizophrenia 385(Q20)
  face recognition 386(Q31)
  obsessive-compulsive disorder 385(Q22), 387(Q42)
  orbitofrontal lobe contracoup injury 391(Q91)
  schizophrenia 375(Q20), 391(Q86)
  sleep and wakefulness 133(Q4)
neurobiology, suicide 244(Q8), 244(Q13), 245(Q18)
neuroblasts 127(Q2)
neurochemistry 141–9
  of arousal and sleep 133–5
  pathways 113–14(Q24), 114(Q25), 114(Q27)
neurocognitive impairment
  first episode schizophrenia 419(Q94)
  in HIV infection 411(Q22)
neurocytoma, central 151–2(Q8)
neurodegeneration, trauma and 151(Q6)
neuroendocrine system 129–31
neuroepithelial tumours, locations 151–2(Q8), 152(Q11)
neurogenesis 127–8
neurohistology 11(Q1)
neuroimaging 155–8
  indications, specific techniques 155(Q1), 156(Q10)
neurokinins 149(A37)
neuroleptic malignant syndrome 249(Q5), 249(Q6), 357(Q50), 359(Q64)
  symptoms 369–70(Q197)
neurology 173–8
neuromelanin 113(Q21)
neuromuscular junction 173(Q2)
neurones 113(Q22)
  action potentials 117(Q4)
  cell body swelling 151(Q1)
  ion concentrations across plasma membrane 117(Q3)
  number in brain 117(Q1)
  organelles 113(Q23)
  structure 11(Q1)
  unipolar 119(A1)
neuropathology 151–3
  Alzheimer's disease 151(Q2)
  Creutzfeldt–Jakob disease (CJD) 151(Q4), 388(Q60), 403(A80)
  Huntington's disease 151(Q7), 398(Q193)
  obsessive-compulsive disorder 385(Q22)
  Parkinson's disease 151(Q1), 151(Q7)
  progressive supranuclear palsy 152(Q10), 398(Q194)
  schizophrenia 152(Q9)
  vCJD 390(Q80)
  Wernicke's encephalopathy 398(Q196)
neuropeptides 145(Q34)
  feeding 146(Q38)
  as neurotransmitters 118(Q6), 145(Q34)
  sources 398(Q199)–398(Q200)

neuropeptide Y (NPY) 146(Q38), 398(Q200)
neurophysiology 117–19
  of arousal and sleep 133–5
  integrated behaviour 121–5
neuropsychiatric investigations 175(Q19)
neuropsychological assessment 357(Q41)
neurosis 195(Q5)
  experimental 68(Q6)
neurotensin (NT) 145–6(Q36)
  receptors 145–6(Q36)
neurotic defences 396(Q159)
neurotic disorders 195–7
  characteristic features 195(Q4)
  gender ratios 195(Q6)
  historical concepts/developments 195(Q5), 196(Q13)
neuroticism 92(Q7), 92(Q12)
neurotransmission 118(Q6)
neurotransmitters 118(Q6), 141(Q2), 141(Q3), 142(Q10)
  inhibitory 143(Q14)
  learning and memory formation 388(Q56)
  metabolites 258(Q15)
  monoamine 141(Q6)
  neuropeptides as 118(Q6), 145(Q34)
  pain perception 122(Q6)
  pharmacology 145(Q31)
  precursors of 258(Q14)
  in psychotropic drug action 258(Q14)
  sleep and 134(Q6)
neurotrophins 146(Q40)
neutropenia 392(Q100)
NHS Plan 327(Q1)
NICE guidelines
  antidepressants for PTSD 410(Q8)
  dementia prevention 410(Q13)
  depression 414(Q48)
  mood stabilizer in bipolar disorder 260(Q31), 367(Q156)
  screening in dementia 317(Q4)
  self-harm risk factors 245(Q20), 245(Q21)
  suicide 245(Q20), 245(Q21)
NICE stepped-care model, depression 192(Q8)
nicotine
  binding sites 301(Q5)
  effect on sleep 238(Q8)
nicotinic receptors 143(Q19)
nidotherapy 205(Q5), 205(Q6)
Nightingale Research Foundation 231(Q1), 231(Q2)
nightmares 237(Q4), 239(Q17), 308(Q10)
night terrors 421(Q120)
nigrostriatal pathway 114(Q27), 141–2(Q7)
nihilistic delusion 357(Q46)
NINCDS-ADRDA 317–18(Q8)
Nissle, Franz 11(Q1)
Nissle body 113(Q23)
Nissl substance 151(Q1)
nitrazepam 237(Q2), 258(Q16)
nitric oxide 228(Q7)
nitric oxide synthase (NOS) 122(Q6)
NMDA receptors 143(Q18), 402(A51)

nociceptors 122(Q6)
nocturnal enuresis 308-9(Q15), 409(Q1), 419(Q98)
nominal data 15(Q1)
nomothetic approach 11(Q6), 91(Q3)
non-accidental injury of children *see* child abuse
non-disjunction 383(Q7)
non-parametric test 20(Q32), 21(Q40)
nonsense mutation 393(Q105)
NO/ONOO hypothesis 228(Q7)
noradrenaline 134(Q6), 142(Q8), 142(Q10)
    reuptake inhibition 260(Q30)
noradrenergic pathway 113-14(Q24), 114(Q25)
normal distribution 18(Q22), 431(A37)
    IQ 313(Q2)
normal-pressure hydrocephalus 182(Q25)
northern blotting 159(Q4), 383(Q2)
NOTCH3 gene 151(Q3), 180(Q11)
NREM sleep 52(Q9), 52(Q10), 54(A14), 133(Q1), 133(Q2), 134(Q7)
    control in depression 238-9(Q14), 239(Q15), 239(Q16)
    in dementia 239(Q18)
    disorders 239(Q19)
    dreams 239(Q23)
    in PTSD 239(Q17)
    recreational drugs affecting 237(Q5), 238(Q8)
    sleep deprivation effect 239(Q16)
NS-SEC 99(Q1)
nuclear magnetic resonance (NMR) 155(Q2), 156(Q11)
nucleic acid bases 159-60(Q7)
nucleolus 113(Q23)
nucleus accumbens 388(Q63)
null hypothesis 19(Q29), 20(Q36), 21(Q39), 417(Q74)
number needed to treat 33-4(Q6), 410-11(Q17)
Nuremberg Code 364(Q111)
nystagmus 355(Q26)
    down-beating 173-4(Q5)
    horizontal 177(A5)

obesity 228(Q8)
objective symptoms 13(A3)
object permanence 87(Q6)
oblimin rotation 21(Q44)
obsessional states, psychotherapy 269(Q2)
obsessions, most common 395(Q147)
obsessive-compulsive disorder (OCD) 196(Q9), 203(Q3), 205(Q1)
    aetiology 196(Q10)
    childhood 308(Q12)
    Down syndrome and 397(Q178)
    features/symptoms 356(Q40), 395(Q145)-395(Q148)
    impulse-control disorders *vs* 336(Q19)
    neuroanatomy 385(Q22), 387(Q42)
    neuropathology 385(Q22)
    prevalence 104(Q11)
    psychological defences 269-70(Q8), 270(Q11)

treatment outcome 395(Q145)-395(Q148)
obstructive sleep apnoea 207(Q2)
occipital cortex, in variant CJD 390(Q80)
oculogyric crisis 249(Q4)
oculomotor nerve 112(Q7), 112(Q8), 112(Q10), 112(Q12)
    palsy 366(Q127)
odds
    of an event 16(Q7)
    post-test 16(Q8)
    pre-test 16(Q8)
odds ratio 31(Q2)
ode-ori 105(Q12), 105(Q13)
oedipal complex 95(Q1)
offenders 418(Q89), 427(Q187)
    age 333(Q2), 333(Q5)
    female 333(Q2), 435-6(A92)
    homicides 419(Q95)
    male 418(Q92)
    mental disorders 334(Q8), 436(A95)
    mentally abnormal 333(Q6), 334(Q7), 334(Q11)
    persistent 333(Q5)
    see also crime; prisoners
offending, minor 334(Q8)
olanzapine 187(Q5), 259(Q18), 359-60(Q70)
    adverse effects 364(Q109)
old-age psychiatry 317-19
    see also elderly people
Old Bailey 343(Q2)
olfactory hallucinations 357-8(Q51)
oligodendrocytes 113(Q22)
oligodendroglioma 151-2(Q8)
one-way ANOVA 423(Q127)
Ontario Child Health Survey 308(Q7)
open-label studies 16(Q10)
ophthalmic nerve 112(Q10)
ophthalmoplegia, bilateral internuclear 179(Q2)
opiates/opioids
    addiction 251(Q4), 390(Q76)
    binding sites 301(Q5)
    detoxification 305(A16)
    injectable heroin 409(Q3)
    receptors 122(Q6), 388-9(Q64)
    relative strengths 251(Q2)
    side-effects 251(Q3)
    withdrawal 302(Q14), 302(Q16), 392(Q95), 409(Q3)
opioid antagonists 390(Q76)
opioid neuropeptides 146(Q37)
opium, introduction (historical) 4(Q11)
oppositional defiant disorder 441(A174)
optic array 79(Q12)
optic canal 111(Q2)
optic disc, swelling 173-4(Q5)
optic nerve 112(Q8), 112(Q9), 112(Q10), 112(Q12)
optic radiation 112(Q6)
oral administration 257(Q7)
oral contraceptives, St John's wort interaction 391(Q85)
orbitofrontal cortex 111(Q3), 123(Q10), 171(A9)
    activation, in OCD 385(Q22), 387(Q42)

contracoup injury 391(Q91)
ordered logistic regression 21(Q42)
ordinal data 15(Q1)
orexin 238(Q9), 383(Q6), 422(Q122)
organelles, neuronal 113(Q23)
organic disorders 179-85
    genetic causes 180(Q9)
    traumatic causes 180(Q12)
organic fugue 201(A1)
'organic mental syndromes' 165(Q6)
organophosphate pesticides 225(Q1), 227(Q3)
orgasms 211(Q3), 211(Q5)
Ornstein, R 52(Q13)
orphenadrine 192(Q7)
oscillopsia 173(Q3)
Osgood, C 95(Q4), 95(Q5)
Osterloh, I 369(Q187)
Oswald, I 52(Q14)
Othello syndrome 337(Q29)
out-of-therapy telephone contact 402(A53)
over-generalization 287-8(Q6)
overweight, factors associated 74(Q7)
oxazepam 388(Q59), 411(Q18)
oxybutynin 176(Q21)
oxyhaemoglobin 157(A6)
oxytocin 129(Q5)

paediatric autoimmune neuropsychiatric disorders 382(A190)
paedophilia 218(Q7), 219(Q13)
    DSM-IV-TR 218(Q7)
pain 122(Q6), 233-5
    anticipatory drugs 252(Q7)
    back and neck 233-4(Q5)
    chronic 233-4(Q5)
        palliative care 251(Q4)
        psychiatric disorders associated 233(Q3)
        suicide risk factors 233(Q4)
    exaggeration 233(Q2)
    gate theory 233(Q1)
    hallucination of 52(Q12)
    historical developments 233(Q1)
    neuropathic 173(Q3), 233-4(Q5)
    perception, mechanisms 233(Q2)
    risk factors 233(Q1)
    threshold 233(Q2)
    in undiagnosed medical condition 233(Q2)
pair-by-pair recall 63(Q3), 63(Q4)
paleostriatum 113(Q15)
palliative care 251-4
palliative coping 57(A8)
palmomental reflex 170(Q11)
panarteritis, systemic segmental 179(Q2)
Pancoast's tumour 412(Q33)
pancreatitis 359(Q69)
panic disorder 195(Q4), 195-6(Q7)
    chromosomal abnormality 160(Q12)
    gender ratio 31(Q4), 195(Q6)
    pain sensitivity 233-4(Q5)
    symptoms 360(Q78)
Papez, circuit of 170(Q5)
Papp-Lantos inclusions 151(Q1)
paracetamol, overdose 227(Q5), 359(Q66)

paradoxical figure 78(Q6)
paraganglioma 152(Q11)
parahippocampal region, connections
  122–3(Q7)
paraldehyde 259(Q24)
parallel processing 63(Q1)
parametric test 20(Q31)
paranoid personality disorder 205(Q3),
  205(Q4), 205(Q6)
paranoid psychoses 187–9
paranoid schizoid position 273(Q4)
paraphasia 371(A10)
paraphilias 217–20
  Scott's analogy 217(Q2), 219(Q13)
paraphrenia 388(Q58)
paraquat 227–8(Q6)
parasuicide 245(Q19)
  epidemiology 244–5(Q16), 245(Q17)
  personality traits/disorders 245(Q19)
  see also self-harm; suicide
parasympathetic nervous system activity
  133(Q2)
paraventricular nucleus 129(Q1)
pareidolia 368(Q170)
parental loss 369(Q193)
parent management training 426(Q170),
  426(Q174)
'parent of origin effect' 371(A13)
parents
  sexual abuse by 426(Q175), 427(Q177)
  suicide risk factors in adolescents
    390(Q79)
  see also mother
parietal lobe lesions 38(Q10), 374(A53)
PARK1, and PARK2 180(Q9)
Parkes, CM 252(Q9), 252(Q11)
parkinsonism 357(Q45)
  Lewy body dementia 318(Q9)
  manganese poisoning leading to
    181(Q15)
Parkinson's disease
  autosomal dominant form 383(Q4)
  case vignette 179–80(Q6)
  genetic causes 180(Q9)
  neuropathology 151(Q1), 151(Q7)
  pathological gambling and 336(Q22)
  symptoms 369–70(Q200)
  therapy, hallucinations associated
    179(Q4)
paroxetine 207(Q5), 239(Q21), 257(Q6),
  386–7(Q40)
paroxysmal hemicrania 176(Q22)
Parsons, T 99–100(Q7)
partition delusions 318(Q11)
partner abuse 336–7(Q28)
part–whole relationship 77(Q1), 77(Q2)
Passingham, RE 51(Q2)
Patau syndrome 160(Q8)
path diagram 21(Q44), 22(Q46)
pathoelaborating effects 104(Q4), 104(Q6)
pathofacilitative effects 104(Q4), 104(Q6)
pathogenic effects 104(Q4), 104(Q6)
pathological crying 420(Q105)
pathological gambling 336(Q20),
  336(Q21), 336(Q22), 336(Q23)
pathological stealing 336(Q25)
pathological triangle 275(Q3), 275–6(Q5)

pathoplastic effects 104(Q4), 104(Q6)
pathoreactive effects 104(Q4), 104(Q6)
pathoselective effects 104(Q4), 104(Q6)
patient, intervention, comparison and
  outcome (PICO) 33(Q1)
Patient Health Questionnaire (PHQ-9)
  428(Q197)
patricide 334(Q12), 435(A89)
Pavlov, Ivan 67(Q2), 67(Q4), 67–8(Q5),
  68(Q6)
PDE5 inhibitors 212(Q7)
peduncular hallucination 368(Q171)
pellagra 180–1(Q14), 366(Q133)
penalty 365(Q123)
Penrose impossible triangle 78(Q6)
Penrose's law 333(Q2)
peptide YY (PYY$_{3-36}$) 123(Q11)
perception 77–81
  apparent movement 78(Q7)
  depth 77(Q3), 77(Q4)
  direct, Gibson's theory 79(Q12)
  Gestalt laws 77(Q1)
  Gregory's theory 79(Q13)
  Neisser's analysis-by-synthesis model
    79(Q14)
  perceiver and stimulus variables
    78(Q10)
  real movement 78(Q8)
  set influencing 78(Q10)
  visual see visual perception
perceptual accentuation 78–9(Q11)
perceptual contrast 95(Q3)
perceptual defence 78–9(Q11)
perceptual illusions 78(Q6)
perceptual set 78(Q10), 78–9(Q11)
Percival, Thomas 356(Q36)
perfectionism 203(Q3)
performance, anxiety relationship
  196(Q13)
perinatal mortality rate 391(Q90)
perinatal psychiatry 207–9
  see also pregnancy
peripheralism 87(Q1)
peripheral neuropathy 412(Q33)
Perls, Fritz 291(Q6)
permuted block randomization 16(Q11)
peroxynitrite 228(Q7)
perphenazine 359–60(Q70)
perseveration 363(Q101), 374(A53)
perseverative utilization behaviour
  37(Q2)
persistent somatoform pain disorder
  199(Q4), 234(Q6)
personal construct therapy 291(Q6),
  291–2(Q7), 292(Q9), 292(Q10)
  key concept 92(Q10), 292(Q11)
personality 91–3
  change in chronic arsenic intoxication
    181(Q16)
  cognitive models 92(Q9)
  definition 91(Q1)
  five-factor model 92(Q8), 92(Q12),
    385(Q27)
  genetics 92(Q12)
  models 91(Q4)
  parasuicide and 245(Q19)
  study of 91(Q3), 92(Q7), 92(Q10)

subjective belief 91(Q2), 91(Q6)
personality disorders 205–6
  admission rates 364(Q107)
  classification by clusters 205(Q1),
    205(Q3)
  cluster C 203(Q3)
  disabling for occupational success
    364(Q105)
  DSM-III-R vs ICD-10 105(Q14)
  DSM-IV-TR axis 165(Q3), 165(Q4)
  formal diagnosis 205(Q2)
  ICD-10 axis 165(Q5)
  parasuicide 245(Q19)
  prevalence 359(Q62)
  somatization disorder and 234(Q6)
  substance misuse in 301(Q2)
  suicide risk and 244(Q11), 245(Q21)
  treatments 205(Q5), 205(Q6)
    dialectical behaviour therapy (DBT)
      269(Q3)
  types 205(Q4)
  see also individual disorders
personality factor (PF) 91(Q4)
personality orders, prevalence 356(Q33)
personalization (cognitive distortion)
  191(Q3), 288(Q7)
personal relationships, interference with
  99(Q5)
person-centred therapy 291(Q6),
  291–2(Q7), 292(Q8), 292(Q10)
persuasion, theories 95(Q3)
pervasive developmental disorders
  308(Q14)
perversion, kleptomania 336(Q26)
petit mal, EEG pattern 394(Q135)
PG-YBOCS, gambling assessment tool
  336(Q23)
phaeochromocytoma 369–70(Q196)
'phantasy' relationship 279(Q2)
pharmacodynamics
  agomelatine 385(Q19)
  buspirone 387(Q45)
  clozapine side-effects 392(Q97)
  cultural aspects 106(Q20)
  mirtazapine 387(Q41)
pharmacokinetics 257(Q1), 257(Q2),
  257(Q3), 258(Q10), 258(Q11),
  385(Q18)
  cultural aspects 106(Q20)
pharmacology, neurotransmitter systems
  145(Q31)
phase I and phase II metabolism 257(Q3)
phenelzine 358(Q52)
phenomenological psychopathology
  11(Q1)
phenomenology 14(A6)
phenothiazines 259(Q18)
phentolamine 389(Q69)
phenylethanolamine-N-methyltransferase
  142(Q8)
phenylketonuria 313(Q3)
phenytoin 175–6(Q20), 259(Q24)
philosophy of science 11–14
Phi phenomenon 78(Q7)
phobia 196(Q11), 196(Q14)
  age of onset 31(Q5)
  gender ratios 195(Q6)

persistence 69(Q18)
   specific (isolated) 195(Q4), 195(Q6),
      196(Q11), 196(Q14)
   see also individual phobias
phobic anxiety 199(Q2)
phonological (articulatory) loop 84(Q8)
phosphodiesterase type 5 (PDE5)
      inhibitors 212(Q7)
phospholipase C (PLC) 144(Q22),
      144(Q26)
phospholipid phosphatidyl
      4,5-bisphosphate (PIP2) 144(Q22)
phosphomonoesters (PME) 156(Q12)
photoreceptors 121(Q1)
phrenology 4(Q8), 4(Q10)
phthalates 227(Q3), 227(Q4), 228(Q8)
physical illness 307(Q2)
   psychiatric assessment of 221–3
physical map, genes 397(Q187)
Piaget, Jean 43(Q1)
   cognitive epistemology model 44(Q9),
      44(Q10)
   egocentric speech 87–8(Q7)
   language and cognitive development
      87(Q1), 87(Q6)
Pibloktoq 357(Q44)
pica 207(Q2), 418(Q84)
Pick's disease 388(Q61)
PICO model 33(Q1)
picrotoxin 145(Q33)
pimozide 199(Q6), 259(Q19)
Pinel, Philippe 3(Q6), 4(Q7), 367–8(Q159)
piperazine phenothiazine 259(Q18),
      259(Q20)
pituitary adenoma 181–2(Q23), 414(Q54)
pituitary gland, infarction 182(Q27)
pituitary tumour 357(Q43)
Plasmodium 181(Q18)
plastic surgery 329(Q3)
platysma 112(Q12)
pleasure principle 73(Q4)
Plutchik, Robert 356(Q31)
Plutchik's emotion wheel 59(Q2), 59(Q3)
POEMS syndrome 435(A80)
point estimate 19(Q28)
point mutations 160(Q11)
poisoning
   arsenic 181(Q16)
   carbon monoxide 180(Q13)
   metal 181(Q15)
   paracetamol 227(Q5)
poisons 227(Q3)
Poisson distribution 18(Q23), 28(A31)
Poisson regression 21(Q42)
polyaromatic hydrocarbons (PAHs)
      227(Q3), 227(Q4)
polydipsia, primary 412(Q29)
polymerase chain reaction (PCR)
      159(Q4), 383(Q2)
pontine-geniculo-occipital (PGO) spikes/
      waves 52(Q8)
pontine raphe group 113–14(Q24)
pontocerebellar tract 114(Q27)
Ponzo illusion 78(Q6)
porphyria, hepatic 181(Q17)
positive predictive value 15(Q6)
positivism 11(Q1), 11(Q2)

positron emission tomography (PET)
   ligands 156(Q9)
   'shivers-down-the-spine' inducing
      music 291(Q4)
postcentral gyrus 385(Q20)
posterior cerebral artery ischaemia
      174–5(Q13)
posterior column 112(Q11)
posterior nucleus, hypothalamus 129(Q3)
postnatal depression 208(Q8)
   follow-up assessment 428(Q198)
   outcome, monitoring 428(Q197)
   risk factors 307(Q1)
   screening 428(Q196)
postpartum delirium 208(Q10)
postpartum depression *see* postnatal
      depression
post-test odds 16(Q8)
post-test probability 16(Q8), 414(Q55),
      415(Q62)
post-traumatic stress disorder (PTSD)
      105(Q14), 196(Q12), 221(Q2)
   CBT in 269(Q5)
   sleep and 239(Q17)
   treatments 234(Q6)
   in young people, sertraline in 410(Q8)
postural hypotension 368(Q54),
      388(Q54), 388(Q54)
potassium ions 117(Q2), 117(Q3), 117(Q4),
      221(Q1)
potency factor, attitudes 95(Q5)
pout reflex 170(Q11)
Powell, Enoch 323(A1)
power (statistics) 19(Q29)
practice effect 356(Q34)
Prader–Willi syndrome 160(Q11),
      314(Q9), 390(Q77)
Pratt, Joseph Hersey 283(Q3)
praxis 170(Q11)
pre-accident driving behaviour 237(Q6)
precentral gyrus, atrophy 152(Q10)
precision, estimates 17–18(Q19)
predictive validity 15(Q5)
prefrontal cortex 111(Q1), 111(Q3),
      134(Q7), 141–2(Q7)
   see also dorsolateral prefrontal cortex
      (DLPFC)
pregnancy 207–9
   anorexia nervosa 414(Q47), 414(Q53)
   antidepressants in 386–7(Q40)
   complications 207(Q2), 208(Q8)
   ectopic 208(Q8)
   substance abuse in 207(Q6),
      428(Q199), 428(Q200)
Premack's principle 365(Q118)
premature ejaculation 165(Q1), 212(Q8),
      212(Q9)
premenstrual syndrome 333(Q3),
      409(Q6)
premotor cortex 111(Q1), 111(Q4)
preoperational stage 44(Q9), 44(Q10),
      359(Q68)
preoptic nucleus 129(Q1)
prepartum anxiety 207(Q3)
prepartum depression 207(Q5)
preplate 128(A2)
pre-post intervention studies 17(Q16)

pre-school problems 308(Q7)
pre-test odds 16(Q8)
pre-test probability 16(Q8), 414(Q55),
      415(Q62)
prevalence 433(A55)
primary consciousness 51(Q1)
primary motor cortex 111(Q1), 111(Q3),
      111(Q4)
priming 169(Q4)
primitive defences 395(Q153)
principal components analysis 21(Q44)
prion protein 151(Q4)
PRISM 419(Q99)
prison
   hospital order *vs* 427(Q188)
   likelihood 322(Q7)
   Mental Health Act 1983 and
      338(Q36)
   transfer from 335(Q17)
prisoners
   aversive conditioning 365(Q120)
   learning disability prevalence
      425(Q154)
   mental disorder prevalence 394(Q130)
   mentally ill 333(Q6)
   psychosis in 427(Q185)
   suicide 243–4(Q7), 244(Q12),
      244(Q15)
   suicide risk 427(Q186)
   see also offenders
Pritchard, James 4(Q10)
probability 19(Q29), 419(Q97)
   heterozygosity, autosomal recessive
      disorder 159(Q1), 159(Q2),
      159(Q3)
   post-test 16(Q8), 414(Q55), 415(Q62)
   pre-test 16(Q8), 414(Q55), 415(Q62)
procedural memory 37(Q6), 84(Q6),
      169(Q4)
   impairment 391(Q87)
process approach 49(Q3), 49(Q4)
process S 133–4(Q5)
Progranulin gene 389(Q65)
progressive multifocal
      leucoencephalopathy 181(Q18)
progressive sampling 424(Q137)
progressive supranuclear palsy 413(Q44)
   case vignette 179–80(Q6)
   neuropathology 152(Q10), 398(Q194)
projection, as defence mechanism
      395(Q153)
projective identification 395(Q153),
      396(Q155)
prolactin 129(Q5), 130(Q11)
   test 419(Q100)
prolonged eye contact technique
      357(Q49)
prophase 159(Q5)
propiobulbar tract 114(Q25)
proprioception 112(Q11)
prosopagnosia 169(Q3)
prospective cohort study 17(Q17)
protein synthesis 134(Q7)
proximity, Gestalt laws of perception
      77(Q1)
pseudobulbar palsy 364(Q110)
pseudocyesis 207(Q1)

pseudodementia 377(A93), 427(Q180)
psoriasis 386(Q39)
psychiatric assessment, in physical illness
    221–3
psychiatric damage, compensation
    344(Q9)
psychiatric disorders
    co-morbid 397(Q175)–397(Q180)
    marriage annulment 343(Q5)
    Mental Capacity Act 2005 and
        344(Q7), 344(Q8)
    morbidity rates 99(Q3)
    prevalence in children 307(Q2),
        389(Q73)
    prevalence in UK 394(Q126)
    in prisoners 394(Q130)
    social inclusion 321(Q2)
psychiatric negligence 344(Q10)
psychiatric service management 327–8
psychoactive drugs see psychotropic
    drugs
psychoanalytically oriented group
    therapy 187(Q6)
psychoanalytical marital therapy
    279(Q2), 279(Q3), 280(Q5), 280(Q6)
psychoanalytic theory 73(Q4)
    motivated-forgetting theory and
        85(A11)
    personality 91(Q4)
psychodrama 291(Q1)
psychodynamic theory 191(Q3)
    of kleptomania 336(Q26)
psychodynamic therapy 396(Q164)–
    396(Q169)
    long-term 269(Q1), 269(Q2)
    marital therapy 279(Q2), 279(Q3),
        280(Q5), 280(Q6)
psychogenic fugue 427(Q183)
psychological assessment 37–40
psychological debriefing 234(Q6)
psychological defences 269–70(Q8),
    270(Q11)
psychological imprinting 354(Q13)
psychological treatment see
    psychotherapy
psychology
    cognitive 49(Q4)
    developmental 49(Q4)
    history 49–50
    social 49(Q4)
psychometrics 37–40
psychopathic inferiority 337(Q31)
psychopathic personality disorder
    337(Q31), 337(Q34)
psychopathic traits 337(Q31)
psychopathology, Tseng's description of
    effects on 104(Q4), 104(Q6)
psychopaths, primary vs secondary
    337(Q32)
psychopathy 337(Q33), 337(Q34)
Psychopathy Checklist -revised (PCL-R)
    337–8(Q35)
psychopharmacology, clinical 257–63
psychosexual medicine 211–13
    key contributions 211(Q3), 212(Q12)
    researchers 211(Q2)
    writers on 211(Q1), 212(Q11)

psychosis
    cycloid 366(Q136)
    first-episode, prognostic factors
        363(Q98)
    in prisoners 427(Q185)
    treatment-resistant 321(Q5)
psychosocial conditions, abnormal
    309(Q17)
psychosocial development, Erikson's
    model 44(Q13), 44(Q14), 44–5(Q15),
    45(Q16), 369(Q178)–369(Q183)
psychosocial factors, DSM-IV-TR axis
    307(Q4)
psychosocial problems
    DSM-IV-TR axis 165(Q3)
    ICD-10 axis 165(Q5)
psychosocial transition, bereavement
    theory 252(Q9)
psychosurgery, consent 338(Q37)
psychotherapy 269–71, 291–3
    effectiveness 297–8
    group see group therapy
    integrated practice with medication
        269(Q6)
    see also individual types
psychoticism 92(Q7)
psychotic symptoms, in medical illness
    221(Q3)
psychotropic drugs 257(Q4)
    Ebstein's anomaly and 208(Q7)
    excretion 385(Q18)
    groups/classification 259(Q18),
        259(Q19)
    mechanism of action 258–9(Q16)
    metabolism 257(Q4), 257(Q6),
        258(Q8)
    neurotransmitters involved in action of
        258(Q14)
    therapeutic drug monitoring 258(Q13)
    volume of distribution 257(Q3)
    see also specific drug groups
ptosis 358–9(Q61)
    partial 173–4(Q5)
puberty, duration 415(Q58)
pulvinar sign 398(Q198), 415(Q59)
punishment, judicial 100(Q13)
purines 159–60(Q7)
putamen 113(Q15)
    atrophy 151(Q7)
pyridostigmine bromide 225(Q1)
pyrimidines 159–60(Q7)
pyrotherapy 4(Q7)

QRS interval 362–3(Q95)
QTc interval prolongation 203(Q6),
    427(Q190)
qualitative studies 17(Q14), 17(Q15)
quality-adjusted life year (QALY) 17(Q18)
questionnaires
    criteria for selection 15(Q6)
    sensitivity 15(Q6)
questions, closed vs open-ended 221(Q2)
quetiapine 187(Q5), 259(Q17), 367(Q154),
    388(Q54)
    hyperprolactinaemia and 414(Q54)
Quick test 37(Q5)
quinoneimine metabolite 227(Q5)

RAAMbo 33(Q5)
randomization
    block 423(Q132)
    methods 16(Q11), 409(Q4), 423(Q131)–
        423(Q133)
    minimization method 423(Q133)
    not possible, trial types used 16(Q13)
    stratified 423(Q131)
randomized controlled trials (RCT)
    16(Q13), 17(Q14), 409(Q4), 420(Q109)
    external validity 416(Q70)
    meta-analysis 413(Q39)
    placebo treatment 420(Q109)
    power of, collaborating centres
        411(Q25), 437(A109)
    psychotherapy 297(Q1)
    statistics 419(Q97)
range 19(Q26), 423(Q130)
rape 218(Q7), 219(Q13)
rapists 218(Q7)
raptophilia 220(A8)
rashes, and low mood 416(Q66),
    421(Q119)
ratio 15(Q1)
rationalization, as defence mechanism
    353(Q5), 395(Q151), 396(Q159)
reaction formation 396(Q159), 396(Q163)
reading disorder 410(Q16)
reasoning, assessment 37(Q3)
reboxetine 386(Q37)
recall 368(Q176)
    types 63(Q3), 63(Q4)
receiver operator curve (ROC) 16(Q9),
    22(Q46), 419(Q96)
recency effect, memory 83(Q4), 84(Q5)
receptive dysphasia 38(Q10)
recidivism 218(Q7), 413(Q43), 418(Q93)
    shoplifting and 427(Q184)
reciprocal determinism 95(Q1)
reciprocal inhibition 365(Q115)
reciprocating a concession 95(Q3)
recognition 368(Q177)
Recognition Memory Test (RMT) 353(Q3)
recollection 368(Q175)
recombination fraction 15(Q4)
'recreational' drugs see drugs of abuse;
    substance abuse/misuse
red nucleus 129(Q1)
reduction mammaplasty 329(Q3)
reflective practice 10(A1)
reflex arcs 174(Q7)
reflexes
    exaggerated (brisk) 174(Q8)
    primitive, in dementia 317(Q2)
reframing, in family therapy 275(Q3)
refusal of treatment 221(Q4)
regression, as defence mechanism
    395(Q153), 395(Q154)
regression analysis 21(Q41), 21(Q42),
    421(Q113)
    model-building 21(Q43)
regression to the mean 17(Q16)
rehabilitation psychiatry 321–3
    assessment tools 321(Q4)
    development 321(Q1)
    focus on function 321(Q3)
    social inclusion 321(Q2), 322(Q7)

rehabilitation service, stages of
    evaluation 321–2(Q6), 322(Q8)
rehearsal, memory 83(Q3)
Reich, Wilhelm 211(Q3), 212(Q11)
reinforcement schedules 68(Q9), 68(Q11),
    68–9(Q12), 69(Q14)
    continuous 68(Q9), 68(Q10)
reinforcers, negative and positive
    69(Q13)
rejection, sensitivity to 95–6(Q7)
relative risk 33–4(Q6), 35(A4)
    reduction 33(Q4), 33–4(Q6)
relearning 368(Q173)
reliability 23(A4), 434(A70)
    split-half 390(Q78)
remand to hospital 335(Q15)
REM sleep 52(Q8), 52(Q10), 54(A14),
    133(Q1), 133(Q3)
    cholinesterase inhibitors effect 237(Q4)
    control in depression 238–9(Q14),
        239(Q15), 239(Q16)
    in dementia 239(Q18)
    disorders 239(Q20)
    dreams 239(Q23)
    drugs affecting 238(Q7)
    in narcolepsy 238(Q9)
    recreational drugs affecting 237(Q5),
        238(Q8)
    sleep deprivation effect 239(Q16)
renal calculi 367(Q152)
renal failure 390–1(Q83), 393–4(Q121)
renal impairment, antipsychotics to be
    avoided 420(Q107)
renal malformations 426(Q165)
renin–angiotensin 123(Q10)
repolarization 117(Q4)
repression, as defence mechanism
    396(Q159)
research methods 15–30
    study designs 16(Q13), 17(Q14),
        17(Q15), 17(Q17)
respiratory rate 52(Q10), 291(Q4)
restless legs syndrome 239(Q21),
    239(Q22)
restoration theory of sleep 52(Q14)
restorative justice 100(Q13)
re-storying 292(Q11)
restricted code, linguistic 87(Q5)
restriction order 335(Q16)
retina 121(Q1)
retinal ganglion cells 121(Q1)
retinal ganglion layer 112(Q9)
retinocochleocerebral vasculopathy
    183(A3)
Retreat (York) 321(Q1)
retrieval-failure theory 84(Q11)
retroactive interference 368(Q174)
retrocollis 249(Q3)
retrograde amnesia 170(Q5), 265(Q6),
    357(Q41)
retrospective cohort study 17(Q17)
Rett syndrome 414(Q49)
reverse learning 54(A14)
Rey-Osterrieth Complex Figure Test
    358(Q53)
rights, of mentally disabled people
    343–4(Q6)

risk assessment 349–50
risk ratio 33(Q4), 33–4(Q6)
risperidone 187(Q5), 257(Q4), 313(Q5),
    366–7(Q146), 426(Q171)
    sexual dysfunction and prolactin levels
        419(Q100)
rivastigmine 259(Q25), 389(Q72)
Rivermead Behavioural Memory Test
    38(Q8)
RNA 159(Q6)
Robertsonian translocation 412(Q35)
Rogers, Carl 91(Q6), 291(Q6)
    client-centred counselling 92(Q11)
    theory of personality 92(Q10)
Rogers-Ramachandran illusion 78(Q8)
role accumulation 99(Q3)
role conflict 99(Q3)
Rosenthal, NE 192(Q13)
Ross, WD 367–8(Q161)
Rotter's Locus of Control Scale 57(A5)
Royal College of Psychiatrists 249(Q1),
    249(Q2), 265(Q5), 363(Q103),
    390(Q78)
Rubin, S 252(Q9)
Rubin's vase 78(Q6)
rubrospinal tract 112–13(Q13)
running commentary 364(Q112)
Rush, Benjamin 335(Q18), 356(Q36)
Ryle, Anthony 205(Q5)

Sabat, Steven 11(Q7)
Sackeim, HA 265(Q2)
sadism 212(Q10)
sadomasochism 212(Q10)
sample size 18(Q19)
sampling methods 424(Q134)–424(Q138)
Sanfilippo syndrome 313(Q3)
sarcoidosis 179(Q3)
Sargant, William 3(Q6)
SCA19 180(Q9)
Schachter and Singer adrenaline
    experiment 59–60(Q6)
Schachter and Wheeler's experiment
    60(Q7)
schema(s) 84(Q10)
    reorganization during sleep 52(Q11)
schema analysis, auditory operational
    processing 122(Q4), 122(Q5)
Schindler, W 369(Q185)
schizoaffective disorder 366(Q140)
schizophrenia 187–9, 369(Q192)
    acute-onset 104(Q8)
    aetiological factors 369(Q192)
    age disorientiation 37(Q1)
    alcohol dependence with 386(Q34)
    birth effect (season) 187(Q2)
    Bleuler and 353(Q1), 354(Q14),
        366(Q139)
    cannabis abuse and 187–8(Q7),
        363(Q97), 411(Q20)
    catatonic 104(Q8), 372(A16)
    cause of increased rates 100(Q11)
    children 308(Q13)
    cognitive impairment 37(Q1)
    cognitive representation 392(Q99)
    DISC1 gene 160(Q16)
    double-bind communications 275(Q3)

    Down syndrome and 397(Q179)
    first episode 363(Q98), 366–7(Q146),
        385(Q20), 397(Q181)–397(Q183)
        neurocognitive impairment
            419(Q94)
    first rank symptoms 353(Q4)
    'four A's' 4(Q9), 187(Q1)
    gender differences 353(Q2)
    gene mutations 369(Q192), 383(Q5)
    hallucinations 104(Q9)
        auditory 104(Q9), 387(Q52)
        functional 355(Q19)
        visual 104(Q9)
    heritability 160(Q15)
        risk in family 366(Q141), 366(Q142),
            366(Q144), 366(Q145),
            397(Q181)–397(Q183)
    historical aspects 4(Q9)
    late-onset, risk 397(Q183)
    learning disability and 425(Q161)
    middle-ear disease and 187–8(Q7)
    movement disorders associated
        353(Q7)
    neologism 356(Q39)
    neuroanatomy 375(Q20), 385(Q20),
        391(Q86)
    neuropathology 152(Q9)
    offenders 334(Q8)
    origin of term 354(Q14)
    outcomes, WHO ten-country study
        104(Q10)
    passivity phenomena 361(Q87)
    postural hypotension in 368(Q54),
        388(Q54)
    prognosis 363(Q98)
    rates 104(Q8), 187–8(Q7)
        among UK immigrants 99(Q4),
            101(A11)
        ethnic groups 100(Q11), 104(Q5),
            187(Q3)
    relapse risk 366–7(Q148)
    risk 366(Q141), 366(Q142), 366(Q143),
        366(Q144), 366(Q145), 397(Q181)–
        397(Q183)
    risk factors 187(Q3), 187–8(Q7)
    sexual dysfunction 419(Q100)
    'simple' 363(Q96)
    'split mind' theory 353(Q1)
    standardized mortality ratio 31(Q5)
    suicide association 244(Q10)
    therapy 187(Q6), 353(Q6), 363(Q102),
        366–7(Q146), 366–7(Q147)
        antipsychotics see antipsychotic
            drugs
        neuroanatomical effects 385(Q20)
        prolactin levels and 419(Q100)
        side-effects 392(Q97)
        treatment-resistant 187(Q5), 392(Q97),
            392(Q100), 396(Q189)
            ECG 397–8(Q189)
    understanding experiences in 14(A8)
    violence and 349(Q1)
    Violence Risk Appraisal Guide (VRAG)
        and 349(Q5)
schizophrenia-like psychosis 417(Q80)
schizotypal personality disorder 205(Q1),
    418(Q87)

school attendance problems 308(Q9)
school refusal 308(Q9)
scotophilia 218(Q8)
Scott's analogy, paraphilias 219(Q13)
screening tools, criteria for selection
    15(Q6), 16(Q9)
seasonal affective disorder (SAD)
    192(Q13)
secobarbital 258(Q12)
secondary consciousness 51(Q1)
secondary sensation (synaesthesia)
    353(Q8)
second opinions 338(Q37), 338(Q38)
sedation
    drug adverse reaction 260(Q34)
    effects of tricyclic antidepressants
        260(Q28)
sedatives 388(Q59)
    alcohol withdrawal and liver disease
        411(Q18)
segregation 103(Q2)
segregation analysis 393(Q110)
seizures
    absence (petit mal), EEG 394(Q135)
    complex partial 389(Q66)
    grand mal, ECT inducing 265(Q1)
    Mozart effect and 291(Q5)
    non-epileptic 386(Q30)
    rTMS side-effect 267(Q2)
    tonic–clonic, EEG 394(Q139)
selection bias 18(Q20)
selective abstraction 288(Q7)
selective attention 63(Q2), 358(Q60)
selective serotonin reuptake inhibitors
    (SSRIs) 262(A30), 386(Q35),
    386–7(Q40)
    childhood/adolescent depression
        308(Q11)
    for elderly 318(Q11)
    mechanism of action 145(Q31)
    neuropathic pain 233–4(Q5)
    OCD 395(Q145)
    persistent somatoform pain disorder
        234(Q6)
    in pregnancy 207(Q5)
    premenstrual syndrome 409(Q6)
    suicide and 244(Q14)
    trial/research methods 16(Q10)
    warfarin and bleeding 392(Q98)
selegeline 429(A13)
self, negative view 287(Q2)
self-actualization 73(Q2), 73(Q3)
    Maslow's theory 91(Q4)
self-consciousness 51(Q1)
self-disclosure, problems, psychotherapy
    269(Q2)
self-esteem
    low 43(Q5)
    in mental health nurses, stress and
        56(Q10)
self-harm (self-injury) 243–7
    dialectical behaviour therapy (DBT)
        269(Q3)
    Down syndrome and 397(Q180)
    NICE guidelines on risk factors
        245(Q20), 245(Q21)
    non-suicidal in adolescents 390(Q82)

recurrent 369(Q191)
repeated 245(Q19)
risk factors 245(Q20)
see also parasuicide
self-poisoning 245(Q17)
self-psychological theory 336(Q26)
self-stories 292(Q8), 293(A9)
sella turcica 111(Q2)
Selye, H 55(Q1)
semantic memory 37(Q6), 84(Q6), 84(Q7),
    169(Q4)
    assessment 37(Q3)
    brain lesion sites 38(Q7)
    loss 442(A183)
    as part of long-term memory 84(Q9)
sensitivity analysis 424(Q143)
sensitivity of test/questionnaire 15(Q6),
    16(Q7)
    plot, versus 1- specificity 419(Q96)
sensitization 379(A125)
sensorimotor stage 44(Q9), 44(Q10)
sensory innervation 112(Q9)
sensory system, development 355(Q20)
sensus communis 12(Q8)
separation, acculturation strategy
    103(Q1)
separation anxiety disorder 308(Q10)
separation differentiation 291(Q2)
serial killers 218(Q10), 334(Q12)
serial processing 63(Q1)
serial recall 63(Q4)
serial sevens 39(A3)
serotonergic pathway 113–14(Q24),
    114(Q25), 114(Q27)
serotonin (5-HT) 134(Q6), 141(Q3)
    $5-HT_{2c}$ antagonist 385(Q19)
    amitriptyline effect 258(Q16)
    MAOI effect on 258(Q16)
    metabolism 387(Q50)
    metabolites 258(Q15)
    precursor 258(Q14)
    receptors 143(Q20), 144(Q26)
        $5-HT_2$ 390(Q75)
        $5-HT_{2A}$ gene 383(Q5), 384(Q16)
        agonist 176(Q22)
        antagonists 387(Q41)
        partial antagonism 387(Q45)
    reuptake inhibition 260(Q30)
    see also selective serotonin reuptake
        inhibitors (SSRIs)
    turnover, in violent offenders
        418(Q89)
serotonin noradrenaline reuptake
    inhibitors (SNRIs) 260(Q30),
    386(Q36)
serotonin syndrome 249(Q8), 354(Q18)
    drugs causing 354(Q18), 356(Q32)
    hyperthermia in 356(Q38)
serotonin transporter (5-HTT)
    244(Q13)
    gene 384(Q16)
sertraline, in PTSD 410(Q8)
set, perception influenced by 78(Q10),
    78–9(Q11)
seven-transmembrane domain (7TM)
    receptors 148(A21)
Sex Offenders Act 1997 218(Q12)

sexual abuse 221(Q2), 369(Q191)
    by family members 426(Q175),
        426(Q176), 427(Q177)
    persistent effects 43(Q5)
sexual acts, interview and filming
    211(Q2)
sexual arousal, female 211(Q4)
sexual assault 410(Q8)
    rape 218(Q7), 219(Q13)
sexual behaviour 123(Q8), 217(Q1)
sexual disorders 212(Q10), 212(Q13),
    217(Q3), 217(Q4)
sexual dysfunction, in schizophrenia
    419(Q100)
sexual energy, blocked 211(Q3)
sexual intercourse, premarital 217(Q1)
sexuality 217(Q4)
    childhood 212(Q12)
    writers on 211(Q1), 212(Q11)
sexual maturation disorder 215(Q2)
sexual offenders 217–20
    exhibitionism 418(Q93)
    legislation 218(Q12)
    prediction of sexual recidivism
        413(Q43)
    risk assessment 218(Q11)
sexual peak 217(Q1)
sexual preference disorders 212(Q10),
    212(Q13), 218(Q8), 218(Q9)
sexual recidivism 413(Q43)
shaking movements 173–4(Q5)
shaping 365(Q114)
shift-work 55(Q2), 55(Q3)
shoplifting 356(Q40), 411(Q19), 435(A92),
    441(A172)
    juvenile delinquency and 426(Q172)
    recidivism and 427(Q184)
short-range motion sensing system
    78(Q8)
short-term memory 83(Q1), 83(Q3)
    see also working memory
sick role 99(Q3), 99–100(Q7), 101(A6),
    361(Q80)
signalling mechanisms, metabotropic
    receptors 144(Q22)
sildenafil 369(Q187)
silent mutation 393(Q103)
similarity, Gestalt laws of perception
    77(Q1)
16PF 91(Q4)
size constancy, after-image 78(Q5)
skewed distribution 413(Q37)
skewness 18(Q19)
Skinner, BF 68(Q8), 69(Q20), 73(Q4)
Skinner box 68(Q8)
Slater, Eliot 3(Q6)
sleep 51(Q4)
    babies 54(A14)
    cholinesterase inhibitor effects 237(Q4)
    chronic loss 51(Q4)
    control 133–4(Q5)
        in depression 238–9(Q14), 239(Q15),
            239(Q16)
    in dementia 239(Q18)
    deprivation 239(Q16)
    drugs affecting 237(Q3), 237(Q4),
        238(Q7)

EEG in 51–2(Q6), 52(Q7)
Hobson's levels 52(Q11), 52(Q12), 52(Q13)
latency 237(Q3), 238(Q8), 239(Q18)
mammalian, advantages 52(Q13)
neuroanatomy 133(Q4)
neurophysiology and neurochemistry 133–5
nocturnal awakenings 238(Q9), 238(Q11)
NREM *see* NREM sleep
in PTSD 239(Q17)
REM *see* REM sleep
restoration theory 52(Q14)
schema reorganization during 52(Q13)
slow-wave 51(Q5)
social/'recreational' drugs effects 237(Q5), 238(Q8)
stages 51(Q5), 51–2(Q6), 52(Q7), 52(Q10)
theories 52(Q13), 52(Q14)
total time 237(Q3), 237(Q5), 238(Q8), 239(Q15)
sleep disorders 237–41, 384(Q10)
caffeine-induced 165(Q1)
drugs associated with 237(Q3)
treatment 238(Q10)
sleep homeostatic drive 135(A5)
sleep hygiene, poor 238(Q13)
sleepiness, pre-accident driving behaviour 237(Q6)
sleep paralysis 238(Q11)
sleep spindles 52(Q6)
sleep–wake cycle 133–4(Q5)
sleepwalking disorder 165(Q1), 416(Q72)
slow acetylators 384(Q14)
slow waves 137(Q3)
Smith–Magenis syndrome 314(Q9)
SNAP-20 218(Q11)
snowball sampling 424(Q138)
social classes 99(Q1)
psychiatric illness and 99(Q2)
separation anxiety disorder 308(Q10)
suicide rates and 243(Q5)
social cognitive theory 419(Q102)
social constructionism 87(Q1)
social defeat hypothesis 100(Q11)
social deprivation, parasuicide and 245(Q17)
social drugs *see* drugs of abuse
social exchange theory 95(Q2)
social functioning, global 309(Q17)
Social Functioning Questionnaire 321(Q4)
social history 358(Q55)
social inclusion, rehabilitation psychiatry 321(Q2), 322(Q7)
socialized speech 87–8(Q7)
social learning 43(Q1)
social learning theory 69(Q21), 95(Q1), 95(Q2)
social motives 74(Q9)
social networks 321(Q2), 322(Q7)
social origins/factors, depression 191(Q4), 363(Q100)
social phobia 195(Q4), 196(Q11), 196(Q14)

elderly 318(Q11)
gender ratios 195(Q6)
psychotherapy 269(Q1)
social problem-solving 205(Q6)
social psychology 49(Q4), 95–7
Social Readjustment Rating Scale (SRRS) 55(Q4)
social science 99–102
social skills 95–6(Q7)
sociocultural psychiatry 99–102
socioeconomic groups
multiple chemical sensitivity and 227(Q2)
parasuicide 245(Q17)
suicide risk and 245(Q20)
sodium ions 117(Q2), 117(Q3), 117(Q4), 221(Q1)
sodium oxybate 146(Q39), 238(Q10)
sodium–potassium pump 117(Q3)
sodium valproate
adverse effects 355(Q28), 359(Q69), 360(Q71)
in bipolar disorder 355(Q28), 367(Q151), 367(Q156)
for breastfeeding mothers 422(Q123)
discovery 369(Q189)
dysphagia 355(Q28)
teratogenicity 362(Q89)
warfarin interaction 384(Q15)
somatization, disorders attributable to 225(Q2)
somatization disorder 199(Q4), 221(Q2)
personality disorders and 234(Q6)
somatoform disorders 199–200(Q7)
gender ratios 199(Q5)
persistent pain, CBT in 234(Q6)
somatoform pain disorder, prevalence 412(Q30)
somatosensory association cortex 111(Q3)
somatostatin 129(Q2)
somnambulism 416(Q72), 417(Q77)
somnolence 179(Q3)
Soranus, of Ephesus 367(Q157)
Southern, Ed 159(Q4)
Southern blotting 159(Q4), 383(Q2)
space occupying lesion, EEG pattern 394(Q134)
spastic paraparesis 174(Q8)
spatial memory 169(Q4)
spatial summation 117–18(Q5)
Spearman–Brown formula 15(Q4)
Spearman's rank correlation coefficient 21(Q40), 416(Q73)
special hospitals, admissions 333(Q1)
special medical services, advice 329–30
specificity of test 15(Q6), 16(Q7), 419(Q96)
SPECT neuroimaging 156(Q8)
speech
developmental delay 356(Q30)
disorders 38(Q10), 175–6(Q20)
egocentric 87–8(Q7)
intensive care unit and 221(Q2)
for self, for others 87–8(Q7)
social origin 87–8(Q7)
see also language

spinal cord
ascending sensory pathways 112(Q11)
descending pathway 112–13(Q13), 113(Q14)
dorsal horn G cells 233–4(Q5)
motor neurone disease 152(Q10)
spinal roots and reflexes 174(Q7)
spinocerebellar ataxias 174(Q8)
SCA19, inheritance 180(Q9)
spinotectal tract 112–13(Q13)
spiral ganglion 121(Q2)
Spitzler, Robert 165(Q6)
split-half reliability 390(Q78)
split-span study 63(Q3), 63(Q4)
splitting, defence of 273(Q1), 395(Q152), 395(Q153)
spouse abuse 336–7(Q28)
spurious associations 26(A20)
Spurzheim, Johann 4(Q10)
'square of crime' 100(Q12)
square root function 20(Q31)
stalking 337(Q29)
standard deviation 19(Q29), 20(Q31), 410(Q9), 417(Q74), 421(Q115)
standard error 19(Q27), 19(Q28), 20(Q31)
standard error of the mean (SEM) 410(Q9)
standardized mortality ratio 18(Q24), 31(Q5)
Stanghellini, Giovanni 11(Q7), 12(Q8)
static understanding 11(Q6), 13(A4)
statistics 15–30, 416(Q69), 423(Q124)–423(Q130)
plots/diagrams 22(Q46)
Statute law 343(Q1)
steady state, pharmacokinetics 258(Q11)
stealing, pathological 336(Q25)
Sternbach, L 369(Q186)
Stevens-Johnson syndrome 175–6(Q20)
stigma 321(Q4), 355(Q23)
enacted 100(Q10)
felt 100(Q10)
stillbirths 391(Q90)
stimulus, conditioned/unconditioned 67(Q3)
stimulus-analysis system (Treisman's model) 64(Q6)
St John's wort 258(Q9), 391(Q85)
St Louis hysteria 199(Q2)
strain theory 100(Q9)
'stranger homicide' 419(Q95)
strangers, fear of 43(Q2)
Strauss, A 99–100(Q7)
streptococcal infection 369(Q190), 416(Q68)
stress 55–7
acute, disorder 363(Q99)
cancer survival and 56(Q10)
job-related 55(Q2), 55(Q3)
life-events 55(A5)
models 55(Q1)
rating scale 361(Q81)
wound healing delayed 56(Q10)
stress-related disorders 195–7
characteristic features 195(Q4)
gender ratios 195(Q6)
historical concepts/developments 195(Q5), 196(Q13)

striate cortex, synaptic density 127(Q5)
striatum 113(Q15), 141–2(Q7)
stroboscopic motion 78(Q7)
stroke
   in CADASIL 180(Q11)
   types 174–5(Q13)
Stroop test 38(Q9), 175(Q18)
structured interview 419(Q99)
Student's *t*-test 417(Q74)
subacute sclerosing panencephalitis
   (SSPE) 181(Q18)
   EEG pattern 137–8(Q6), 394(Q125)
subdural haematoma 180(Q12)
subjective symptoms 11(G3)
sublimation 396(Q160)
subplate neurones 128(A4)
substance abuse/misuse 105(Q14),
   361(Q85)
   binding sites 301(Q1), 301(Q5)
   diagnosis, DSM-IV-TR 302(Q8)
   drug classification 301(Q3), 301(Q4)
   learning disability and 313(Q4)
   management, FRAMES 303(Q18)
   medical in-patients 329(Q1)
   mental illness due to 335(Q14)
   in personality disorder 301(Q2)
   in pregnancy 207(Q6), 428(Q199),
      428(Q200)
   PRISM for 419(Q99)
   suicide and 244(Q9)
   urinary tract symptoms 416(Q71)
   see also alcohol; *individual drugs*
substance dependence, DSM-IV-TR,
   diagnosis 302(Q9)
substance P 146(Q37)
substantia nigra 113–14(Q24), 116(A17),
   141–2(Q7)
   pallor 152(Q10)
substituted benzamide 259(Q18),
   259(Q19)
substitution mutation 393(Q101)
suicide 243–7
   adolescents 390(Q79)
   age-specific rates 105(Q17)
   anomic 360(Q79)
   anxious personality disorder and
      420(Q111)
   attempted 244(Q14), 244–5(Q16),
      358(Q56), 362–3(Q95)
      psychiatric negligence and 344(Q10)
      rate 361(Q82)
   in bipolar disorder 192(Q13)
   culture and 105(Q16)
   drugs affecting 244(Q14), 244(Q15)
   epidemiology 243(Q4), 243(Q5),
      244(Q12)
   gender ratio 31(Q4)
   in Huntington's disease 415(Q57)
   mental disorders associated 244(Q9),
      244(Q10)
   methods 243(Q3), 243–4(Q7),
      244(Q15), 436(A95)
   neurobiology 244(Q8), 244(Q13),
      245(Q18)
   after parasuicide 245(Q19)
   personality disorders and 244(Q11),
      420(Q111)

prisoners 243–4(Q7), 244(Q12),
   244(Q15)
psychiatric negligence and 344(Q10)
rates 243(Q2), 243(Q4), 245(Q22)
   Japan 105(Q16)
   UK 105(Q17), 419(Q95)
   USA 105(Q18)
risk factors 245(Q20), 390(Q79)
   in chronic pain 233(Q4)
   NICE guidelines 245(Q20), 245(Q21)
risk groups (by occupation) 243(Q6)
risk in prisoners 427(Q186)
risk in widows/widowers 252(Q10)
as social phenomenon 243(Q1)
see also parasuicide
sulci, medial temporal lobe 113(Q19)
sulpiride 258(Q11), 259(Q18)
summation 357(Q49)
sundowning 239(Q18)
superimposition, depth cues 77(Q4)
superior colliculus 113(Q21), 121(Q2)
superior olivary complex 121(Q2)
superior temporal sulcus 113(Q19)
superoxide 228(Q7)
supinator, reflex, spinal root transmitting
   174(Q7)
suppression, in grief 396(Q157)
suprachiasmatic nuclei 133–4(Q5)
supraoptic nucleus 129(Q3)
Supreme Court of the UK 343(Q2)
surface dyslexia 170(Q8)
survival analysis methods 21(Q38)
survival curves, statistics 21(Q38)
Susac's syndrome 179(Q3)
suspension-bridge experiment (Dutton
   and Aron) 60(Q10)
susto 105(Q13)
Sweden
   child protection 307–8(Q6)
   suicides 243(Q5)
Sydenham's chorea 416(Q68)
Sylvian fissure 111(Q4)
symmetry, facial/body 96(Q8)
sympathetic stimulation 123(Q10)
synacthen 130(Q9)
synaesthesia 353(Q8)
synapses 117–18(Q5)
   elimination, and numbers 127(Q5)
synaptic density 127(Q5)
synaptic plasticity 146(Q40)
synaptogenesis 127(Q5)
syndrome of inappropriate antidiuretic
   hormone (SIADH) 418(Q91)
synpraxic speech 88(Q8)
syntax 44(Q11)
α-synuclein 399(A4), 435(A86)
α-synuclein immunoreactive Papp–
   Lantos inclusions 151(Q1)
α-synucleinopathy 151(Q1)
syphilis
   screening 317(Q4)
   secondary 434(A66)
systematic desensitization 195(Q5),
   365(Q116)
systematic retrieval 9(Q3)
systemic lupus erythematosus (SLE)
   179(Q3)

systemic marital therapy 279(Q2),
   279(Q3), 279–80(Q4), 280(Q5),
   280(Q6)
systems theory 277(A5)
Szasz, Thomas 99–100(Q7), 356(Q36)

T4 and T3 hormones 130(Q8)
tachykinin proteins 149(A37)
tactile hallucinations, schizophrenia
   104(Q9)
taijinkyofusho 105(Q12), 105(Q13)
Taiwan
   depression prevalence 104(Q11)
   OCD prevalence 104(Q11)
Takezaki, H 369(Q184)
Tanner's growth charts 43(Q1)
TAPS study 321(Q1)
Tarasoff, T 375(A72)
tardive dyskinesia 384(Q16), 386(Q33)
taste hallucinations 52(Q11), 112(Q9),
   179(Q4)
tau correlation coefficient 21(Q40),
   416(Q73)
Tau gene 388(Q61)
tau protein 387(Q49)
t-distribution 19(Q29)
teams 360(Q76)
   unconscious processes 270(Q9),
      270(Q10)
tectobulbar tract 112–13(Q13)
tectospinal tract 112–13(Q13)
teenage mothers 307(Q1)
telomeres 385(Q23)
temazepam 302–3(Q17)
temperament, childhood 43(Q6), 44(Q8)
   difficult children 43(Q6), 44(Q7)
temperature
   body *see* body temperature
   sensation 112(Q11)
temporal lobe 112(Q6)
   ECT effect 265(Q3)
   posterior superior, lesion 38(Q10)
temporal lobe epilepsy 357–8(Q51)
temporal neocortex, dominant, lesions
   38(Q7)
temporal summation 119(A5)
tension headache 173(Q1)
TEOSS study 187(Q5)
teratogenicity 362(Q89)
tertiary circular reactions 359(Q68)
testamentary capacity 343(Q4)
testosterone 123(Q8)
test-retest 15(Q3), 15(Q4)
tetrabenazine 145(Q31)
texts
   classic, in psychiatry 3(Q4)–3(Q6)
   on sexuality 211(Q1)
texture gradient 77(Q4)
thalamus, ECT effect 265(Q3)
theory of mind 171(A9)
therapeutic alliance 279–80(Q4)
therapeutic communities 295–6
therapeutic drug monitoring 258(Q13)
therapeutic factors
   hope as 273(Q5)
   Yalom's 273(Q5), 283(Q4)
therapeutic window 384–5(Q17)

therapist factors 297(Q3)
theta waves 52(Q6)
thiamine deficiency 174(Q11)
thinking, changes in, CBT and 287(Q2)
thioxanthines 259(Q19)
Thorndike puzzle-box 69(Q13)
thought(s) 87–9
    interference 377(A87)
    language relationship 87(Q1), 87(Q6)
    pioneers in 87(Q6)
    spoken out loud 357(Q47)
thought-action clinics 283(Q3)
thought blocking 361(Q87)
thought broadcasting 363–4(Q104)
Thurstone scales 95(Q4)
thymine 159(Q6), 159–60(Q7)
thyroid disorders 181–2(Q23)
thyroid hormones 130(Q8), 181–2(Q23),
    203(Q6)
thyroid stimulating hormone (TSH)
    129(Q5), 130(Q8), 181–2(Q23)
thyrotoxicosis 181–2(Q23)
thyrotrophin-releasing hormone (TRH)
    130(Q8), 181–2(Q23)
thyroxine 123(Q9), 130(Q8), 181–2(Q23)
tics 173(Q4), 180(Q7)
    in Gilles de la Tourette's syndrome
        180(Q7), 411(Q23), 434(A67)
    motor 180(Q7), 196(Q10)
tip-of-the-tongue phenomenon 84(Q11)
tobacco, in pregnancy 428(Q200)
tocophobia 207(Q3), 208(Q8)
token economy 365(Q119)
Tolosa–Hunt syndrome 432(A40)
tongue muscles 112(Q12)
tonic-clonic attacks, EEG pattern
    394(Q139)
topiramate 175–6(Q20), 259(Q23),
    259(Q24), 360(Q71), 367(Q152)
    discovery 369(Q188)
    renal calculi and 367(Q150)
    weight loss 385(Q22)
tort, committing 343–4(Q6)
total institution 99–100(Q7), 100(Q9)
Tourette's syndrome see Gilles de la
    Tourette's syndrome
Tower of London, test 38(Q9)
toxic disorders 181(Q17)
Toxoplasma gondii 181(Q19)
toxoplasmosis 181(Q19)
Training in Community Living (TCL)
    programme 361(Q83)
trait model, personality 91(Q4), 91(Q5),
    91(Q6)
transactional model 55(Q1)
transcortical sensory dysphasia 170(Q7)
transcranial magnetic stimulation 267–8
    response rates 267(Q2)
    side-effects 267(Q1)
transference 269(Q7)
    interpretation 396(Q169)
transgenderism 217(Q5)
transient amnesic syndrome 170(Q5)
transient global amnesia 410(Q15)
transitional objects 273(Q2), 357(Q49)
transition mutations 393(Q102)
translation 383(Q1)

transsexualism 215(Q2), 217(Q5)
    ICD-10 215(Q3)
transvestism 217(Q5)
tranylcypromine 259(Q26)
Treisman's attenuation model 64(Q6),
    66(A8)
tremor 173(Q4), 301(Q7), 357(Q45)
triangle of person 269(Q7)
triangulation 276(Q6)
triceps, reflex, spinal root transmitting
    174(Q7)
tricyclic antidepressants
    antihistaminergic action 260(Q28)
    MAOI combination 358(Q52)
    overdose, ECG 397–8(Q188)
    in pregnancy 207(Q5)
    side-effects 260(Q28)
trigeminal nerve 112(Q7), 112(Q8),
    112(Q9), 112(Q12)
trigeminal neuralgia 173(Q3)
triggers to action (Zola) 99–100(Q7)
triiodothyronine 130(Q8)
tri-iodothyronine, thyrotoxicosis
    181–2(Q23)
trimipramine 358(Q52)
triptan drug group 176(Q22)
trisomy 13 160(Q8)
trisomy 18 160(Q8)
trisomy 21 see Down syndrome
trochlear nerve 112(Q7)
    palsy 173(Q2), 366(Q129)
Tropheryma whippelii 181(Q18),
    442(A195)
trust versus mistrust 369(Q178)
tryptophan, melatonin synthesis 142(Q9)
L-tryptophan, as neurotransmitter
    precursor 258(Q14)
tryptophan hydroxylase 141(Q3), 244(Q8)
t-test 20(Q32), 20(Q36), 417(Q74)
    independent sample 416(Q69),
        417(Q74)
    paired 416(Q69), 417(Q74), 423(Q124)
tuberculous meningitis 175(Q16),
    175(Q17)
tuberose sclerosis 313(Q3), 314(Q10)
Tuke, Daniel Hack 3(Q4), 3(Q5)
Tuke, William 321(Q1)
Turner syndrome 160(Q8), 426(Q164),
    426(Q165), 426(Q166), 426(Q167)
twin studies 393(Q108)
twisted card illusion 78(Q6)
two-factor theory of avoidance learning
    69(Q15), 69(Q16)
Two-Track Model of Bereavement
    252(Q9), 252(Q10)
two-way ANOVA 423(Q128)
type I error 15–16(Q7)
tyramine-rich foods 259(Q27), 389(Q69)
Tyrer, Peter 205(Q5)
tyrosine 142(Q8)
L-tyrosine 258(Q14)
tyrosine hydroxylase 142(Q8), 142(Q10)

ubiquitin inclusions 174(Q8)
UK
    age of criminal responsibility 334(Q9)
    attempted suicide rate 361(Q82)

criminology 333(Q3)
dementia prevalence 105(Q15)
epidemiology of mental disorders
    394(Q126)–394(Q130)
immigrants
    psychiatric symptom rate 104(Q7)
    schizophrenia rates 99(Q4), 101(A11)
legal aspects, psychiatric care 343–5
parasuicide 245(Q17)
partner abuse 336–7(Q28)
suicide methods in 243(Q3)
suicide rates 243(Q5), 244(Q12)
ultimatum game 96(Q8)
uncertainty 9(Q2), 9(Q3), 437(A109)
    PICO model 33(Q1)
unconscious processes (Freud) 270(Q9)
understanding, forms 13(A4)
undoing, defence mechanism 395(Q150),
    396(Q159)
'unexplained' symptoms 225(Q2)
uniparental disomy 160(Q11)
universality 283–4(Q5)
upper motor neurone lesions 174(Q6)
uracil 159(Q6)
uraemia 181(Q17)
urinary incontinence 173–4(Q5),
    249(Q6)
urinary tract symptoms, ketamine and
    416(Q71)
uroxicide 334(Q12)
USA
    suicide methods in 243(Q3)
    suicide rates 105(Q18)
utilitarian approach 358(Q58)
utilization behaviour 37(Q2)

vaginal adenocarcinoma 227–8(Q6)
vaginismus 212(Q9)
vagus nerve 112(Q8), 112(Q9)
    dysfunction 174(Q6)
    stimulation 267–8
validity 15(Q5), 362(Q92), 416(Q70)
    content 15(Q5)
    criterion 15(Q5)
    discriminant 15(Q5)
    external, of RCT 416(Q70)
    face 15(Q5)
    predictive 15(Q5)
values
    diversity 14(A9)
    perceptual accentuation 78–9(Q11)
values-based practice 12(Q9)
variable ratio reinforcement 69(Q21)
variance (statistics) 20(Q31), 20(Q33),
    21(Q39)
variant CJD (vCJD) 175(Q19), 390(Q80)
    hockey-stick sign 398(Q195)
    neuropathology 390(Q80)
    pulvinar sign 398(Q198), 415(Q59)
varimax rotation 21(Q44)
vascular dementia 317(Q2), 427(Q179)
vascular disorders, age of onset 180(Q10)
vasculopathy-related genes 151(Q3)
vasoconstriction 123(Q10)
vegetative state 169(Q2)
velocardiofacial syndrome (VCFS)
    160(Q10), 366(Q143), 393(Q113)

venlafaxine 262(A30), 414(Q48), 418(Q83)
ventral anterior nucleus, hypothalamus 129(Q3)
ventral tegmental area 141–2(Q7), 387(Q48)
ventrolateral prefrontal cortex (VLPFC) 111(Q1)
ventromedial cortex 170(Q9)
verapamil 391(Q88), 422(Q121)
verbal memory, impairment, schizophrenia 419(Q94)
verbal response, Glasgow Coma Scale 169(Q1)
vermilion border 207(Q4)
vesicles 118(Q6), 145(Q34)
vibration, sensation 112(Q11)
vigabatrin 259(Q24)
violence
    interventions 426(Q170)
    mental disorder and 349(Q1)
    premenstrual 333(Q3)
Violence Risk Appraisal Guide (VRAG) 349(Q2), 349(Q5)
violent offenders 418(Q89)
viral meningitis 175(Q16), 175(Q17)
virtue ethics 356(Q35)
visual analogue pain score, interval scale 15(Q2)
visual attention 64–5(Q8)
visual cortex 112(Q6)
visual hallucinations
    delirium 221(Q3), 317(Q7)
    Lewy body dementia 318(Q9)
    Parkinson's disease therapy and 179(Q4)
    schizophrenia 104(Q9)
visual hyperaesthesia 368(Q167)
visual impairment 221(Q2)
visual pathway 121(Q1)
visual perception
    Gibson's theory 79(Q12)
    of movement 78(Q8)
visual system 78(Q8)
visuomotor coordination test 176(Q23)
visuospatial impairment 318(Q9)
vitamin B, effect on cannabis screen 411(Q20)
vitamin B1 deficiency 174(Q11)

vitamin B12 deficiency 179(Q1)
vitamin deficiency, dementia and 317(Q3)
vitamin model 55(Q1)
voltage-gated ion channel 117(Q2), 117(Q4), 143(Q18)
volume of distribution 257(Q2), 257(Q3), 258(Q10), 384(Q17)
voluntary manslaughter 334–5(Q13)
Von Krafft-Ebbing, R 3(Q6), 211(Q1), 211(Q3), 212(Q12)
voting rights 343(Q3)
voyeurism 212(Q10), 217(Q2)
vulnerability factors 100(Q8)
Vygotsky, LS 87(Q1), 87(Q6), 88(Q8)
    egocentric speech 87–8(Q7)

Wagner-Jauregg, Julius 4(Q7)
WAIS see Wechsler Adult Intelligence Scale (WAIS)
wakefulness
    caffeine effect 237(Q5)
    control 133–4(Q5)
    neuroanatomy 133(Q4)
Wall, PD 233(Q1)
warfarin 384(Q15), 392(Q98)
warmth, impression of stranger 95(Q6)
Warnock, Sir Geoffrey (GJ Warnock) 12(Q8)
water deprivation test 412(Q29)
Watson, John B 49(Q2), 87(Q1), 195(Q5)
Watzlawick, Paul 275–6(Q5)
waving 170(Q11)
Weakland, J 275(Q2)
Wechsler Adult Intelligence Scale (WAIS) 37(Q5), 391(Q89)
    subtests 175(Q18), 176(Q23)
Wechsler Memory Test (WMT) 353(Q3)
weighted kappa 15(Q4)
weight gain, drugs associated 259(Q21), 259(Q23)
weight loss 385(Q21)
    anorexia nervosa 203(Q3)
    causes 428(Q192)–428(Q195)
Weigl Colour–Form Sorting Test (WCFST) 353(Q3)
Wernicke's area 112(Q6)
    lesion 38(Q10)
Wernicke's dysphasia 170(Q7), 170(Q8)

Wernicke's encephalopathy 174(Q11), 207(Q2), 302(Q12)
    neuropathology 398(Q196)
Whipple's disease 181(Q18), 428(Q195)
White, Michael 291(Q6)
Whorf's linguistic determinism 87(Q6)
Whytt, Robert 196(Q13)
Widdershoven, Guy 11(Q7)
wife battering 336–7(Q28)
Wilcoxon signed rank test 20(Q32)
Wilcoxon's rank-sum test 423(Q125), 423(Q130)
wills, testamentary capacity and 343(Q4)
Wilson's disease 174(Q12), 180(Q8), 182(Q26)
Windelband, Wilhelm 11(Q6)
windigo 105(Q13), 368(Q165)
Winnicott, Donald 273(Q2), 273(Q3)
Wisconsin Card Sorting Test 38(Q9)
WISC-R 37(Q5)
withdrawal syndrome
    alcohol 302(Q11), 411(Q18)
    opiate 302(Q14), 302(Q16), 392(Q95), 409(Q3)
    substance dependence 302(Q9)
Wolpe, J 195(Q5)
Woodworth, Robert 73(Q4)
Worden, JW 252–3(Q13)
working alliance 273(Q1)
working memory 37(Q6), 84(Q8), 169(Q4)
    assessment 37(Q3), 37(Q6)
    Baddeley's model 65(Q11)
    see also short-term memory
World Health Organization (WHO), analgesic ladder 251(Q1)
wound healing, stress and 56(Q10)
Wundt, Wilhelm 49(Q1)

Yalom, Irving 273(Q5), 283(Q2), 283(Q3)
Yates correction 420(Q106)
Yerkes-Dodson relationship 197(A13)

zaleplon 258(Q8)
ziprasidone 187(Q5)
Zola, I 99–100(Q7)
zolpidem 237(Q2), 257(Q4), 301(Q4)
zopiclone 260(Q33), 389(Q68)
z-score 19(Q28)
zuclopenthixol 259(Q19)

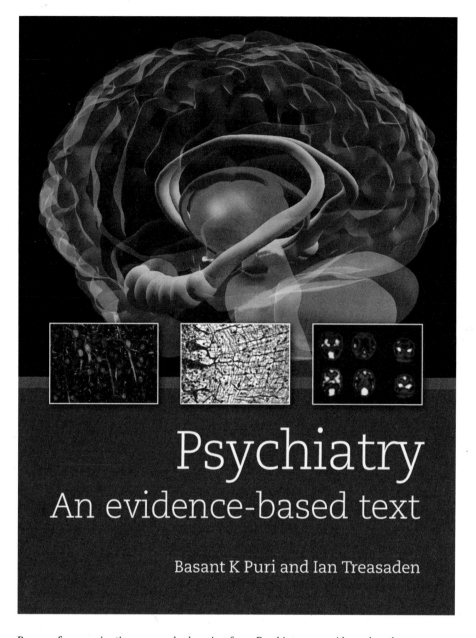

Psychiatry
An evidence-based text

Basant K Puri and Ian Treasaden

Prepare for examination success by learning from *Psychiatry: an evidence-based text.*

Then test your knowledge and skills by working through the questions in *Revision MCQs and EMIs for the MRCPsych.*

Psychiatry: an evidence-based text is succinct, user-friendly and thoroughly referenced. Chapters are written by leading experts from the UK and around the world. Following the structure and syllabus of the MRCPsych exam, the textbook is sequenced to build upon the basic sciences underpinning psychiatry, through to an in-depth description of pharmacological and psychological treatments used. The evidence-based approach helps you relate theory and research to clinical practice.

To find out more about the book or purchase online visit www.hodderarnold.com